Advanced Principles and Practice of Dialysis

Advanced Principles and Practice of Dialysis

Edited by Sean Eastwood

hayle medical

New York

Hayle Medical,
750 Third Avenue, 9th Floor,
New York, NY 10017, USA

Visit us on the World Wide Web at:
www.haylemedical.com

ISBN: 978-1-63241-664-3

The publisher's policy is to use permanent paper from mills that operate a sustainable forestry policy. Furthermore, the publisher ensures that the text paper and cover boards used have met acceptable environmental accreditation standards.

Printed in China.

Cataloging-in-Publication Data

Advanced principles and practice of dialysis / edited by Sean Eastwood.
p. cm.
Includes bibliographical references and index.
ISBN 978-1-63241-664-3
1. Hemodialysis. 2. Dialysis. 3. Blood--Filtration. 4. Nephrology. I. Eastwood, Sean.
RC901.7.H45 A38 2019
617.461 059--dc23

Table of Contents

Preface

The process of removing toxins, excess water and solutes from the blood is known as dialysis. It is performed for individuals whose kidneys are unable to perform these functions naturally. Dialysis is usually a temporary treatment for patients suffering from acute kidney injury or awaiting a transplant of the kidney. It may also be a permanent measure for patients whose condition does not allow for a transplant of the kidney. The three primary types of dialysis are hemodialysis, hemofiltration and peritoneal dialysis. Hemodiafiltration and intestinal dialysis are the two secondary types of dialysis. This book is a compilation of chapters that discuss the most vital and emerging trends in the area of dialysis. In this book, using case studies and examples, constant effort has been made to make the understanding of dialysis as easy as possible, for the readers.

The researches compiled throughout the book are authentic and of high quality, combining several disciplines and from very diverse regions from around the world. Drawing on the contributions of many researchers from diverse countries, the book's objective is to provide the readers with the latest achievements in the area of research. This book will surely be a source of knowledge to all interested and researching the field.

In the end, I would like to express my deep sense of gratitude to all the authors for meeting the set deadlines in completing and submitting their research chapters. I would also like to thank the publisher for the support offered to us throughout the course of the book. Finally, I extend my sincere thanks to my family for being a constant source of inspiration and encouragement.

Editor

Continuous Quality Improvement in Daily Clinical Practice: A Proof of Concept Study

Jonathan A. Lorch[1], Victor E. Pollak[2,3]*

1 Department of Medicine, Weill Cornell Medical College and The Rogosin Institute, New York, New York, United States of America, 2 Department of Medicine, University of Colorado Health Sciences Center, Aurora, Colorado, United States of America, 3 MIQS, Inc., Boulder, Colorado, United States of America

Abstract

Continuous Quality Improvement (CQI) is an iterative process of: planning to improve a product or process, plan implementation, analyzing and comparing results against those expected, and corrective action on differences between actual and expected results. It is little used in clinical medicine. Anemia, a complex problem in End Stage Renal Disease patients, served to test the ability of an unique electronic medical record (EMR) optimized for daily care to empower CQI in practice. We used data collected during daily care, stored in the EMR, and organized to display temporal relationships between clinical, laboratory, and therapeutic events. Our aims were optimal hemoglobin with minimum epoetin, and maintaining stable hemoglobin and epoetin. The study was done on 250 patients treated by maintenance hemodialysis (HD), receiving epoetin prior to February 1, 2010 and followed to July 31, 2011. Repleting iron, ensuring iron sufficiency, slow epoetin reduction, and decision support tools enabling data display over long periods in patient-centered reports were key elements. Epoetin dose, adjusted 6–8 weekly, was based on current clinical conditions and past responses. Hemoglobin increased by months 1–2; epoetin decreased from month 4. By months 16–18, epoetin had decreased 42% to 9,720 units/week while hemoglobin increased 8% to 123.6 g/L. Hemoglobin and epoetin were stable from month 7 onward. New epoetin orders decreased 83%. Transferrin saturation increased after the study start. Individual patient hemoglobin variation decreased by 23%, range by 27%. Mortality, 11.78 per 100 patient years, was 42% less than United States dialysis patient mortality. Allowable epoetin charges decreased by $15.33 per treatment and were $22.88 less than current Medicare allowance. The study validates the hypothesis that an EMR optimized for daily patient care can empower CQI in clinical medicine and serve to monitor medical care quality and cost.

Editor: Mercedes Susan Mandell, University of Colorado, United States of America

Funding: VEP received salary support from MIQS, Inc. The funders had no role in study design, data collection and analysis, decision to publish, or preparation of the manuscript.

Competing Interests: VEP is Founder, Member of the Board of Directors, owner of stock, and fulltime employee of MIQS, Inc. JAL is owner of stock of MIQS, Inc.

* E-mail: vpollak@miqs.com

Introduction

The statistical approach to continuous quality improvement (CQI) was invented by Shewhart over 50 years ago [1], and applied in industrial manufacturing and service industries by W. Edwards Deming [2]. He demonstrated repeatedly its capacity to improve quality and reduce costs of manufacturing and services. CQI is an iterative and continuing process of improvement that involves: (1) planning to improve a product or process, (2) implementation of the plan, (3) analyzing results and comparing results against those expected, and (4) taking corrective action on significant differences between actual and expected results. Critical to effective CQI implementation are, among others: deciding to adopt the CQI philosophy, constancy of purpose toward improvement of service, leadership to help people do a better job, training to achieve that end, and an education and self-improvement program [2]. At its heart, CQI concerns itself with taming variability. In industry the focus is on processes that affect quality of the final product, whereas in clinical medicine it is on the varied responses to therapeutic interventions determined at least in part by the biology of individual patients, their co-morbidities, and details of their illnesses.

Care of chronic diseases that now predominate in medical practice accounts for >75% of US medical care costs [3]. In chronic disease, Fries wrote over 35 years ago "a major failure of the traditional chart is its inability to indicate adequately complex temporal relationships between clinical, laboratory, and therapeutic events" [4]. One of us (VEP) postulated that "successful management and treatment of patients and the important individual manifestations of a chronic disease require complex feedback systems that relate therapeutic interventions to clinical and laboratory information relevant to multi-organ systems over prolonged periods" [5]. Although testing this postulate seems to us to depend at least in part on collecting and viewing relevant data sequentially over time, this process is far from routine. We found little literature on CQI in clinical medicine, and sparse reports on the effect of electronic medical records (EMRs) on quality improvement in any chronic disease [6].

The patient-centered, comprehensive, coded, analyzable EMR used herein, first developed 30 years ago, was designed specifically to enable CQI in medical practice [5,7]. Discrete practice details for diseases affecting multiple organ systems were transformed into coded data, enabling rearrangement of data elements at the point-of-care to facilitate clinical practice and observations over many years.

End Stage Renal Disease (ESRD) is complex, costly, and affects >600,000 patients in the United States [8]. Because ESRD is highly regulated with mandated criteria to start dialysis treatment and frequent State and Federal oversight, ESRD has unique advantages as a model for a proof of concept study. Treatments, devices, drugs used, and dialysis procedures are largely standardized, but outcomes vary greatly between dialysis facilities [9] even though standardized treatment protocols are used widely.

In protocol-driven health care delivery some individuals will not benefit from the parameters of the protocol; without individual scrutiny of care choices patients could actually be harmed. Increasing epoetin alfa (EPO) given to HD patients has led to administration of very large amounts, now acknowledged to adversely affect survival at least in patients with moderate anemia (Hb 100–130 g/L) [10,11].

For the present study we examine the effects of treatment of anemia, a chronic condition in HD patients with ESRD. Underlying causes include deficiency of iron stores and the erythrocyte stimulating hormone erythropoetin. EPO has played a major role in anemia treatment for >20 years [12]. Adequate iron stores are needed for optimal EPO response [13]. Iron deficiency is common in patients treated by HD [14] and those with decreased renal function not on dialysis [15]. Yet many studies of EPO use in chronic renal failure were done on patients iron deficient when EPO was administered [16–18]. When EPO is administered to patients deficient or marginally sufficient in iron, demands for iron for hemoglobin (Hb) production are likely to deplete iron available for other essential metabolic processes.

We have reported favorable effects of treatment with IV iron but not with oral iron [14]. Later, retrospective analysis of clinical practice from 1998 to 2007 clearly demonstrated the importance of iron in long-term survival of HD patients, and that survival was better with relatively low EPO doses [19]. The practice at that time was to administer EPO using a standardized protocol in doses aimed to maintain patient Hb within the 100–120 g/L range; to decrease or withhold EPO solely on when the latest patient Hb was >125 or >130 g/L; and to resume and even increase EPO administration when Hb had not responded or when the latest Hb decreased to <90 or <100 g/L [20].

Analysis showed that this approach was associated with wide Hb swings and frequent prolonged periods with low Hb levels. We therefore developed a prospective patient-centered CQI approach, and report on its design and testing under the leadership of one of the authors (JAL). We made use of patient-specific data collected during daily care and stored in the EMR. Our objectives were: to achieve optimal Hb with minimum required EPO, and maintain stable Hb and EPO dose.

Methods

The Participants

The study was done on all 264 patients treated by maintenance in-center HD in one of three dialysis unit managed by The Rogosin Institute (New York, NY) and affiliated with New York Presbyterian Hospital and Weill Medical College of Cornell University. Before February 2010, intravenous (IV) iron and EPO had been prescribed using a protocol consistent with the Kidney Disease Outcomes Quality Initiative (KDOQI) guidelines [20], and influenced by Centers for Medicare and Medicaid Services (CMS) mandates. The 250 patients, who had been receiving EPO in October 2009 to February 2010, are the subjects of this analysis. They were followed until July 31, 2011.

The EMR

The EMR (MIQS Inc, Boulder, CO) employs a relational database (SAP Sybase Adaptive Server Enterprise, SAP AG, Walldorf, Germany), running on a server computer (Oracle, Redwood Shores CA). Its architecture is shown diagrammatically in Figure 1. It is accessed using a custom toolset (4D, Inc., San Jose, CA) from client personal computers in dialysis units and other practice sites [21]. All clinical, administrative, and financial data are immediately accessible at all times on patients ever entered into the database. Subject to security considerations, lifetime patient data relevant to pertinent caregiver needs are accessed whenever and wherever needed.

Coded data elements include diagnoses, procedures, symptoms, signs, medications, allergies, and hospitalizations. HD treatment screens record all details at the time of treatment. HD orders and medications to be given during HD automatically populate treatment screen fields.

Accuracy and completeness of data on EPO and IV iron administered during HD treatments are facilitated and ensured by full software integration of billing and clinical information. Accuracy and completeness of data on hospital admissions are also facilitated and ensured by software integration of billing and clinical information.

To provide clinically useful point-of-care reports MIQS-designed embedded query tools are incorporated. They provide classes of reports (including single patient tabular, multi-patient tabular, and aggregate reports) to organize data quickly in any way desired over any time span, to make knowledge available about individual patients, and groups. User created reports can be updated and organized at the point-of-care, and are designed to facilitate clinical decisions based on timely, complete, relevant,

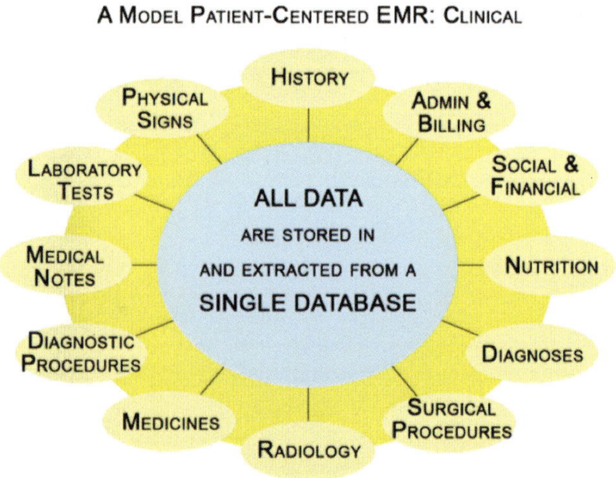

Figure 1. A model of a patient-centered EMR that, with a single database, accommodates multiple clinical functions and domains of information. As shown these include symptoms, physical signs, laboratory tests, medicines, diagnoses, diagnostic and surgical procedures, radiology, medical notes, nutrition, and social work. The single database also accommodates and includes the needs of: caregivers and other staff; data entry and reporting of physicians, nurses, dietitians, social workers, pharmacists, administrators, and clerical, billing, and accounting staff; multiple locations including main and remote dialysis units, peritoneal dialysis unit, home HD, chronic kidney disease, renal and other transplant, physician office, hospital outpatient; non-clinical functions such as insurance, fee tables, charges, physician billing, dialysis unit billing, electronic remittance and explanation of benefits.

patient-specific, time-oriented data. Individual patient reports include contemporaneous medications and laboratory tests, comprehensive lifetime lists of diagnoses, surgical procedures, diagnostic procedures, allergies, adverse drug reactions, immunizations, and hospitalizations.

The Framework for the CQI Study

Based on our previous study [19] we developed a framework for hematinic medication administration in individual patients treated by HD. It was not a protocol to be applied uniformly to a heterogeneous patient population. Rather, the elements of the framework represented goals that had been shown to result in optimum patient survival using a minimum amount of EPO. To achieve the desired goals required knowledge of each patient, familiarity with factors causing apparent EPO resistance, and visual access in a single report to the domains of data that might effect application of the framework in individual patients.

The goals within the framework included: Iron replete patients were to receive IV iron 200 mg monthly as a single dose. Patients not iron sufficient (TSAT <25% and/or serum ferritin <300 μg/L) were to receive iron 200 mg during 5 consecutive HD treatments, thereafter 200 mg monthly. EPO and iron dose changes were to be evaluated monthly. EPO changes were to be made only 6–8 weekly as normal erythrocyte lifespan is ~120 days [22], and because we had observed that large Hb variations accompanied frequent EPO changes.

Other details were:

- Patients with Hb<120 g/L and/or EPO>27,000 units/week were examined and data reviewed to determine possible cause(s) for EPO resistance. If considered resistant EPO dose was held unchanged until resistance judged by clinical examination, increased serum albumin and decreased C reactive protein, was considered unlikely.
- In patients unresponsive to EPO, the dose was reduced stepwise to the last level at which a response to EPO occurred.
- Before EPO was increased, a previously responsive patient with stable Hb<115 g/L was evaluated for inflammatory states and other possible reasons for unresponsiveness.
- If Hb was <110 g/L, EPO dose changes were made to try to attain a new goal of 120 g/L.
- If not iron sufficient, IV iron was given to achieve iron sufficiency, leaving EPO dose unchanged. EPO dose was changed only after iron sufficiency was established and maintenance iron initiated.
- If Hb was >125 g/L on 3 consecutive occasions EPO was reduced by 20%, but never to 0 (zero).
- EPO dose was not to be raised to >27,000 units/week without close consideration.
- When iron sufficient, EPO naive patients received EPO 90 units/Kg/week initially. The dose was not adjusted for 6–8 weeks, and the starting dose was not changed before there was evidence of iron sufficiency. Once a response was achieved (Hb 115–125 g/L), EPO was reduced by 20%. With assurance of iron repletion and sufficiency, EPO dose was then modified as in EPO established patients.

Implementation

Implementation required a new approach to prescribing hematinic drugs and managing the process. The prevailing practice had been that the medical director or attending physicians signed EPO orders previously written by designated nurses. Guiding the protocol used for EPO prescription was the then current CMS policy that penalized reimbursement when the Hb was >130 g/L. The prevailing widely used practice was that EPO dose could be increased, decreased, or discontinued every two weeks based only on the most currently available Hb. In addition, individual physicians might also write anemia medication orders. We found by retrospective data analysis that this practice had had an adverse effect on patient Hb (Figure 2).

To enable the new CQI study framework EPO administration was brought under the anemia management team, a core group of caregivers charged with reviewing all patients with a clear understanding of the clinical condition and past response to EPO doses of each patient. Prior to the start, the results of the retrospective analysis and the rationale underlying the new framework were communicated to and discussed with the team by one of the authors (JAL). Orders were to be written only by the anemia management team. Orders by individual physicians were stopped. Senior management endorsed the process to ensure that it was carried out.

Patient-centered EPO administration required first-hand knowledge of each patient and data that might affect the response. Therapeutic decisions were made systematically at one-month intervals by caregivers knowledgeable about each patient's course. These included physicians, nurses and nurse practitioners. Also participating were the unit administrator, nurse manager and physician responsible for implementation of the CQI framework.

To review individual patients, data from HD treatments, medications administered, and laboratory domains were aggregated monthly for the prior 18-months using the aggregate class of reports. Projection on a 140 cm television screen wall mounted in a conference room enabled all team members to see the data simultaneously and participate in decision making. Adjustments to IV iron and EPO were made as needed, consistent with the CQI framework. For acute problems, data aggregated weekly were displayed over a shorter time span. For chronic and perplexing problems, data were aggregated quarterly over several years.

Controls

The other two other dialysis units administered by The Rogosin Institute served as contemporaneous controls. Both used the EMR in daily practice, were aware of the approach undertaken by the study unit, and of the desirability of reducing EPO administered in view of the upcoming changes in HD treatment reimbursement. An EPO dosing strategy was not imposed, but was left to each unit. Physicians and clinical staff had no training in the processes of CQI.

Data Analysis

For analysis, the aggregate report was used to abstract data monthly for the historical period 12 months before and the CQI period 18 months after start of the study. Data captured included the number of HD treatments, mean post dialysis weight, Hb, TSAT, serum ferritin, serum albumin, C reactive protein and number of injections, total given, and mean dose of EPO and iron. Mean EPO/week, EPO/Kg/week, IV iron/month, and iron/Kg/month were calculated (Figure 3). Other reports abstracted new and discontinued EPO and IV iron orders. All Hb, TSAT, EPO and iron administration values were exported to JMP software (SAS Institute Inc., Cary, NC) to calculate monthly patient means and percentiles.

Using the Lab - Multiple Patients report, Hb values were abstracted for the two historical 6-month periods before and three 6-month periods after the study start. Data were exported to SAS JMP. Means, standard deviations (SD), coefficients of variation

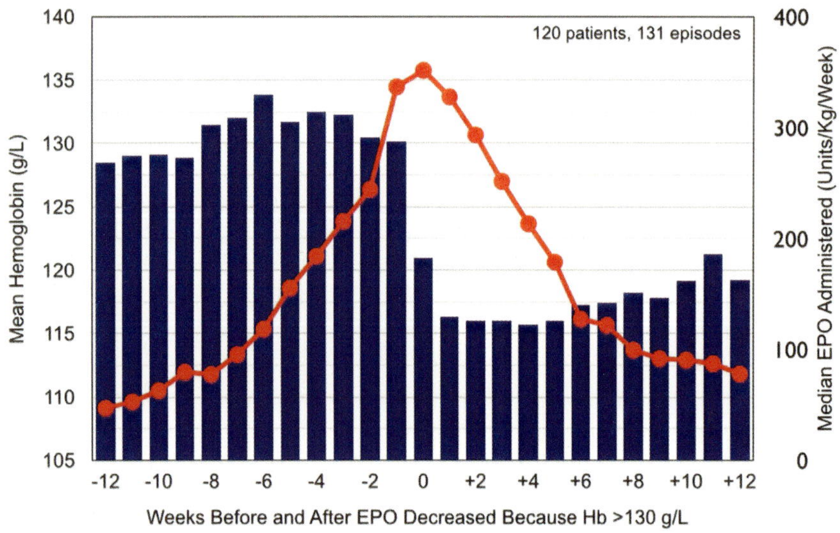

Figure 2. Summary of findings for 12 weeks before and after EPO administration was decreased because Hb was >130 g/L in 120 patients (131 episodes) in the study dialysis unit during the protocol period in calendar year 2009. EPO reduction (blue bars) was followed by pronounced and prolonged reduction of Hb (red dots) to <115 g/L. Similar observations were made in 2 other dialysis units that deployed the EMR.

year-month	**2009-11**	**2009-12**	**2010-1**	**2010-2**	**2010-3**	**2010-4**	**2010-5**	**2010-6**	**2010-7**	**2010-8**
HD Treatments & Lab Tests										
HD Treatments	13	13	13	12	14	13	12	13	13	13
HD Duration (min)	206	212	209	207	209	207	212	212	209	209
Blood processed (L)	65.9	73.8	77.6	70.9	67.7	70.7	68.5	65.1	66.7	66.3
Weight (kg) Post-HD	56.0	57.7	57.5	59.0	57.8	59.2	58.4	59.2	59.8	59.9
Serum creatinine (umol/L)	787	707	734	787	1,078	712	999	866	999	782
Kt/V	1.95	1.48	1.44	1.48	1.04	2.69	1.44	1.44	3.17	1.40
Serum albumin (g/L)	36	33	37	42	43	40	43	41	42	43
C Reactive Protein (mg/L)				11.3	2.5	2.0	5.4	35.1	1.6	10.4
Hemoglobin (g/L)	**88**	**100**	**115**	**118**	**140**	**132**	**132**	**150**	**135**	**147**
RBC (10^12/L)	2.86	3.38	3.71	3.72	4.65	4.38	4.26	5.19	4.71	4.77
Hematocrit (%)	28.7	32.6	37.6	37.3	44.6	41.8	41.2	47.5	43.8	47.1
MCV (fl)	91.0	89.0	92.0	90.0	90.0	97.4	93.0	96.1	93.0	99.4
MCH (pg)	28.4	26.1	27.7	28.8	28.1	30.8	29.7	30.5	30.4	31.7
MCHC (g/L)	312	294	300	320	314	317	318	318	326	320
TSAT (%)	33	20	35	12	18	33	20	55	44	39
Serum ferritin (ug/L)			280			455			672	
Platelet count (10^9/L)	442	292	251	170	194	149	221	165	181	202
Medications Given during HD										
EPO units (count)	12	13	13	12	13	13	12	13	13	10
EPO units (total)	48,400	93,500	100,100	92,400	100,100	91,300	79,200	66,000	39,600	22,000
EPO units (mean)	4,033	7,192	7,700	7,700	7,700	7,023	6,600	5,077	3,046	2,200
EPO units/Week (mean)	**10,275**	**19,850**	**21,252**	**21,252**	**19,734**	**19,383**	**18,216**	**14,013**	**8,407**	**4,671**
EPO units (mean) /Kg/Week	184	344	370	360	342	327	312	237	141	78
Venofer mg iron (count)	0	5	0	5	6	1	6	1	1	1
Venofer mg iron (total)		1,000		1,000	1,200	200	1,200	200	200	200
Venofer mg iron (mean)		200		200	200	200	200	200	200	200
Total iron counts	0	5	0	5	6	1	6	1	1	1
Total iron given (mg)	0	1,000	0	1,000	1,200	200	1,200	200	200	200
Iron given mg (mean/injection)		200		200	200	200	200	200	200	200
Total iron (mean/HD)	0	77	0	83	86	15	100	15	15	15
Total iron given (mg/month)	**0**	**939**	**0**	**1,018**	**1,047**	**188**	**1,221**	**188**	**188**	**188**
Total iron given (mg/Kg/month)	0.0	16.3	0.0	17.3	18.1	3.2	20.9	3.2	3.1	3.1

Figure 3. Aggregate report used for CQI in a 44 year old female patient treated by dialysis for 23 years. Although the report was run monthly for the latest 18-months, for clarity only a 10-month time span is shown. This report automatically calculated data for monthly intervals during 2009. Displayed are HD treatments, data relevant to the erythron and iron status, and the EPO and IV iron administered. In November 2009 to January 2010, despite EPO administration of 355–445 units/Kg/week, hemoglobin was low and falling; the low TSAT and relatively low MCH pointed to iron insufficiency. She received 3.4 g of iron intravenously between February and May 2010. An increase in Hb, TSAT, MCH, and serum albumin was evident in May, and continued.

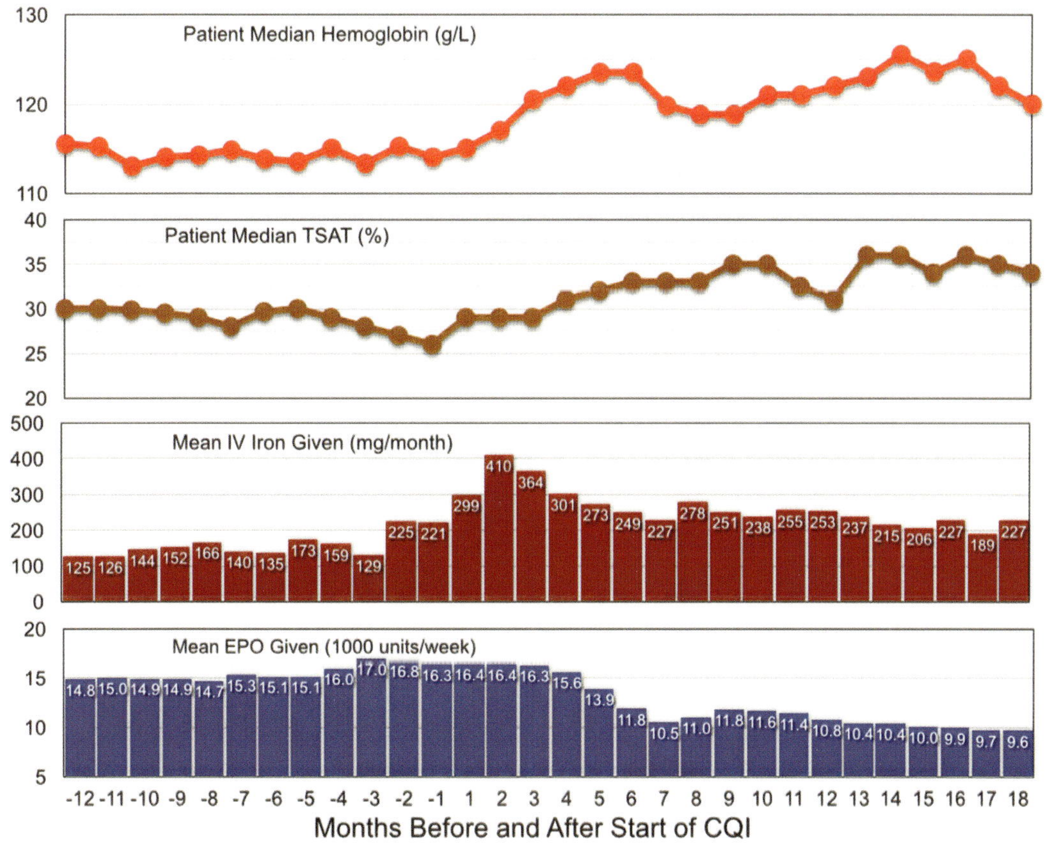

Figure 4. For all study patients, patient median Hb, median TSAT, mean IV iron and mean EPO administered in the protocol period 12 months before study start and the 18-month CQI period.

and ranges were calculated as measures of variability, for Hb values of each patient during each 6-month period. Means, medians, SD, ranges, and coefficients of variation were then calculated for all patients.

Mortality per 100 patient years was calculated as is done by USRDS [8], by dividing the number of deaths by the total time in years that the patients were treated by HD, and multiplying by 100.

Medicare Part B allowable charges for EPO and IV iron were calculated using Centers for Medicare and Medicaid Services (CMS) published data and from the amount of each drug given during any month divided by the number of HD treatments during that month. Included were treatments both for patients studied longitudinally and for all others treated in that month.

Study Approval

The Institutional Review Board did not require informed consent as (1) the study of quality improvement was considered to be a part of routine clinical care of the patients, and (2) the data were analyzed anonymously. The study was approved by the Institutional Review Board of Weill Medical College of Cornell University.

Results

Mean patient age was 59±16.2 years; 55% were male, 34% White, 46% Black, 20% of other ethnic groups. Primary renal disease was: glomerulonephritis in 35%, hypertension in 30%, diabetic nephropathy in 21%. From February 1, 2010 to July 31, 2011, 17 patients received a kidney transplant, 9 were transferred to peritoneal and nocturnal home HD, 22 to another dialysis unit, and one was lost to follow up.

In the 12-month historical period prior to study start, patient monthly median Hb varied between 113.0 and 115.5 g/L, TSAT between 26% and 30%, with the lowest values immediately before study start (Figure 4). IV iron given varied between 124 mg and 159 mg per month, with larger amounts in the last two months before study start. EPO administration varied between 14,800 and 17,000 units per week.

IV iron administered increased in month 1, peaked at 410 mg/month in month 2, and decreased to ≈250 mg/month by month 6. In months 13–18, an average of 215 mg was given monthly. Hb increased in month 1, and was consistently higher thereafter. In months 13–18 patient monthly median Hb was 120 to 125 g/L. EPO administered decreased slightly in month 4, and further in months 5 and 6. In months 16–18 mean EPO dose was 9,720 units/week.

To provide more details of changes over time, percentiles of TSAT, serum ferritin, Hb, and EPO administered are displayed monthly. Median serum ferritin, measured 3-monthly, increased from 552 μg/L before study start to 1148 μg/L in months 13–18 (Figure 5a). TSAT levels increased steadily from CQI months 1 to 9 for all percentiles (Figure 5b). In months 13–18, the 10th and 25th percentiles were 23.7% and 29,1% respectively, indicating that iron insufficiency was then uncommon. Hb levels increased steadily from CQI month 1 onward (Figure 5c). In months 13–18, levels were 142.7 g/L for the 90th percentile, 132.5 g/L for the

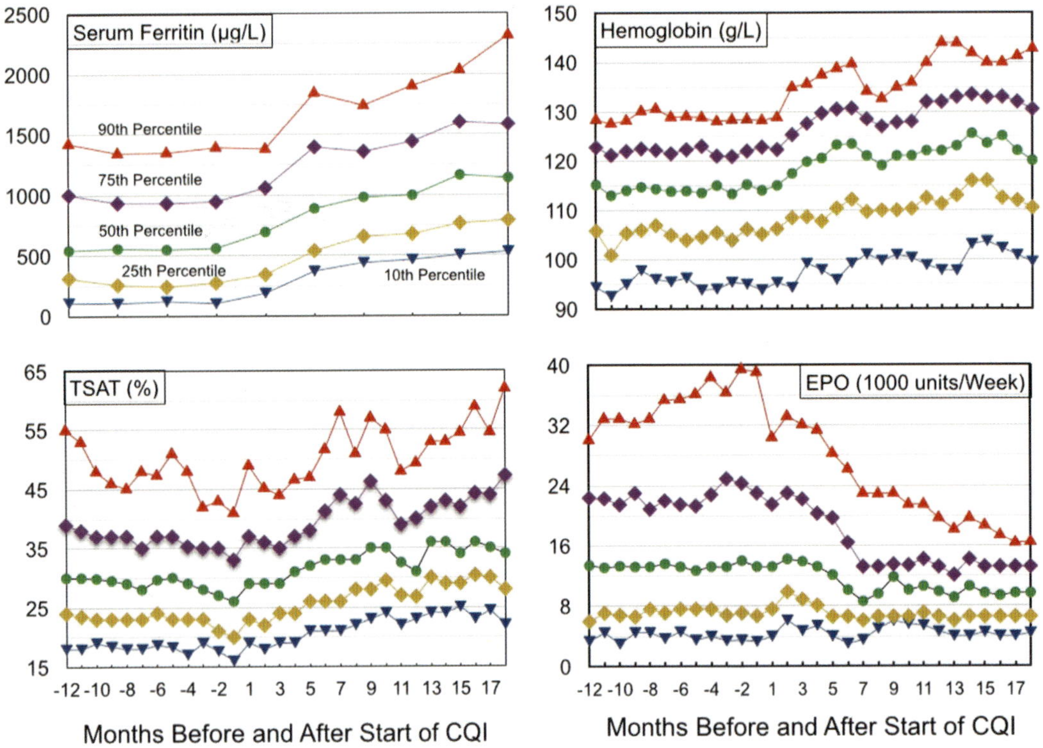

Figure 5. Percentiles of patients by (a) serum ferritin, (b) TSAT, (c) hemoglobin, and (d) administered EPO for 12 months before and 18 months after study start.

75th, 122.7 g/L for the 50th, 113.3 g/L for the 25th, and 101.2 g/L for the 10th percentile. EPO administration levels decreased steadily from CQI months 3 to 6, indicating that administered EPO decreased whether initially very high or more modest (Figure 5d). The most striking decreases occurred in the 90th and 75th percentiles. The 50th percentile changed negligibly in months 1–4, and decreased to an average of 9,786 units/week (134 units/Kg/week) in months 13–18.

There were 2.10 new and 2.08 discontinued IV iron orders per patient year in the historical period (Figure 6). New IV iron orders doubled in the first 6 CQI months and then decreased to 1.44 per year in months 13–18, when discontinued orders were 0.86 per patient year. New EPO orders, 6.77 per patient year in the

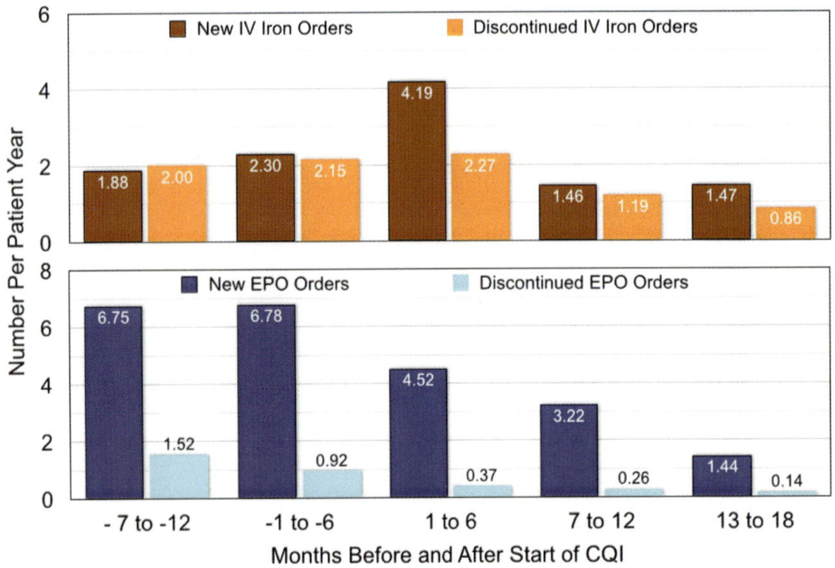

Figure 6. New orders and discontinued orders for IV iron and for EPO for two 6-month periods before and three 6-month periods after the start of the CQI process.

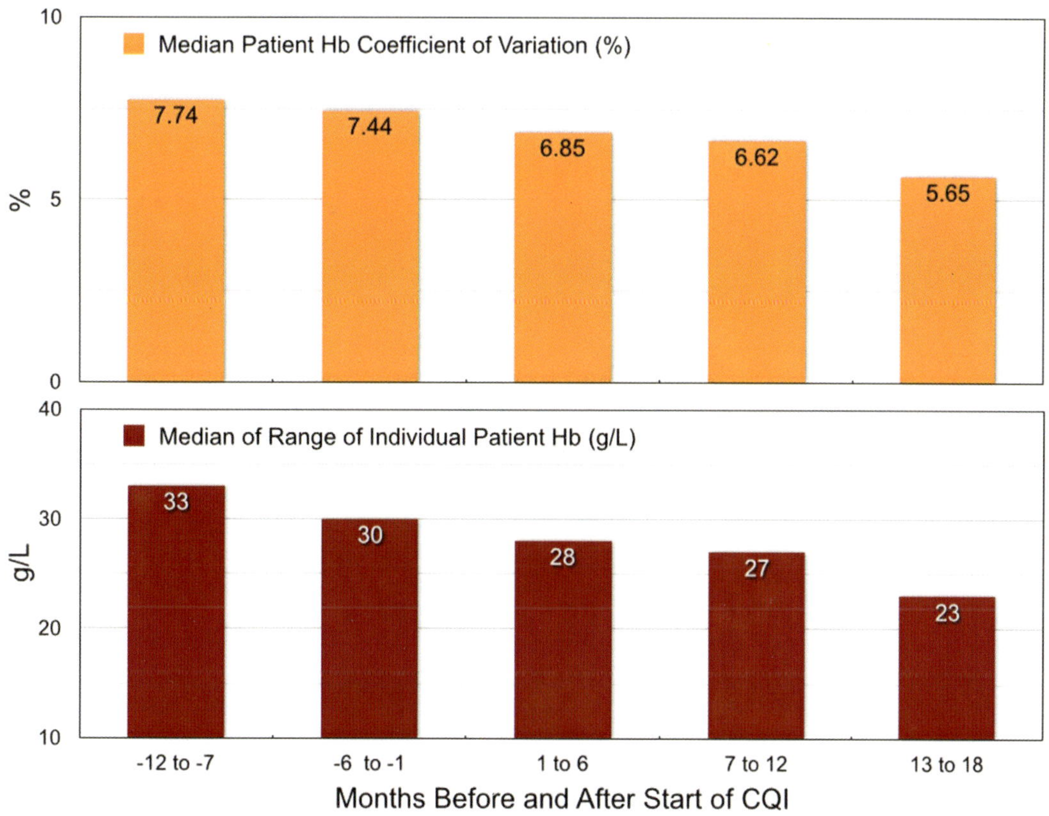

Figure 7. Patient median Hb coefficients of variation and median Hb ranges for two 6-month periods before and three 6-month periods after the start of the CQI process.

historical period, decreased 83% in CQI months 13–18 to 1.12. EPO discontinuation orders, 1.20 per patient year in the historical period, decreased 84% in CQI months 13–18 to 0.19.

With 3 caregivers reviewing the data, 12 caregiver hours were needed at study start for the review of 250 patients; another 3 hours were needed for one caregiver to enter new and changed orders. With experience and increased stability of Hb and TSAT, and of EPO and IV iron orders, fewer caregiver hours were needed: in CQI months 13–18, 6 caregiver hours for the monthly review, and 1.5 caregiver hours to enter new and changed orders. Thus anemia management which consumed 15 caregiver hours per month at study start required only 7.5 caregiver hours per month at the end of the CQI study.

The individual patient coefficient of variation and range of Hb values in individual patients were analyzed in five 6-month periods (Figure 7). The coefficient of variation and range decreased after the study start and were least in CQI months 13–18. Coefficients of variation for all Hb measurements for each individual patient, 7.53% (IQR 5.68, 10.63) in the historical period, decreased by 23% to 5.82% (IQR 4.13, 9.04) in CQI months 13–18. The variation of Hb measurements decreased by 27% from 31.5 g/L to 23 g/L.

Table 1. Selected data on patients in the study unit who died and who were alive at the end of the study.

	Died (n = 35)	Alive (n = 215)	p
Age at study start (years)	70.6±14.4	58.6±14.7	<0.001
Admissions per patient year	4.65	1.27	<0.001
Hb (g/L)	112.5 (100.5, 120.5)	121.0 (114.0, 126.0)	<0.001
TSAT (%)	29.5 (23.5, 35.1)	33.0 (29.0, 37.4)	<0.01
Serum ferritin (μg/L)	1080 (607, 1305)	922 (568, 1328)	NS
Serum albumin (g/L)	37.0 (33.0, 38.5)	40.5 (38.0, 42.0)	<0.001
C-reactive protein (mg/L)	12.3 (6.1, 36.0)	6.33 (2.65, 13.10)	<0.005
EPO given (1000 units/week)	13.53 (7.59, 18.98)	10.25 (6.58, 15.75)	<0.05

Laboratory test results and EPO administered are median values and interquartile range (IQR).

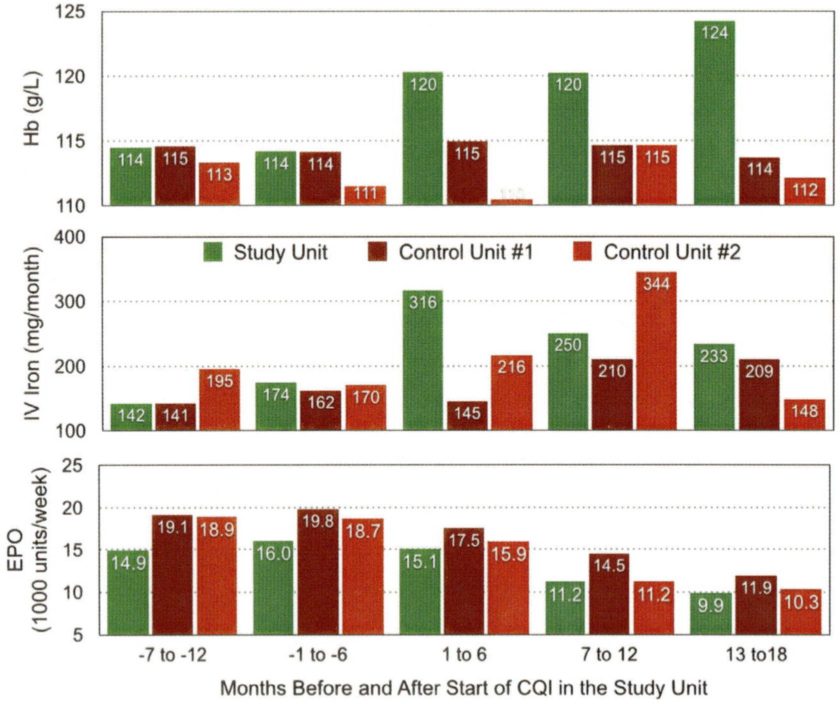

Figure 8. Patient median Hb and mean IV iron and EPO administered in the CQI study and two control units. Data are summarized for two 6-month periods before and three 6-month periods after start of the CQI process in the CQI study unit.

Using data from all patients treated in the unit from 2004 to 2011 with 10 or more Hb values per year, we analyzed by calendar year the per patient range of Hb levels. This historical perspective showed that from 2004–2009 the range was ≤20 g/L in only 4% of patients, and ≤30 g/L in 15%. In 2011, by contrast, the proportion meeting these low ranges had increased to 9% and 33% respectively.

In the 12 months before CQI start patients were followed for a total of 219.77 years and there were 331 hospital admissions (1.51 per year). During the 18-month CQI period the patients were followed for a total of 297.06 years, and there were 422 admissions to hospital (1.42 per year).

Thirty-five patients died during the CQI study. The mortality rate, 11.78 per 100 patient years, was 42% less than the 2009 United States rate for all dialysis patients of 19.95 per 100 years

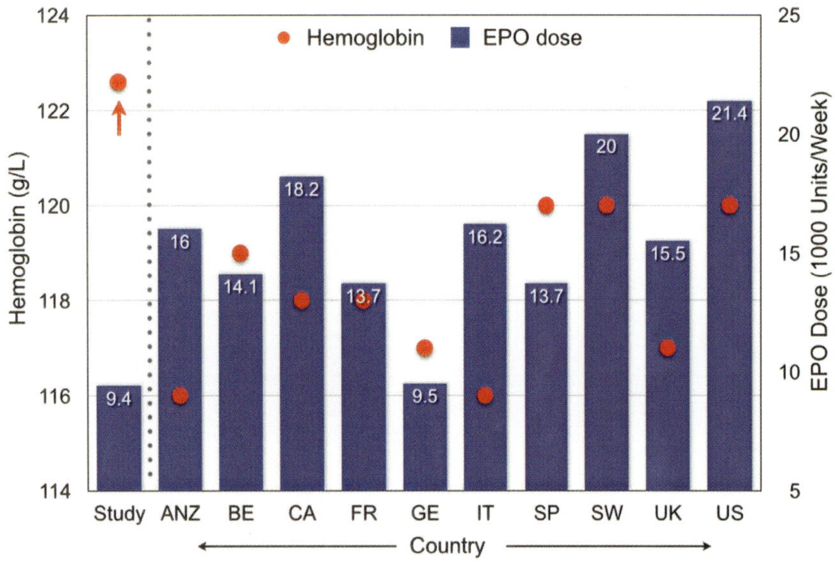

Figure 9. EPO dose and Hb in 2005–2008 in ten countries [26] and in the study unit (Study) in February–July, 2011. (Abbreviations: ANZ= Australia and New Zealand; BE= Belgium; CA= Canada; Fr= France; GE= Germany; IT= Italy; SP= Spain; SW= Sweden; UK= United Kingdom; US= United States).

Table 2. Selected data on patients in the study and two control units in months 13–18 after start of CQI in the study unit.

	Study Unit	Control Unit #1	Control Unit #2
Hemoglobin			
Patient median Hb (g/L)	123.6	114	112
Change from 6 months before CQI start in study unit	+8.8%	0%	+1%
Median patient coefficient of variation (%)	5.65%	6.51%	7.55%
EPO			
EPO administered (units/week)	9,867	11,874	10,264
Change from 6 months before CQI start in study unit	−35.5%	−37.7%	−45.5%
EPO new orders per patient year	1.44	7.91	6.44
IV iron			
IV iron administered (mg/month)	233	209	148
IV iron new orders per patient year	1.47	7.04	7.30

[8] and did not differ significantly from that before study start. Compared with those who survived the 35 patients who died were 12 years older, had lower serum albumin, lower TSAT, higher C-reactive protein, and a more frequent rate of hospital admission (Table 1). Slightly more EPO was administered in those who died.

In control units #1 and# 2 there were 202 and 175 patients, average age 63.1 and 64.0 years, who received EPO in the 4 months before February 2010. During 216 and 170 years of follow up, deaths were respectively 14.2 and 18.8 per 100 patient years. Little attention was paid to iron administration and EPO was reduced without a defined plan; in unit #2 EPO was reduced in the first 6 months before IV iron administration was increased (Figure 8). TSAT increased to 30.7% and 36.0% by months 13–18 in the two units, serum ferritin to 854 and 1,170 µg/L, but Hb was unchanged (Figure 9). EPO was reduced to a comparable level in all 3 units. New orders for EPO per patient year in months 13–18 were 5.4 and 4.5 times more frequent in the control units than in the study unit; new orders for IV iron were 4.8 and 5.0 times more frequent (Table 2). The median coefficient of variation of Hb was 15% and 34% higher in the control than in the study units.

The allowable charges for the hematinic medications administered to all patients in the study unit were summarized in five 6-month periods. The allowable charges for EPO administered, $48.99 per HD treatment in the 12-month historical period before CQI start, decreased to $33.69 per treatment in the 13–18 months after CQI start. That of IV iron increased from $4.50 to $7.19.

For comparison, the Medicare 2012 per treatment "bundle" allowance was $56.82 for erythrocyte stimulating agents (EPO and darbepoetin alfa) per HD treatment and $6.54 for IV iron. Thus the allowable charges of $40.88 for CQI study patient use of these two hematinic drugs in months 13–18 was $22.88 (34.8%) less than the Medicare "bundle" allowance.

Discussion

Standardized protocols are used widely in the United States, where recent EPO use has decreased 40%, with a 6.7% decrease in Hb from 120 to 112 g/L [23]. In the present study the control units used the same EMR as the CQI study unit, but continued a protocol-based approach to anemia treatment. Over 18 study months, EPO administration decreased 41% with little change in Hb. In the CQI study unit, by contrast, EPO administration decreased 42%, but Hb increased by 8.8%; there was also less Hb variation than in the controls (Table 2). EPO administered weekly in the CQI study unit was also much less than that in 9 countries in a recent study of a randomly selected group of 300 patients from each of 10 countries [24]. Yet, Hb in the CQI unit was 2.6 to 6.6 g/L higher than in each of these 10 countries.

There have been concerns about adverse effects of Hb>120 g/L in renal failure [16–18]. Re-analysis, however, showed the lowest mortality was associated with the highest achieved Hb [25,26]. In other studies, patient mortality was highest with Hb≤ 110 g/L, lowest with Hb>120 g/L [27–31]. In the CQI study

Table 3. Percentage of patients with various TSAT levels in the last 3 months of three studies over 14 years from 1997 to 2011.

IV iron administration	Years of Study	CQI	TSAT (%)			
			≤15	≤20	≤25	≤30
Previous Studies						
Iron insufficient at study start, prospective [12]	1996–1997	Yes	1	9	30	48
Clinical practice, retrospective [17]	1998–2007	No	5	16	29	51
Present Study						
CQI Study Unit	2009–2011	Yes	1	5	11	26
Control Unit #1	2009–2011	No	5	17	40	62
Control Unit #2	2009–2011	No	5	11	27	45

unit, patient median Hb was 121.0 g/L in survivors, 112.5 g/L in those who died. Hospital admissions were 3.66 times more frequent in those who died. Arranged in ranks (≤100; 100.1–110; 110.1–120; >120 g/L) Hb distribution differed in the two groups ($\chi^2_{[3]} = 19.6$, $p<0.0003$). These data are consistent with an association of mortality with age and morbidity rather than with high Hb.

We investigated the importance of iron and effect of Hb on survival in a 9.5-year retrospective study of 1774 patients [19]. Multifactorial analysis demonstrated the favorable effect of Hb> 120 g/L. As compared with the 442 patients with Hb>120 g/L, the hazard ratios for death for Hb 110–120, 100–110, and < 100 g/L were respectively 1.67, 2.69, and 2.83. In the last 3 months of the present study, TSAT was ≤20% in 5%, ≤25% in 11% of patients in the CQI study unit, (Table 3), while in control units #1 and #2 respectively the proportions were higher: ≤20% in 17% and 11% of patients, ≤25% in 40% and 27%.

This suggested that the conventional method of IV iron administration in intermittent courses, without systematic feedback, was associated with suboptimal results; patients were probably cycling between iron deficiency and repletion, without being continuously iron sufficient. In the CQI study group only 6% of patients had TSAT ≤20% in the last 3 months, suggesting that continuous long-term modulation of interrelationships between IV iron, EPO dose and Hb was probably enabled by the CQI process.

In contrast to the current widely used approach that strongly encourages application of population-based guidelines or protocols to individual patient care, CQI enables clinicians to assess variables such as severity of symptoms, illness, comorbidity, and other clinical nuances [32] with clinically pertinent reports immediately available at the point-of-care. Skilled clinicians can thereby generate patient and practice specific knowledge on a day-to-day basis for each patient as an individual, and practice medicine based on scientific judgment conditioned by the totality of available up-to-date evidence of the state of the patient [33].

The application to patient care of protocols without critical oversight of details of individual patients neither promotes nor enables consideration by caregivers of details of the patient illness; it may result in treating patients without regard specifically to factors such as age, race, gender, and co-morbid conditions that may impair or enhance treatment responses. This is particularly so with protocols based on ensuring that certain predetermined numbers are met. By contrast, the CQI process promotes and enables attention to many details of care of patients as individuals, and as individual members of a patient population. It enables caregivers to inquire of the reasons why therapeutic objectives were not met, promotes correction of underlying problems or complications, and does so repeatedly and particularly.

We have shown that a disciplined, classic CQI process wedded to an appropriately designed EMR can lead to better outcome and reduce cost. Neither alone suffices. To facilitate decisions repeatedly over long time spans access serially to relevant time-oriented information including laboratory tests and medications is essential; these data must be organized to display feedback over time between treatments and their effects. Without an EMR that so displays data in spreadsheet (or graphic) metaphor the task is personnel intensive and overwhelming. Needed for introduction and implementation of CQI is clinical and administrative leadership and education and encouragement of physicians, nurses, and other caregivers.

The present study has limitations. It was applied to a single clinical problem, and needs testing with others. It was tested in a dialysis unit treating patients with chronic renal failure, and requires testing in other populations and practice environments. It should also be tested with other EMRs that display feedback over time between treatments and their effects.

Conclusions

Medical therapies are often based on randomized studies where patient variability is intentionally filtered out, or protocols assembled from relevant literature; these are rarely tested in diverse populations. Physicians are also bereft of tools and techniques to apply randomized study results or protocols to each particular individual patient. CQI is an iterative process to understand and contain the effects of variability that, in clinical medicine, stems from the biologic uniqueness of individual patients and their co-morbid conditions.

A recent Institute of Medicine report concluded: "Although unprecedented levels of information are available, patients and clinicians often lack access to guidance that is relevant, timely, and useful for the circumstances at hand. Overcoming this challenge will require applying computing capabilities and analytic approaches to develop real-time insights from routine patient care, disseminating knowledge using new technological tools, and addressing the regulatory challenges that can inhibit progress" [34].

The CQI process is sustainable, practical and appropriate for most complex, expensive therapies now used in chronic disease patient care. We suggest that it provides a model to address both the issues raised by the recent Institute of Medicine report, and an approach to design of methodologies to optimize physician decision making for individual patient care in heterogeneous patient populations.

Acknowledgments

The authors wish to thank John P. Flynn whose work in software design over the past 20 years enabled this study.

Author Contributions

Conceived and designed the experiments: JAL VEP. Performed the experiments: JAL. Analyzed the data: VEP. Wrote the paper: VEP.

References

1. Shewhart W (1986) Statistical Method from the Viewpoint of Quality Control. Mineola, NY: Dover.
2. Deming WE (1982) Out of the Crisis. Cambridge, England: Cambridge University Press.
3. Heffler S, Smith S, Keehan S, Borger C, Clemens MK, et al. (2005) U.S. health spending projections for 2004–2014. Health Aff (Millwood) Suppl Web Exclusives: W5-74-W5-85.
4. Fries JF (1972) Time-oriented patient records and a computer data bank. JAMA 222: 1536–1542.
5. Pollak VE, Buncher CR, Donovan ER (1977) On-line computerized data handling system for treating patients with renal disease. Arch. Int. Med 137: 446–456.
6. Buntin MB, Burke MF, Hoaglin MC, Blumenthal D (2011) The benefits of health information technology: a review of the recent literature shows predominantly positive results. Health Aff (Millwood) 30: 464–471.
7. Pollak VE (1985) The computer in medicine: its application to medical practice, quality control, and cost containment. JAMA 253: 62–68.
8. U.S. Renal Data System, USRDS (2011) Annual Data Report: Atlas of Chronic Kidney Disease and End-Stage Renal Disease in the United States, National Institutes of Health, National Institute of Diabetes and Digestive and Kidney Diseases, Bethesda, MD, 2011. U.S. Renal Data System, USRDS 2011.
9. Goodkin DA, Bragg-Gresham JL, Koenig KG, Wolfe RA, Akiba T, et al (2003) Association of comorbid conditions and mortality in hemodialysis patients in

Europe, Japan, and the United States: the Dialysis Outcomes and Practice Patterns Study (DOPPS). J Am Soc Nephrol 14: 3270–3277.
10. Weinhandl ED, Gilbertson DT, Collins AJ (2011) Association of Mean Weekly Epoetin Alfa Dose with Mortality Risk in a Retrospective Cohort Study of Medicare Hemodialysis Patients. Am J Nephrol 34: 298–308.
11. Servilla KS, Singh AK, Hunt WC, Harford AM, Miskulin D, et al. (2009) Anemia Management and Association of Race with Mortality and Hospitalization in a Large Not-for-profit Dialysis Organization." Am J Kidney Dis 54: 498–510.
12. Eschbach JW, Egrie JC, Downing MR, Browne JK, Adamson JW (1987) Correction of the anemia of end-stage renal disease with recombinant human erythropoietin. Results of a combined phase I and II clinical trial. N Engl J Med 316: 73–78.
13. Eschbach JW (1991) Erythropoietin 1991—an overview. Am J Kidney Dis 18: 3–9.
14. Pollak VE, Lorch JA, Means RTJ (2001) Unanticipated favorable effects of correcting iron deficiency in chronic hemodialysis patients. J Investig Med 49: 173–183.
15. Hsu CY, McCulloch CE, Curhan GC (2002) Iron status and hemoglobin level in chronic renal insufficiency. J Am Soc Nephrol 13: 2783–2786.
16. Besarab A, Bolton WK, Browne JK, Egrie JC, Nissenson AR, et al (1998) The effects of normal as compared with low hematocrit values in patients with cardiac disease who are receiving hemodialysis and epoetin. N Engl J Med 339: 584–590.
17. Drueke TB, Locatelli F, Clyne N, Eckardt KU, Macdougall IC, et al (2006) Normalization of Hemoglobin Level in Patients with Chronic Kidney Disease and Anemia. N Engl J Med 355: 2071–2084.
18. Singh AK, Szczech L, Tang KL, Barnhart H, Sapp S, et al (2006) Correction of Anemia with Epoetin Alfa in Chronic Kidney Disease. N Engl J Med 355: 2085–2098.
19. Pollak VE, Lorch JA, Shukla R, Satwah S (2009) The importance of iron in long-term survival of maintenance hemodialysis patients treated with epoetin-alpha and intravenous iron: analysis of 9.5 years of prospectively collected data. BMC Nephrol 10: 6.
20. (2006) KDOQI Clinical Practice Guidelines and Clinical Practice Recommendations for Anemia in Chronic Kidney Disease. Am J Kidney Dis 47: S11–145.
21. Pollak VE, Lorch JA (2007) Effect of electronic patient record use on mortality in End Stage Renal Disease, a model chronic disease: retrospective analysis of 9 years of prospectively collected data. BMC Med Inform Decis Mak 7: 38.
22. Eschbach JW, Funk D, Adamson J, Kuhn I, Scribner BH, et al. (1967) Erythropoiesis in patients with renal failure undergoing chronic dialysis. N Engl J Med 276: 653–658.
23. Fuller DS, Pisoni RL, Bieber BA, Robinson BM (2013) The DOPPS Practice Monitor for US Dialysis Care: Trends Through December 2011. Am J Kidney Dis 61: 342–346.
24. McFarlane PA, Pisoni RL, Eichleay MA, Wald R, Port FK, et al. (2010) International trends in erythropoietin use and hemoglobin levels in hemodialysis patients. Kidney Int 78: 215–223.
25. Besarab A, Frinak S, Yee J (2009) What is so bad about a hemoglobin level of 12 to 13 g/dL for chronic kidney disease patients anyway? Adv Chronic Kidney Dis 16: 131–142.
26. Agarwal R (2010) Individualizing decision-making—resurrecting the doctor-patient relationship in the anemia debate. Clin J Am Soc Nephrol 5: 1340–1346.
27. Ofsthun N, Labrecque J, Lacson E, Keen M, Lazarus JM (2003) The effects of higher hemoglobin levels on mortality and hospitalization in hemodialysis patients. Kidney Int 63: 1908–1914.
28. Hampl H, Hennig L, Rosenberger C, Amirkhalily M, Gogol L, et al (2005) Effects of Optimized Heart Failure Therapy and Anemia Correction with Epoetin Beta on Left Ventricular Mass in Hemodialysis Patients. Am J Nephrol 25: 211–220.
29. Regidor DL, Kopple JD, Kovesdy CP, Kilpatrick RD, McAllister CJ, et al (2006) Associations between Changes in Hemoglobin and Administered Erythropoiesis-Stimulating Agent and Survival in Hemodialysis Patients. J Am Soc Nephrol 17: 1181–1191.
30. Portoles J, Lopez-Gomez JM, Aljama P (2007) A prospective multicentre study of the role of anaemia as a risk factor in haemodialysis patients: the MAR Study. Nephrol Dial Transplant 22: 500–507.
31. Fort J, Cuevas X, García F, Pérez-García R, Lladós F, et al (2010) Mortality in incident haemodialysis patients: time-dependent haemoglobin levels and erythropoiesis-stimulating agent dose are independent predictive factors in the ANSWER study. Nephrol Dial Transplant 25: 2702–2710.
32. Feinstein AR, Horwitz RI (1997) Problems in the "evidence" of "evidence-based medicine". Am J Med 103: 529–535.
33. Rawlins M (2009) De testimonio: on the evidence for decisions about the use of therapeutic interventions. Lancet 372: 2152–2161.
34. National Research Council (2012) Best Care at Lower Cost: The Path to Continuously Learning Health Care in America. Washington, DC: The National Academies Press.

2

Patients' Perceptions of Information and Education for Renal Replacement Therapy: An Independent Survey by the European Kidney Patients' Federation on Information and Support on Renal Replacement Therapy

Wim Van Biesen[1]*, Sabine N. van der Veer[2], Mark Murphey[3], Olga Loblova[4,5], Simon Davies[6]

1 Renal Division, Ghent University Hospital, Ghent, Belgium, **2** Department of Medical Informatics, Academic Medical Center, Amsterdam, The Netherlands, **3** Irish Kidney Association, Dublin, Ireland, **4** A&R Edelman, London, United Kingdom, **5** Department of Public Policy, Central European University, Budapest, Hungary, **6** Department of Nephrology, University Hospital of North Staffordshire, Stoke on Trent, United Kingdom

Abstract

Background: Selection of an appropriate renal replacement modality is of utmost importance for patients with end stage renal disease. Previous studies showed provision of information to and free modality choice by patients to be suboptimal. Therefore, the European Kidney Patients' Federation (CEAPIR) explored European patients' perceptions regarding information, education and involvement on the modality selection process.

Methods: CEAPIR developed a survey, which was disseminated by the national kidney patient organisations in Europe.

Results: In total, 3867 patients from 36 countries completed the survey. Respondents were either on in-centre haemodialysis (53%) or had a functioning graft (38%) at the time of survey. The majority (78%) evaluated the general information about kidney disease and treatment as helpful, but 39% did not recall being told about alternative treatment options than their current one. Respondents were more often satisfied with information provided on in-centre haemodialysis (90%) and transplantation (87%) than with information provided on peritoneal dialysis (79%) or home haemodialysis (61%), and were more satisfied with information from health care professionals vs other sources such as social media. Most (75%) felt they had been involved in treatment selection, 29% perceived they had no free choice. Involvement in modality selection was associated with enhanced satisfaction with treatment (OR 3.13; 95% CI 2.72–3.60). Many respondents (64%) could not remember receiving education on how to manage their kidney disease in daily life. Perceptions on information seem to differ between countries.

Conclusions: Kidney patients reported to be overall satisfied with the information they received on their disease and treatment, although information seemed mostly to have been focused on one modality. Patients involved in modality selection were more satisfied with their treatment. However, in the perception of the patients, the freedom to choose an alternative modality showed room for improvement.

Editor: Giuseppe Remuzzi, Mario Negri Institute for Pharmacological Research and Azienda Ospedaliera Ospedali Riuniti di Bergamo, Italy

Funding: Baxter Healthcare provided logistical and financial support for this initiative through an unrestricted scientific grant to CEAPIR. The funders had no role in study design, data collection and analysis, decision to publish, or preparation of the manuscript.

Competing Interests: Wim Van Biesen has received travel fees on different occasions from Baxter, Fresenius and Gambro, and serves as a steering committee member of a Fresenius sponsored study (IPOD-PD). Olga Lo¨blova´ has been employed by A&R Edelman and has received consultancy fees from A&R Edelman and Baxter. Simon Davies has received research funding and honoraria for lecturing and advisory board participation from Baxter and Fresenius.

* Email: wim.vanbiesen@ugent.be

Introduction

Clinical practice guidance for treatment of kidney disease worldwide advocate the provision of information and education to patients, as well as patient involvement in the process of selecting a treatment modality [1–3]. Timely and adequately informing and educating kidney patients may result in a more balanced modality selection [4–6], promote independence and encourage self-management [7], and may be linked to a better prepared start of dialysis [8].

Previous studies suggested that the majority of patients wants to be given information on different treatment options, and that they want to participate in treatment selection [9,10]. Still, the quality, comprehensibility and completeness of information and education provided to kidney patients seem to be suboptimal at best [11–14]. This may partly explain why some patients have little knowledge of their disease as well as a limited awareness of their different treatment options [15,16]. Also, it has been reported that many kidney patients perceive a lack of choice in whether to start renal replacement therapy (RRT), or in which modality to select [12,17]. Study results like these raised concerns among the members of the executive committee of the European Kidney Patients' Federation (CEAPIR).

CEAPIR was founded in 1981 and is a non-profit umbrella organization for 23 national kidney patients' associations in European countries ranging from Norway to Portugal, and from the United Kingdom to Latvia. CEAPIR's main aims are to promote the prevention of kidney disease, establish access to treatment for all European kidney patients, and set a European quality standard for treatment of kidney disease. This quality standard states –among other things– that clear information for and education of patients is necessary to fully inform patients' choices and decisions (www.ceapir.org).

To inform and support a plan of action to improve attainment of this standard across Europe, CEAPIR wanted to explore the current perception of information provision and education amongst patients in Europe, as the scarce available evidence is largely USA based [12,13,18].

Therefore, CEAPIR initiated a European project with the aim to explore patients' perceptions and satisfaction with regard to information and education in general and on different modalities, and their involvement in the modality selection process.

Methods

Survey development and dissemination

The executive committee of CEAPIR – consisting of kidney patients and carers– initiated the survey. They framed and selected the preliminary questions in English based on consensus during a face-to face meeting, followed-up by several discussions via e-mail. They started from CEAPIR's minimal requirement regarding the necessity of "clear and precise *information* and *education* of patients at every stage of the treatment cycle to fully inform patients on their *choices and decisions* on all available treatment options" (www.ceapir.org). The preliminary questions were then circulated to the national patient societies with a request for feedback. This formed the basis for a draft English, electronic survey that was pilot tested among members of the Irish Kidney Association, and revised accordingly.

For dissemination, CEAPIR asked the national patient societies to translate the survey in their local language, and subsequently distribute it among their members. Societies were encouraged to choose a dissemination strategy that matched their organisation's infrastructure and ongoing activities. Examples of strategies included a paper version of the survey in the society's periodical magazine (Germany and Poland), sending it via e-mail while combining it with another survey that was already planned on a related topic (United Kingdom), or launching it on a society's website.

Data collection and analyses

A professional data management company collected the data from November 2010 to November 2011; they also arranged data entry and storage. Our primary data analysis consisted of descriptive statistics, for which we presented results as valid percentages. In order to investigate the association between treatment decision making (being somewhat or very involved yes/no; having a treatment choice yes/no) and overall satisfaction with received kidney care (being very satisfied yes/no) we calculated odds ratios (OR) and 95% confidence intervals (CI).

We explored the influence of recall bias (i.e., a systematic error due to differences in accuracy or completeness of remembering past experiences) on respondents' recollection of receiving information or education at the start of RRT we performed a χ^2 test comparing responses of respondents who had been on their current modality 2 years or less versus more than 2 years. P-values below.05 were considered to indicate a statistically significant difference between these groups.

To address large differences between countries regarding the number of respondents, we performed a separate analysis for countries with more than 20% of respondents (i.e. Poland and Germany) vs other countries using χ^2 test, with reporting of Odds ratios and 95% confidence intervals.

All statistical analyses were performed using IBM SPSS Statistics 22 by OL, WVB and SVDV.

The protocol and accompanying information for patients of this retrospective study were evaluated by the ethical committee of the Amsterdam Medical Centre (W14_126#14.17.0160), which waived the need for ethical approval. Patient identification data were anonymized for data storage by CEAPIR and data were de-identified before data analysis. The fact that patients completed and send back the questionnaire, after being informed on the purpose and scope of the survey, was considered equivalent to informed consent.

Results

In total, 3867 patients from 36 different countries responded to the survey. Table 1 displays their characteristics. Germany and Poland each contributed more than 20% of the respondents. The majority of completed questionnaires were received by postal mail through the national societies (58.6%), whereas 17.7, 15.6 and 8.1% were received via e-mail, the CEAPIR website and other (social) media, respectively.

Information on kidney disease and treatment modalities

The majority of respondents (73.8%) reported to have been provided with information on reduced kidney function in the year prior to starting RRT, while 44.9% recalled receiving diet-related information. More than one third (39.3%) did not remember anyone speaking to them about alternative treatment options than their current one or the possibility of changing treatments (Germany = 34.6%, OR 1.03 (95% CI 0.88–1.20) and Poland = 45.9%, 0R 1.65 (95% CI 1.40–1.99) versus other countries). This did not differ between respondents who had been on their current modality ≤2 versus >2 years ($\chi^2 = 0.059$, $p = 0.8$).

In general, respondents evaluated the information they got about kidney disease or treatment options as very (46.1%) or somewhat (32.3%) helpful; 11% answered they did not receive or could not remember receiving any information (very useful: Germany = 32.5%, OR 0.43 (95% CI 0.37–0.50) and Poland = 40.9%, OR 0.60 (95% CI 0.52–0.73) versus respondents from other nationalities). For those who said to have received information, the appreciation differed between sources and modalities: Figure 1 shows that health care professionals were more frequently scored as a helpful information source than patient organisations, websites or social media. Furthermore, respondents were more often satisfied with information provided on in-centre haemodialysis and transplantation compared to information on home-based therapies, with which approximately a third of respondents reported to be (very) unsatisfied (Figure 2).

Table 1. Respondents' characteristics (total n = 3867).

Characteristics	**Respondents**[a)]
Age (years)	
18 to 29	245 (6.7)
30 to 49	990 (27.2)
50 to 69	1828 (50.2)
70 or older	579 (15.9)
Gender	
Male	1944 (53.9)
Country of residence [b)]	
Germany	1063 (29.9)
Poland	772 (21.7)
Ireland	269 (7.6)
Hungary	187 (5.3)
Portugal	186 (5.2)
Austria	183 (5.1)
Lithuania	136 (3.8)
Finland	120 (3.4)
United Kingdom	114 (3.2)
Italy	93 (2.6)
Current employment status	
Employed	1340 (37.6)
Not employed	992 (27.8)
Retired	1145 (32.1)
Other	91 (2.6)
Time between kidney disease diagnosis and start of first treatment	
Less than 3 months	973 (26.6)
3 to 12 months	548 (15.0)
More than 12 months	2137 (58.4)
Treatment modality at the time of survey completion	
In-centre haemodialysis	1988 (52.6)
Home haemodialysis	91 (2.4)
Peritoneal dialysis (APD, CAPD)	276 (7.3)
Transplanted	1427 (37.7)
Being prepared for dialysis	257 (6.8)
Time on current modality	
Less than 1 year	151 (25.9)
1 or 2 years	190 (32.5)
3 to 5 years	122 (20.9)
More than 5 years	121 (20.7)
Currently listed on transplant waiting pool	
Yes	871 (35.2)
No	1498 (60.6)
Don't know	101 (4.1)

Abbreviations: APD, automated peritoneal dialysis; CAPD, continuous ambulatory peritoneal dialysis; RRT, renal replacement therapy.
a) Numbers in this column refer to number of respondents (valid %).
b) Top 10 countries with most respondents, together holding 87.8% of all respondents. Other countries were Azerbaijan, Belarus, Belgium, Bosnia and Herzegovina, Bulgaria, Croatia, Cyprus, Denmark, Estonia, France, Georgia, Greece, Iceland, Latvia, Norway, Romania, Russia, San Marino, Slovakia, Slovenia, Spain, Sweden, Switzerland, The Netherlands, Turkey, Ukraine.

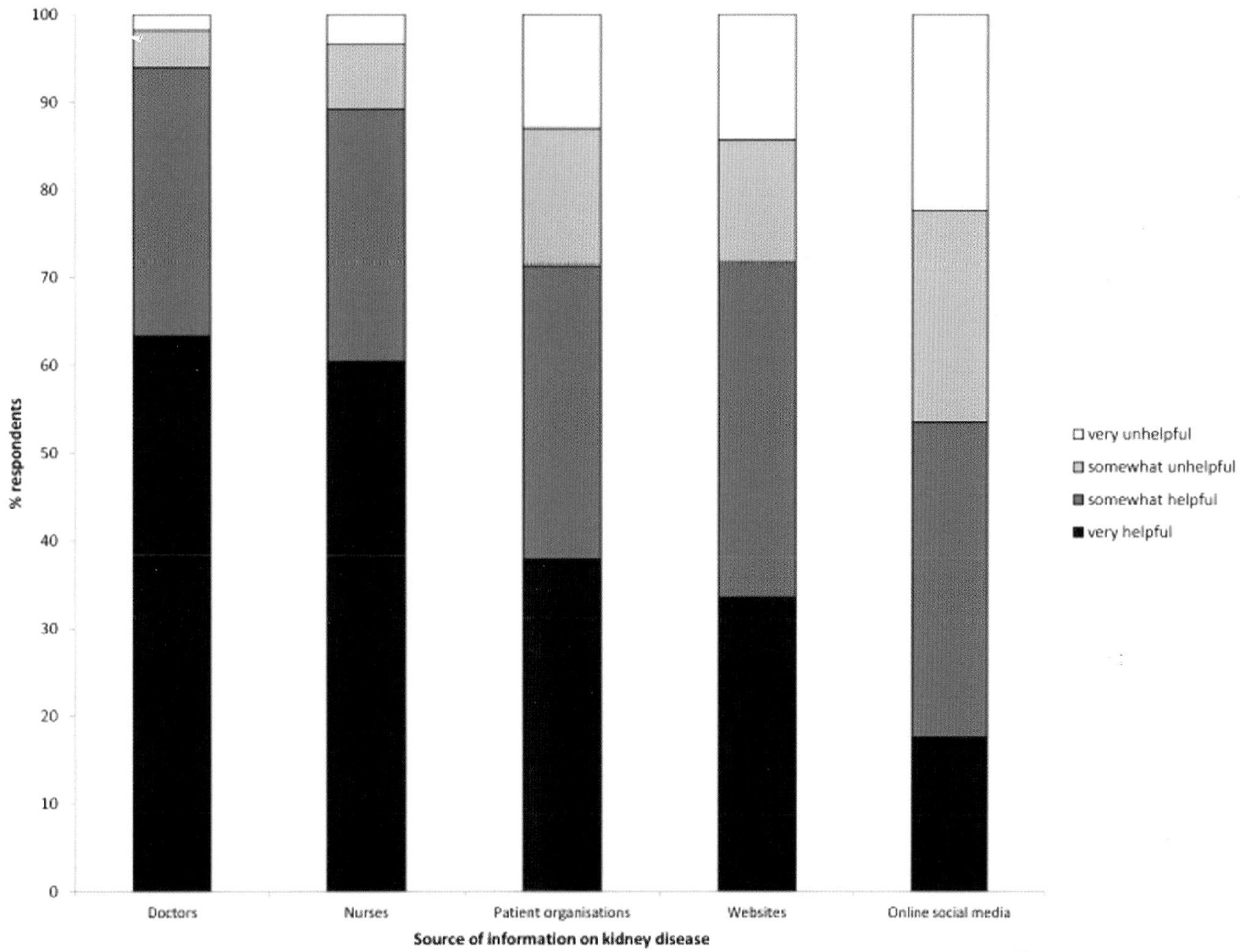

Figure 1. Respondents' scores on how helpful different information sources on kidney disease have been. Abbreviations: HD, haemodialysis, PD, peritoneal dialysis.

Treatment decision making

Almost half of respondents indicated that they had been very much (46.7%) involved in the process of selecting a RRT modality (Germany = 46.9%, OR 1.12 (95% CI: 0.96–1.30) and Poland = 31.6%, OR 0.58 (95% CI 0.49–0.70) vs other countries) or somewhat (28.2%) involved. A little more than half (51.2%) perceived they could choose their treatment method (Germany: 57.9%, OR: 1.31; 95% CI 1.12–1.52 and Poland 44.8%, OR 0.77; 95% CI: 0.65–0.91 versus other countries), whereas 48.8% explicitly stated they could not or did not know. Examples of reasons for not having a choice, which respondents provided as free text comments, were that not all modalities were provided in their centre (mostly for home-based therapies), or presence of medical contra-indications. Almost one fourth (22.8%) remembered the medical team suggesting at some time that their social circumstances (e.g., living conditions, work) were a contra-indication for a certain RRT modality (Germany = 24.8%, OR 1.14 (95% CI 0.96–1.35) and Poland = 16.7%, OR 0.69 (95% CI 0.56–0.86) versus other countries).

Almost all respondents were somewhat (31%) or very (63.2%) satisfied with the overall level of their kidney care (very satisfied: Germany = 77.8%, OR 2.51 (95% CI 2.12 to 2.97) and Poland = 42.1%, OR 0.52 (95% CI 0.44 to 0.61) versus other countries). It appeared that participants who felt they had been involved in the modality selection process were more likely to be very satisfied than those who had not been involved (OR 3.13 (95% CI 2.72–3.60); Germany: OR 2.43 (95% CI 1.78–3.31) and Poland: OR 3.30 (95% CI 2.72–3.60). We found a similar association between perceptions of having a choice of treatment and overall satisfaction with care (OR 2.25 (95% CI 1.97–2.56; Germany: OR 1.79 (95% CI 1.34–2.40) and Poland: OR 2.10 (95% CI 1.57–2.81). Time since start dialysis being <2 or >2 years did not influence any of these results.

Education and support

More than half of the respondents (64.2%) did not receive or could not remember receiving education on how to manage kidney disease in their daily life (Germany = 84.8%, OR 2.50 (95% CI: 2.00–3.00) and Poland = 36.4%, OR 0.25 (95% CI 0.21–0.30) versus other countries). We found no difference between participants who had been on their current modality $\leq$ 2 versus >2 years ($\chi^2 = 3.3$, $p = 0.07$).

Regarding respondents' employment status at the time they first started RRT, 27.8% were retired and 3% unemployed. Of the remaining respondents, 22.1% indicated that starting RRT did not affect their employment status. However, 48.4% stopped

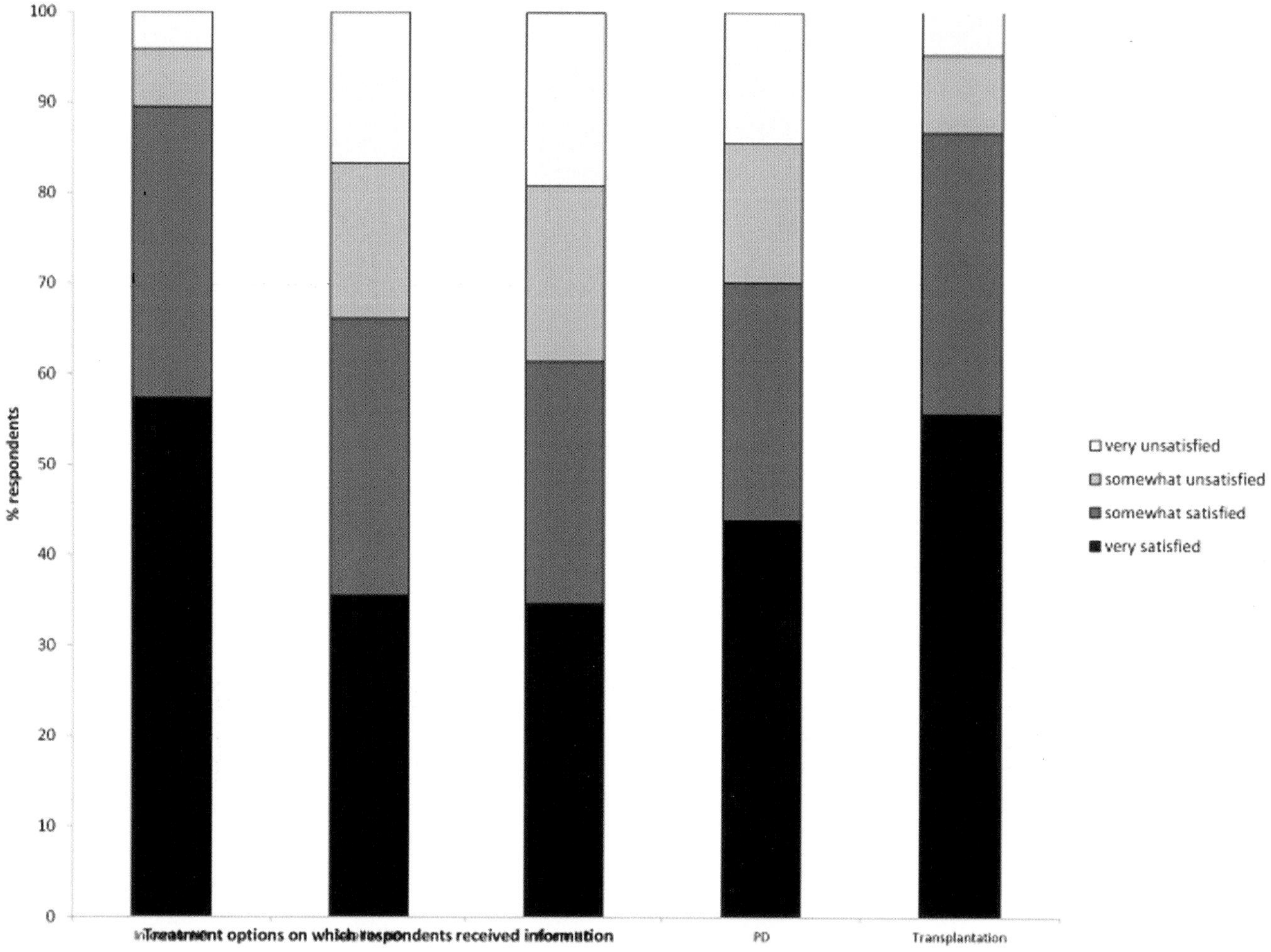

Figure 2. Respondents' satisfaction with information they had on treatment options.

working, 20.7% reduced their working hours, and 8.7% changed their job. Of respondents who stopped working or changed their job due to their kidney disease, only 22.8% received a training or education to support them with finding a new job.

When asked how satisfied they were with the level of access to a dietician, most participants appeared to be somewhat (34.9%) or very (36.7%) satisfied, while for 9.6% support from a dietician was completely not available (very satisfied: Germany = 60.4%, OR 1.09 (95% CI 0.94–1.27) and Poland = 63.3%, OR 1.24 (95% CI 1.04–1.47) versus other countries). For social workers these percentages were comparable (34.3%, 32.3%, and 12.2%)(very satisfied: Germany = 35.7%, OR 0.56 (95% CI 0.48–0.65) and Poland = 70.1%, OR 2.36 (95% CI 1.98–2.82) versus other countries).

Up to 40.2% of participants did not know whom to address a complaint to, should they ever be dissatisfied with their treatment.

Overall, 20.0% indicated that financial cost was a barrier for optimal treatment for them (Germany = 11.9%, OR 0.78 (95% CI: 0.62–0.98) and Poland = 23.4% (95% CI 1.44–2.17), versus other countries). Patients reporting a financial barrier tended to be less satisfied with their overall care (all respondents OR 0.42 (95% CI 0.35–0.50); Germany: OR 0.30 (95% CI 0.20–0.44) and Poland OR 0.65 (95% CI 0.46–0.92)).

Discussion

This paper reports the results of a CEAPIR initiated survey that succeeded in involving nearly 4,000 kidney patients from 36 European countries. In general, survey participants reported to be satisfied with the information they received on their disease and treatment, and felt they had been involved in selecting their treatment modality. Moreover, we found being involved to be positively related to overall treatment satisfaction. Nevertheless, more than half of respondents perceived they could not freely choose their modality, and information to facilitate selection of alternative modalities seemed suboptimal, with half of respondents not remembering being presented another modality than their current one. Also education to support the management of kidney disease in patients' daily and professional lives was perceived suboptimal.

Modality selection: a free and informed choice?

A substantial part of our respondents did not recall that they were provided with information on alternative modalities. This confirms previous research reporting similar percentages of patients who felt that different therapies were not presented equally for selecting a modality [12,18]; a systematic review of qualitative studies [13] found that patients did not have the information they wanted on treatment options. Our finding that participants were more satisfied with information on in-centre HD than with home-based therapies is also in line with other studies [5,12,18], as was the proportion of respondents perceiving a lack of choice when selecting a modality [12].

There are several potential explanations for the process of modality selection being suboptimal with regard to information and freedom of choice. First, not all potential modalities may be available in a centre, which was also brought forward as a reason by some of our respondents. Morton et al. [13] found that resources often formed the basis of treatment decisions, and that limited access to centre-based dialysis was a consistent reason for choosing home-based therapies. A Danish study suggested that a genuine offer of out-of-centre dialysis would be needed to encourage greater use of modalities other than in-centre haemodialysis [10]. These findings, together with our study results, may warrant future research to investigate to what extent different modalities are actually being offered to kidney patients in European countries. This would inform health policy makers on if and how to stimulate centres to offer all modalities to their patients. It does not necessarily imply that all modalities should be provided in each centre because this may hamper building of experience. Instead, it may be better to, for example, create collaborative structures in which patients can be referred for training on home-based therapies to one central location, and organisational (and financial) barriers to such referrals are addressed.

Secondly, also late referral may jeopardise a free choice of treatment modality. Late referral has been suggested to negatively influence the selection of home based modalities [19], and to contribute to an unbalanced modality mix [20]. More than half of our survey participants recalled the time between the diagnosis of their kidney disease and the start of RRT to be less than three months. Even if we assume that part of these respondents underestimated this time period [12], still for many of them the time would be considered too short for optimal preparation of the patient, e.g., to create an arterio-venous fistula. However, several authors have demonstrated that in centres with dedicated programmes, free modality choice can be offered despite late referral [21–23]. Future research may explore the availability of such programmes across Europe.

Thirdly, some health care professionals may refrain from providing information on a particular modality due to their perception of the presence of contra-indications [24], most of which are not absolute [3] and often based on psycho-social concerns [13,25]. Also in our survey we found medical as well as social contra-indications as perceived reasons for not being offered a certain treatment option. Yet, several studies demonstrated that health care professionals' perceptions may vary widely, depending upon their experience, background, training and personal beliefs [26,27]. Consequently, part of the kidney patients may be denied a fully free choice based on the presumptions of their healthcare workers. Application of a tool guaranteeing presentation of all available treatment options in a systematic way to patients rather than a tool asking (dichotomous) questions, or the opinion of the educator on what might be of interest to the patient, might help to assure optimal and unprejudiced provision of information.

Patient involvement in modality selection

We found that a large majority of kidney patients participating in our survey felt that they had been involved in the process of selecting a treatment modality, which appeared to be associated with higher levels of satisfaction with current treatment. Based on their qualitative study, Lee et al. [10] suggested that patients want to participate in choice of modality, but that especially for those on in-centre haemodialysis, selection of alternative modalities was often not facilitated. In general, patients seem increasingly willing to, and asking for, being involved in clinical decisions [28]. At the same time, the model proposed by Flyn et al. [9] made a distinction between patients' preferences regarding receiving information, deliberating that information, and making the final treatment decision. From that study it appeared that all patients want to be informed, but that their preferences for being involved in the deliberation and decision process may vary. Additionally, there is debate on to what extent it is ethical to leave treatment decisions entirely to patients [29]. Nevertheless, health policy makers increasingly advocate patient involvement in decision making, which asks for ways to further optimise this in clinical practice.

One way may be to provide patients with information on experience from other patients, which may strongly influence their decision making [13]. In line with this, Winterbottom *et al.* [*30*]. concluded based on a study among students that information provided by patients was considered more influential than when obtained from healthcare professionals. Participants in the CEAPIR survey gave most value to physicians and nurses as a source of information on kidney disease, but unfortunately it was not specifically asked to value information coming from other patients.

Another potential field of focus is the development of tools to engage kidney patients in the decision-making process with their care providers [31,32]. For renal replacement modality selection, such decision aids should at least mention and explain all available options, taking into account that therapies might be valued differently by different patients for different reasons [33]. Furthermore, the format of clinical practice guidelines should be constructed in a way that stimulates an equal conversation between patient and healthcare worker, rather than just providing a unidirectional flow of information from the clinical perspective [34].

Information on impact of aspects of disease and treatment on daily living

More than half of the patients in our survey did not remember receiving advise or information on how to manage their kidney disease in their daily life. In the systematic review by Morton et al. [13], the majority of studies indicated that patients and family members were concerned about how to handle practicalities of treatment in their daily life. In most of the included studies, patients judged that provided information was too little focused on minimising impact on daily activities such as working, hobbies, care for children and grandchildren, and too much on length of survival. So, although about 2 out of 3 patients in our survey indicated they satisfied with the availibility of a dietician or a social worker, it is unclear in how far the advice provided by these professionals was really helpful to solve the problems of daily living of attributable to the disease. It is remarkable for example that only one out of four patients in need for a new job indicated they had received assistance for this important aspect of their care.

Strengths and weaknesses of the study

To our knowledge, this survey is the first to explore the topic of information and education among such a large number of kidney patients. Furthermore, no previous study managed to involve so many different countries, making this survey the first project to explore this topic on a broad international level.

Despite being a relatively small sample from all kidney patients in Europe, our respondents appeared to be representative with regard to treatment modality. For countries participating in the

ERA-EDTA registry the percentages of prevalent patients receiving HD in 2011 ranged from 23.8 to 83.6%, 3.7 to 11.3% were treated with PD, and 6.6 to 71.9% had a functioning graft [35]. In our survey, these percentages were 55%, 7.3% and 37.7% for the respective treatment modalities. With regard to the age distribution, our cohort might have been slightly overrepresented in the middle age class (50–69 years) and underrepresented in the age category of 70 years and older. It is unclear from the current survey whether the use of paper survey vs electronic survey only has resulted in more patient participation. However, it is clear that countries were the survey was also available as a paper version are overrepresented in this survey.

We were not able to further investigate the representativeness of our survey participants due to the unsolicited and sometimes indirect nature of the national dissemination strategies, an aspect that might induce selection bias. This prevented us from determining the size and characteristics of the original study population. Apart from impeding calculation of the survey's response rate, it also hampered a precise comparison between responders and non-responders. In general, younger patients with higher education levels and better health status are more likely to participate in a study like ours than their older, sicker and less educated counterparts [18,36]. Previous studies suggested that including healthier patients tend to report higher levels of satisfaction with care, which may lead to a too positive picture based on our results. At the same time younger, higher educated participants may have the opposite effect. So, we assume that ultimately the potential selection bias did not significantly influence our results [36,37].

At the time of initiating the survey, CEAPIR did not intend it to be a research project, but rather an exploration of perceptions among the patients they represent. Although they made an effort to incorporate feedback from national patient organisations and pilot-tested the survey among Irish patients, a strict methodology to ensure unambiguous interpretation of the questions was lacking. On one hand, uniform interpretation may have been further jeopardised by having the survey translated locally without resources to apply a validated method [38]. On the other hand, this most likely decreased selection bias, which in turn increased the representativeness of the study. Also, the survey captured patient perceptions rather than actual practices of information provision and education across Europe. While our results may provide valuable pointers for selecting areas for further research, we cannot use them to determine whether information or education was not provided, or whether it was provided and patients did not recognise it as such or did not remember it. Even though our analyses suggested no effect of recall bias on our findings, these limitations warrant caution when drawing conclusions based on our study results.

Future research

Based on our study findings, we suggest that it is worthwhile to further investigate the extent to which dialysis centres in Europe offer all modalities to their patients. Additionally, future research may explore the availability of dedicated vascular access programmes in European countries, as well as their effect on the freedom of modality choice for European kidney patients.

CEAPIR delegated the translation and dissemination of the survey to national patient organisations. We assume that having the survey translated in patients' own language greatly increased the number of respondents. However, future initiatives should try to formalise translation by allocating resources to facilitate the use of accepted methods. This will contribute to the methodological rigour of survey-based studies, and improve interpretation of the results. Interestingly, countries that choose to distribute the survey on paper managed to involve a large number of patients. Although we cannot calculate actual response rates, we hypothesize that using paper-based questionnaires may be a way of increasing response and decreasing selection bias in patient populations that are relatively old and with a high disease burden. Further research on this topic is of high relevance. Similar future initiatives should therefore consider to provide surveys on paper in addition to electronic formats.

An analysis of the data separate for Germany and Poland (the two largest contributors) versus other nationalities, demonstrated that for some topics, perceptions seem to be country-specific, however without substantial change in the general interpretation of the data. It would be interesting to further explore which characteristics (of patients, culture, the health care system, etc.) contribute to these differences across Europe.

Lastly, many of our survey participants provided additional information and explanations as free comments. In the view of the richness and magnitude of these data, we are considering to summarize these individual comments in a representative by means of a future qualitative, thematic analysis.

Conclusions

This study suggests that part of the gap between desired and observed modality mix of renal replacement therapies in Europa may be due to suboptimal information provision to patients, as well as to patients not being offered the full range of treatment options in an equal and unbiased manner. There was an association between involvement in modality selection and patient satisfaction. Health care providers, researchers and guideline developers should focus on developing and applying tools to facilitate the engagement of patients in modality selection.

Acknowledgments

The authors and CEAPIR want to thank all those who contributed to this project, first of all the patients who participated, but also all the volunteers and nurses that facilitated the survey's distribution.

Author Contributions

Conceived and designed the experiments: WVB SVDV MM OL. Performed the experiments: MM OL. Analyzed the data: WVB SVDV OL. Contributed reagents/materials/analysis tools: OL MM. Contributed to the writing of the manuscript: WVB SVDV OL SD.

References

1. Caring for Australians with Renal Impairment (CARI). Acceptance onto dialysis guidelines. CARI 2005. Available: http://www.cari.org.au/Dialysis/dialysis%20acceptance/Predialysis_education_aug-2005.pdf. Accessed 2014 Feb 23.
2. Moss AH (2001) Shared decision-making in dialysis: the new RPA/ASN guideline on appropriate initiation and withdrawal of treatment. American journal of kidney diseases: the official journal of the National Kidney Foundation 37: 1081–1091.
3. Covic A, Bammens B, Lobbedez T, Segall L, Heimburger O, et al. (2010) Educating end-stage renal disease patients on dialysis modality selection: clinical advice from the European Renal Best Practice (ERBP) Advisory Board. Nephrology, dialysis, transplantation: official publication of the European Dialysis and Transplant Association - European Renal Association 25: 1757–1759.
4. Van Biesen W, De Vecchi A, Dombros N, Dratwa M, Gokal R, et al. (1999) The referral pattern of end-stage renal disease patients and the initiation of dialysis: a European perspective. Peritoneal dialysis international: journal of the International Society for Peritoneal Dialysis 19 Suppl 2: S273–275.

5. Kurella Tamura M, Li S, Chen SC, Cavanaugh KL, Whaley-Connell AT, et al. (2013) Educational programs improve the preparation for dialysis and survival of patients with chronic kidney disease. Kidney international.
6. Mehrotra R, Marsh D, Vonesh E, Peters V, Nissenson A (2005) Patient education and access of ESRD patients to renal replacement therapies beyond in-center hemodialysis. Kidney international 68: 378–390.
7. Curtin RB, Mapes DL (2001) Health care management strategies of long-term dialysis survivors. Nephrology nursing journal: journal of the American Nephrology Nurses' Association 28: 385–392; discussion 393–384.
8. Stehman-Breen CO, Sherrard DJ, Gillen D, Caps M (2000) Determinants of type and timing of initial permanent hemodialysis vascular access. Kidney international 57: 639–645.
9. Flynn KE, Smith MA, Vanness D (2006) A typology of preferences for participation in healthcare decision making. Soc Sci Med 63: 1158–1169.
10. Lee A, Gudex C, Povlsen JV, Bonnevie B, Nielsen CP (2008) Patients' views regarding choice of dialysis modality. Nephrology, dialysis, transplantation: official publication of the European Dialysis and Transplant Association - European Renal Association 23: 3953–3959.
11. Winterbottom A, Conner M, Mooney A, Bekker HL (2007) Evaluating the quality of patient leaflets about renal replacement therapy across UK renal units. Nephrology, dialysis, transplantation: official publication of the European Dialysis and Transplant Association - European Renal Association 22: 2291–2296.
12. Song MK, Lin FC, Gilet CA, Arnold RM, Bridgman JC, et al. (2013) Patient perspectives on informed decision-making surrounding dialysis initiation. Nephrology, dialysis, transplantation: official publication of the European Dialysis and Transplant Association - European Renal Association 28: 2815–2823.
13. Morton RL, Tong A, Howard K, Snelling P, Webster AC (2010) The views of patients and carers in treatment decision making for chronic kidney disease: systematic review and thematic synthesis of qualitative studies. BMJ 340: c112.
14. van der Veer SN, Jager KJ, Visserman E, Beekman RJ, Boeschoten EW, et al. (2012) Development and validation of the Consumer Quality index instrument to measure the experience and priority of chronic dialysis patients. Nephrology, dialysis, transplantation: official publication of the European Dialysis and Transplant Association - European Renal Association 27: 3284–3291.
15. Finkelstein FO, Story K, Firanek C, Barre P, Takano T, et al. (2008) Perceived knowledge among patients cared for by nephrologists about chronic kidney disease and end-stage renal disease therapies. Kidney international 74: 1178–1184.
16. Wright JA, Wallston KA, Elasy TA, Ikizler TA, Cavanaugh KL (2011) Development and results of a kidney disease knowledge survey given to patients with CKD. American journal of kidney diseases: the official journal of the National Kidney Foundation 57: 387–395.
17. Morton RL, Snelling P, Webster AC, Rose J, Masterson R, et al. (2012) Dialysis modality preference of patients with CKD and family caregivers: a discrete-choice study. American journal of kidney diseases: the official journal of the National Kidney Foundation 60: 102–111.
18. Fadem SZ, Walker DR, Abbott G, Friedman AL, Goldman R, et al. (2011) Satisfaction with renal replacement therapy and education: the American Association of Kidney Patients survey. Clinical journal of the American Society of Nephrology: CJASN 6: 605–612.
19. Lameire N, Van Biesen W (1999) The pattern of referral of patients with end-stage renal disease to the nephrologist–a European survey. Nephrology, dialysis, transplantation: official publication of the European Dialysis and Transplant Association - European Renal Association 14 Suppl 6: 16–23.
20. Lameire N, Wauters JP, Teruel JL, Van Biesen W, Vanholder R (2002) An update on the referral pattern of patients with end-stage renal disease. Kidney international Supplement: 27–34.
21. Lobbedez T, Verger C, Ryckelynck JP, Fabre E, Evans D (2013) Outcome of the sub-optimal dialysis starter on peritoneal dialysis. Report from the French Language Peritoneal Dialysis Registry (RDPLF). Nephrology, dialysis, transplantation: official publication of the European Dialysis and Transplant Association - European Renal Association 28: 1276–1283.
22. Lobbedez T, Lecouf A, Ficheux M, Henri P, Hurault de Ligny B, et al. (2008) Is rapid initiation of peritoneal dialysis feasible in unplanned dialysis patients? A single-centre experience. Nephrology, dialysis, transplantation: official publication of the European Dialysis and Transplant Association - European Renal Association 23: 3290–3294.
23. Povlsen JV (2009) Unplanned start on assisted peritoneal dialysis. Contributions to nephrology 163: 261–263.
24. Oliver MJ, Garg AX, Blake PG, Johnson JF, Verrelli M, et al. (2010) Impact of contraindications, barriers to self-care and support on incident peritoneal dialysis utilization. Nephrology, dialysis, transplantation: official publication of the European Dialysis and Transplant Association - European Renal Association 25: 2737–2744.
25. Jager KJ, Korevaar JC, Dekker FW, Krediet RT, Boeschoten EW (2004) The effect of contraindications and patient preference on dialysis modality selection in ESRD patients in The Netherlands. American journal of kidney diseases: the official journal of the National Kidney Foundation 43: 891–899.
26. Hingwala J, Diamond J, Tangri N, Bueti J, Rigatto C, et al. (2013) Underutilization of peritoneal dialysis: the role of the nephrologist's referral pattern. Nephrology, dialysis, transplantation: official publication of the European Dialysis and Transplant Association - European Renal Association 28: 732–740.
27. Tennankore KK, Hingwala J, Watson D, Bargman JM, Chan CT (2013) Attitudes and perceptions of nephrology nurses towards dialysis modality selection: a survey study. BMC nephrology 14: 192.
28. Chewning B, Bylund CL, Shah B, Arora NK, Gueguen JA, et al. (2012) Patient preferences for shared decisions: a systematic review. Patient education and counseling 86: 9–18.
29. Muthalagappan S, Johansson L, Kong WM, Brown EA (2013) Dialysis or conservative care for frail older patients: ethics of shared decision-making. Nephrology, dialysis, transplantation: official publication of the European Dialysis and Transplant Association - European Renal Association 28: 2717–2722.
30. Winterbottom AE, Bekker HL, Conner M, Mooney AF (2012) Patient stories about their dialysis experience biases others' choices regardless of doctor's advice: an experimental study. Nephrology, dialysis, transplantation: official publication of the European Dialysis and Transplant Association - European Renal Association 27: 325–331.
31. Ameling JM, Auguste P, Ephraim PL, Lewis-Boyer L, DePasquale N, et al. (2012) Development of a decision aid to inform patients' and families' renal replacement therapy selection decisions. BMC medical informatics and decision making 12: 140.
32. Stiggelbout AM, Van der Weijden T, De Wit MP, Frosch D, Legare F, et al. (2012) Shared decision making: really putting patients at the centre of healthcare. BMJ 344: e256.
33. Van Biesen W, van der Veer SN, Jager KJ, Fouque D, Wanner C, et al. (2013) What guidelines should or should not be: implications for guideline production. Nephrology, dialysis, transplantation: official publication of the European Dialysis and Transplant Association - European Renal Association 28: 1980–1984.
34. van der Weijden T, Pieterse AH, Koelewijn-van Loon MS, Knaapen L, Legare F, et al. (2013) How can clinical practice guidelines be adapted to facilitate shared decision making? A qualitative key-informant study. BMJ quality & safety 22: 855–863.
35. http://www.era-edta-reg.org/files/annualreports/pdf/AnnRep2011.pdf lva.
36. Crow R, Gage H, Hampson S, Hart J, Kimber A, et al. (2002) The measurement of satisfaction with healthcare: implications for practice from a systematic review of the literature. Health Technol Assess 6: 1–244.
37. van der Veer SN, Arah OA, Visserman E, Bart HA, de Keizer NF, et al. (2012) Exploring the relationships between patient characteristics and their dialysis care experience. Nephrology, dialysis, transplantation: official publication of the European Dialysis and Transplant Association - European Renal Association 27: 4188–4196.
38. Streiner DL, Norman GR (2008) Health measurement scales. A practical guide to their development and use. 4th ed. Oxford, NY: Oxford university press.

3

Erectile Dysfunction and Risk of End Stage Renal Disease Requiring Dialysis: A Nationwide Population-Based Study

Yuan-Chi Shen[1,2], Shih-Feng Weng[3,4], Jhi-Joung Wang[3], Kai-Jen Tien[5,6]*

1 Department of Urology, Kaohsiung Chang Gung Memorial Hospital, Kaohsiung, Taiwan, **2** Cheng Shiu University, Kaohsiung, Taiwan, **3** Department of Medical Research, Chi Mei Medical Center, Tainan, Taiwan, **4** Department of Hospital and Health Care Administration, Chia Nan University of Pharmacy and Science, Tainan, Taiwan, **5** Division of Endocrinology and Metabolism, Department of Internal Medicine, Chi Mei Medical Center, Tainan, Taiwan, **6** The Center of General Education, Chia Nan University of Pharmacy and Science, Tainan, Taiwan

Abstract

Background: Previous studies have suggested that erectile dysfunction (ED) is an independent risk factor for macrovascular disease. Very few studies have evaluated the relationship between ED and risk of end stage renal disease (ESRD) requiring dialysis.

Methods: A random sample of 1,000,000 individuals from Taiwan's National Health Insurance database was collected. We selected the control group by matching the subjects and controls by age, diabetes, hypertension, coronary heart disease, hyperlipidemia, area of residence, monthly income and index date. We identified 3985 patients with newly-diagnosed ED between 2000 and 2008 and compared them with a matched cohort of 23910 patients without ED. All patients were tracked from the index date to identify which patients subsequently developed a need for dialysis.

Results: The incidence rates of dialysis in the ED cohort and comparison groups were 10.85 and 9.06 per 10000 person-years, respectively. Stratified by age, the incidence rate ratio for dialysis was greater in ED patients aged <50 years (3.16, 95% CI: 1.62–6.19, $p = 0.0008$) but not in aged 50–64 (0.94, 95% CI: 0.52–1.69, $p = 0.8397$) and those aged ≥ 65 (0.69, 95% CI: 0.32–1.52, $p = 0.3594$). After adjustment for patient characteristics and medial comorbidities, the adjusted HR for dialysis remained greater in ED patients aged <50 years (adjusted HR: 2.08, 95% CI: 1.05–4.11, $p<0.05$). The log-rank test revealed that ED patients <50-years-old had significantly higher cumulative incidence rates of dialysis than those without ($p = 0.0004$).

Conclusion: Patients with ED, especially younger patients, are at an increased risk for ESRD requiring dialysis later in life.

Editor: Chih-Pin Chuu, National Health Research Institutes, Taiwan

Funding: The authors have no support or funding to report.

Competing Interests: The authors have declared that no competing interests exist.

* Email: cmmctkj@gmail.com

Introduction

Erectile dysfunction (ED) is defined as the inability to achieve or maintain an erection sufficient for sexual performance [1]. ED is an important worldwide issue, affecting 152 million men in 1995 and 322 million men in 2025 and negatively impacts life quality, self-esteem, and intimacy [2,3]. One telephone survey of ED prevalence in Taiwan reported that nearly thirty percent of men over 30 years had ED [4]. This medical problem has been associated with endothelial dysfunction and low-grade vascular inflammation and often clusters with hypertension, diabetes mellitus, hyperlipidemia, obesity, and metabolic syndrome [5,6,7]. In addition, it has been reported ED as an independent risk factor for macrovascular diseases such as coronary heart disease, cerebrovascular disease (CVD), and peripheral artery disease [8,9,10,11,12,13].

ED has been extensively studied in relation to metabolic disease and CVD but rarely in relation to microvascular diseases such as end stage renal disease (ESRD). Although ED is commonly found in patients in a late stage of chronic kidney disease (CKD) [14], little attention has been paid to whether it is related to the progression of kidney disease. Several studies have found that there is strong association between CVD and ESRD and that the interaction between the two diseases is bidirectional and complex [5,15,16,17]. Because CVD and ESRD may share a common pathophysiological pathway, it is possible that ED might also be associated with the development of ESRD. One cross-sectional study by Hermans et al., investigating the relationship between ED and microangipathy in diabetes, found ED to be associated with retinopathy but not with level of estimated glomerular filtration rate (eGFR) [18], though another cross-sectional investigation by

Table 1. Demographic characteristics and comorbid medical disorders for patients with and without erectile dysfunction (ED) in Taiwan.

Category	Subcategory	Patients with ED (N = 3985)	Patients without ED (N = 23910)	P-value
Age	0–49	1654(41.51%)	10063(42.09%)	0.7350
	50–64	1475(37.01%)	8818(36.88%)	
	≥65	856(21.48%)	5029(21.03%)	
Diabetes	Yes	541(13.58%)	3058(12.79%)	0.1704
	No	3444(86.42%)	20852(87.21%)	
Hypertension	Yes	905(22.71%)	5422(22.68%)	0.9628
	No	3080(77.29%)	18488(77.32%)	
Coronary heart disease	Yes	327(8.21%)	1935(8.09%)	0.8090
	No	3658(91.79%)	21975(91.91%)	
Hyperlipidemia	Yes	370(9.28%)	2079(8.70%)	0.2233
	No	3615(90.72%)	21831(91.30%)	
Area	North	2143(53.78%)	13387(55.99%)	0.0640
	Central	740(18.57%)	4267(17.85%)	
	South	1003(25.17%)	5729(23.96%)	
	East	99(2.48%)	527(2.20%)	
Income	NT<15840	1801(45.19%)	10646(44.53%)	0.4754
	NT 15841~25000	988(24.79%)	5858(24.50%)	
	NT>25001	1196(30.01%)	7406(30.97%)	

Chuang et al. reported it to be associated with both albuminuria and eGFR [19]. In a meta-analysis by Navaneethan et al., the prevalence of ED in chronic kidney disease was 70%, though one of the limitations with that review was that the studies reviewed were of small sample sizes and had cross-sectional designs [20].

In this longitudinal follow-up study, we used a population-based national insurance dataset in Taiwan to examine the relationship between ED and the risk of ESRD requiring dialysis.

Methods

Data sources

Taiwan launched a single-payer National Health Insurance (NHI) program on March 1, 1995. The NHI database covers nearly all of Taiwan's population, and is one of the largest and most complete population-based datasets in the world. The data used in this study came from the Longitudinal Health Insurance Database 2000 (LHID2000), which is a sub-set of NHI database that contains all claims data (from 1996 to 2011) of one million beneficiaries. This sample was systemic-randomly selected in 2000. There are no significant differences in age, gender and health care costs between the sample group and all enrollees in the NHI program. The LHID2000 provides encrypted patient identification numbers, gender, date of birth, dates of admission and discharge, the ICD-9-CM (International Classification of Diseases, Ninth Revision, Clinical Modification) codes of diagnoses and procedures, details of prescriptions, registry of Catastrophic Illness Patient Database, as well as costs covered and paid for by NHI. The institutional review board of Chi Mei Medical Center approved the protocol of this study. Informed consent was not required because the datasets were devoid of identifiable personal information.

Study sample

A retrospective cohort study was conducted with two study groups: a newly onset ED (erectile dysfunction) group and a matched non-ED control group during the recruitment period of 2000–2008. ED was defined in a patient if he had (1) at least two outpatient service claims with the codes of ED (ICD-9-CM code 60784) at any hospital or local medical clinic or (2) any one single hospitalization with ED listed among the five claims diagnosis codes. Patients diagnosed as having ED before 2000 were excluded. CKD is a well-known strong predictor for ESRD requiring dialysis. To evaluate the true association between ED and ESRD requiring dialysis, any patient with a diagnosis of renal function impairment (ICD9CM code: 582, 583, 585, 586, 588) was excluded. Because the outcome of interest was the occurrence of ESRD requiring dialysis, we also excluded patients identified in the registry of Catastrophic Illness Patient Database as being diagnosed as having chronic kidney disease (ICD-9-CM code 585), which would indicate that they were receiving dialysis for ESRD before their diagnosis of ED.

For each ED patient, six patients not diagnosed with ED were randomly selected from the dataset as a control group match. ED patients were matched with members of the control group by age, diabetes, hypertension, coronary heart disease, hyperlipidemia, area of residence, monthly income and index date. The index date for the ED subjects was the date of their first registration. The year of that index date was used to create the index date for each comparison subject. Demographic data such as gender, age, geographic area of Taiwan, and monthly income (record as NT$) were collected. Baseline co-morbidities of these patients were also recorded. These included diabetes mellitus (ICD9CM code:250), hypertension (ICD9CM code:401–405), coronary heart disease (ICD9CM code:410–414), and hyperlipidemia (ICD9CM code:272), because these co-morbidities are known to affect the risk of ESRD. We counted any of these comorbid conditions if the

Table 2. Risk for end stage renal disease (ESRD) requiring dialysis in patients with and without erectile dysfunction (ED).

		Patients with ED				Patients without ED				IRR (95% CI)	P value
		N	ESRD requiring dialysis	PY#	Rate*	N	ESRD requiring dialysis	PY#	Rate*		
All		3985	33	30412.37	10.85	23910	162	178837.16	9.06	1.20(0.82–1.74)	0.3445
Age	<50	1654	13	12530.70	10.37	10063	25	76264.65	3.28	3.16(1.62–6.19)	0.0008
	50–64	1475	13	11206.17	11.60	8818	80	64914.22	12.32	0.94(0.52–1.69)	0.8397
	≥65	856	7	6675.50	10.49	5029	57	37658.29	15.14	0.69(0.32–1.52)	0.3594
Follow up years	0–2	3985	1	7942.73	1.26	23910	14	47482.70	2.95	0.43(0.06–3.25)	0.4110
	2–4	3955	7	7694.23	9.10	23566	39	45660.37	8.54	1.07(0.48–2.38)	0.8778
	≥4	3575	25	14775.41	16.92	21114	109	85694.09	12.72	1.33(0.86–2.05)	0.1982

#PY, person-years.
*Rate: per 10000 person-years.

condition was diagnosed in an inpatient setting or in three or more ambulatory care claims coded one year before the index medical care date. Follow-up time in person-years (PY) was calculated for each person until diagnosis of ESRD requiring dialysis, death, or the end of 2011.

Statistical Analyses

All statistical operations were performed using the SAS 9.3.1 statistical package (SAS Institute, Inc., Cary, North Carolina, USA). Pearson's $\chi 2$ tests was used to compare differences in the baseline characteristics, co-morbid medical disorders and socio-demographic status between the study and control cohort. The incidence rate was calculated as the number of ESRD requiring dialysis cases during the follow-up, divided by the total person-years for each group by age and duration. The risk of being diagnosed as having ESRD requiring dialysis was compared between the ED group and the control group by estimating the incidence rate ratio using Poisson regression. Moreover, stratified Cox proportional hazard regression (stratified by age group <50 and ≥50) analysis was used to compute the adjusted hazard ratio for developing ESRD requiring dialysis between patients with and without ED after adjusting for possible confounding factors (diabetes, hypertension, coronary heart disease, hyperlipidemia, geographic area and monthly income). Kaplan-Meier analysis was also used to calculate the cumulative incidence rates of ESRD requiring dialysis between two cohorts, and the log-rank test was used to analyze the differences between the survival curves. A two sided P value <0.05 was considered significant.

Results

As can been seen in Table 1, a summary of the baseline characteristics and comorbid conditions of the two groups, 3985 male ED patients and 23910 non-ED patients were enrolled in the study. Because we selected the control group by matching with patients' characteristics and comorbidities, there were no significant differences in diabetes, hypertension, coronary heart disease, hyperlipidemia, geographic area and income.

Table 2 shows the risk for ESRD requiring dialysis in all patients stratified by age and number at risk of follow-up years. During the follow-up period, the incidence rates for ESRD requiring dialysis for the ED and non-ED cohorts were 10.85 and 9.06 per 10000 person-years, respectively. Stratified by age, the younger group <50 years has the most pronounced (IRR = 3.16, 95% CI = 1.62–6.19, p = 0.0008). We found no group differences in risk for ESRD requiring dialysis in the age groups 50–64 years and ≥65 years (IRR = 0.94, 95% CI = 0.52–1.69, p = 0.8397 and IRR = 0.69, 95% CI = 0.32–1.52, p = 0.3594, respectively). Analyzing by number at risk of follow up years, we found that the IRR for ESRD requiring dialysis increased progressively but not significantly along with the duration of ED.

We further analyzed the crude and adjusted HR for ESRD requiring dialysis in patients aged <50 years and those aged ≥50 (Table 3). After adjusting for age, gender, DM, HTN, CHD, hyperlipidemia, geographic area and monthly income, we found ED patients aged <50 years to be 2.08 times more likely to develop ESRD requiring dialysis (adjusted HR = 2.08, 95% CI = 1.05–4.11, P<0.05). There were no group differences in crude and adjusted HRs for ESRD requiring dialysis in those aged ≥ 50 years.

The results of Kaplan-Meier analysis revealed that ED patients <50 years old had a higher cumulative incidence rate for ESRD requiring dialysis than the comparison cohort (log-rank test P = 0.0004) (Figure 1).

Table 3. Crude and adjusted hazard ratios (HR) for the development of end stage renal disease (ESRD) requiring dialysis among the sample patients stratified by age.

		Age <50		Age ≥ 50	
		Crude HR (95% CI)	Adjusted HR (95% CI)	Crude HR (95% CI)	Adjusted HR (95% CI)
Erectile dysfunction	Yes	3.17*(1.62–6.19)	2.08*(1.05–4.11)	0.83(0.52–1.33)	0.85(0.53–1.37)
	No	1.00	1.00	1.00	1.00

*P-value <0.05.
Adjusted for diabetes, hypertension, coronary heart disease, hyperlipidemia, geographic area and monthly income.

Discussion

Many studies have reported ED to be associated with macrovasclular disease, but few have investigated the impact of ED on the progression of a microvascular disease such as kidney disease. This study represents the first nationwide population-based study to investigate the relationship between ED and risk for ESRD requiring dialysis in an Asian population. We found the incidence rate for ESRD requiring dialysis to be 10.85 per 10000 person-years in patients with ED. The risk was especially greater in younger ED patients of age <50 years. After adjusting for patient characteristics and medical comorbidities, we did not find an association between ED and increased risk in patients of age ≥50. The crude and adjusted HR for ESRD dialysis was 3.17-times and 2.08-times higher risk in ED patients of age <50 years than it was in the comparison cohort, respectively. Although the HR decreased after adjustment, ED patients remained at significantly higher risk.

Several studies have investigated the association between ED and microvascular disorders. One cross-sectional study by Siu et al., investigating the prevalence and risk factors of ED in diabetic patients [21], found a significant association between ED and microangiopathy and reported the odd ratios for retinopathy, microalbuminuria, clinical proteinuria and sensory neuropathy to be 2.27, 1.68, 2.27, and 2.05, respectively. Another small cross-sectional study involving 82 male diabetics in Japan reported an association between ED and proteinuria [22], though that study did not address the relationship between ED and eGFR. One study of 221 male diabetes reported an association between ED prevalence of elevated albuminuria [18], but found no difference in eGFR level between patients with ED and those without. Chuang et al., conducting a cross-sectional study to evaluate the association between ED and severity of albuminuria [19], reported that not only was ED associated presence of albuminuria and low eGFR level, but it had a stronger association on the presence of macroalbuminuria than microalbuminuria (odd ratios 4.49 and 2.28, respectively). ED is a common feature of CKD and ESRD. Two studies have closely correlated ED to the stage of CKD [14,20]. Although their results differed somewhat, both studies reported an association between ED and microangiopathy and suggested that it might have an impact on the disease progression.

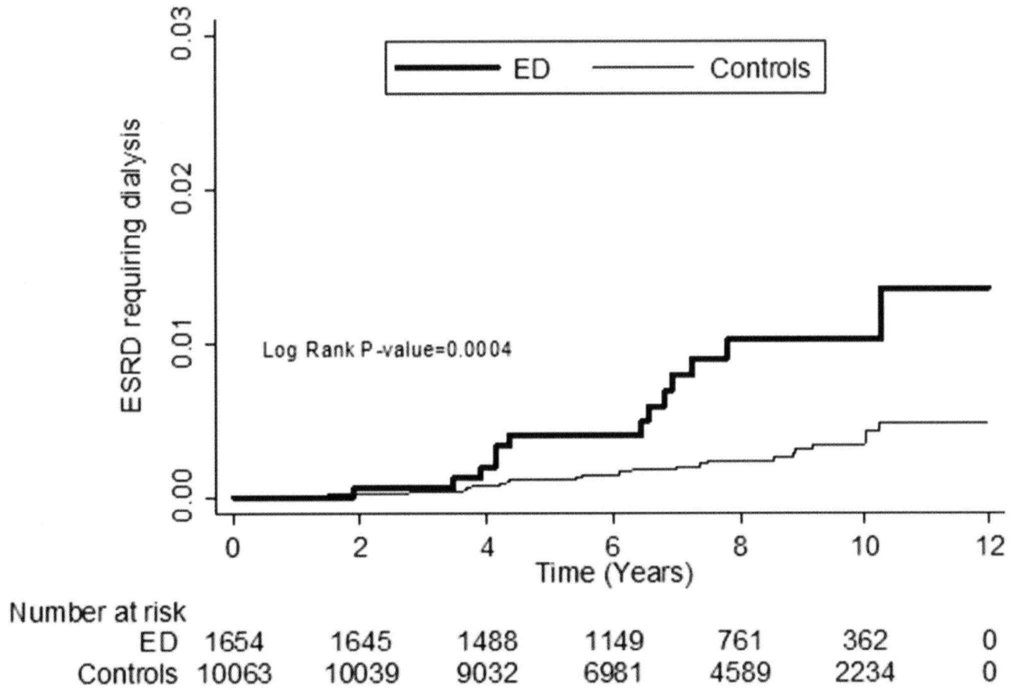

Figure 1. The cumulative incidence rate for end stage renal disease (ESRD) requiring dialysis for patients <50 years of age with erectile dysfunction (ED) and without ED (log-rank P value =0.0004).

ED is generally thought to be secondarily increased in subjects with CKD and ESRD. However, a cross-sectional study design cannot be used to infer directionality. One important step to clarify the direction of the putative ED-ESRD association is the performance of a longitudinal study of individuals initially free of ESRD at baseline. Because CKD is an extremely strong predictor for ESRD requiring dialysis, we also excluded patients diagnosed as having any form kidney disease. Our study used ESRD requiring regular dialysis as the end point to evaluate the influence of ED on the progression of kidney disease.

Although the underlying mechanism contributing to the association between ED and risk of ESRD requiring dialysis is likely complex, there are some possible explanations that can be considered. First, metabolic comorbidities and cardiovascular disease are highly prevalent in ED patients. One national database in United States reported the crude prevalence rates to be 41.6% for hypertension, 42.4% for hyperlipidemia and 20.2% for diabetes in ED patients [5]. These metabolic comorbidities are the traditional risk factors that can deteriorate renal function. Since metabolic comorbidities were matched and adjusted for in the present study, the relationship between ED and ESRD requiring dialysis survived. The association between ED and ESRD may be in part due to these metabolic comorbidities, but they cannot explain the entire relationship between ED and ESRD. Second, ED is considered as a surrogate marker of endothelial damage, which is an important pathologic change in ED [23]. The hallmark of endothelial dysfunction is reduced synthesis of nitric oxide (NO), increased vasoconstrictor peptide endothelin-1 (ET-1), and increased production of the asymmetric dimethylarginine (ADMA) and inflammatory cytokines, including interleukin-6 (IL-6), C-reactive protein (CRP) and tumor necrosis factor-a (TNF-a) [24]. NO reduction was found to result in increased glomerular capillary pressure, vascular resistance and decreased capillary ultrafiltration in one animal study [25], suggesting that long term endothelial dysfunction might result in irreversible kidney damage. One study by Ravani and colleagues suggested that ADMA is inversely related to GFR and represents a strong and independent marker for progression to ESRD [26]. A population-based cohort study of up to 4926 patients with 15 years of follow-up reported that elevations of most inflammation markers, including TNF-a receptor 2 and IL-6 level, could predict risk of CKD [27]. Therefore, ED might be considered as an early marker and factor predisposing an individual to ESRD and not just diseases secondary to ESRD only.

In the current study, individuals who were diagnosed with ED later in life were at much less risk for ESRD requiring dialysis. The reason for this difference is not known. We speculate this lack of association in an elderly population may be due to several reasons. Compared with ED, the traditional risk factors for ESRD, which include hypertension, hyperlipidemia and diabetes, may have more impact on the disease progression. Marumo et al. evaluated the age-related prevalence of ED and the comorbidities to be common in ED patients in a cross-sectional study [28], and found the prevalence of hypertension, hyperlipidemia and diabetes to be dramatically increased after the age of 50 years. In the present study, the lack of association between ED and ESRD in elderly population may be due to by our adjustment for confounders in our model or may be due to the fact that elderly people with ESRD in Taiwan often refuse chronic dialysis therapy. In addition, the incidence of ESRD requiring dialysis may be underestimated in the elderly population.

This study has some limitations. First, the diagnosis of ED was based on diagnostic codes recorded by the physician in the NHI claims forms; therefore, some registration bias might be involved. The identification of ED and ESRD requiring dialysis diagnoses were based on diagnoses listed in an administrative database and therefore may be less accurate than diagnoses undertaken individually following standard procedures. In Taiwan, the self-administered International Index of Erectile Dysfunction (IIEF-5) questionnaire is usually used to assess and quantify the patients' subjective symptoms of ED. The diagnosis as well as the severity of ED can be evaluated based on the results of self-administered IIEF-5 questionnaire. Because the patients' raw questionnaire scores were not available in the administrative database, we defined ED by ICD-9-CM codes. To ensure the accuracy of these diagnostic codes, only the ED patients diagnosed by two patient claims records citing ED a primary diagnosis were recorded. ESRD requiring dialysis is definitely registered in Catastrophic Illness Patient Database in Taiwan. Patients identified in the registry of Catastrophic Illness Patient Database as having diagnosis of chronic kidney disease (ICD-9-CM code 585), which would indicate that they were receiving dialysis for ESRD. Therefore, registration bias was minimized as much as possible in this study. Another limitation may be related to lack of willingness to discuss possible ED problems in Taiwan. It is possible that some of the controls may have ED but not yet diagnosed. If this were the case, our results would have been biased toward the null leading to a more conservative estimate of association. Another limitation is that disease severity could not be assessed from our dataset. Still another limitation was claims records do not include smoking, Chinese herbal medicine, occupation, and family histories. Nor are environmental data recorded. Despite these limitations, the study is strong because it has a longitudinal, large population-based design and covers nearly all of Taiwan's residents. As such, both referral and selection biases are minimized.

In conclusion, patients with ED, which is conventionally considered as a risk factor of cardiovascular disease, are at increased risk for ESRD, especially in younger adults. Patients with early diagnosed ED are at an increased risk for ESRD with dialysis later in life. Further studies are needed to evaluate the possible underlying mechanisms between these two conditions.

Acknowledgments

This study is based in part on data from the National Health Insurance Research Database provided by the Bureau of National Health Insurance, Department of Health and managed by the National Health Research Institutes (Registered number 100057). The interpretation and conclusions contained herein do not represent those of the Bureau of National Health Insurance, Department of Health, or the National Health Research Institutes. We thank James F. Steed (Di Jian-shi) for editing the English language and reviewing the manuscript.

Author Contributions

Conceived and designed the experiments: YCS KJT. Performed the experiments: YCS SFW JJW KJT. Analyzed the data: SFW KJT. Contributed reagents/materials/analysis tools: YCS SFW JJW KJT. Contributed to the writing of the manuscript: YCS KJT.

References

1. Lewis RW, Fugl-Meyer KS, Corona G, Hayes RD, Laumann EO, et al. (2010) Definitions/Epidemiology/Risk Factors for Sexual Dysfunction. Journal of Sexual Medicine 7: 1598–1607.

2. O'Leary MP, Althof SE, Cappelleri JC, Crowley A, Sherman N, et al. (2006) Self-esteem, confidence and relationship satisfaction of men with erectile dysfunction treated with sildenafil citrate: a multicenter, randomized, parallel

group, double-blind, placebo controlled study in the United States. The Journal of urology 175: 1058–1062.
3. McKinlay JB (2000) The worldwide prevalence and epidemiology of erectile dysfunction. Int J Impot Res 12 Suppl 4: S6–S11.
4. Hwang TI, Tsai TF, Lin YC, Chiang HS, Chang LS (2010) A survey of erectile dysfunction in Taiwan: Use of the erection hardness score and quality of erection questionnaire. The journal of sexual medicine 7: 2817–2824.
5. Seftel AD, Sun P, Swindle R (2004) The prevalence of hypertension, hyperlipidemia, diabetes mellitus and depression in men with erectile dysfunction. The Journal of urology 171: 2341–2345.
6. Viigimaa M, Doumas M, Vlachopoulos C, Anyfanti P, Wolf J, et al. (2011) Hypertension and sexual dysfunction: time to act. Journal of hypertension 29: 403–407.
7. Weinberg AE, Eisenberg M, Patel CJ, Chertow GM, Leppert JT (2013) Diabetes severity, metabolic syndrome, and the risk of erectile dysfunction. The journal of sexual medicine 10: 3102–3109.
8. Blumentals W, Gomez-Caminero A, Joo S, Vannappagari V (2003) Is erectile dysfunction predictive of peripheral vascular disease? The Aging Male 6: 217–221.
9. Chew KK, Finn J, Stuckey B, Gibson N, Sanfilippo F, et al. (2010) Erectile Dysfunction as a Predictor for Subsequent Atherosclerotic Cardiovascular Events: Findings from a Linked-Data Study. The journal of sexual medicine 7: 192–202.
10. Ma RC-W, So W-Y, Yang X, Yu LW-L, Kong AP-S, et al. (2008) Erectile Dysfunction Predicts Coronary Heart Disease in Type 2 Diabetes. Journal of the American College of Cardiology 51: 2045–2050.
11. Ponholzer A, Temml C, Obermayr R, Wehrberger C, Madersbacher S (2005) Is erectile dysfunction an indicator for increased risk of coronary heart disease and stroke? European urology 48: 512–518.
12. Salem S, Abdi S, Mehrsai A, Saboury B, Saraji A, et al. (2009) ORIGINAL RESEARCH—ERECTILE DYSFUNCTION: Erectile Dysfunction Severity as a Risk Predictor for Coronary Artery Disease. The journal of sexual medicine 6: 3425–3432.
13. Thompson IM, Tangen CM, Goodman PJ, Probstfield JL, Moinpour CM, et al. (2005) Erectile dysfunction and subsequent cardiovascular disease. Jama 294: 2996–3002.
14. Bellinghieri G, Santoro D, Mallamace A, Savica V (2008) Sexual dysfunction in chronic renal failure. J Nephrol 21 Suppl 13: S113–117.
15. Stenvinkel P (2010) Chronic kidney disease: a public health priority and harbinger of premature cardiovascular disease. Journal of internal medicine 268: 456–467.
16. Uhlig K, Levey AS, Sarnak MJ (2002) Traditional cardiac risk factors in individuals with chronic kidney disease. pp. 118–127.
17. Zoccali C, Goldsmith D, Agarwal R, Blankestijn PJ, Fliser D, et al. (2011) The complexity of the cardio–renal link: taxonomy, syndromes, and diseases. Kidney International Supplements 1: 2–5.
18. Hermans MP, Ahn SA, Rousseau MF (2009) Erectile dysfunction, microangiopathy and UKPDS risk in type 2 diabetes. Diabetes & metabolism 35: 484–489.
19. Chuang YC, Chung MS, Wang PW, Lee WC, Chen CD, et al. (2012) Albuminuria is an independent risk factor of erectile dysfunction in men with type 2 diabetes. J Sex Med 9: 1055–1064.
20. Navaneethan SD, Vecchio M, Johnson DW, Saglimbene V, Graziano G, et al. (2010) Prevalence and Correlates of Self-Reported Sexual Dysfunction in CKD: A Meta-analysis of Observational Studies. American Journal of Kidney Diseases 56: 670–685.
21. Siu S, Lo SK, Wong K, Ip K, Wong Y (2001) Prevalence of and risk factors for erectile dysfunction in Hong Kong diabetic patients. Diabetic medicine 18: 732–738.
22. Yamasaki H, Ogawa K, Sasaki H, Nakao T, Wakasaki H, et al. (2004) Prevalence and risk factors of erectile dysfunction in Japanese men with type 2 diabetes. Diabetes Research and Clinical Practice 66: S173–S177.
23. Shamloul R, Ghanem H (2013) Erectile dysfunction. The Lancet 381: 153–165.
24. Aversa A, Bruzziches R, Francomano D, Natali M, Gareri P, et al. (2010) Endothelial dysfunction and erectile dysfunction in the aging man. International Journal of Urology 17: 38–47.
25. Reckelhoff J, Manning R (1993) Role of endothelium-derived nitric oxide in control of renal microvasculature in aging male rats. American Journal of Physiology-Regulatory, Integrative and Comparative Physiology 265: R1126–R1131.
26. Ravani P (2005) Asymmetrical Dimethylarginine Predicts Progression to Dialysis and Death in Patients with Chronic Kidney Disease: A Competing Risks Modeling Approach. Journal of the American Society of Nephrology 16: 2449–2455.
27. Shankar A, Sun L, Klein BEK, Lee KE, Muntner P, et al. (2011) Markers of inflammation predict the long-term risk of developing chronic kidney disease: a population-based cohort study. Kidney International 80: 1231–1238.
28. Marumo K, Nakashima J, Murai M (2001) Age-related prevalence of erectile dysfunction in Japan: Assessment by the International Index of Erectile Function. International Journal of Urology 8: 53–59.

4

A Meta-Analysis of Mortality in End-Stage Renal Disease Patients Receiving Implantable Cardioverter Defibrillators (ICDs)

Tien-Hsing Chen[1,2]*, Hung-Ta Wo[1], Po-Cheng Chang[1], Chun-Chieh Wang[1], Ming-Shien Wen[1], Chung-Chuan Chou[1]

1 Department of Cardiology, Chang-Gung Memorial Hospital, Linko, Taiwan, **2** Department of Cardiology, Chang-Gung Memorial Hospital, Xiamen, China, Chang Gung University College of Medicine, Kaohsiung, Taiwan

Abstract

Data on the effectiveness of implantable implantable cardioverter defibrillators (ICDs) with respect to reducing mortality in patients with chronic kidney disease (CKD) and end-stage renal disease (ESRD) are lacking. The purpose of this meta-analysis was to compare the mortality of patients with ESRD who have received and not received an ICD. A search was conducted on January 31, 2013 of Medline, Cochrane, EMBASE, and Google Scholar. Studies were selected for inclusion based on the following criteria. 1) Randomized controlled trial. 2) ESRD patients with heart failure. 3) Device therapy (ICD, CRT-defibrillator [CRT-D]) used to treat heart failure. 4) Primary outcome is survival analysis. 5) Retrospective study if survival analysis was performed. The primary outcome was overall survival (OS), and the secondary outcome was 2-year survival. Odds ratios (ORs) with 95% confidence intervals (CI) were calculated, and a χ^2-based test of homogeneity was performed. Three studies were included in the analysis. The combined OR for OS was 2.245 (95% CI 1.871 to 2.685, $P<0.001$), indicating that patients with an ICD had a significantly higher OS than those without an ICD. The combined OR for 2-year survival was 2.312 (95% CI 1.921 to 2.784, $P<0.001$), indicating that patients with an ICD had a significantly higher 2-year survival rate than those without an ICD. The use of ICD in patients with ESRD is associated with an increase in the OS and the 2-year survival rate.

Editor: Thomas Berger, Medical University Innsbruck, Austria

Funding: The authors have no support or funding to report.

Competing Interests: The authors have declared that no competing interests exist.

* Email: skyheart0826@gmail.com

Introduction

The number of patients with end-stage renal disease (ESRD) receiving dialysis is increasing worldwide. It is estimated that in the United States alone more than 2 million people will be receiving dialysis by 2020 [1]. Patients receiving dialysis have approximately 8-fold greater all-cause mortality as compared to the general population, with cardiovascular disease accounting for approximately 43% of the mortality [1,2]. Individuals with chronic kidney disease (CKD) are at a markedly increased risk of death from cardiovascular causes, including sudden cardiac death (SCD) due to arrhythmias [3,4].

Implantable implantable cardioverter defibrillators (ICDs) have been shown to reduce mortality and the risk of SCD in patients with severe heart failure as a result of ischemic and nonischemic cardiomyopathy, and in patients with arrhythmias [5–8]. However, data on the effectiveness of ICDs in patients with CKD and ESRD are lacking, and sometimes conflicting [9–14]. This is in part because patients with renal disease were often excluded from ICD studies [15,16]. It has been proposed that the survival advantage of ICDs in patients with renal disease as suggested by some studies may be negated as a result of comorbidities such as anemia, diabetes, and hypertension in these patients [15].

Tompkins et al. [17] reported that bleeding and ICD device-related complications were significantly more common in patients with ESRD. Alsheikh-Ali et al. [18] categorized patients by New York Heart Association (NYHA) class and estimated glomerular filtration rate (eGFR). The analysis suggested that the benefits of ICDs in patients with more advanced disease may be limited by the greater frequency of deaths due to causes other than arrhythmias. Bilchick et al. [19] found that CKD was associated with increased mortality rate in patients undergoing ICD implantation for the primary prevention of SCD (hazard ratio [HR] = 2.33). Similarly, a meta-analysis performed by Korantzopoulos et al. [20] in 2009 suggested that CKD is associated with increased mortality in patients who receive ICD therapy.

Given the increase in mortality rate of patients with CKD and ESRD, and the paucity of data regarding the outcome of ICD implantation in this group of patients, further investigation is warranted. The purpose of this study was to perform a meta-analysis to compare the mortality of ESRD patients receiving device therapy (ICD) with those who did not received device therapy.

Methods

Literature Search Strategy

A search was conducted of Medline, Cochrane, EMBASE, and Google Scholar using combinations of the search terms: chronic kidney disease, end-stage renal disease, dialysis, heart failure,

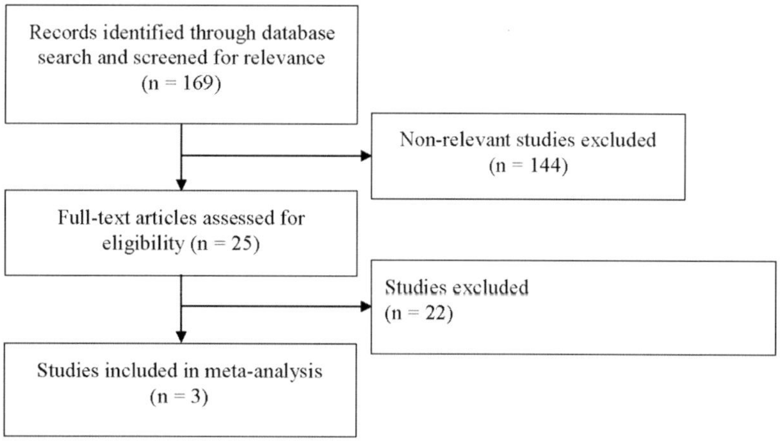

Figure 1. Flow diagram of study selection.

mortality, survival, device therapy, implantable cardioverter-defibrillator/ICD, cardiac resynchronization therapy defibrillator/CRT-D. The search date was January 31, 2013. Each publication was carefully examined, including the names of all authors, to avoid duplication of data.

Selection criteria

Studies were selected for analysis based on the following inclusion criteria. 1) Randomized controlled trial. 2) ESRD patients with heart failure. 3) Device therapy (ICD, CRT-defibrillator [CRT-D]) used to treat heart failure. 4) Primary outcome is survival analysis. 5) Retrospective study if the survival analysis was performed. Exclusion criteria for this analysis were as follows. 1) Study participants were not ESRD patients. 2) The study was not designed for ESRD patients with/without device therapy. 3) Studies that investigated if ESRD is risk factor/predictor of the prognosis for heart failure patients with device therapy (ICD, CRT-D). 4) Survival rate was not part of the analysis.

Data extraction

Studies were identified by two independent reviewers using the aforementioned search strategy. A third reviewer was consulted when there was uncertainty regarding eligibility.

The following data were extracted from studies that met the inclusion criteria: name of the first author, year of publication, study design, number of participants in each treatment group, participants' age and gender, overall survival (OS) rate, median OS time, 2-year survival rate, rate of comorbidities related to heart failure

Data analysis

The primary outcome was OS, and the secondary outcome was 2-year survival rate. The primary outcome, OS was used to evaluate treatment efficacy. Odds ratios (ORs) with 95% confidence intervals (CI) were calculated for binary outcomes and compared between patients with and without device therapy. A χ^2-based test of homogeneity was performed, and the inconsistency index (I^2) statistic was determined. If I^2 was >50% or >75%, the trials were considered to be heterogeneous or highly heterogeneous, respectively. An I^2<25% indicated homogeneity among the studies. When heterogeneity existed between studies (I^2>50%) a random-effects model was calculated. Otherwise, fixed-effects models were calculated. Pooled summary statistics for ORs of the individual studies were reported. Sensitivity analysis was performed based on the leave-one-out approach. Publication bias analysis was not performed because the number of studies was too few to detect an asymmetric funnel [21]. All analyses were performed using Comprehensive Meta-Analysis statistical software, version 2.0 (Biostat, Englewood, NJ). A value of $P<0.05$ was considered to indicate statistical significance.

Results

Literature search

After applying the inclusion and exclusion criteria, a total of 3 studies were included in this meta-analysis [22–24]. A flowchart of the study selection is shown in Figure 1. The 3 studies included in the meta-analysis are summarized in Table 1. Two studies included only ESRD patients [22,24], whereas one study included both CKD and ESRD patients [23]. For the purposes of this analysis, only data of ESRD patients from the study by Khan et al. [23] were used in the analysis.

Study characteristics and clinical outcomes

The ORs for OS of the 3 studies ranged from 1.164 to 2.317 (Fig. 2). There was homogeneity in the combined OR among the 3 studies ($Q=1.976$, $I^2=0\%$, $P=0.372$); therefore a fixed-effects model of analysis was used. Examination of the combined OR revealed a significant difference between ICD and no-ICD therapy. The combined OR was 2.245 (95% CI 1.871 to 2.685, $P<0.001$), indicating that patients with an ICD had a significantly higher OS than those without ICD therapy.

The ORs for the 2-year survival rate of the 3 studies ranged from 1.688 to 3.500 (Fig. 3). There was homogeneity in the 2-year survival rate between the studies when the data were pooled for analysis ($Q=1.067$, $I^2=0.00\%$, $P=0.586$); therefore a fixed-effects model of analysis was used. Examination of the combined OR revealed a significant difference between ICD and no-ICD therapy. The combined OR was 2.312 (95% CI 1.921 to 2.784, $P<0.001$), indicating that patients with an ICD had a significantly higher 2-year survival rate than those without ICD therapy.

Table 1. Summary of the 3 studies included in the meta-analysis.

1st Author	Year of Publication	Study Type	Group	Number of Patients	Age (y)	Sex (male)	OS rate	Median OS time	2-year Survival Rate	Rate of heart failure-related comorbidity
Hiremath[22]	2010	Retrospective	ICD	50	70.3±10.0	84%	60%	8 years	84%	ND
			Non-ICD	50	69.9±9.7	84%	42%	3.1 years	60%	ND
Khan*[23]	2010	Retrospective	ICD	14	64±12	93%	35.7%	ND	55%	100%
			Non-ICD	31	63±15	68%	32.3%	ND	42%	100%
Herzog[24]	2005	Retrospective	ICD	460	63.1±13.1	57%	51%	ND	53%	60.4%
			Non-ICD	5582	63.1±14.2	46%	31%	ND	33%	55.8%

Age data are presented as mean ± standard deviation.
OS, overall survival; ND, not derived.
*Only data of patients with end-stage renal disease were used in the analysis.

Figure 4 shows the results of the meta-analysis of OS with one study removed in turn. The results indicate that the direction and magnitude of the combined estimates did not have a large variation. This finding indicates that the results of the meta-analysis exhibits good reliability.

Discussion

The results of this meta-analysis indicate that the use of ICD in patients with ESRD is associated with an increase in the OS and the 2-year survival rate.

Data from prospective, randomized studies examining the effect of ICD therapy in patients with CKD/ESRD are lacking, and thus there is no general consensus on the use of device therapy in these patients. An ongoing trial (ICD2 trail) is randomizing dialysis patients, regardless of left ventricular function, to receive ICD therapy or not; however, study results are not expected until 2017 [25]. Most small retrospective studies have failed to show that patients with CKD or ESRD derive any survival benefit from ICD implantation [9,11–14]. A subgroup analysis of data from the MADIT-II study showed a survival benefit of ICD implantation in patients with an eGFR >35 mL/min, but not in those in which the eGFR was ≤35 mL/min [9,10]. Studies have reported a 1-year survival of patients with CKD with ICD implantation of 61% [12] and median survival of 6.3 years [14], and a median survival of ESRD patients with an ICD of 1.1 to 3.2 years [12,13].

Three studies were included in this meta-analysis. Herzog et al. [24] examined dialysis patients hospitalized from 1996 to 2001 for ventricular fibrillation/cardiac arrest who received ICD implantation within 30 day of admission. In the cohort, there were 460 patients (7.6%) who received ICD implantation and 5,582 (92.4%) that did not. The estimated 1-, 2-, 3-, 4-, and 5-year survival rates in the ICD group were 71%, 53%, 36%, 25%, and 22%, respectively, and in the no-ICD group were 49%, 33%, 23%, 16%, and 12% ($P<0.0001$). Analysis of the data showed that ICD implantation was independently associated with a 42% reduction in the risk of death (relative risk [RR] = 0.58). The authors concluded that in addition to the improvement in survival, ICD therapy was underutilized in this population. Khan et al. [23] studied 78 patients with moderate to severe CKD (45 patients with ESRD) with a left ventricular ejection fraction (LVEF) ≤35%, of whom 32 had an ICD, for an average follow-up of 2.7±2.3 years. In the group receiving dialysis (n = 45), ICD placement did not impact survival. In the patients with CKD who were not receiving dialysis (n = 33), survival was significantly better in patients with an ICD (2-year survival 80% vs. 54%, P = 0.027) after adjustment for sex, race, GFR, digoxin use, and presence of coronary disease, heart failure, or hypertension (OR = 0.23). Hiremath et al. [22] compared the outcomes of 50 patients with ESRD who had received ICD implantation with 50 patients with ESRD who did not have ICDs. The mean LVEF was similar between the 2 groups (approximately 29%). Median OS in the full cohort was 4.7 years with 20 deaths in the ICD group and 29 deaths in the no-ICD group. The median survival in the ICD group was 8.0 years, and 3.1 years in the no-ICD group. The multivariable analysis indicated that all-cause mortality was significantly less in the ICD group than in the no-ICD group (HR = 0.40).

The benefits of ICDs have been shown to be reduced in patients with advanced renal disease [9,10,26]. Furthermore, the complication rate of ICD implantation is higher in patients with ESRD than in patients without ESRD [27-29]. Patients with CKD have increased mortality from non-cardiac causes, cardiac non-SCD, SCD, and infections and while ICD implantation may decrease the risk of SCD it will not affect the risk of death from non-cardiac

Study (year)	Statistics for each study: Odds ratio	Lower limit	Upper limit	*Z* value	*P* value	Relative weight
Hiremath (2010)	2.071	0.933	4.597	1.790	0.073	5.25
Khan (2010)	1.164	0.449	3.013	0.312	0.755	3.69
Herzog (2005)	2.317	1.913	2.805	8.603	0.000	91.06
Total (Fixed)	2.245	1.871	2.695	8.680	0.000	

Q value=1.976, I-square=0%, *P* value=0.372

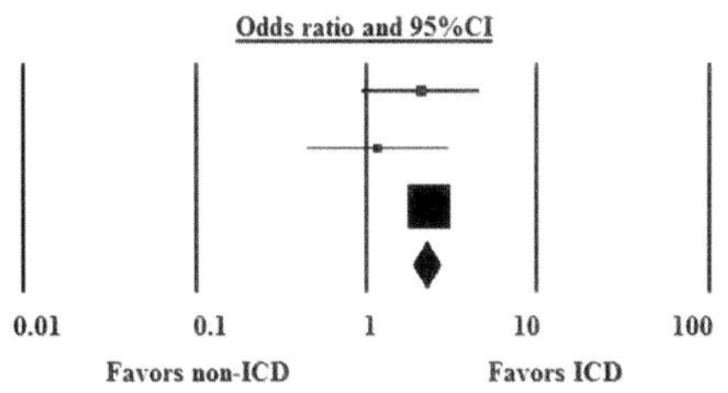

Figure 2. Forest plot of odds ratios (ORs) with 95% confidence intervals (CIs) for overall survival (OS) of the included studies. P<0.05 indicates a statistically significant difference.

causes such as infection, and there is increased risk of complications from device placement. The risk of SCD increases as renal function deteriorates, and this increase in risk is multifactorial in origin. The incidences of coronary artery disease, left ventricular hypertrophy, and left ventricular dysfunction are all increased in patients with ESRD. In addition, dialysis can lead to the development of interstitial fibrosis, endothelial dysfunction, and atheroma formation, which all can worsen the aforementioned conditions. The above highlight the competing causes of death in patients with CKD; conditions that are not affected by ICD placement.

The difference in survival between patients receiving dialysis and those not receiving dialysis as reported by Khan et al. [23] may be because in CKD patients ventricular arrhythmias can be terminated with ICD therapy [30]. In patients receiving dialysis, however, comorbidities which are not affected by ICD therapy may be present [31,32]. It has also been suggested that the defibrillation threshold may be increased in patients with ESRD, and thus optimal conversion of arrhythmias may not occur [33]. Despite the use of an ICD, the OS of patients with CKD is lower as compared to patients with normal kidney function [34]. On the other hand, CKD patients with an ICD still benefit from improved survival with ICD placement. For example, Amin et al. [35] showed in patients with stage 1 and 2 CKD, ICD implantation reduces mortality; however, in more advanced stages of CKD the benefit is less significant and age dependent. The authors attribute this finding to the fact that patients with more advanced CKD having a higher procedural risk and decreased life expectancy. When average procedural mortality was taken into account, the authors found that ICD implantation is favored at <80 years of age for stage 3 CKD, at <75 years of age for stage 4 CKD, and at <65 years of age for ESRD.

ICD therapy appears to be underutilized in patients with CKD, although patients with ESRD are at high risk for ventricular arrhythmias and SCD. Herzog et al. [24] reported a 42% reduction in overall death risk in dialysis patients, yet only 8% of eligible patients received an ICD. Other data [1] and studies [36] have also indicated that the use of ICD therapy in patients with CKD and ESRD is low. Therapies such as aspirin, beta blockers, and angiotensin converting enzyme inhibitors are used less frequently in patients with more severe renal failure [37], and thus physicians may be less likely to use other therapies (i.e., ICD) as well. There is also the concern of increased complications of ICDs in patients with renal failure [17]. Finally, as previously discussed; there is lack of data from well-designed clinical studies for this group of patients. Interestingly, the 2013 American College of Cardiology Foundation (ACCF) guidelines for the use of implantable ICDs and CRT include patients with CKD and ESRD [38].

The primary limitation of this meta-analysis is the small number of included studies. However, the inclusion criteria were strict by design to include only studies that were high quality and relevant to addressing the research question. In addition, only patients with ESRD were included. It remains to be determined if the results are also applicable to patients with CKD, but not ESRD.

Conclusions

In conclusion, the results of this meta-analysis indicate that the use of an ICD in patients with ESRD is associated with an increase in the OS and the 2-year survival rate. Based on these results, the use of ICD therapy in these patients is warranted.

Study (year)	Statistics for each study: Odds ratio	Lower limit	Upper limit	*Z* value	*P* value	Relative weight
Hiremath (2010)	3.500	1.361	8.999	2.600	0.009	3.86
Khan (2010)	1.688	0.473	6.021	0.807	0.420	2.13
Herzog (2005)	2.289	1.891	2.772	8.482	0.000	94.01
Total (Fixed)	2.312	1.921	2.784	8.853	0.000	

Q value=1.067, I-square=0%, *P* value=0.586

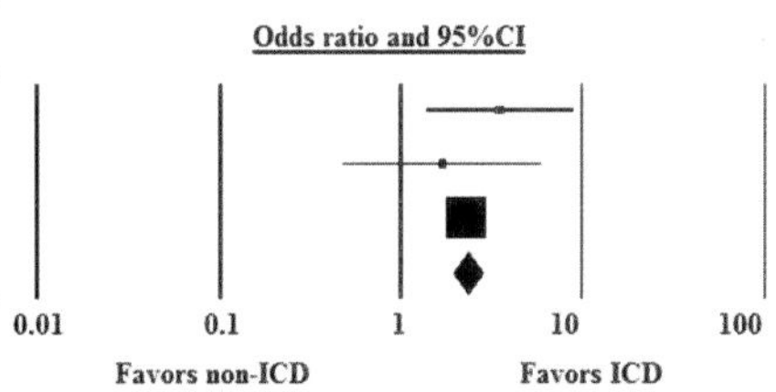

Figure 3. Forest plot of odds ratios (ORs) with 95% confidence intervals (CIs) for 2-year survival of the included studies. P<0.05 indicates a statistically significant difference.

Removed Study (year)	Statistics with study removed				
	Odds ratio	Lower limit	Upper limit	*Z* value	*P* value
Hiremath S (2010)	2.255	1.870	2.721	8.495	0.000
Khan (2010)	2.303	1.912	2.774	8.783	0.000
Herzog (2005)	1.633	0.886	3.008	1.573	0.116
Total (Fixed)	2.245	1.871	2.695	8.680	0.000

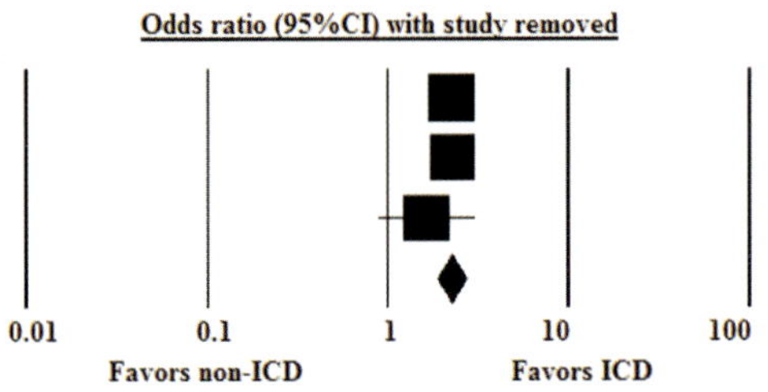

Figure 4. Sensitivity analysis for the influence of individual studies on pooled estimates by the leave-one-out approach for overall survival (OS). Data are presented as odds ratio (OR) with the 95% confidence interval (CI). P<0.05 indicates a statistically significant difference.

Author Contributions

Conceived and designed the experiments: T-HC C-CW. Performed the experiments: T-HC H-TW P-CC. Analyzed the data: T-HC M-SW C-CC. Contributed reagents/materials/analysis tools: T-HC. Wrote the paper: T-HC.

References

1. US Renal Data System 2012 Annual Data Report: Atlas of Chronic Kidney Disease and End-Stage Renal Disease in the United States. Bethesda, National Institutes of Health, National Institute of Diabetes and Digestive and Kidney Diseases, 2012. Available at: http://www.usrds.org/atlas.aspx. Accessed August 1, 2013.
2. Herzog CA, Mangrum JM, Passman R (2008) Sudden cardiac death and dialysis patients. Semin Dial 21:300–307.
3. Eknoyan G, Beck GJ, Cheung AK, Daugirdas JT, Greene T, et al. (2002) Effect of dialysis dose and membrane flux in maintenance hemodialysis. N Engl J Med 347:2010–2019.
4. Wanner C, Krane V, Marz W, Olschewski M, Mann JF, et al. (2005) Atorvastatin in patients with type 2 diabetes mellitus undergoing hemodialysis. N Engl J Med 53:238–248.
5. Bardy GH, Lee KL, Mark DB, Poole JE, Packer DL, et al. (2005) Amiodarone or an implantable cardioverter-defibrillator for congestive heart failure. N Engl J Med 352:225–237.
6. Kadish A, Dyer A, Daubert JP, Quigg R, Estes NA, et al. (2004) Prophylactic defibrillator implantation in patients with nonischemic dilated cardiomyopathy. N Engl J Med 350:2151–2158.
7. Moss AJ, Hall WJ, Cannom DS, Daubert JP, Higgins SL, et al. (1996) Improved survival with an implanted defibrillator in patients with coronary disease at high risk for ventricular arrhythmia. Multicenter Automatic Defibrillator Implantation Trial Investigators. N Engl J Med 335:1933–1940.
8. Moss AJ, Zareba W, Hall WJ, Klein H, Wilber DJ, et al. (2002) Prophylactic implantation of a defibrillator in patients with myocardial infarction and reduced ejection fraction. N Engl J Med 346:877–883.
9. Goldenberg I, Moss AJ, McNitt S, Zareba W, Andrews ML, et al. (2006) Relations among renal function, risk of sudden cardiac death, and benefit of the implanted cardiac defibrillator in patients with ischemic left ventricular dysfunction. Am J Cardiol 98:485–490.
10. (2002) K/DOQI Clinical Practice Guidelines for Chronic Kidney Disease: Evaluation, Classification, and Stratification Part 4. Definition and classification of stages of chronic kidney disease. Am J Kidney Dis 39:S46–S75.
11. Chen-Scarabelli C, Scarabelli TM (2007) Chronic renal insufficiency is an independent predictor of mortality in implantable cardioverterdefibrillator recipients. Pacing Clin Electrophysiol 30:371–376.
12. Cuculich PS, Sanchez JM, Kerzner R, Greenberg SL, Sengupta J, et al. (2007) Poor prognosis for patients with chronic kidney disease despite ICD therapy for the primary prevention of sudden death. Pacing Clin Electrophysiol 30:207–213.
13. Robin J, Weinberg K, Tiongson J, Carnethon M, Reddy M, et al. (2006) Renal dialysis as a risk factor for appropriate therapies and mortality in implantable cardioverter-defibrillator recipients. Heart Rhythm 3:1196–1201.
14. Turakhia MP, Varosy PD, Lee K, Tseng ZH, Lee R, et al. (2007) Impact of renal function on survival in patients with implantable cardioverter- defibrillators. Pacing Clin Electrophysiol 30:377–384.
15. O'Shaughnessy MM, Lappin DW, Reddan DN (2012) Sudden cardiac death in dialysis: do current guidelines for implantable cardioverter defibrillator therapy apply to patients with end-stage kidney disease? Semin Dial 25:272–276.
16. Cannizzaro LA, Piccini JP, Patel UD, Hernandez AF (2011) Device therapy in heart failure patients with chronic kidney disease. J Am Coll Cardiol 58:889–896.
17. Tompkins C, McLean R, Cheng A, Brinker JA, Marine JE, et al. (2011) End-stage renal disease predicts complications in pacemaker and ICD implants. J Cardiovasc Electrophysiol 22:1099–1104.
18. Alsheikh-Ali AA, Trikalinos TA, Ruthazer R, Terrin N, Wong JB, et al. (2011) Risk of arrhythmic and nonarrhythmic death in patients with heart failure and chronic kidney disease Am Heart J 161:204–209.e1.
19. Bilchick KC, Stukenborg GJ, Kamath S, Cheng A (2012) Prediction of mortality in clinical practice for medicare patients undergoing defibrillator implantation for primary prevention of sudden cardiac death. J Am Coll Cardiol 60:1647–155.
20. Korantzopoulos P, Liu T, Li L, Goudevenos JA, Li G (2009) Implantable cardioverter defibrillator therapy in chronic kidney disease: a meta-analysis. Europace 11:1469–175.
21. Sutton AJ, Duval SJ, Tweedie RL, Abrams KR, Jones DR (2000) Empirical assessment of effect of publication bias on meta-analyses. BMJ 320:1574–1577.
22. Hiremath S, Punnam SR, Brar SS, Goyal SK, Gardiner JC, et al. (2010) Implantable defibrillators improve survival in end-stage renal disease: results from a multi-center registry. Am J Nephrol 32:305–310.
23. Khan F, Adelstein E, Saba S (2010) Implantable cardioverter defibrillators confer survival benefit in patients with renal insufficiency but not in dialysis-dependent patients. J Interv Card Electrophysiol 28:117–123.
24. Herzog CA, Li S, Weinhandl ED, Strief JW, Collins AJ, et al. (2005) Survival of dialysis patients after cardiac arrest and the impact of implantable cardioverter defibrillators. Kidney Int 68:818–825.
25. de Bie MK, Lekkerkerker JC, van Dam B, Gaasbeek A, van Buren M, et al. (2008) Prevention of sudden cardiac death: rationale and design of the Implantable Cardioverter Defibrillators in Dialysis Patients (ICD2) Trial – a prospective pilot study. Curr Med Res Opin 24:2151–2157.
26. Williams ES, Shah SH, Piccini JP, Sun AY, Koontz JI, et al. (2011) Predictors of mortality in patients with chronic kidney disease and an implantable defibrillator: an EPGEN substudy. Europace 13:1717–122.
27. Aggarwal A, Wang Y, Rumsfeld JS, Curtis JP, Heidenreich PA (2009) Clinical characteristics and in-hospital outcome of patients with end-stage renal disease on dialysis referred for implantable cardioverter-defibrillator implantation. Heart Rhythm 6:1565–1571.
28. Dasgupta A, Montalvo J, Medendorp S, Lloyd-Jones DM, Ghossein C, et al. (2007) Increased complication rates of cardiac rhythm management devices in ESRD patients. Am J Kidney Dis 49:656–663.
29. Teruya TH, Abou-Zamzam AM Jr, Limm W, Wong L, Wong L (2003) Symptomatic subclavian vein stenosis and occlusion in hemodialysis patients with transvenous pacemakers. Ann Vasc Surg 17:526–529.
30. Hreybe H, Ezzeddine R, Bedi M, Barrington W, Bazaz R, et al. (2006) Renal insufficiency predicts the time to first appropriate defibrillator shock. Am Heart J151:852–856.
31. Grothe C, Belasco A, Bettencourt A, Diccini S, Vianna L, et al. (2009) Lethality of endocarditis due to S. aureus among patients on hemodialysis. Nephrol Nurs J 36: 613–619.
32. Thomson P, Stirling C, Traynor J, Morris S, Mactier R (2010) A prospective

observational study of catheter-related bacteraemia and thrombosis in a haemodialysis cohort: Univariate and multivariate analyses of risk association. Nephrol Dial Transplant 25:1596–1604.

33. Wase A, Basit A, Nazir R, Jamal A, Shah S, et al. (2004) Impact of chronic kidney disease upon survival among implantable cardioverter-defibrillator recipients. J Interv Card Electrophysiol 11:199–204.
34. Cuculich PS, Sánchez JM, Kerzner R, Greenberg SL, Sengupta J, et al. (2007) Poor prognosis for patients with chronic kidney disease despite ICD therapy for the primary prevention of sudden death. Pacing Clin Electrophysiol 30:207–213.
35. Amin MS, Fox AD, Kalahasty G, Shepard RK, Wood MA, et al. (2008) Benefit of primary prevention implantable cardioverter-defibrillators in the setting of chronic kidney disease: a decision model analysis. J Cardiovasc Electrophysiol 19:1275–1280.
36. Voigt A, Ezzeddine R, Barrington W, Obiaha-Ngwu O, Ganz LI, et al. (2004) Utilization of implantable cardioverter-defibrillators in survivors of cardiac arrest in the United States from 1996 to 2001. J AmColl Cardiol 44:855–858.
37. Berger AK, Duval S, Krumholz HM (2003) Aspirin, beta-blocker, and angiotensin-converting enzyme inhibitor therapy in patients with end-stage renal disease and an acute myocardial infarction. J Am Coll Cardiol 42:201–208.
38. Russo AM, Stainback RF, Bailey SR, Epstein AE, Heidenreich PA, et al. (2013) ACCF/HRS/AHA/ASE/HFSA/SCAI/SCCT/SCMR 2013 appropriate use criteria for implantable cardioverter-defibrillators and cardiac resynchronization therapy: a report of the American College of Cardiology Foundation appropriate use criteria task force, Heart Rhythm Society, American Heart Association, American Society of Echocardiography, Heart Failure Society of America, Society for Cardiovascular Angiography and Interventions, Society of Cardiovascular Computed Tomography, and Society for Cardiovascular Magnetic Resonance. J Am Coll Cardiol 61:1318–1368.

5

The Relationship between Renal Function and Plasma Concentration of the Cachectic Factor Zinc-Alpha2-Glycoprotein (ZAG) in Adult Patients with Chronic Kidney Disease

Caroline C. Pelletier[1,2,3]❡, Laetitia Koppe[1,2,3]❡, Pascaline M. Alix[1,2,3]❡, Emilie Kalbacher[1,2,3], Marine L. Croze[1,2], Aoumeur Hadj-Aissa[1,4], Denis Fouque[1,2,5], Fitsum Guebre-Egziabher[1,2,3], Christophe O. Soulage[1,2]*

1 Université de Lyon, F-69600, Oullins, France, **2** INSERM, U1060, CarMeN, INSA-Lyon, Univ. Lyon-1, Villeurbanne, France, **3** Hospices Civils de Lyon, Service de Néphrologie, Hôpital E Herriot, Lyon, France, **4** Hospices Civils de Lyon, Exploration Fonctionnelle Rénale et Métabolique, Hôpital E Herriot, Lyon, France, **5** Hospices Civils de Lyon, Service de Néphrologie, Centre Hospitalier Lyon-SUD, Pierre-Bénite, France

Abstract

Zinc-α2-glycoprotein (ZAG), a potent cachectic factor, is increased in patients undergoing maintenance dialysis. However, there is no data for patients before initiation of renal replacement therapy. The purpose of the present study was to assess the relationship between plasma ZAG concentration and renal function in patients with a large range of glomerular filtration rate (GFR). Plasma ZAG concentration and its relationship to GFR were investigated in 71 patients with a chronic kidney disease (CKD) stage 1 to 5, 17 chronic hemodialysis (HD), 8 peritoneal dialysis (PD) and 18 non-CKD patients. Plasma ZAG concentration was 2.3-fold higher in CKD stage 5 patients and 3-fold higher in HD and PD patients compared to non-CKD controls ($P<0.01$). The hemodialysis session further increased plasma ZAG concentration (+39%, $P<0.01$). An inverse relationship was found between ZAG levels and plasma protein ($r_s=-0.284$; $P<0.01$), albumin ($r_s=-0.282$, $P<0.05$), hemoglobin ($r_s=-0.267$, $P<0.05$) and HDL-cholesterol ($r_s=-0.264$, $P<0.05$) and a positive correlation were seen with plasma urea ($r_s=0.283$; $P<0.01$). In multiple regression analyses, plasma urea and HDL-cholesterol were the only variables associated with plasma ZAG ($r^2=0.406$, $P<0.001$). In CKD-5 patients, plasma accumulation of ZAG was not correlated with protein energy wasting. Further prospective studies are however needed to better elucidate the potential role of ZAG in end-stage renal disease.

Editor: Leighton R. James, University of Florida, United States of America

Funding: This study was supported by two governmental institutions from France, INSERM and INSA-Lyon, and by the Fédération Nationale d'Aide aux Insuffisants Rénaux (FNAIR). CC.PELLETIER and PM. ALIX held grants from "Société Française de Néphrologie," E KALBACHER was the recipient of a grant from "Académie de Médecine" and L. KOPPE held a fellowship from "Fondation pour la Recherche Médicale". ML CROZE held a grant from the French "Ministère de l'Enseignement Supérieur et de la Recherche." The authors have no competing financial interests to disclose. The funders had no role in study design, data collection and analysis, decision to publish, or preparation of the manuscript.

Competing Interests: The authors have declared that no competing interests exist.

* Email: Christophe.Soulage@insa-lyon.fr

❡ These authors contributed equally to this work.

Introduction

Chronic kidney disease (CKD) and especially end-stage renal disease (ESRD) are associated with increased plasma concentration of numerous adipokines presumably as the result of a decreased glomerular filtration and/or a blunted renal degradation. Indeed, plasma concentrations of leptin [1], adiponectin [2,3], fibroblast growth factor 21 (FGF-21) [4], retinol binding protein 4 (RBP-4) [5], chemerin [6] were found to be increased in ESRD patients. Zinc-α2-glycoprotein (thereafter referred to as ZAG) is a 43-kDa soluble glycoprotein first isolated from human plasma [7] and proposed as a tumour-derived cancer cachexia factor [8,9]. Indeed, ZAG is overexpressed in many malignant tumours and is strongly associated with adipose tissue atrophy in cancer cachexia [10]. ZAG is however also produced by many non-malignant tissues, including white adipose tissue (WAT) and epithelia cells from liver, breast, gastrointestinal tract as well as sweat glands [11]. ZAG is described as a lipid-mobilizing factor in adipose tissue [12]. The biological activity of ZAG is linked to a cyclic AMPc-mediated signalling system through interaction with a β3/β2 adrenoreceptors [9,10,13,14]. ZAG displays both lipolytic and antilipogenic effects on adipose tissue [9,15] and stimulates uncoupling protein-1 (UCP-1) expression in brown adipose tissue, increasing thermogenesis and lipid utilization [16]. Currently, only few data are available on ZAG metabolism in kidney disease. Philipp et al [17] and Leal et al [18,19] recently showed an increased plasma ZAG concentration in chronic hemodialysis patients, suggesting a defect of its renal clearance. However, there is no data regarding the actual plasma level of ZAG in CKD patients before initiation of renal replacement therapy. It therefore remains unclear whether the plasma accumulation of ZAG simply results from the decrease in glomerular filtration rate (GFR). The purpose of this cross-sectional study was therefore to prospectively assess the relationship between plasma ZAG concentration and GFR in patients with a large range of renal function. Plasma ZAG concentration was measured in a cohort of 71 CKD patients from stage 1 to 5, 18 non-CKD patients and correlations were explored with clinical and biochemical markers of renal function and metabolism. Plasma ZAG was further measured in 17 hemodialysis (HD) and 8 peritoneal dialysis (PD) patients.

Materials and Methods

Ethic statement

This research was approved by the local institutional review committee (reference D-09-17, Comité de Protection des Personnes - Recherche Biomédicale, CPP Lyon Sud-Est IV) and conducted in accordance with its ethical standards and the principles of the Declaration of Helsinki. All subjects involved in the research signed written informed consent forms prior to enrolment.

Subjects

From November 2010 to March 2013, a total of 89 subjects (43 men and 46 women), among which 18 non-CKD subjects, were recruited from Nephrology department and Unité de Jour d'Exploration Rénale et Néphrologie (UJERN) (E. Herriot University hospital Lyon, France). Glomerular filtration rate (eGFR) was estimated using the CKD EPI formula [20,21] and CKD stages were determined according to K/DOQI guidelines [22]. Seventeen chronic HD and 8 PD patients on renal replacement therapy for more than 6 months were further recruited at the Nephrology/Hemodialysis unit (E. Herriot University hospital, Lyon, France). Patients with severe conditions including systemic inflammation or known malignant active diseases were excluded from the study. People were classified into 8 groups: Healthy volunteers, CKD stage 1, CKD stage 2, CKD stage 3, CKD stage 4, CKD stage 5 - no renal replacement therapy, CKD stage 5 - hemodialysis, CKD stage 5 - peritoneal dialysis.

Anthropometric and clinical measurements

Body weight was measured in light clothing without shoes to the nearest 100 g on a digital scale, corresponding to dry weights for HD patients. Height was measured in standard position with a portable stadiometer. Body mass index (BMI) was calculated as body weight divided by squared height. Body fat mass was calculated according to Deurenberg et al (1991) using the following formula: Body fat (%) = (1.20×BMI)+(0.23×Age)−(10.8×Gender) where male gender = 1, female gender = 0 [23]. CKD patients were considered having PEW if they presented at least 3 out of 4 of the following criterions, BMI<23 kg/m^2, Albumin<38 g/L (bromcresol green assay), Pre-albumin < 300 mg/L or Protein intake<0.6 g/kg.24 h according to Fouque et al (2008) [24].

Blood sampling

After an overnight fast, blood samples were obtained by venipuncture, except for HD blood samples that were obtained immediately before and after dialysis from arterial line of the mechanical bloodstream. Blood samples were centrifuged at 3500×g for 10 min to isolate plasma supernatant which was snap frozen in liquid nitrogen and stored at −20°C until use.

Glomerular filtration rate measurements (mGFR)

In a subset of 42 CKD stage 1 to 4 subjects, GFR was measured by the gold standard method, i.e. the urinary inulin clearance (ml/min per 1.73 m^2), as described previously [25]. Briefly, inulin (Polyfructosan[inutest], Laevosan, Linz, Austria) was infused continuously for 4 hours after a priming dose. Blood and urine were collected every 30 minutes by peripheral venous catheter and spontaneous voiding, respectively. Inulin was measured by the enzymatic method [26]. GFR was calculated with the UV/P formula with U = urine inulin concentration, V = urinary volume and P = plasma inulin concentration.

ZAG immunoassay

Plasma ZAG concentrations were determined with a commercially available ZAG Enzyme Immunoassay (RayBiotech Inc, Tebu-Bio, Le-Perray-en-Yvelines, France) according to the manufacturer's instructions. The detection limit was 21 pg/ml and intra and inter-assay coefficient was 3.6% and 3.2% respectively. Measurements were performed at least in duplicate. Post-dialysis ZAG concentrations were corrected for hemoconcentration using plasma protein concentrations assayed according to the method of Bradford [27] with bovine serum albumin as standard. The correction was performed using the following equation: $[ZAG]_{Corrected} = ([Proteins]_{pre\text{-}HD}/[Proteins]_{post\text{-}HD}) \times [ZAG]_{post\text{-}HD}$ with $[Proteins]_{pre\text{-}HD}$, plasma protein concentration before haemodialysis session, $[Proteins]_{post\text{-}HD}$ and $[ZAG]_{post\text{-}HD}$, plasma protein and plasma ZAG concentrations after haemodialysis session, respectively.

Other biochemical measurements

Plasma urea, bicarbonate, hemoglobin, protein, glucose, HDL and LDL cholesterol, triglycerides, and C-reactive protein (CRP) were measured by standard laboratory methods in a certified laboratory. Albumin was measured by immunonephelometry. Creatinine assay was performed by enzymatic method (Roche, Meylan, France), with calibrators assigned by an isotope-dilution mass spectrometry. Plasma glycerol concentration (an index of white adipose tissue lipolysis) was measured using a colorimetric enzymatic assay (Glycerol assay, R-Biopharm, Saint-Didier, France) and normalized to body fat mass as described by Axelsson et al (2011) [28].

Statistical analysis

Data were analysed using Graphpad Prism 5.0 (GraphPad softwares, La Jolla, USA) and Statview 4.5 (Abacus concept, Berkeley, USA) softwares. The data are expressed as mean±1 standard deviation (SD) or as median (interquartile range [IQR]) when variable were not normally distributed. Distributions were tested for normality using d'Agostino-Pearson test. Differences between groups were assessed by Kruskall & Wallis test followed when appropriate by Dunn tests. Simple comparisons were made using Mann & Whitney U test. Sex ratio and medications between groups were compared using Chi-square test. Univariate analysis was performed using the Spearman rank correlation method. A multivariate linear regression analysis was used to define the variables most predictive of circulating ZAG concentration after selection of the measures found to be associated with ZAG by univariate analysis (i.e. urea, plasma proteins, hemoglobin and HDL-cholesterol). A P<0.05 was considered as statistically significant in all analysis.

Table 1. Baseline characteristics of non CKD, CKD, hemodialysis and peritoneal dialysis patients involved in the study (N = 114).

	Non CKD	CKD stage					HD	PD	P-value
		1	2	3	4	5			
Sex, male/female	9/9	2/6	8/12	11/7	7/5	6/7	8/9	4/4	P = 0.777
Age, y	52 (28–63)	31 (20–48)	59(48–70)	69 (58–76)	67 (54–76)	61 (58–66)	66 (53–86)	58 (46–71)	P = 0.001
Weight, kg	67.0 (53.0–73.8)	59.5 (48.2–74.5)	65.0 (58.5–76.3)	75.0 (64.5–92.3)	74.0 (64.0–85.8)	71.0 (60.0–87.5)	65.0 (55.0–77.8)	63.9 (55.5–76.8)	P = 0.156
BMI, kg/m^2	23.4 (21.2–25.6)	20.8 (18.5–25.6)	25.3 (22.1–27.2)	26.7 (23.4–32.9)	26.2 (24.3–31.8)	24.0 (22.9–30.8)	25.8 (21.9–30.3)	23.9 (20.7–29.5)	P = 0.100
Creatinine, μM	58.5 (50.8–62.3)	53.5 (42.0–72.0)	82.5 (72.5–93.5)	137 (122–171)	301 (198–368)	456 (382–639)	643 (450–815)	641 (498–846)	P<0.001
eGFR, ml/min.1.73 m^2	109 (99–138)	124 (94–134)	75 (68–88)	43 (33–45)	16 (14–24)	9 (8–12)	N/A	N/A	P<0.001
Urea, mM	4.7 (3.9–5.7)	4.2 (3.6–6.8)	6.1 (5.0–7.7)	13.6 (9.5–15.3)	20.7 (14.3–24.5)	24.0 (17.2–28.5)	21.4 (18.3–28.2)	16.6 (14.7–21.2)	P<0.001
Bicarbonates, mM	25.0 (23.2–27.1)	25.9 (23.9–30.5)	26.8 (24.5–28.3)	23.3 (22.1–25.8)	21.9 (18.6–25.8)	24.8 (21.8–26.8)	24.1 (22.5–25.0)	26.9 (24.4–28.7)	P = 0.002
Proteins, g/L	70.0 (65.8–76.5)	70.5 (54.3–75.8)	70.0 (66.5–75.8)	73.0 (70.3–79.3)	73.5 (70.3–75.0)	72.0 (65.0–76.0)	68.0 (66.0–72.0)	74.5 (65.5–78.0)	P = 0.385
Albumin, g/L	41.5 (37.0–42.9)	37.0 (17.0–41.0)	41.8 (37.0–43.7)	36.9 (35.0–42.5)	38.0 (33.0–40.0)	32.0 (26.5–34.5)	38.0 (33.5–40.5)	35.0 (27.0–36.0)	P = 0.009
Hemoglobin, g/L	127 (117–144)	126 (107–140)	130 (122–138)	119 (102–134)	112 (101–122)	118 (102–122)	116 (102–122)	125 (104–136)	P = 0.003
Glucose, mM	4.8 (4.3–5.4)	4.8 (4.2–5.4)	5.0 (4.5–5.7)	5.9 (4.4–7.0)	5.3 (4.8–6.3)	5.6 (4.8–6.9)	5.4 (4.4–5.8)	4.9 (4.7–8.1)	P = 0.129
Triacylglycerols, mM	0.76 (0.55–1.33)	1.74 (1.44–3.02)	1.30 (1.00–1.97)	1.46 (1.08–2.21)	1.37 (1.21–2.60)	1.61 (1.33–2.16)	1.87 (1.04–2.38)	1.32 (0.71–2.84)	P = 0.038
HDL cholesterol, mM	1.10 (0.95–1.32)	1.10 (0.91–1.57)	1.29 (0.98–1.86)	1.19 (1.00–1.36)	1.14 (0.90–1.24)	1.01 (0.87–1.1)	1.18 (0.99–1.56)	1.48 (0.69–4.03)	P = 0.449
LDL cholesterol, mM	2.38 (1.87–3.22)	2.25 (1.73–5.02)	2.83 (2.20–3.84)	1.61 (1.33–2.01)	1.44 (1.26–2.79)	2.18 (1.64–2.67)	2.02 (1.42–3.68)	2.18 (1.68–2.52)	P = 0.044
CRP, mg/L	2.9 (2.9–3.2)	3.0(2.9–7.2)	2.9 (2.9–3.1)	4.5 (2.9–7.0)	2.9 (2.9–9.6)	3.2 (2.9–11.3)	4.4 (2.9–9.2)	2.9 (2.9–2.9)	P = 0.067
Anti diabetic therapy,%	0.0	12.5	5.0	50.0	77.7	23.1	17.6	50.0	P<0.001
Lipid-lowering therapy,%	5.9	12.5	30.0	66.7	80.0	38.5	47.0	50.0	P = 0.001
RAA inhibitors,%	11.8	37.5	25.0	88.9	60.0	77.0	41.2	62.5	P<0.001
Beta blockers, %	0	0	22.2	47.1	27.3	30.8	58.8	37.5	P = 0.005

Continuous data are expressed as median (interquartile range) and compared using Kruskall & Wallis test. Categorical data are expressed as the frequency (%) and compared using Chi square test. Abbreviations: CKD, chronic kidney disease, BMI, body mass index, eGFR estimated glomerular filtration rate, HD, hemodialysis, N/A, not applicable, PD, peritoneal dialysis, RAA, renin angiotensin aldosterone. eGFR was calculated using CKD EPI formula. Differences were considered significant at P<0.05.

Table 2. Dialysis adequacy for HD and DP patients.

	Hemodialysis	Peritoneal Dialysis
Dialysis modality	9 HD/8 HDF	5 CAPD/3 CCPD
Catheter/Fistula/not documented, n =	3/12/2	NA
Time of dialysis (h/week)	12.27±0.61	NA
Blood flow (ml/mn)	340.91±24.27	NA
Kt/V	1.67±0.31	NA
Weekly Kt/V urea	NA	2.43±0.51
Weekly peritoneal clearance (L/week/1.73 m^2)	NA	89.18±22.53
Residual renal fonction (L/week/1.73 m^2)	NA	48.3±25.01

Data are expressed as means ± one standard deviation. Abbreviations: CAPD, continuous ambulatory peritoneal dialysis, CCPD continuous cyclic peritoneal dialysis, HD, hemodialysis; HDF, hemodiafiltration, NA, not applicable.

Results

Patient data

We recruited 71 patients with CKD from stage 1 to end-stage 5 (aged 57±17 years), 18 non-CKD patients (aged 48±19 years), 17 HD patients (aged 66±17 years) and 8 PD patients (aged 58±14 years). Their renal diseases were glomerulonephritis (N = 32 including 19 diabetes), renovascular disease (N = 22, including 14 nephroangiosclerosis), 9 tubulointerstitial disease, 5 cystic kidney diseases and of other or unknown aetiologies in 28 patients. Non-CKD patients were referred of renal function evaluation for urinary lithiasis exploration or before kidney donation. Out of the 96 CKD, HD and PD patients, 54 were on antihypertensive drugs (56.8%), 45 on lipid lowering drugs (47.3%), 32 were on beta-

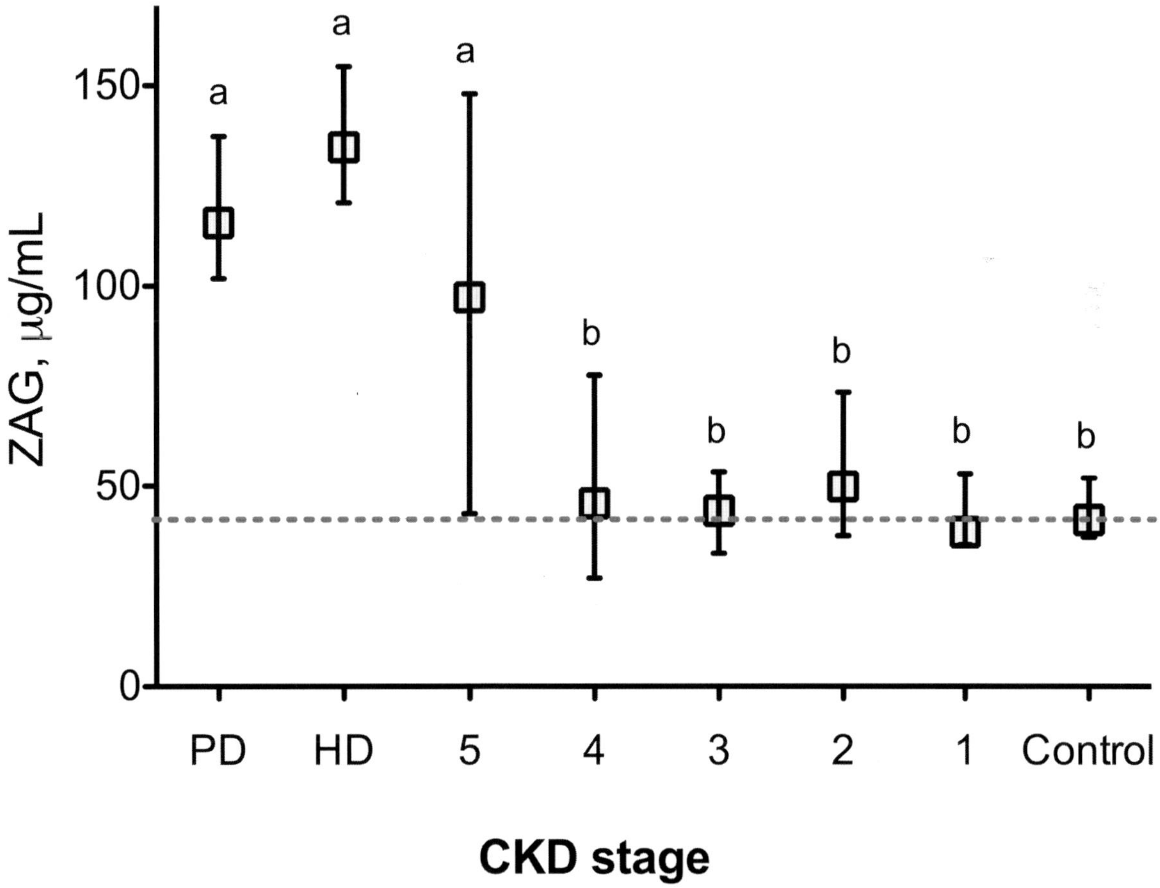

Figure 1. Plasma ZAG concentration is increased in end stage renal disease patients. ZAG concentration was quantified in plasma from non-CKD subjects (N = 18), chronic kidney disease (CKD stage 1 to 5, N = 71), hemodialysis (HD, N = 17) and peritoneal dialysis (PD, N = 8) patients by enzyme immunoassay. eGFR was estimated using CKD EPI formula as described in methods. Data are presented as median (interquartile range). Different letters indicate a significant difference at the P<0.05 level.

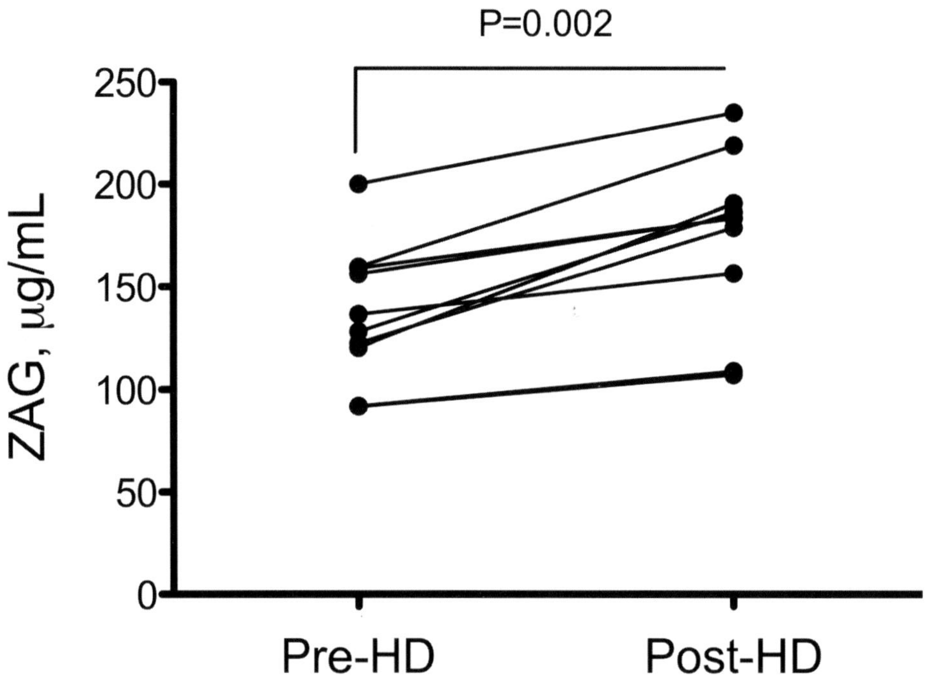

Figure 2. Plasma ZAG concentration increases during hemodialysis session. ZAG concentration was quantified by enzyme immunoassay before and after an hemodialysis session in ESRD patients (N = 8). ZAG concentrations were corrected for hemoconcentration as described in methods. Differences between pre and post dialysis concentrations were considered significant at the $P<0.05$ level (Wilcoxon test for paired samples). Abbreviation: HD, hemodialysis.

blockers (33.3%) and 30 on antidiabetic drugs (31.5%, amongst which 24 used insulin and 6 oral antidiabetics). The main clinical, anthropometric and biochemical characteristics of the cohort are summarized in **Table 1** and dialysis adequacy is described in **Table 2**. As expected, eGFR (estimated by CKD EPI, $P<0.001$), plasma creatinine ($P<0.001$) and urea ($P<0.001$) were different between groups.

Plasma ZAG concentration increases in ESRD patients

Surprisingly, plasma ZAG concentration did not gradually increase from CKD stage 1 to CKD stage 4 when compared to non-CKD patients (**Figure 1**). Plasma ZAG concentration was however 2.3-fold higher in CKD 5 (ESRD) patients as compared with non-CKD patients or CKD stage 1 to 4 patients (Kruskall & Wallis test, $P<0.005$). The plasma ZAG concentration was 41.5 (interquartile range (IQR), 37.3–52.0) µg/ml for non-CKD

Table 3. Univariate correlations with ZAG concentrations.

	rho	P-value	
Age, y	0.103	0.340	
BMI, kg.m^{-2}	0.112	0.296	
CRP, mg L^{-1}	0.088	0.507	
Protein, g.L^{-1}	−0.284	0.008	**
Albumin, g.L^{-1}	−0.282	0.016	*
Hemoglobin, g.L^{-1}	−0.264	0.015	*
Bicarbonate, mM	−0.001	0.905	
Urea, mM	0.283	0.008	**
Creatinine, µM	0.274	<0.01	**
Proteinuria, g.24 h^{-1}	0.257	0.061	
Glucose, mM	0.138	0.200	
HDL-cholesterol, mM	−0.265	0.034	*
LDL-cholesterol, mM	−0.097	0.448	
Triacylglycerols, mM	0.119	0.340	

Abbreviations: BMI: Body mass index, CRP: C-reactive protein, eGFR: estimated glomerular filtration rate. Correlations were significant at P<0.05 level.

Table 4. Multiple linear regression showing association with plasma ZAG concentration ($r^2 = 0.406$, P<0.001).

Dependent variable: plasma ZAG

Independent variable	β coefficient	Standard error	P-value	
Urea	2.024	0.583	<0.005	***
Proteins	−1.346	0.571	0.023	*
Hemoglobin	−0.195	0.264	0.465	
HDL-cholesterol	−27.217	11.739	0.025	*
Intercept	181.182	54.338		

Correlations were significant at P<0.05 level.

patients and 97.2 (43.1–147.9) µg/ml for CKD 5 subjects (P< 0.01). No significant difference in ZAG concentration could be demonstrated depending on gender (male vs female: 56 (33–126) vs 40 (31–100) µg/ml, P = 0.096) or diabetic status (non diabetes mellitus *vs* diabetes mellitus, 46 (33–115) vs 48 (27–110) µg/ml, P = 0.908). Plasma ZAG concentration was not significantly different from non-dialyzed CKD 5 patients neither in HD patients (134.6 (120.7–154.7) µg/ml) nor in PD patients (134.6 (98.2–137.3) µg/ml). To get further insight, GFR was measured in a subset of patients (CKD 1 to CKD 5, N = 42) by the gold standard method, i.e. the urinary inulin clearance. In good agreement, no correlation was found between GFR assessed by inulin clearance and plasma ZAG concentration in patients with CKD stage 1 to 4 (Spearman $r_s = 0.174$, P = 0.283).

HD patients exhibited a further increase in plasma ZAG concentration after the dialysis session. The mean plasma ZAG concentration was 132.3 (113.3–159.2) µg/ml before and 196.1 (168.8–217.9) µg/ml after haemodialysis session (+48%, P = 0.002). Hemodialysis resulted in a significant hemoconcentration evidenced by the increased plasma protein concentration (68.3±6.1 vs 74.8±7.8 g/L, before and after HD, respectively, + 9%, P = 0.015). However, the post-dialysis increase in ZAG concentration did not only result from hemoconcentration since normalization of ZAG concentration to plasma protein concentration did not abolish this difference (**Figure 2**). Corrected ZAG concentration after haemodialysis session was 183.7 (144.7–197.7) µg/ml (+39%, P = 0.008).

Table 5. Characteristics of CKD-5 patients with PEW.

	No PEW	PEW	
Sex, male/female	14/12	6/5	P = 0.969
Age, y	63 (54–73)	62 (47–84)	P = 0.947
Weight, kg	68.0 (57–78)	55 (51–77)	P = 0.122
BMI, kg/m^2	27.4 (23.0–30.0)	21.8 (19.2–24.0)	P = 0.021*
Creatinine, µM	589.5 (443.3–822.5)	613.0 (407.0–683.0)	P = 0.921
Urea, mM	21.0 (17.0–27.8)	18.5 (17.1–26.9)	P = 0.642
Bicarbonates, mM	24.5 (22.8–26.0)	24.0 (22.0–25.0)	P = 0.393
Proteins, g/L	69.5 (66.8–76.3)	64.0 (59–77.0)	P = 0.079
Albumin, g/L	36.0 (33.5–39.2)	27.0 (26.0–33.1)	P = 0.001***
Prealbumin, mg/L	0.31 (0.28–0.39)	0.22 (0.18–0.32)	P = 0.013*
Hemoglobin, g/L	116.5 (103.5–123.3)	116.0 (103.0–121.0)	P = 0.907
Glucose, mM	5.5 (4.8–6.6)	5.4 (4.5–6.0)	P = 0.505
Triacylglycerols, mM	1.75 (1.29–1.56)	1.45 (1.01–1.39)	P = 0.290
HDL cholesterol, mM	1.13 (0.86–1.32)	1.04 (0.98–1.57)	P = 0.816
LDL cholesterol, mM	2.15 (1.69–3.59)	1.76 (1.32–2.56)	P = 0.113
CRP, mg/L	3.2 (2.9–9.1)	2.9 (2.9–12.0)	P = 0.912
Anti diabetic therapy, %	30.8	18.2	P = 0.668
Lipid-lowering therapy, %	45.5	46.2	P = 1.000
RAA, %	45.4	57.7	P = 0.860
Beta blocking agents, %	45.4	42.3	P = 1.000

Continuous data are expressed as median (interquartile range) and compared using Mann & Whitney U test. Categorical data are expressed as the frequency (%) and compared using Chi square test. Abbreviations: CKD, chronic kidney disease, CRP, C-reactive protein, BMI, body mass index, PEW, protein-energy wastng, RAA, renin angiotensin aldosterone.

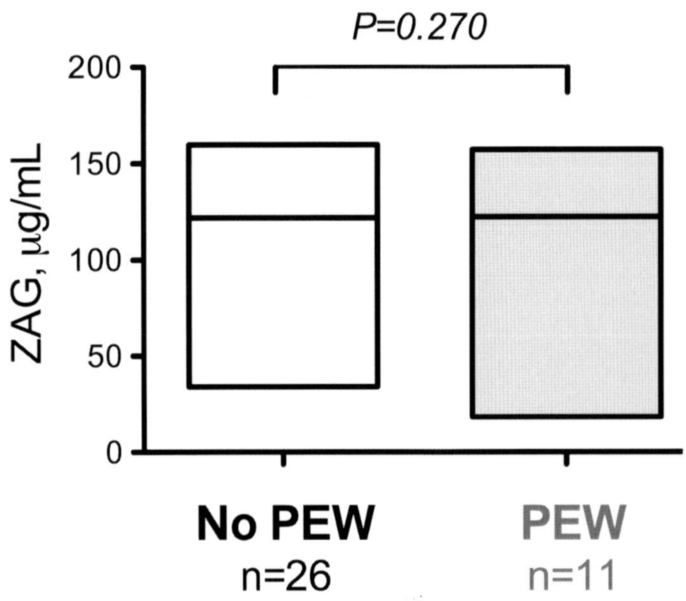

Figure 3. Plasma ZAG concentration in CKD-5 patients with a diagnostic of protein-energy wasting. The boxes indicate the range (i.e. min to max) and the line indicate the median. Note that no difference was found to be significant at the $P<0.05$ level. Abbreviation: PEW, protein-energy wasting.

Relationships between plasma ZAG Concentration and clinical or biochemical parameters

The results of the univariate correlation analysis are summarized in **Table 3**. In CKD patients stage 1 to 5, plasma ZAG concentrations negatively correlated with plasma protein concentration ($r_s = -0.284$, $P<0.01$), albumin ($r_s = -0.282$, $P<0.05$) hemoglobin ($r_s = -0.264$, $P<0.05$), urea ($r_s = 0.283$, $P<0.01$) and HDL-cholesterol ($r_s = -0.265$, $P<0.05$). Multiple regression analysis (**Table 4**) including urea, protein, haemoglobin and HDL-cholesterol indicated that only urea ($P<0.005$) and HDL-cholesterol ($P<0.05$) were associated with ZAG plasma concentration. Urea, proteins, haemoglobin and HDL-cholesterol explained 41% of the variance of plasma ZAG concentration ($P<0.001$). Out of the 38 patients CKD-5, HD or PD, 11 (29%) presented PEW according to the criterions described in the method section (see patient characteristics in **Table 5**). We therefore re-analyzed the plasma ZAG concentrations of CKD-5, HD and PD patients presenting or not PEW. No significant difference in plasma ZAG concentration was noticed between these 2 sub-groups (**Figure 3**) suggesting that ZAG accumulates in CKD but does not have any relation with PEW. Since ZAG was described to exert potent lipolytic activity, plasma glycerol was measured in a subset of 39 patients (17 non CKD and 22 CKD) as an index of lipolysis. We did not observe any difference in plasma glycerol concentration between HV and CKD patients (**Figure 4**). Additionally, no significant correlation was found between ZAG and plasma glycerol concentration.

Discussion

Zinc alpha2-glycoprotein is a soluble glycoprotein acting as a cachexia factor through its activity on adipose tissue. Few studies [17–18,19] recently demonstrated that plasma ZAG concentration was increased in chronic hemodialysis patients, suggesting a defect of its renal clearance. However, there is no data reporting the actual concentration of ZAG in CKD patients before initiation of renal replacement. We report in the present study that plasma ZAG concentration sharply increases in CKD 5 patients, as in patients with renal replacement therapy, but is poorly correlated to the decrease in GFR.

The CKD stage 5 patients included in the present investigation exhibited a marked elevation of plasma ZAG concentration (2.3-fold, $p<0.005$) that was also observed for PD patients, pre- and post-dialysis HD patients. ZAG accumulation in CKD 5 can result from a decrease of its renal clearance, an increased secretion rate by epithelia cells or both. In a pioneering work, Eckman et al suggested that the kidney could play a key role in the catabolism of ZAG [29]. Because of its rather small molecular weight (43 kDa) and size (Stokes radius 3.24 nm), a fraction of plasma ZAG normally passes through the glomerular membrane after which it is totally reabsorbed at the tubular level. They reported that impairment of renal function, with either decreased GFR or decreased tubular reabsorption, results in a rise in ZAG/creatinine clearance ratio [29]. In the present study, we did not find a strong correlation between plasma ZAG and GFR since ZAG concentration only rises in CKD stage 5. It is well known that glomerular filtration rate estimated by the CKD EPI formula may not accurately reflect renal function [30]. We therefore confirmed these findings with the direct measurement of GFR using the gold standard method of inulin clearance that yielded similar results.

To the best of our knowledge there is only scarce data in the literature regarding the fate of ZAG in the body. The actual turnover rate of ZAG in plasma is to date unknown. Many works documented the increase in plasma concentration of cytokines and hormones such as adiponectin and leptin in ESRD subjects [1–3,31]. Indeed, leptin is cleared from the bloodstream by the kidney through glomerular filtration followed by metabolic degradation in the renal tubules [32]. Normal renal function removes 12% of circulating leptin while in patients with CKD, there is virtually no renal uptake of leptin [32]. If ZAG breakdown occurs as it has been described for leptin in renal tubules, a decrease in GFR and/ or tubular reabsorption could explain the rise of plasma ZAG concentration observed in CKD patients. An alternative hypothesis is that ZAG secretion could be specifically increased in uremic

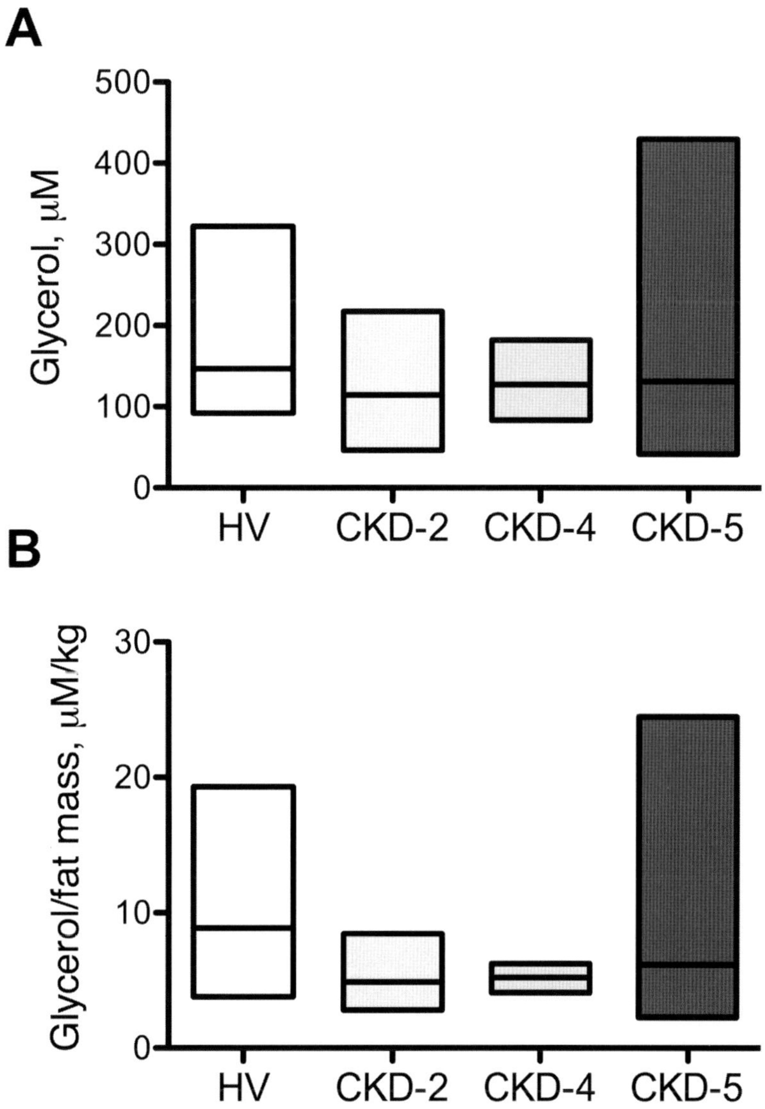

Figure 4. Plasma glycerol concentration in non-CKD and CKD patients. Plasma glycerol was measured as an index of lipolysis in 17 non-CKD patients, 6 CKD-2, 4 CKD-4 and 12 CKD-5 patients. **A)** plasma glycerol concentration **B)** Plasma glycerol, concentration normalized to body fat mass as described in methods. No difference was found to be significant at the $P<0.05$ level using Kruskall & Wallis test.

subjects. Supporting this idea, we recently demonstrated that uremic plasma stimulates ZAG production by adipocytes *in vitro* and that 5/6 nephrectomized rodents exhibited a significantly increased ZAG protein content in WAT associated with a significant decrease in WAT deposition [33]. We further showed that subcutaneous white adipose tissue biopsies from patients with end-stage renal disease exhibited a higher content of ZAG (5.7 folds) than age-matched controls [33], raising the hypothesis that deregulation of ZAG secretion could also contribute to the increased plasma ZAG concentration reported ESRD patients. Although Ryden et al reported that there was no significant contribution of WAT to the circulating levels of ZAG [34], we can hypothesize that an up-regulation of ZAG production by some tissues could contribute to the increased plasma ZAG concentration. We noticed that plasma ZAG concentration increased during HD independently of hemoconcentration (**Figure 3**) suggesting that additional ZAG is secreted in the organism during HD process. Inflammation, shear stress, oxidative stress, catecholamine secretion or lack of biocompatibility, associated with HD could enhance ZAG secretion. In good agreement, we found a significant increase in plasma ZAG concentration in post-HD patient compared to PD patients ($P = 0.004$). This result suggests that the increase in circulating ZAG that occurs during HD process is related to factors that are lacking in PD. Glucocorticoids are described to increase ZAG secretion [35,36]. And cortisol level has been shown to be increased by hemodialysis session [37] suggesting that glucocorticoids could enhance ZAG secretion and contribute to the perdialytic increase in plasma ZAG concentration. In contrast, inflammatory cytokines such as TNF-alpha were shown to decreased ZAG secretion [38–40]. The hemodialysis procedure has been associated with enhanced sympathetic activity (recently reviewed in [41]). When the plasma concentration of norepinephrine (NE) was used as a measure of sympathetic outflow, plasma NE was shown to be increased above values in 45% of hemodialysis patients [42]. Beta agonists were described to increase ZAG secretion in white adipose tissue, sympathetic overactivity/catecholamine release could therefore contribute to the perdialytic increase in ZAG. Tedeschi et al (2012) indeed reported a relationship between plasma norepinephrine and ZAG in heart failure patients [43].

The physiological consequences of increased ZAG concentration in renal failure remain to be elucidated. Axelsson et al [28] reported that plasma glycerol concentration (normalized to body fat mass) was increased in CKD stage 5 suggesting an increased lipolytic activity from their white adipose tissue (WAT). In contrast, we failed to show any increase of plasma glycerol in CKD patients (with or without normalization to body fat mass) or any relationship between plasma glycerol and ZAG concentrations. From our data, there is therefore no line of evidence that ZAG accumulation could contribute to PEW in CKD patients as observed in patients with cancer cachexia. ZAG could however contribute to metabolic disturbances since Philipp et al [17] reported that ZAG serum levels negatively correlated with fasting insulin and homeostasis model assessment of insulin resistance (HOMA-IR). Olofsson et al [44] also noticed that ZAG serum levels correlated with serum levels of cholesterol in healthy subjects. Thus, as described in patients with cancer [45], ZAG could contribute to CKD-associated metabolic disturbances, such as insulin resistance and dyslipidemia.

A negative correlation was found between ZAG concentration and plasma albumin ($r_s = -0.282$, $p<0.05$) and positive correlation between ZAG and urea ($r_s = 0.283$, $P<0.01$). We however failed to find a significant correlation between plasma albumin level and urea ($r_s = -0.005$, $P = 0.953$) that does not support an association with wasting. The significant correlation found between plasma ZAG and urea could be explained by the fact that level of urea reflects the accumulation of many uremic toxins that could stimulate ZAG production in CKD [33]. In an animal study, ZAG was further described to exert antiproliferative activity on epithelial tubular cells after acute kidney injury [46] suggesting that accumulation of ZAG could maybe compound renal dysfunction. Further studies are however needed to decipher the pathophysiological role of ZAG in ESRD.

In conclusion, in this study, we report that ZAG protein accumulates in plasma in ESRD and hemodialysis patients but this increase is not directly correlated to the decrease in GFR. In our study, plasma ZAG concentration was not associated with PEW. The main limitation of the present study is however that it is observational and therefore that it is difficult to make causal inference. Further prospective studies are needed to better elucidate the potential role of ZAG in end-stage renal disease.

Acknowledgments

The authors gratefully acknowledge Dr Bertrand CARE, PhD and Assoc. Prof. Hédi A SOULA, PhD (CarMeN Lab, INSERM U1060, Lyon, France) for mathematical and statistical assistance.

Author Contributions

Conceived and designed the experiments: CCP LK DF COS. Performed the experiments: CCP LK PA MLC EK. Analyzed the data: CCP FGE AHA DF COS. Wrote the paper: CCP FGE COS. Recruited patients and collected clinical data: CCP LK EK AHA FGE. Discussed, reviewed and edited the manuscript: LK PA EK MLC FGE AHA DF.

References

1. Merabet E, Dagogo-Jack S, Coyne DW, Klein S, Santiago JV, et al (1997) Increased plasma leptin concentration in end-stage renal disease. J Clin Endocrinol Metab 82: 847–850.
2. Zoccali C, Mallamaci F, Tripepi G, Benedetto FA, Cutrupi S, et al (2002) Adiponectin, metabolic risk factors, and cardiovascular events among patients with end-stage renal disease. J Am Soc Nephrol 13: 134–141.
3. Guebre-Egziabher F, Bernhard J, Funahashi T, Hadj-Aissa A, Fouque D (2005) Adiponectin in chronic kidney disease is related more to metabolic disturbances than to decline in renal function. Nephrol Dial Transplant 20: 129–134.
4. Stein S, Bachmann A, Lössner U, Kratzsch J, Blüher M, et al (2009) Serum levels of the adipokine FGF21 depend on renal function. Diabetes Care 32: 126–128.
5. Ziegelmeier M, Bachmann A, Seeger J, Lossner U, Kratzsch J, et al (2007) Serum levels of adipokine retinol-binding protein-4 in relation to renal function. Diabetes Care 30: 2588–2592.
6. Pfau D, Bachmann A, Lössner U, Kratzsch J, Blüher M, et al (2010) Serum levels of the adipokine chemerin in relation to renal function. Diabetes Care 33: 171–173.
7. Burgi W, Schmid K (1961) Preparation and properties of Zn-alpha 2-glycoprotein of normal human plasma. J Biol Chem 236: 1066–1074.
8. Sánchez LM, Chirino AJ, Bjorkman Pj (1999) Crystal structure of human ZAG, a fat-depleting factor related to MHC molecules. Science 283: 1914–1919.
9. Russell ST, Zimmerman TP, Domin BA, Tisdale MJ (2004) Induction of lipolysis in vitro and loss of body fat in vivo by zinc-alpha2-glycoprotein. Biochim Biophys Acta 1636: 59–68.
10. Bing C (2011) Lipid mobilization in cachexia: mechanisms and mediators. Curr Opin Support Palliat Care 5: 356–360.
11. Tada T, Ohkubo I, Niwa M, Sasaki M, Tateyama H, et al (1991) Immunohistochemical localization of Zn-alpha 2-glycoprotein in normal human tissues. J Histochem Cytochem 39: 1221–1226.
12. Hirai K, Hussey HJ, Barber MD, Price SA, Tisdale MJ (1998) Biological evaluation of a lipid-mobilizing factor isolated from the urine of cancer patients. Cancer Res 58: 2359–2365.
13. Russell ST, Tisdale MJ (2012) Role of β-adrenergic receptors in the anti-obesity and anti-diabetic effects of zinc-α2-glycoprotien (ZAG). Biochim Biophys Acta 1821: 590–599.
14. Russell ST, Hirai K, Tisdale MJ (2002) Role of beta3-adrenergic receptors in the action of a tumour lipid mobilizing factor. Br J Cancer 86: 424–428.
15. Gong F-Y, Zhang S-J, Deng J-Y, Zhu H-J, Pan H, et al (2009) Zinc-alpha2-glycoprotein is involved in regulation of body weight through inhibition of lipogenic enzymes in adipose tissue. Int J Obes (Lond) 33: 1023–1030.
16. Sanders PM, Tisdale MJ (2004) Effect of zinc-alpha2-glycoprotein (ZAG) on expression of uncoupling proteins in skeletal muscle and adipose tissue. Cancer Lett 212: 71–81.
17. Philipp A, Kralisch S, Bachmann A, Lossner U, Kratzsch J, et al (2011) Serum levels of the adipokine zinc-α2-glycoprotein are increased in chronic hemodialysis. Metab Clin Exp 60: 669–672.
18. Leal VO, Lobo JC, Stockler-Pinto MB, Farage NE, Abdalla DSP, et al (2012) Is zinc-α2-glycoprotein a cardiovascular protective factor for patients undergoing hemodialysis? Clin Chim Acta 413: 616–619.
19. Leal VO, Lobo JC, Stockler-Pinto MB, Farage NE, Velarde GC, et al (2012) Zinc-α2-glycoprotein: is there association between this new adipokine and body composition in hemodialysis patients? Ren Fail 34: 1062–1067.
20. Levey AS, Bosch JP, Lewis JB, Greene T, Rogers N, et al (1999) A more accurate method to estimate glomerular filtration rate from serum creatinine: a new prediction equation. Modification of Diet in Renal Disease Study Group. Ann Intern Med 130: 461–470.
21. Stevens LA, Schmid CH, Greene T, Zhang YL, Beck GJ, et al (2010) Comparative performance of the CKD Epidemiology Collaboration (CKD-EPI) and the Modification of Diet in Renal Disease (MDRD) Study equations for estimating GFR levels above 60 mL/min/1.73 m2. Am J Kidney Dis 56: 486–495.
22. K/DOQI clinical practice guidelines for chronic kidney disease: evaluation, classification, and stratification (2002). Am J Kidney Dis 39: S1–266.
23. Deurenberg P, Weststrate JA, Seidell JC (1991) Body mass index as a measure of body fatness: age- and sex-specific prediction formulas. Br J Nutr 65: 105–114.
24. Fouque D, Kalantar-Zadeh K, Kopple J, Cano N, Chauveau P, et al (2008) A proposed nomenclature and diagnostic criteria for protein-energy wasting in acute and chronic kidney disease. Kidney Int 73: 391–398.
25. Buron F, Hadj-Aissa A, Dubourg L, Morelon E, Steghens J-P, et al (2011) Estimating glomerular filtration rate in kidney transplant recipients: performance over time of four creatinine-based formulas. Transplantation 92: 1005–1011.
26. Dubourg L, Hadj-Aïssa A, Ferrier B (2010) Adaptation of an enzymatic polyfructosan assay to clinical practice. Anal Biochem 405: 266–268.
27. Bradford MM (1976) A rapid and sensitive method for the quantitation of microgram quantities of protein utilizing the principle of protein-dye binding. Anal Biochem 72: 248–254.
28. Axelsson J, Aström G, Sjölin E, Qureshi AR, Lorente-Cebrián S, et al (2011) Uraemic sera stimulate lipolysis in human adipocytes: role of perilipin. Nephrol Dial Transplant 26: 2485–2491.
29. Ekman R, Johansson BG, Ravnskov U (1976) Renal handling of Zn-alpha2-glycoprotein as compared with that of albumin and the retinol-binding protein. J Clin Invest 57: 945–954.
30. Cirillo M, Anastasio P, De Santo NG (2005) Relationship of gender, age, and body mass index to errors in predicted kidney function. Nephrol Dial Transplant 20: 1791–1798.

31. Guebre-Egziabher F, Bernhard J, Geelen G, Malvoisin E, Hadj-Aissa A, et al (2005) Leptin, adiponectin, and ghrelin dysregulation in chronic kidney disease. J Ren Nutr 15: 116–120.
32. Cumin F, Baum HP, de Gasparo M, Levens N (1997) Removal of endogenous leptin from the circulation by the kidney. Int J Obes Relat Metab Disord 21: 495–504.
33. Pelletier CC, Koppe L, Croze ML, Kalbacher E, Vella RE, et al (2013) White adipose tissue overproduces the lipid-mobilizing factor zinc α2-glycoprotein in chronic kidney disease. Kidney Int 83: 878–886.
34. Rydén M, Agustsson T, Andersson J, Bolinder J, Toft E, et al (2012) Adipose zinc-α2-glycoprotein is a catabolic marker in cancer and noncancerous states. J Intern Med 271: 414–420.
35. Russell ST, Tisdale MJ (2005) The role of glucocorticoids in the induction of zinc-alpha2-glycoprotein expression in adipose tissue in cancer cachexia. Br J Cancer 92: 876–881.
36. Hassan MI, Waheed A, Yadav S, Singh TP, Ahmad F (2008) Zinc alpha 2-glycoprotein: a multidisciplinary protein. Mol Cancer Res 6: 892–906.
37. Letizia C, Mazzaferro S, De Ciocchis A, Cerci S, Morabito S, et al (1996) Effects of haemodialysis session on plasma beta-endorphin, ACTH and cortisol in patients with end-stage renal disease. Scand J Urol Nephrol 30: 399–402.
38. Bao Y, Bing C, Hunter L, Jenkins JR, Wabitsch M, et al (2005) Zinc-alpha2-glycoprotein, a lipid mobilizing factor, is expressed and secreted by human (SGBS) adipocytes. FEBS Lett 579: 41–47.
39. Gao D, Trayhurn P, Bing C (2010) Macrophage-secreted factors inhibit ZAG expression and secretion by human adipocytes. Mol Cell Endocrinol 325: 135–142.
40. Mracek T, Gao D, Tzanavari T, Bao Y, Xiao X, et al (2010) Downregulation of zinc-{alpha}2-glycoprotein in adipose tissue and liver of obese ob/ob mice and by tumour necrosis factor-alpha in adipocytes. J Endocrinol 204: 165–172.
41. Rubinger D, Backenroth R, Sapoznikov D (2013) Sympathetic nervous system function and dysfunction in chronic hemodialysis patients. Semin Dial 26: 333–343.
42. Zoccali C, Mallamaci F, Parlongo S, Cutrupi S, Benedetto FA, et al (2002) Plasma norepinephrine predicts survival and incident cardiovascular events in patients with end-stage renal disease. Circulation 105: 1354–1359.
43. Tedeschi S, Pilotti E, Parenti E, Vicini V, Coghi P, et al (2012) Serum adipokine zinc α2-glycoprotein and lipolysis in cachectic and noncachectic heart failure patients: relationship with neurohormonal and inflammatory biomarkers. Metab Clin Exp 61: 37–42.
44. Olofsson LE, Olsson B, Lystig T, Jacobson P, Jernås M, et al (2010) Preliminary report: Zn-alpha2-glycoprotein genotype and serum levels are associated with serum lipids. Metab Clin Exp 59: 1316–1318.
45. Mracek T, Stephens NA, Gao D, Bao Y, Ross JA, et al (2011) Enhanced ZAG production by subcutaneous adipose tissue is linked to weight loss in gastrointestinal cancer patients. Br J Cancer 104: 441–447.
46. Schmitt R, Marlier A, Cantley LG (2008) Zag expression during aging suppresses proliferation after kidney injury. J Am Soc Nephrol 19: 2375–2383.

6

Early Nephrology Referral Reduces the Economic Costs among Patients Who Start Renal Replacement Therapy: A Prospective Cohort Study in Korea

Jeonghwan Lee[1,2], Jung Pyo Lee[2,3], Ji In Park[2,4], Jin Ho Hwang[2,5], Hye Min Jang[2,6], Ji-Young Choi[2,7], Yong-Lim Kim[2,7], Chul Woo Yang[2,8], Shin-Wook Kang[2,9], Nam-Ho Kim[2,10], Yon Su Kim[2,4], Chun Soo Lim[2,3,4]*, CRC for ESRD investigators[2]

1 Department of Internal Medicine, Hallym University Hangang Sacred Heart Hospital, Seoul, Korea, **2** Clinical Research Center for End Stage Renal Disease (CRC for ESRD), Daegu, Korea, **3** Department of Internal Medicine, Seoul National University Boramae Medical Center, Seoul, Korea, **4** Department of Internal Medicine, Seoul National University College of Medicine, Seoul, Korea, **5** Department of Internal Medicine, Chung-Ang University Hospital, Seoul, Korea, **6** Department of Statistics, Kyungpook National University, Daegu, Korea, **7** Department of Internal Medicine, Kyungpook National University School of Medicine, Daegu, Korea, **8** Department of Internal Medicine, The Catholic University of Korea College of Medicine, Seoul, Korea, **9** Department of Internal Medicine, Yonsei University College of Medicine, Seoul, Korea, **10** Department of Internal Medicine, Chonnam National University Medical School, Gwangju, Korea

Abstract

Background: The nature of cost-saving effects of early referral to a nephrologist in patients with chronic kidney disease (CKD) is not fully evaluated. We evaluated the health care costs before and after dialysis according to the referral time.

Methods: A total of 879 patients who were newly diagnosed as having end-stage renal disease from August 2008 to June 2011 were prospectively enrolled. The early referral (ER) group was defined as patients who were referred to a nephrologist more than a year before dialysis and had visited a nephrology clinic 2 or more times. Patients whose referral time was less than a year were considered the late referral (LR) group. Information about medical costs was acquired from the claim data of the Korea Health Insurance Review and Assessment Service.

Results: The total medical costs during the first 12 months after the initiation of dialysis were not different between the 526 ER patients and the 353 LR patients. However, the costs of the ER patients during the first month were significantly lower than those of the LR patients (ER vs. LR: 3029±2219 vs. 3438±2821 US dollars [USD], P = 0.025). The total 12-month health care costs before the initiation of dialysis were significantly lower in the ER group (ER vs. LR: 6206±5873 vs. 8610±7820 USD, P<0.001). In the multivariate analysis, ER significantly lowered the health care costs during the 12 months before (2534.0±436.2 USD, P<0.001) and the first month (428.5±172.3 USD, P = 0.013) after the initiation of dialysis.

Conclusions: The ER of patients with CKD to a nephrologist is associated with decreased medical costs during the pretreatment period of renal replacement therapy and the early period of dialysis initiation.

Editor: Leighton R. James, University of Florida, United States of America

Funding: This study was supported by a grant of the Korea Healthcare technology R&D Project, Ministry of Health and Welfare, Republic of Korea. (HI10C2020). The funders had no role in study design, data collection and analysis, decision to publish, or preparation of the manuscript.

Competing Interests: The authors have declared that no competing interests exist.

* Email: cslimjy@snu.ac.kr

Introduction

Chronic kidney disease (CKD) is a major public health problem that is continually growing worldwide. The overall prevalence of CKD around the world is 10–16% [1–3]. In the United States, the prevalence estimate for CKD rose from 12.3% to 14.0% over the past 20 years [4]. Kidney function progressively declines in a proportion of CKD patients without adequate therapy, eventually progressing to devastating end-stage renal disease (ESRD) [5]. In accordance with the increasing prevalence of CKD, the prevalence of ESRD has also increased. The total treated ESRD population in the United States rose from 450,000 in 2004 to 593,086 in 2010 [4]. In Korea, the overall number of ESRD patients was 56,396, and the prevalence was 738.3 per million population, at the end of 2009 [6]. The prevalence increased by approximately 12% during the period 2000–2009.

Along with the increase in ESRD prevalence, the economic costs resulting from the care of these patients have increased. In the United States, the annual medical cost of dialysis patients borne by the Centers for Medicare and Medicaid in 2008 was 26.8 billion USD, which was 5.9% of the total costs of the entire population, and the annual increase rate reached 13.2% [7]. Among patients starting dialysis, the proportion of elderly patients and those with diabetes have increased compared with the past [8], and thus the economic burden of patients on dialysis is serious.

Therefore, proper management or intervention of CKD patients is required to improve clinical outcomes and reduce medical costs.

The late referral (LR) of patients to a nephrologist in the course of CKD progression has increased the morbidity and mortality [9–19]. The timely referral of CKD patients to a nephrologist is associated with a higher quality of care before the start of renal replacement therapy [20–26] and with improved outcomes after the initiation of dialysis [27–31]. The increased morbidity of patients referred late to a nephrologist is likely to result in a greater usage of health care resources. Our previous investigation revealed that timely referral (1 year before dialysis) to a nephrologist integrated with education about dialysis was associated with reduced usage of temporary vascular catheters and improved survival [32]. Although early referral (ER) has been suggested to produce cost savings in addition to the health benefits for the patient, there are few reports that have directly analyzed the effects of referral time on medical costs before and after the start of dialysis. To evaluate the economic benefits of ER to a nephrologist, we investigated the difference in the economic burden according to the referral time using national health insurance claim data in a prospective cohort ESRD patients.

Methods

Cohort Description

This study was nested within an ongoing cohort study (Clinical Research Center for End Stage Renal Disease, CRC for ESRD) of patients with ESRD in South Korea. The CRC for ESRD is a nationwide multi-center web-based comprehensive prospective cohort of CKD patients on dialysis whose aim is to analyze the treatment effects on survival or quality of life and cost-effectiveness by dialysis modality [32,33]. All enrolled patients are adults aged 20 years old or older and who started dialysis for ESRD without a schedule for kidney transplantation within 3 months. The patients began to be registered in July 2008, and 31 hospitals in Korea are currently participating in the CRC for ESRD cohort study. Until September 2012, a total of 1620 CKD patients who had newly started dialysis and 2917 patients who had already been on dialysis had been enrolled. All patients provided their written consent to participate voluntarily in this study. The study was approved by the institutional review board at each center [The Catholic University of Korea, Bucheon St. Mary's Hospital; The Catholic University of Korea, Incheon St. Mary's Hospital; The Catholic University of Korea, Seoul St. Mary's Hospital; The Catholic University of Korea, St. Mary's Hospital; The Catholic University of Korea, St. Vincent's Hospital; The Catholic University of Korea, Uijeongbu St. Mary's Hospital; Cheju Halla General Hospital; Chonbuk National University Hospital; Chonnam National University Hospital; Chung-Ang University Medical Center; Chungbuk National University Hospital; Chungnam National University Hospital; Dong-A University Medical Center; Ehwa Womens University Medical Center; Fatima Hospital, Daegu; Gachon University Gil Medical Center; Inje University Pusan Paik Hospital; Kyungpook National University Hospital; Kwandong University College of Medicine, Myongji Hospital; National Health Insurance Corporation Ilsan Hospital; National Medical Center; Pusan National University Hospital; Samsung Medical Center, Seoul; Seoul National University, Boramae Medical Center; Seoul National University Hospital; Seoul National University, Bundang Hospital; Yeungnam University Medical Center; Yonsei University, Severance Hospital; Yonsei University, Gangnam Severance Hospital; Ulsan University Hospital; Wonju Christian Hospital (in alphabetical order)]. All clinical investigators followed the Ethics for Medical Research and conducted this study in accordance with the guidelines of the 2008 Declaration of Helsinki.

Study Participants

We selected and studied 1011 adult patients who were newly diagnosed as having ESRD and started dialysis between August 2008 and June 2011 from the new patient registry in the CRC for ESRD cohort. Of the 132 patients who were excluded, the data regarding visits to a nephrologist were missing for 61 patients, and data regarding the type of initial dialysis were unknown for 33 patients. In addition, 38 patients were excluded due to the lack of cost data because of an unmatched identifier. The early referral group (ER) was defined as patients who were referred to a nephrologist more than 1 year before dialysis initiation and who had visited a nephrology clinic 2 or more times; the remaining patients whose referral time was less than a year were considered the late referral group (LR) [32].

Clinical Data Acquisition

Information about the participants was primarily collected from the data server of the CRC for ESRD for analysis. All traceable identifiers were removed prior to the analysis to ensure patient confidentiality. The clinical and laboratory data had been stored in the form of web-based medical questionnaires. The questionnaire items were filled in by data coordinators, who were trained in each center to collect patient data by a combination of chart reviews and direct interviews using a standardized form. The questionnaires included data on demographics, previous medical history, laboratory results, dialysis modality and prescription, type of permanent access used for the first dialysis, and medications. The estimated glomerular filtration rate (eGFR) was calculated by CKD-EPI equations [34]. The modified Charlson co-morbidity index (CCI) and Davies co-morbidity index (DCI) at the initiation of dialysis were recorded for each patient. The modified CCI and DCI values were calculated using the method described in a previous study [35–37]. The patients were asked to respond to the questionnaire when they first visited a nephrologist before starting dialysis.

Health Care Costs

Information about the medical costs during the 1 year periods just before and after the initiation of dialysis was acquired from the claim data of the Korea Health Insurance Review and Assessment Service (HIRA). In Korea, government-initiated public health insurance is mandatory, and private health insurance without national health insurance is not allowed for direct medical costs. All populations are obligatorily registered in the national health insurance service, and almost all legitimate medical costs are controlled and reimbursed via the Korea HIRA. We calculated the medical costs by an official request for the claim data of medical costs from the Korea HIRA and data integration by the coded identifiers of patients in the CRC for ESRD. To determine the economic cost of an illness, three types of costs should be considered: direct costs, indirect costs (productivity loss), and intangible costs. In this study, we evaluated direct medical expenditures, including physician visit costs, admission costs, surgery costs, physical therapy costs, and total medicine costs. The following costs were excluded: traffic costs, which are considered a direct non-medical cost; traditional Chinese herbal medicine costs; indirect costs; and intangible costs, which cannot be directly collected through the claim data of the Korea HIRA. All of the costs were calculated in the currency unit of the Korean Won (KRW) (US$1 = 1,100 KRW in 2013).

Statistical Analysis

In the descriptive analysis of the demographic and clinical characteristics and laboratory results, continuous variables were expressed as the mean and standard deviation, and categorical variables were described numerically with a percentage. Comparisons between the groups based on referral time were performed using a t-test for continuous variables and Chi-square or Fisher's exact tests for categorical variables when appropriate. We presented the mean with the standard error of the mean for the entire cost. The associations between medical costs and independent parameters were assessed using univariate and multivariate linear regression methods. Variables in the univariate models were selected *a priori* and by clinical significance, and included the type of referral, age, sex, type of dialysis modality, body mass index, causes of underlying kidney disease, hemoglobin level, and serum albumin level. Multivariate model included variables that were proved to be associated (P value <0.10) with the total medical costs. SAS/STAT 9.2 (SAS Institute Inc., Cary, NC, USA) was used in the analysis of the medical costs, and IBM SPSS ver. 20.0 was used to compare the demographic and clinical parameters. A P value <0.05 was considered statistically significant.

Results

Patients Characteristics by Referral Pattern

The patients' clinical and laboratory characteristics are summarized in Table 1. The mean age was 55.8±14.1 years old, and 59.5% of patients were male. Of the 879 patients enrolled in the cost analysis, 526 patients were in the ER group, and 353 were in the LR group. The time from referral to dialysis was significantly longer in the ER group than in the LR group (63.9±62.1 months vs. 2.7±3.4 months, P<0.001). In the LR group, the proportion of patients who visited a nephrologist less than 2 times before dialysis initiation reached up to 34.8%. The most common cause of renal disease was diabetic nephropathy in both groups.

At the time of the referral to a nephrologist, ages were younger, the blood pressure (BP) and serum creatinine level were lower, and the hemoglobin level and eGFR were higher in the ER group than in the LR group. At the time of dialysis initiation, most findings, including the age, sex, co-morbidity index, serum creatinine, eGFR, hemoglobin levels, calcium and phosphate levels, urate levels, and total cholesterol levels were similar in both groups. However, diastolic BP (77.5±13.4 vs. 79.5±14.8 mmHg, P=0.041) and LDL cholesterol levels (89.9±39.0 vs. 98.7±58.6 mmHg, P=0.018) were lower in the ER group.

Medical Costs

The monthly medical costs before and after the initiation of dialysis are summarized in table 2 and figure 1. The total medical costs during the first 12 months after the initiation of dialysis were not different between the two groups (ER vs. LR: 18947±11864 vs. 19104±11501 USD, P=0.845). However, the costs of the ER patients during the first month were significantly lower than those of the LR patients (ER vs. LR: 3029±2219 vs. 3438±2821 USD, P=0.025). The total 12-month health care costs before the initiation of dialysis were significantly lower in the ER group (ER vs. LR: 6206±5873 vs. 8610±7820 USD, P<0.001).

We evaluated the impact of various clinical and laboratory parameters on medical costs by univariate and multivariate analyses. Table 3 summarizes the results of the costs during the first month after dialysis initiation. The referral type (ER) reduced the costs (409.1±174.3 USD, P=0.019) and the dialysis modality (hemodialysis) increased the medical costs (823.8±184.3 USD, P< 0.001) during the first month in the univariate analysis. The patients' age, gender, body mass index, causes of renal disease, hemoglobin level, and serum albumin level were not associated with the medical costs. In the multivariate analysis, ER significantly reduced the medical costs (428.5±172.3 USD, P=0.013) during the first month after dialysis initiation.

The univariate and multivariate analyses on the costs during the 1 year before dialysis also showed a significant association of the referral time with the medical costs (Table 4). In the univariate analysis, ER (2404.1±447.4 USD, P<0.001) and the cause of renal disease reduced the costs, and age (30.1±15.7 USD, P=0.055) and hemoglobin level (89.9±47.3 USD, P=0.057) showed an association with increased medical costs. In the multivariate analysis, ER was also proved to be significantly associated with reduced medical costs (2534.0±436.2 USD, P< 0.001).

Medications and Vascular Access

Frequency of medication use, including antihypertensive drug, antiplatelet agents, anticoagulants, vitamin D, and phosphate binders, were not different between the two groups. Erythropoiesis-stimulating agents use was more (68.0 vs. 59.3%, P=0.007) in the ER group. In the ER group, frequency of native arteriovenous fistula was higher (30.7% vs. 20.1%, P=0.003) and temporary tunneled-catheter use was lower (40.2% vs. 49.0%, P=0.031).

Discussion

We evaluated the benefit of ER to a nephrologist with respect to economic costs in a prospective cohort of patients who started dialysis for ESRD. We found that ER to a nephrologist significantly reduced medical costs during the periods of 1 year before and 1 month after the initiation of renal replacement therapy using national health insurance claim data. Patients with advanced CKD are frequently complicated with anemia, electrolyte imbalances, hypertension, mineral bone disorders, and other risk factors of cardiovascular diseases. Therefore, correcting and reversing the causes of renal impairment and managing the comorbidities in CKD are important to improve clinical outcomes and patient survival. Education of CKD patients about dialysis can reduce the incidence of emergent hemodialysis via a central venous catheter [38,39]. Recently, we reported that the timely referral of patients with CKD to a nephrologist is associated with the reduced usage of a central venous catheter for hemodialysis, improved patient survival, and decreased cardiovascular mortality [32]. The participants of this study are slightly different from our previous investigation in that the duration of patients' enrollment of this study was shorter by about 4 months and the definition of the ER group was defined as patients who had been referred 1 year before dialysis and who had visited nephrology clinic at least two times irrespective to the status of education about dialysis. In this study, we also proved that early referral to a nephrologist could reduce the usage of temporary vascular catheter for hemodialysis, and improve patients' blood pressure and lipid level control. The economic benefits of ER to a nephrologist were expected due to reduced morbidities and improved patient survival. To date, there have been several reports that ER to a nephrologist is cost-effective. However, those studies were retrospective analyses or included indirect estimations of medical costs [21,25,40,41]. In this study, we directly proved the cost-saving effect of ER by the integration of the clinical data of patients who started dialysis for ESRD from a prospective cohort and the claim data of a national health insurance organization.

Despite the various benefits of early nephrology referral, there are still many patients who are referred to a nephrology clinic too

Table 1. Patient characteristics by referral pattern at the time of referral and dialysis initiation.

	Total ESRD			
	Total	Early referral	Late referral	P Value
	(*N*=879)	**(*N*=526)**	**(*N*=353)**	
Age at the time of referral (year)	52.5±15.1	50.6±15.1	55.4±14.6	<0.001
Findings at the time of referral to nephrologist				
Underlying kidney disease (%)				0.003
Diabetes mellitus	48.7	49.6	47.4	
Hypertension	17.4	15.4	20.5	
Glomerulonephritis	16.4	18.7	12.9	
Polycystic kidney disease	2.5	3.5	1.1	
Others	10.5	9.3	12.1	
Unknown	4.5	3.5	5.9	
Systolic BP (mmHg)	146.3±26.8	142.9±25.1	150.2±28.1	0.001
Diastolic BP (mmHg)	84.4±16.6	83.4±16.0	85.4±17.1	0.132
Serum creatinine (mg/dL)	4.94±4.50	2.82±2.70	7.41±4.90	<0.001
eGFR (mL/min/1.73 m^2)	23.9±23.3	34.3±25.2	11.8±12.7	<0.001
Hemoglobin (g/dL)	10.1±5.3	11.3±6.8	8.8±1.8	<0.001
Number of visits to a nephrologist from referral to dialysis (%)				<0.001
None	7.1	0	17.7	
1 time	6.9	0	17.1	
2 times or more	86.0	100	65.2	
Time from referral to dialysis (month)	39.2±56.6	63.9±62.1	2.7±3.4	<0.001
Age at the time of dialysis (year)	55.8±14.1	55.9±13.8	55.6±14.6	0.761
Gender (male, %)	59.5	59.2	60.1	0.774
Findings at the time of dialysis				
Modified Charlson co-morbidity index	5.1±2.6	5.2±2.6	5.0±2.5	0.337
Davies co-morbidity index2	1.0±0.9	1.0±0.9	1.0±1.0	0.836
Systolic BP (mmHg)	139.7±22.2	138.9±22.2	140.8±22.1	0.222
Diastolic BP (mmHg)	78.3±14.0	77.5±13.4	79.5±14.8	0.041
BMI (kg/m^2)	23.1±3.5	23.1±3.3	23.1±3.7	0.882
Serum creatinine (mg/dL)	8.48±4.41	8.48±4.17	8.48±4.73	0.996
eGFR (mL/min/1.73 m^2)	7.6±7.4	7.3±6.6	7.9±8.4	0.214
Hemoglobin (g/dL)	8.8±1.7	8.9±1.7	8.8±1.6	0.287
Uric acid (mg/dL)	8.1±2.6	8.0±2.6	8.1±2.5	0.593
Calcium (mg/dL)	7.8±1.0	7.8±1.0	7.7±1.1	0.368
Phosphate (mg/dL)	5.4±1.8	5.4±1.8	5.5±1.9	0.672
Total cholesterol (mg/dL)	161.3±53.6	158.6±49.9	165.5±58.6	0.063
LDL cholesterol (mg/dL)	93.5±48.1	89.9±39.0	98.7±58.6	0.018

Values for continuous variables are expressed as the means ± standard deviation; values for categorical variables are expressed as proportions.
BMI, body mass index; BP, blood pressure; eGFR, estimated glomerular filtration rate; HDL, high-density lipoprotein; LDL, low-density lipoprotein

late for impending renal replacement therapy. The problems related to LR are common in many countries, and the proportion of patients who are referred when facing the impending dialysis is up to 31–38% [9,42,43]. The LR of CKD patients to a nephrologist can increase the medical costs due to increased mortality and comorbidities. The increased incidence of emergent hemodialysis and the frequent use of a temporary central venous catheter for hemodialysis contribute to the increased medical costs associated with LR [23,44]. Moreover, the increased duration of admission for the first dialysis is an important factor for the increased economic burden [16]. Although we could not compare the duration of admission between the two groups, more patients in the ER group started hemodialysis with their own native arteriovenous fistula without insertion of temporary central venous catheter. Reduced catheter usage contributed to the cost-saving effects in the ER group. The increased medical costs in the LR group may have resulted from the increased number or severity of the comorbidities associated with rapidly aggravating renal dysfunction. However, in this study, the cost-saving effects of ER were independent of comorbid conditions because we could not find a difference in the severity of illness between the ER and LR groups. Cost-saving effects of ER did not persist more than 1 months after dialysis start. It can be possible that main factors influencing on the decreased medical costs of ER work on during the predialysis period or early period of dialysis initiation. Detrimental effects of LR have been reported to be influential on 3 months short-term mortality, but not on long-term mortality [45]. After dialysis start, all patients are treated by nephrologists, patterns of clinical practice affecting on medical costs necessarily come to be similar between the ER and LR groups. Interestingly, medical costs in the ER groups were remarkably decreased before dialysis start. Advanced CKD patients are complicated with various medical problems, including hypertension, dyslipidemia, diabetes, and mineral bone disease. If patients were not referred to a nephrologist at the right time, inappropriate or overlapped laboratory tests would increase the medical costs in the LR group. In addition, detailed and appropriate medical therapy in the ER group would decrease the morbidities and medical costs before dialysis initiation. In this study, although more patients in the ER group were prescribed erythropoiesis-stimulating agents and the usage of antihypertensive drugs was not different between the two groups, blood pressure and lipid level were better controlled and medical costs were decreased through cost-effective care in the ER group.

There are several causes of the LR of patients with CKD to a nephrologist despite the clinical benefits of ER. With respect to clinicians or medical facilities, the lack of communication between doctors or hospitals, the absence of definite guidelines for the referral time to a nephrologist, and ambivalent opinions about dialysis in the elderly or high risk patients are factors that affecting LR [46]. With respect to patients, the refusal of dialysis, a lack of knowledge about CKD and dialysis, and economic poverty might function as factors that affect LR. Economic difficulties have been reported several times as the main cause of LR [29,47]. When patients with CKD are referred late due to economic difficulties, adequate treatment and preparation for dialysis are inevitably delayed. Increased metabolic complications related to ESRD eventually raise the medical costs related to dialysis and hospital admission, which in turn deteriorate the patients' economic status. The timely referral of patients with CKD, especially those with a poor socioeconomic status, to a nephrologist is necessary to prevent delayed dialysis due to a lack of knowledge and negative thinking about renal replacement therapy and to reduce the unnecessary medical expenses related to delayed referral.

Despite the unique findings and advantages, this study has several limitations. At first, there can be concerns about the lead time bias that patients in the ER group had better renal function, lower blood pressure, less severe anemia, and lower LDL cholesterol levels at the time of referral, and these reduced comorbidities could influence to the reduced medical costs in the ER group. These facts that patients in the ER group showed better clinical conditions are not surprising because they were referred about 5 years earlier than those in the LR group. At least, almost all parameters including age and co-morbidity index at the time of dialysis were similar between the ER and LR groups, and it is hard to say that patients in the ER group had better renal function or lesser comorbidities at the same time 6 or 12 months before dialysis initiation. If we could adjust parameters at the 12 months before dialysis instead of parameters at the time of dialysis initiation, multivariate regression model would be more accurately fitted to predict medical costs during the 12 months before dialysis initiation. However, due to the limited data collection in this cohort study, we could not gather clinical parameters or laboratory data at the 12 months before dialysis initiation, but only get data at the time of referral and at the time of dialysis initiation. Secondly, we only analyzed and compared the medical costs during the 12 months before and after dialysis initiation, not the whole or average medical costs from referral to dialysis initiation. Considering the 5 year mean duration from referral to dialysis in the ER group, if we could have compared the total 5 year medical costs or yearly medical costs during the 5 years between the two groups, the cost-saving effects of ER would be proved apparently without bias. The reasons why we focused on the medical costs during the 12 months before dialysis initiation were that we had divided the ER and LR groups by the referral time of 12 months and aimed to compare the medical costs around the time just before and after dialysis initiation. Actually, during the 12 months before dialysis initiation, monthly medical costs and the difference of medical costs between the ER and LR groups increased steadily. A considerable part of cost-saving effects of ER derived from the reduced medical costs during the several months of impending dialysis. It is still important that patients in the LR group spend much more medical costs probably due to the increased length of hospital stay and increased use of temporary vascular catheters immediately before dialysis initiation. Lastly, we could not investigate the relationship between medical costs and other clinical and laboratory parameters including eGFR, co-morbidity index, blood pressure, and cholesterol levels in univariate analysis. However, it might not lessen the strength of our results because these parameters were similar between the two groups.

The care of patients with CKD requires not only evaluation and treatment of decreased renal function but also a multidisciplinary

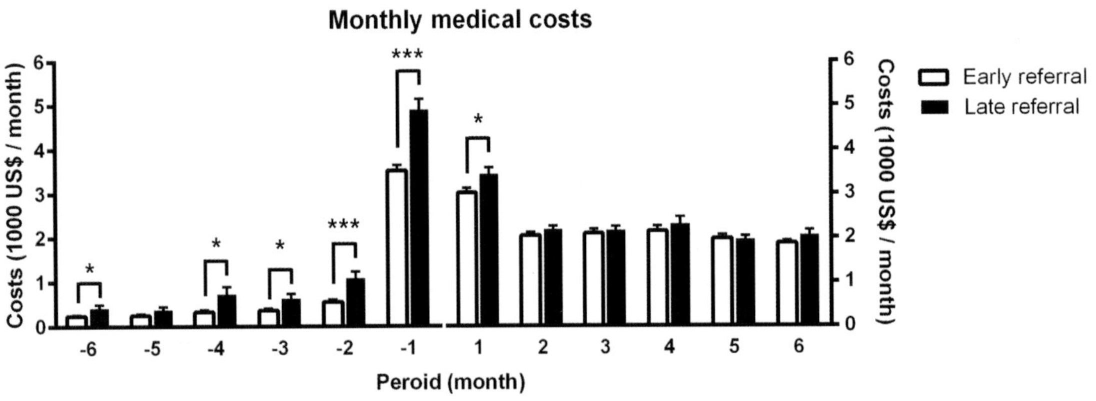

Figure 1. Monthly medical costs before and after the initiation of dialysis. The monthly medical costs are represented, comparing 'early referral' and 'late referral' according to the time period. The values (unit: US dollars) are expressed as the mean ± SEM. *P<0.05, ***P<0.001.

Table 2. Medical costs during the first year before and after dialysis therapy.

	Periods	Costs (USD)		
		Early referral	Late referral	P Value
After dialysis initiation (month)	0~1	3029±2219	3438±2821	0.025
	1~2	2044±1679	2181±1515	0.223
	2~3	2091±2087	2162±1669	0.597
	3~4	2148±2317	2301±3079	0.456
	4~5	1975±1623	1953±1258	0.844
	5~6	1871±1148	2046±2086	0.215
	0~12	18947±11864	19104±11501	0.845
Before dialysis initiation (month)	−1~0	3529±2696	4896±4629	<0.001
	−2~−1	555±1297	1092±2624	<0.001
	−3~−2	367±922	635±1779	0.015
	−4~−3	333±1003	725±3092	0.032
	−5~−4	259±705	382±1180	0.108
	−6~−5	247±520	417±1352	0.042
	−6~0	4926±3811	7162±6762	<0.001
	−12~0	6206±5873	8610±7820	<0.001

Costs are expressed as the mean ± standard deviation values.

approach, including proper blood pressure control, appropriate selection of medications and their dosages, the avoidance of nephrotoxic drugs, education about diet, preparation for renal placement therapy, psychological consultations, and economic evaluations. Timely referral is essential to improve patient outcomes and survival, but a considerable proportion of patients are referred late to dialysis for various reasons, including a lack of knowledge, negative preconceptions about dialysis, and economic difficulties. In this study, we demonstrated that the ER of CKD patients could reduce economic costs during the period before and after the initiation of renal replacement therapy. Considering the benefits of ER to a nephrologist in both economic and clinical terms, clinicians should focus on the timely referral of patients with CKD.

Acknowledgments

A proportion of this work was selected for oral presentation and presented at Kidney Week 2013, American Society of Nephrology Annual Meeting, on November 9 at the Georgia World Congress Center in Atlanta, GA. We express our gratitude to all participants and investigators of the cohort study (Clinical Research Center for End Stage Renal Disease, CRC for ESRD) in South Korea. Jeonghwan Lee (Hallym University Hangang Sacred Heart Hospital, Seoul, Korea), Jung Pyo Lee, Chun Soo Lim (Seoul National University Boramae Medical Center, Seoul, Korea), Ji In Park, Yon Su Kim (Seoul National University College of Medicine, Seoul, Korea), Jin Ho Hwang (Chung-Ang University Hospital, Seoul, Korea), Hye Min Jang, Ji-Young Choi, Yong-Lim Kim (Kyungpook National University, Daegu, Korea), Chul Woo Yang (The Catholic University of Korea College of Medicine, Seoul, Korea), Shin-Wook Kang (Yonsei University College of Medicine, Seoul, Korea), Nam-Ho Kim (Chonnam

Table 3. Multivariate analysis for the medical costs during the first month after dialysis initiation.

	Univariate model		Multivariate model	
Variables	Parameter estimates	P Value	Parameter estimates	P Value
Type of referral (early referral)	−409.1±174.3	0.019	−428.5±172.3	0.013
Age (years)	−1.2±6.1	0.846		
Gender (female)	53.9±175.3	0.759		
Type of dialysis (hemodialysis))	823.8±184.3	<0.001	845.7±184.8	<0.001
BMI	−26.7±22.0	0.226		
Causes of renal disease				
Diabetes mellitus	−197.2±236.0	0.404		
Glomerulonephritis	−571.9±295.5	0.053		
Hypertension	−285.0±302.6	0.347		
Hemoglobin (g/dL)	−14.0±22.4	0.532		
Serum albumin (g/dL)	−4.1±6.1	0.503		

Parameter estimates (unit: USD) are expressed with β ± standard error values.

Table 4. Multivariate analysis for medical costs during the 1 year before dialysis initiation.

	Univariate model		Multivariate model	
Variables	**Parameter estimates**	**P Value**	**Parameter estimates**	**P Value**
Type of referral (early referral)	−2404.1±447.4	<0.001	−2534.0±436.2	<0.001
Age (years)	30.1±15.7	0.055	27.9±15.7	0.076
Gender (female)	−431.4±449.8	0.338		
Type of dialysis (hemodialysis)	389.2±478.5	0.416		
BMI	8.1±55.3	0.883		
Causes of renal disease				
Diabetes mellitus	−637.6±571.5	0.265	−860.2±596.7	0.150
Glomerulonephritis	−2520.9±720.0	<0.001	−2247.6±749.5	0.003
Hypertension	−1507.3±717.3	0.036	−1814.4±737.1	0.014
Hemoglobin (g/dL)	89.9±47.3	0.057	81.4±46.3	0.080
Serum albumin (g/dL)	7.2±8.8	0.412		

Parameter estimates (unit: USD) are expressed with β ± standard error values.

National University Medical School, Gwangju, Korea) are participating CRC for ESRD, and Chun Soo Lim (email: cslimjy@snu.ac.kr) is the lead author of this article.

Author Contributions

Conceived and designed the experiments: JL JPL YSK CSL. Performed the experiments: JPL JIP JHH JYC YLK CWY SWK NHK YSK. Analyzed the data: JL JPL HMJ JYC CSL. Contributed reagents/materials/analysis tools: YLK CSL. Wrote the paper: JL JPL CSL.

References

1. Levey AS, Coresh J (2012) Chronic kidney disease. Lancet 379: 165–180.
2. James MT, Hemmelgarn BR, Tonelli M (2010) Early recognition and prevention of chronic kidney disease. Lancet 375: 1296–1309.
3. Kim S, Lim CS, Han DC, Kim GS, Chin HJ, et al. (2009) The prevalence of chronic kidney disease (CKD) and the associated factors to CKD in urban Korea: a population-based cross-sectional epidemiologic study. J Korean Med Sci 24 Suppl: S11–21.
4. Collins AJ, Foley RN, Herzog C, Chavers B, Gilbertson D, et al. (2013) US Renal Data System 2012 Annual Data Report. Am J Kidney Dis 61: A7, e1–476.
5. Keith DS, Nichols GA, Gullion CM, Brown JB, Smith DH (2004) Longitudinal follow-up and outcomes among a population with chronic kidney disease in a large managed care organization. Arch Intern Med 164: 659–663.
6. Jin DC (2011) Current status of dialysis therapy in Korea. Korean J Intern Med 26: 123–131.
7. Collins AJ, Foley RN, Herzog C, Chavers B, Gilbertson D, et al. (2009) United States Renal Data System 2008 Annual Data Report. Am J Kidney Dis 53: S1–374.
8. Seok SJ, Kim JH, Gil HW, Yang JO, Lee EY, et al. (2010) Comparison of patients starting hemodialysis with those underwent hemodialysis 15 years ago at the same dialysis center in Korea. Korean J Intern Med 25: 188–194.
9. Hommel K, Madsen M, Kamper AL (2012) The importance of early referral for the treatment of chronic kidney disease: a Danish nationwide cohort study. BMC Nephrol 13: 108.
10. Chan MR, Dall AT, Fletcher KE, Lu N, Trivedi H (2007) Outcomes in patients with chronic kidney disease referred late to nephrologists: a meta-analysis. Am J Med 120: 1063–1070.
11. Innes A, Rowe PA, Burden RP, Morgan AG (1992) Early deaths on renal replacement therapy: the need for early nephrological referral. Nephrol Dial Transplant 7: 467–471.
12. Arora P, Obrador GT, Ruthazer R, Kausz AT, Meyer KB, et al. (1999) Prevalence, predictors, and consequences of late nephrology referral at a tertiary care center. J Am Soc Nephrol 10: 1281–1286.
13. Jungers P, Zingraff J, Page B, Albouze G, Hannedouche T, et al. (1993) Detrimental effects of late referral in patients with chronic renal failure: a case-control study. Kidney Int Suppl 41: S170–173.
14. Metcalfe W, Khan IH, Prescott GJ, Simpson K, MacLeod AM (2000) Can we improve early mortality in patients receiving renal replacement therapy? Kidney Int 57: 2539–2545.
15. Ifudu O, Dawood M, Homel P, Friedman EA (1996) Excess morbidity in patients starting uremia therapy without prior care by a nephrologist. Am J Kidney Dis 28: 841–845.
16. Jungers P, Zingraff J, Albouze G, Chauveau P, Page B, et al. (1993) Late referral to maintenance dialysis: detrimental consequences. Nephrol Dial Transplant 8: 1089–1093.
17. Stack AG (2003) Impact of timing of nephrology referral and pre-ESRD care on mortality risk among new ESRD patients in the United States. Am J Kidney Dis 41: 310–318.
18. Roderick P, Jones C, Drey N, Blakeley S, Webster P, et al. (2002) Late referral for end-stage renal disease: a region-wide survey in the south west of England. Nephrol Dial Transplant 17: 1252–1259.
19. Kazmi WH, Obrador GT, Khan SS, Pereira BJ, Kausz AT (2004) Late nephrology referral and mortality among patients with end-stage renal disease: a propensity score analysis. Nephrol Dial Transplant 19: 1808–1814.
20. Yokoyama Y, Yamazaki S, Hasegawa T, Wakita T, Hayashino Y, et al. (2009) Impact of early referral to nephrologist on mental health among hemodialysis patients: a Dialysis Outcomes and Practice Patterns Study (DOPPS). Nephron Clin Pract 113: c191–197.
21. Levin A, Lewis M, Mortiboy P, Faber S, Hare I, et al. (1997) Multidisciplinary predialysis programs: quantification and limitations of their impact on patient outcomes in two Canadian settings. Am J Kidney Dis 29: 533–540.
22. Winkelmayer WC, Glynn RJ, Levin R, Owen W Jr, Avorn J (2001) Late referral and modality choice in end-stage renal disease. Kidney Int 60: 1547–1554.
23. Astor BC, Eustace JA, Powe NR, Klag MJ, Sadler JH, et al. (2001) Timing of nephrologist referral and arteriovenous access use: the CHOICE Study. Am J Kidney Dis 38: 494–501.
24. Avorn J, Winkelmayer WC, Bohn RL, Levin R, Glynn RJ, et al. (2002) Delayed nephrologist referral and inadequate vascular access in patients with advanced chronic kidney failure. J Clin Epidemiol 55: 711–716.
25. Schmidt RJ, Domico JR, Sorkin MI, Hobbs G (1998) Early referral and its impact on emergent first dialyses, health care costs, and outcome. Am J Kidney Dis 32: 278–283.
26. Stehman-Breen CO, Sherrard DJ, Gillen D, Caps M (2000) Determinants of type and timing of initial permanent hemodialysis vascular access. Kidney Int 57: 639–645.
27. Smart NA, Titus TT (2011) Outcomes of early versus late nephrology referral in chronic kidney disease: a systematic review. Am J Med 124: 1073–1080.
28. Chen SC, Hwang SJ, Tsai JC, Liu WC, Hwang SC, et al. (2010) Early nephrology referral is associated with prolonged survival in hemodialysis patients even after exclusion of lead-time bias. Am J Med Sci 339: 123–126.
29. Kinchen KS, Sadler J, Fink N, Brookmeyer R, Klag MJ, et al. (2002) The timing of specialist evaluation in chronic kidney disease and mortality. Ann Intern Med 137: 479–486.
30. Avorn J, Bohn RL, Levy E, Levin R, Owen WF Jr, et al. (2002) Nephrologist care and mortality in patients with chronic renal insufficiency. Arch Intern Med 162: 2002–2006.

31. Winkelmayer WC, Glynn RJ, Levin R, Mittleman MA, Pliskin JS, et al. (2002) Late nephrologist referral and access to renal transplantation. Transplantation 73: 1918–1923.
32. Kim do H, Kim M, Kim H, Kim YL, Kang SW, et al. (2013) Early referral to a nephrologist improved patient survival: prospective cohort study for end-stage renal disease in Korea. PLoS One 8: e55323.
33. Choi JY, Jang HM, Park J, Kim YS, Kang SW, et al. (2013) Survival advantage of peritoneal dialysis relative to hemodialysis in the early period of incident dialysis patients: a nationwide prospective propensity-matched study in Korea. PLoS One 8: e84257.
34. Levey AS, Stevens LA, Schmid CH, Zhang YL, Castro AF 3rd, et al. (2009) A new equation to estimate glomerular filtration rate. Ann Intern Med 150: 604–612.
35. Charlson ME, Pompei P, Ales KL, MacKenzie CR (1987) A new method of classifying prognostic comorbidity in longitudinal studies: development and validation. J Chronic Dis 40: 373–383.
36. Davies SJ, Russell L, Bryan J, Phillips L, Russell GI (1995) Comorbidity, urea kinetics, and appetite in continuous ambulatory peritoneal dialysis patients: their interrelationship and prediction of survival. Am J Kidney Dis 26: 353–361.
37. Chae JW, Song CS, Kim H, Lee KB, Seo BS, et al. (2011) Prediction of mortality in patients undergoing maintenance hemodialysis by Charlson Comorbidity Index using ICD-10 database. Nephron Clin Pract 117: c379–384.
38. Caskey FJ, Wordsworth S, Ben T, de Charro FT, Delcroix C, et al. (2003) Early referral and planned initiation of dialysis: what impact on quality of life? Nephrol Dial Transplant 18: 1330–1338.
39. Jones C, Roderick P, Harris S, Rogerson M (2006) Decline in kidney function before and after nephrology referral and the effect on survival in moderate to advanced chronic kidney disease. Nephrol Dial Transplant 21: 2133–2143.
40. Ledoux F, Rasamimanantsoa D, Moulin B, Hannedouche T (2001) From the first symptoms to terminal renal failure: need for a nephrologic follow-up. Rev Med Interne 22: 245–254.
41. Smith DH, Gullion CM, Nichols G, Keith DS, Brown JB (2004) Cost of medical care for chronic kidney disease and comorbidity among enrollees in a large HMO population. J Am Soc Nephrol 15: 1300–1306.
42. Roderick P, Jones C, Tomson C, Mason J (2002) Late referral for dialysis: improving the management of chronic renal disease. QJM 95: 363–370.
43. Roubicek C, Brunet P, Huiart L, Thirion X, Leonetti F, et al. (2000) Timing of nephrology referral: influence on mortality and morbidity. Am J Kidney Dis 36: 35–41.
44. Eadington DW (1996) Delayed referral for dialysis. Nephrol Dial Transplant 11: 2124–2126.
45. Kessler M, Frimat L, Panescu V, Briancon S (2003) Impact of nephrology referral on early and midterm outcomes in ESRD: EPidemiologie de l'Insuffisance REnale chronique terminale en Lorraine (EPIREL): results of a 2-year, prospective, community-based study. Am J Kidney Dis 42: 474–485.
46. Ismail N, Neyra R, Hakim R (1998) The medical and economical advantages of early referral of chronic renal failure patients to renal specialists. Nephrol Dial Transplant 13: 246–250.
47. Obialo CI, Ofili EO, Quarshie A, Martin PC (2005) Ultralate referral and presentation for renal replacement therapy: socioeconomic implications. Am J Kidney Dis 46: 881–886.

7

Role of Far Infra-Red Therapy in Dialysis Arterio-Venous Fistula Maturation and Survival

Khalid Bashar[1]*, Donagh Healy[1], Leonard D. Browne[2], Elrasheid A. H. Kheirelseid[1], Michael T. Walsh[2], Mary Clarke - Moloney[1], Paul E. Burke[1], Eamon G. Kavanagh[1], Stewart Redmond Walsh[3]

1 Department of vascular surgery, University Hospital Limerick, Limerick, Ireland, **2** Centre for Applied Biomedical Engineering Research (CABER), Department of Mechanical, Aeronautical & Biomedical Engineering, Materials and Surface Science Institute, University of Limerick, Limerick, Ireland, **3** Department of surgery, National University of Ireland, Galway, Ireland

Abstract

Introduction: A well-functioning arteriovenous fistula (AVF) is the best modality for vascular access in patients with end-stage renal disease (ESRD) requiring haemodialysis (HD). However, AVFs' main disadvantage is the high rate of maturation failure, with approximately one third (20%–50%) not maturing into useful access. This review examine the use of Far-Infra Red therapy in an attempt to enhance both primary (unassisted) and secondary (assisted) patency rates for AVF in dialysis and pre-dialysis patients.

Method: We performed an online search for observational studies and randomised controlled trials (RCTs) that evaluated FIR in patients with AVF. Eligible studies compared FIR with control treatment and reported at least one outcome measure relating to access survival. Primary patency and secondary patency rates were the main outcomes of interest.

Results: Four RCTs (666 patients) were included. Unassisted patency assessed in 610 patients, and was significantly better among those who received FIR (228/311) compared to (185/299) controls (pooled risk ratio of 1.23 [1.12–1.35], p = 0.00001). In addition, the two studies which reported secondary patency rates showed significant difference in favour of FIR therapy-160/168 patients - compared to 140/163 controls (pooled risk ratio of 1.11 [1.04–1.19], p = 0.003).

Conclusion: FIR therapy may positively influence the complex process of AVF maturation improving both primary and secondary patency rates. However blinded RCTs performed by investigators with no commercial ties to FIR therapy technologies are needed.

Editor: Daniel Schneditz, Medical University of Graz, Austria

Funding: The authors have no support or funding to report.

Competing Interests: The authors have declared that no competing interests exist.

* Email: khalidbashar@rcsi.ie

Introduction

The number of patients with end stage renal disease (ESRD) requiring haemodialysis (HD) is steadily rising, a trend that is expected to continue [1]. Vascular access is a critical component in successful HD. A well-functioning arteriovenous fistula (AVF) is the best modality for HD vascular access [2–6]. AVF maturation is a complex process of remodelling. The newly formed fistula has to form a low resistance circuit capable of dilation to accommodate the increased blood flow required for HD. The AVF also has to be cannulated repeatedly with ease. The need for re-intervention to maintain patency should be minimal [2–4,6,7].

AVFs' main disadvantage is the high rate of maturation failure, with approximately one third (20%–50%) not maturing into useful access [8–10]. AVFs have higher primary failure rates to mature compared to grafts [8,11,12]. However they last longer, and with exclusion of fistulas that fail to mature primarily, the cumulative patency from formation to permanent failure is superior to grafts. AVFs also require fewer secondary interventions in the form of angioplasty, stenting or thrombectomy [8,13–16]. AVFs are associated with fewer complications compared to AVG and CVC in terms of infection, death, vascular access salvage procedures and hospitalizations [15,16]. Also, a mature AVF has a lower incidence of thrombosis and stenosis. This translates into prolonged patency rates and lower risk for infection [1,17–20].

Maturation of AVF depends on variable biomechanical forces. Remodelling of the arterial limb is characterised by vessel dilatation and outward hypertrophic remodelling of the intimal layer. Remodelling at the venous end can be accompanied by aggressive intimal thickening resulting in inward hypertrophic remodelling. Intimal hyperplasia (IH) is defined as the abnormal migration and proliferation of vascular smooth muscle cells provoked by injury, inflammation or stretch with associated

Table 1. Results of the study quality assessment.

Included study	Domain	Support for judgement	DH's judgement
Lai 2013 ESVS [37]	Random sequence generation	The method of generating the random sequence was not described.	Unclear
	Allocation concealment	No description of methods for maintaining allocation concealment.	Unclear
	Blinding of participants and personnel	Participants and personnel were not blinded. Dysfunctional access signs and other referral criteria could have a subjective component.	High risk of bias
	Blinding of outcome assessment	Outcome assessors were not blinded. Dysfunctional access signs and other referral criteria could have a subjective component.	High risk of bias
	Incomplete outcome data	Loss to follow up was minimal. Analysis was not by intention to treat. 9/59 control group patients crossed over to the intervention group potentially leading to bias in favour of the intervention	Unclear
	Selective reporting	No link to the protocol was given	Unclear
	Other sources of bias	None	Not available
Lin 2007 J Am Soc Neph [35]	Random sequence generation	A computerised minimisation algorithm was used	Low risk of bias
	Allocation concealment	Allocation sequence was kept by a study nurse who would not disclose allocations until time of intervention. Diagnosing malfunction in a fistula could have had a subjective element.	Unclear
	Blinding of participants and personnel	Participants and personnel were not blinded.	High risk of bias
	Blinding of outcome assessment	Outcome assessors were not blinded. Diagnosing malfunction in a fistula could have had a subjective element.	High risk of bias
	Incomplete outcome data	Loss to follow up was minimal and was similar between groups and was unlikely to influence results	Low risk of bias
	Selective reporting	Protocol was not available.	Unclear
	Other sources of bias	None	Not available
Lin 2013 AJKD [38]	Random sequence generation	A computer generated sequence was used	Low risk of bias
	Allocation concealment	Sealed opaque envelope were used to conceal allocation. There was no information in the manuscript or protocol on who had access to the envelopes and whether they were opened sequentially	Unclear
	Blinding of participants and personnel	No blinding. Diagnosing malfunction in a fistula could have had a subjective element.	High risk of bias
	Blinding of outcome assessment	Ultrasonographers were blinded however patients were not blinded. Diagnosing malfunction in a fistula could have had a subjective element.	High risk of bias
	Incomplete outcome data	Loss to follow up was similar between groups and unlikely to influence results	Low risk of bias
	Selective reporting	Link to protocol was provided (NCT01138254). Trial was not prospectively registered and there were several changes made including changes to outcomes.	High risk of bias
	Other sources of bias	None	Not available
Lin 2013 Neph Dial Transplant [36]	Random sequence generation	A computer generated sequence was used	Low risk of bias

Table 1. Cont.

Included study	Domain	Support for judgement	DH's judgement
	Allocation concealment	Sealed opaque envelope were used to conceal allocation. Two study nurses had access to the envelopes and there was no information in the manuscript or protocol on whether they were opened sequentially	Unclear
	Blinding of participants and personnel	No blinding. Diagnosing malfunction in a fistula could have had a subjective element.	High risk of bias
	Blinding of outcome assessment	No blinding. Diagnosing malfunction in a fistula could have had a subjective element.	High risk of bias
	Incomplete outcome data	Loss to follow up was similar between groups and unlikely to influence results	Low risk of bias.
	Selective reporting	All outcomes that were mentioned in the protocol were reported. The subgrouping based on polymorphisms of heme oxygenase-1 was not prespecified	Low risk of bias
	Other sources of bias	None	Not available

deposition of extracellular matrix in the intimal layer of the vein [21–23].

Far infra-red FIR therapy, which is a form of heat therapy, has been implicated in improvement of endothelial function and haemodynamics in coronary arteries, probably through up-regulating endothelial nitric oxide synthase (eNOS) expression in arterial endothelium leading to improved cardiac function in patients with chronic heart diseases [24]. Repeated leg hyperthermia using FIR has been shown to reduce oxidative stress in bed ridden type II diabetics [25].

FIR has also been reported to show encouraging results in phantom limb pain control [26], stimulation of the secretion of TGF-beta1 and activation of fibroblasts which may promote better wound healing independent of skin blood flow and skin temperature [27,28], reduction of both stress and fatigue levels of patients with end stage renal disease (ESRD) and stimulates the autonomic nervous system in those who are receiving regular haemodialysis (HD) [29].

This review was designed to examine the effect of FIR on AVF maturation using primary and secondary patency rates as the main outcomes of interest.

Methods

This systematic review and meta-analysis were conducted according to the Preferred Reporting Items for Systematic Review and Meta-Analysis (PRISMA) guidelines [30].

Eligibility Criteria

We included observational studies or randomised controlled trials (RCTs) that examined FIR therapy in patients with AVFs and ESRD. Eligible studies reported on AVF patency rates in FIR and non-FIR groups at one year or more following initiation of FIR therapy. Cases series and case reports were excluded. There was no restriction with regard to publication status or language.

Search strategy

A search of the literature for relevant studies was conducted in March 2014. We searched Medline without date restriction using the free text "far infra-red". Additionally we used the strategy (["far infra-red" OR "far infrared" OR "post conditioning"] AND ["arteriovenous fistula" "dialysis" OR "end stage renal disease" OR "dialysis access" OR "access survival" OR "primary patency" OR "secondary patency" OR "fistula maturation]") to search CINAHL, EMBASE, the Cochrane library and Google Scholar. Bibliographies of included studies were searched for additional studies.

Abstracts of the relevant titles were subsequently obtained and evaluated for eligibility (KB, DH). Any remaining uncertainty was resolved by examination of the full article (KB, DH). Discussion with a third author (SRW) resolved discrepancies in cases of disagreement regarding eligibility.

The relevant outcomes for this review were primary patency – defined as unassisted AVF patency rates after at least 12 months of follow up - and secondary patency – defined as assisted patency rates after at least 12 months of follow up. The incidence of salvage procedures (endoluminal procedures or surgical procedures) for dysfunctional fistulas during follow up was a secondary outcome.

Data Collection

Data were extracted and checked for accuracy by two reviewers (KB, DH) independently and recorded on a Microsoft Excel spreadsheet. Any disagreements in extracting data were discussed between two reviewers (KB, DH), and if not settled this was resolved by consulting with a third reviewer (SRW). The following information regarding participant characteristics were recorded: age, sex, presence of co-morbidities, start of HD, primary and secondary patency rates, AVF salvage procedures, underlying cause of ESRD, definition of first AVF malfunction and overall access survival. The trials' inclusion and exclusion criteria were also recorded.

Quality assessment for risk of bias

The risk of bias for each study was assessed according to the criteria outlined in the in the Cochrane Handbook for Systematic Reviews of Interventions [31]. For each included study; the method used to perform random sequence generation, allocation concealment and blinding was described. The study was then

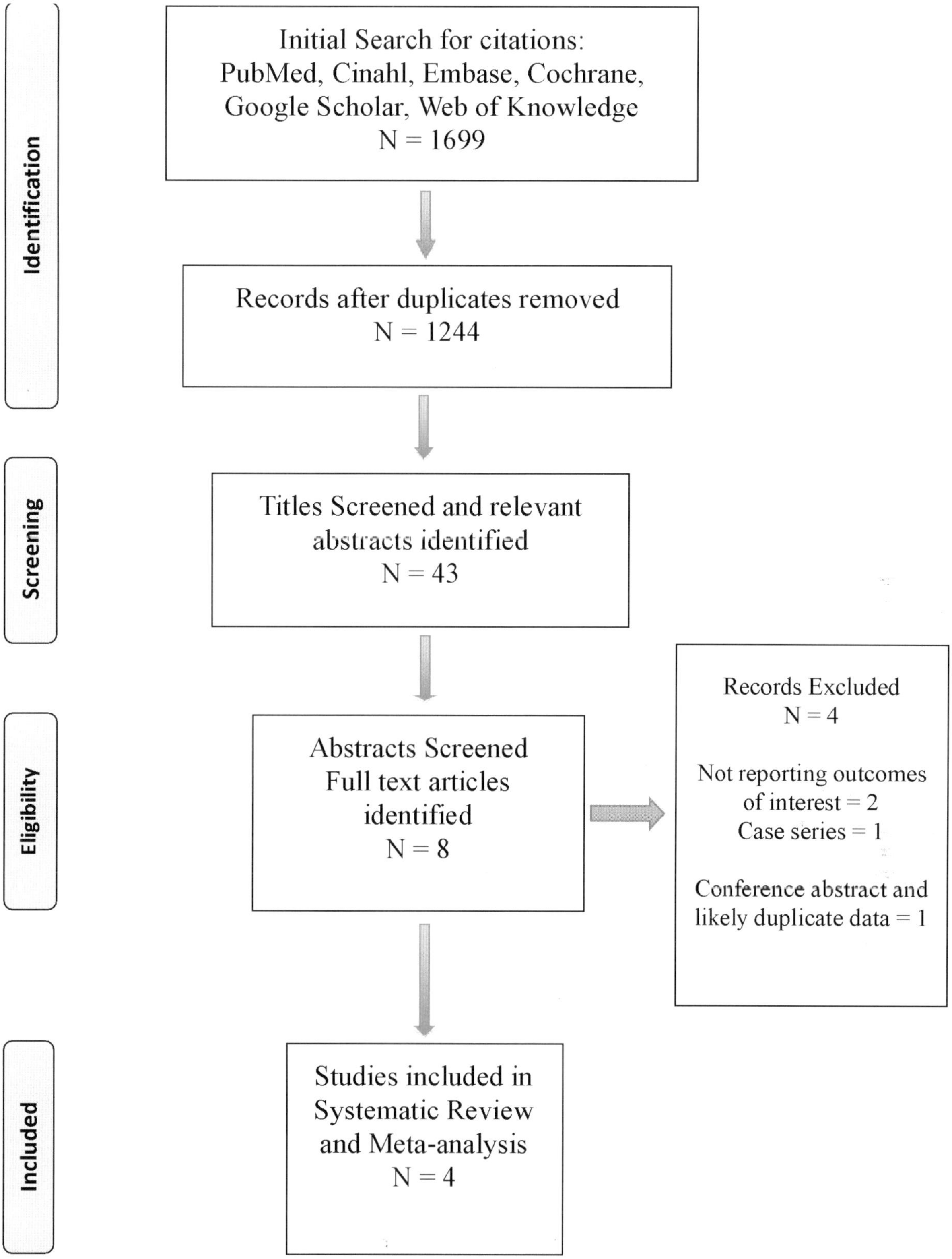

Figure 1. PRISMA 2009 Flow Diagram.

scrutinised for incomplete data outcomes, selective reporting and other potential sources of bias. Where possible, study protocols were obtained from trial registries to ascertain whether there was selective reporting within studies [Table 1].

Data analysis

Statistical analyses were performed using Review Manager version 5.2.8 [32]. Pooled risk ratios were calculated using the random effects model of DerSimonian and Laird [33]. For

Table 2. Inclusion & exclusion criteria and definition of AVF malfunction for included studies.

Study	Inclusion criteria	Exclusion criteria	Definition of AVF malfunction
Lin 2007 [35]	(1) Receiving 4 h of maintenance HD therapy three times weekly for at least 6 months at Taipei Veterans General Hospital, (2) Using a native AVF as the current vascular access for more than 6 months, without interventions within the last 3 months, and (3) Creation of AVF by cardiovascular surgeons in our hospital with the standardized surgical procedures of venous end-to-arterial side anastomosis in the upper extremity.	During the 1-yr follow-up, patients would be excluded from the study because of the following censoring criterion: (1) Renal transplantation, (2) Death with a functioning access, (3) Shifting to peritoneal dialysis, and (4) Loss of follow-up.	The need for any interventional procedure (surgery or angioplasty) to correct an occlusive or malfunctioning AVF that cannot sustain an extracorporeal blood flow >200 ml/min during HD after exclusion of the following stenosis-unrelated events: Infectious complication, progressive aneurysmal formation, or steal syndrome.
Lin 2013_AJKD [38]	(1) Aged 18–80 years, (2) Had CKD with estimated glomerular filtration rate (eGFR) of 5–20 mL/min/1.73 m^2, (3) Were not anticipated to receive dialysis or kidney transplantation within the next 3 months, and (4) Were undergoing AVF creation with venous end-to-arterial side anastomosis in the upper extremity.	(1) Those receiving an arteriovenous graft or cuffed tunnelled double-lumen catheter as the type of permanent vascular access, (2) Heart failure of New York Heart Association functional class III or IV, and (3) Episode of cardio- or cerebrovascular event or receiving intervention therapy within 3 months prior to screening.	The need for any interventional procedure (surgery or angioplasty) to correct an occlusive or malfunctioning fistula which could not sustain an extracorporeal blood flow >200 mL/min during HD after excluding the following stenosis-unrelated events, such as infectious complication, progressive aneurysmal formation or steal syndrome.
Lai_2013 [37]	(1) Received two or more PTA on the target lesions at upper extremities, with the last PTA successfully performed within the week before patient enrolment, and (2) After successful completion of at least 1 week of HD treatment, the patients with AVF or AVG were consecutively enrolled and randomly assigned to either a post-PTA FIR radiation group or a control group receiving the usual form radiation therapy at a 1:1 ratio.	(1) Received HD treatments other than three times a week, (2) Had previously received FIR radiation Therapy, (3) Received implantation of an endovascular stent, (4) Had multiple lesions that a single radiation field did not cover or the central lesion was considered too deep to be irradiated, (5) Missed FIR radiation treatments exceeding 10%, (6) Underwent renal transplantation, (7) Switched to peritoneal dialysis treatments, and (8) Had any severe disease with an estimated life expectancy of less than 1 year.	A significant lesion was defined as a lumen loss of 50% or more compared with adjacent normal vessel on angiography following dysfunctional diagnosis based on clinical signs suggestive of stenosis.
Lin_2013_NDT [36]	(1) Receiving 4 h of maintenance HD therapy three times weekly for at least 6 months at Taipei Veterans General Hospital, (2) Using a native AVF as the present vascular access for >6 months, without interventions within the last 3 months, and (3) Creation of AVF by cardiovascular surgeons in our hospital with the standardized surgical procedures of venous end-to-arterial side anastomosis in the upper extremity.	Received an AV graft as the first vascular access.	The need for any interventional procedure (surgery or angioplasty) to correct an occlusive or malfunctioning fistula which could not sustain an extracorporeal blood flow >200 mL/min during HD after excluding the following stenosis-unrelated events, such as infectious complication, progressive aneurysmal formation or steal syndrome.

continuous outcome variables the weighted mean difference (WMD) was calculated. The presence of statistical heterogeneity between studies was evaluated using the Cochran's Q statistic. P-values less than 5% were considered as statistically significant. Publication bias was assessed visually using a funnel plot, and additionally by comparing fixed and random effects modelling in a sensitivity analysis – this is a recognised method that can detect the influence of small-study effects [34].

Results

Study Selection

The results of the study selection process are summarized in the PRISMA flow diagram (Figure 1). The initial search yielded a total of 1669 citations, with 1244 citations remaining following removal of duplicates. The titles of these citations were screened with a total of 43 titles deemed potentially relevant. The abstracts of those titles were examined and eight full text articles were subsequently retrieved and examined. After assessing for eligibility

Table 3. Patients' Characteristics across included studies.

Study	Patients		Age		Gender M:F		Diabetes		Hypertension		Hx of AVF failure		Time on HD		Withdrawals
	FIR	Control	FIR	Control	FIR	Control	FIR	Control	FIR	Control	FIR	Control	FIR	Control	
Lin 2007 [35]	63/72	64/73	61.9±14.4	59.2±19.0	37:35	38:35	25	24	40	39	33	34	85.2±41.1	79.2±42.2	Creation of another vascular access because of the poor response to angioplasty: 1 patient receiving FIR therapy and four patients in control group. Patients were censored in case of: Renal transplantation ($n = 3$), death with a functioning access ($n = 5$), shifting to peritoneal dialysis ($n = 4$) or loss of follow-up ($n = 1$).
Lin 2013_AJKD [38]	60	62	63.2±18.5	63.0±14.4	32:28	35:27	28	23	18	20	-	-	Pre-dialysis	Pre-dialysis	Lost to F/U: FIR = 1; Control = 1. Shifting to PD: FIR = 1; Control = 1. Death e AVF: FIR = 2; Control = 3. Renal transplantation: FIR = 1. New AVF (Infection): Control = 1. D/C intervention: FIR = 2; Control = 1.
Lin 2013_NDT [36]	119/139	120/141	61.3±14.1	62.8±15.9	79:60	71:70	45	47	80	90	47	45	66.0±59.1	75.9±58.0	Underwent creation of another vascular access due to non-stenotic lesions: 3 patients receiving FIR therapy and 2 patients in the control group. Patients were censored in case of: Renal transplantation (n = 5), death with a functioning access (n = 15), shift to peritoneal dialysis (n = 5) or loss of follow-up (n = 9).
Lai 2013 [37]	69	50	62.7±10.9	63.1±12.5	32:37	24/26	42	28	48	38	All	All	50.4±42.0	58.8±56.4	Crossover patients: 9 from Control to FIR.

Study or Subgroup	FIR Events	FIR Total	Control Events	Control Total	Weight	Risk Ratio M-H, Random, 95% CI	Year
Lin 2007	55	64	46	68	23.2%	1.27 [1.05, 1.54]	2007
Lai 2013	17	69	9	50	1.6%	1.37 [0.67, 2.82]	2013
Lin 2013_AJKD	52	59	43	61	24.3%	1.25 [1.04, 1.51]	2013
Lin 2013_NDT	104	119	87	120	50.9%	1.21 [1.06, 1.37]	2013
Total (95% CI)		**311**		**299**	**100.0%**	**1.23 [1.12, 1.35]**	
Total events	228		185				

Heterogeneity: $Tau^2 = 0.00$; $Chi^2 = 0.33$, df = 3 (P = 0.96); $I^2 = 0\%$
Test for overall effect: Z = 4.45 (P < 0.00001)

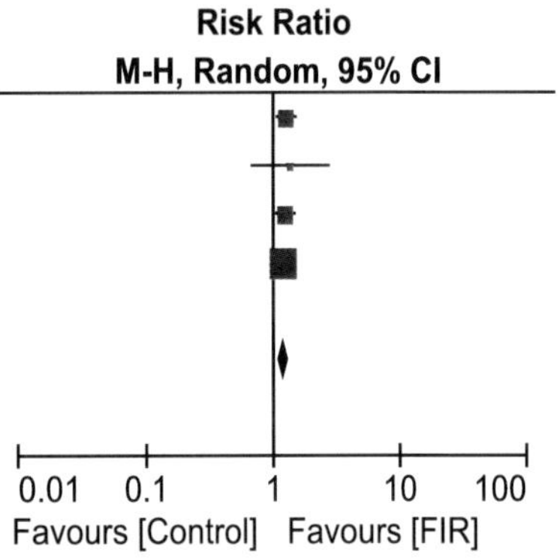

Figure 2. Forest Plot showing Primary AVFs patency at 12 months.

criteria, four RCT's were included in the review [35–38]. Three of those studies reported on patients with history of previous AVF who had been on HD prior to FIR therapy [35–37], while one study reported on patients with newly formed AVF not on HD [38]. We were not able to include another study by Lin et al [39] with a follow up of 3 months for primary patency rates as it was a conference abstract only, also we had concerns that the data in this study was used in another study by the same author [36] that has already been included in this review. Three studies were excluded from the final analysis after going through the full articles. Shipley et al followed their patients for six months in a case series of 20 patients – no control group - and reported maturation in 10 of those patients [40]. Two studies did not report on the outcomes of interest to the author of this systematic review [29,41].

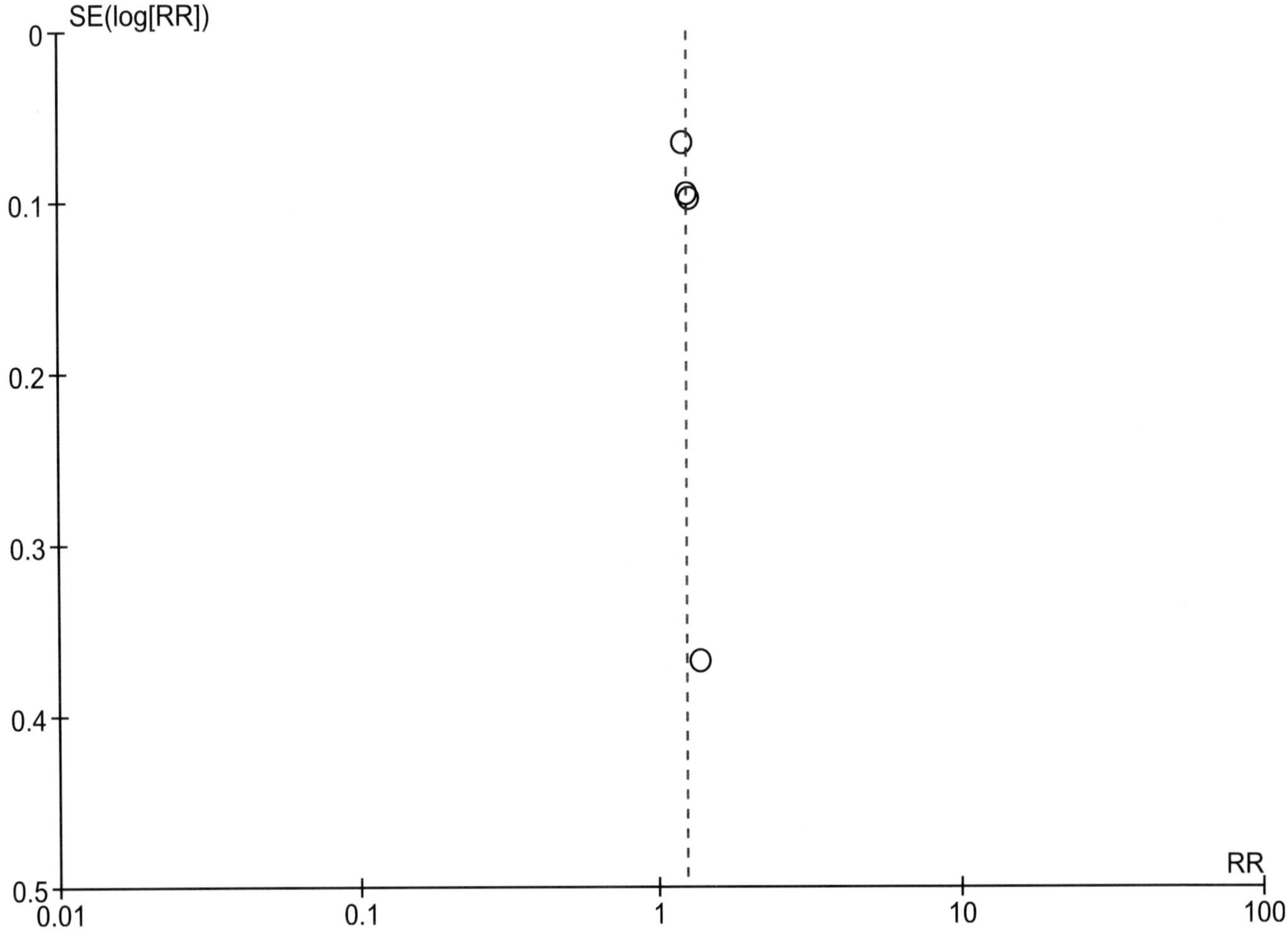

Figure 3. Funnel plot for Primary AVFs patency at 12 months.

Study or Subgroup	FIR Events	FIR Total	Control Events	Control Total	Weight	Risk Ratio M-H, Random, 95% CI	Year
Lin 2007	55	64	46	68	30.6%	1.27 [1.05, 1.54]	2007
Lin 2013_NDT	104	119	87	120	67.2%	1.21 [1.06, 1.37]	2013
Lai 2013	17	69	9	50	2.2%	1.37 [0.67, 2.82]	2013
Total (95% CI)		**252**		**238**	**100.0%**	**1.23 [1.10, 1.37]**	
Total events	176		142				

Heterogeneity: Tau² = 0.00; Chi² = 0.31, df = 2 (P = 0.86); I² = 0%
Test for overall effect: Z = 3.79 (P = 0.0001)

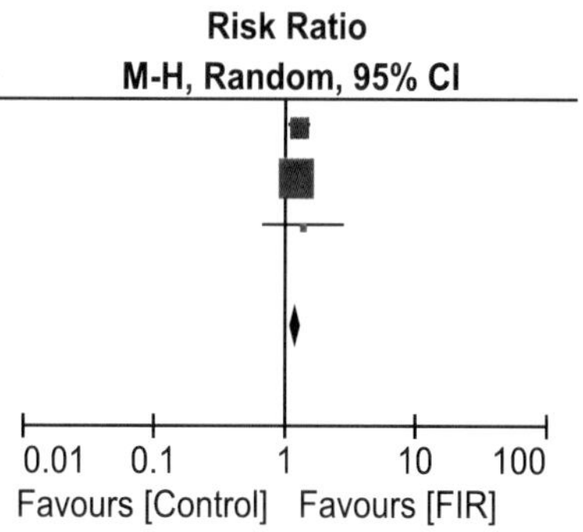

Figure 4. Forest Plot showing Primary AVFs patency at 12 months, Lin et al RCT on new AVFs excluded.

Characteristics of included studies

Far Infrared (FIR) technique. All studies included used the same technique for delivering of FIR therapy. WS TY101 FIR emitter (WS Far Infrared Medical Technology Co., Ltd., Taipei, Taiwan) was used in all studies which generates electromagnetic waves with wavelengths in the range between 5 and 25 (peak at 5–8.2 μm). The top radiator was set at a height of 20–30 cm above the surface of the AVF with the treatment time set at 40 min during HD three times per week.

Participants

The four studies included 666 patients, with 340 patients randomised to receive FIR therapy – median age 62.3±14.5 SD, while 326 were randomised to the control group – median age 62.0±14.5 SD. 348 patients were males–180 in FIR group and 168 in the control group, while females were 318, of those 160 received FIR therapy and 158 were controls.

Inclusion and exclusion criteria of studies are outlined in [Table 2], along with the definition of AVF malfunction for each of the included studies.

Apart from Lin et al who evaluated the effects of FIR in pre-dialysis patients with newly formed AVFs [38], the remaining RCTs included patients who already started HD. Mean time on HD in months for Lin et al [35] was 85.2±41.1 for FIR group and 79.2±42.2 for the control group, for Lai et al [37] FIR = 50.4±42 and control = 58.8±56.4 and for Lin et al in 2013 [36] FIR = 66.0±59.1 and control = 75.9±58.0. All patients in included trials received FIR therapy for 40 minutes per session three times a week for the duration of the study.

Lai et al studied patients with history of dysfunctional AVFs and repeated angioplasty. The mean life of the AVFs for their patients was 21.8±23.0 months for FIR group and 23.5±22.6 months for the controls [37]. 33 patients from 72 had history of AVF malfunction and 14 patients required surgical intervention, while 20 patients had a total of 49 angioplasty procedures in the FIR group compared to 34 patients from 73 with history of AVF malfunction, 13 of those required surgical intervention and 20 patients with total of 46 angioplasty procedures in the control group, in the RCT by Lin et al in 2007 [35]. Similarly, 47 patients had history of AVF malfunction with 12 patients requiring surgery from 139 and 35 patients underwent 79 angioplasty procedures in the FIR group, compared to 45 patients with history of malfunction, 13 patients of those required surgery and 32 patients underwent angioplasty as a salvage procedure in the control group in the study by Lin et al in 2013 [36]. All patients in both FIR and control groups had angioplasty procedures prior to recruitment in the study by Lai et al [37], while none of the patients included by Lin et al had a history of either surgical or angioplasty salvage procedures since they were all first time AVFs [38]. Lai et al had 9 of their patients who were initially randomised to the control group crossing over to the FIR group based on their request [37]. Clinical maturation was reported in 49 (81.7%) patients of 60 who received FIR therapy by Lin et all, compared to 37 (59.7%) from the 62 control subjects [38]. Sub –group analysis by age, gender and diagnosis of hypertension was not possible as this was not included in studies, and we did not have access to the raw data used by the authors. Other patients' characteristics are detailed in [Table 3].

Primary - unassisted - patency rates at 1 year

All of the 4 included studies (610 patients) reported on unassisted – primary – patency rate after 12 months of follow-up on the FIR therapy. 228/311 patients in FIR group had primarily patent AVFs at 12 months compared to 185/299 patients in the

Study or Subgroup	FIR Events	FIR Total	Control Events	Control Total	Weight	Risk Ratio M-H, Random, 95% CI
Lin 2013_AJKD	58	59	52	61	41.2%	1.15 [1.03, 1.29]
Lin 2013_NDT	102	109	88	102	58.8%	1.08 [0.99, 1.19]
Total (95% CI)		**168**		**163**	**100.0%**	**1.11 [1.04, 1.19]**
Total events	160		140			

Heterogeneity: Tau² = 0.00; Chi² = 0.71, df = 1 (P = 0.40); I² = 0%
Test for overall effect: Z = 2.97 (P = 0.003)

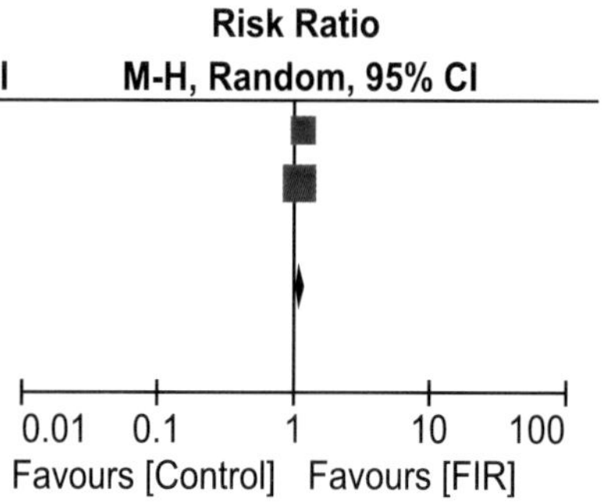

Figure 5. Forest plot showing assisted patency rates at 12 months.

	FIR		Control			Risk Ratio		Risk Ratio
Study or Subgroup	Events	Total	Events	Total	Weight	M-H, Random, 95% CI	Year	M-H, Random, 95% CI
Lin 2007	7	63	16	64	67.4%	0.44 [0.20, 1.01]	2007	
Lin 2013_AJKD	4	60	7	62	32.6%	0.59 [0.18, 1.91]	2013	
Total (95% CI)		**123**		**126**	**100.0%**	**0.49 [0.25, 0.95]**		
Total events	11		23					
Heterogeneity: Tau² = 0.00; Chi² = 0.15, df = 1 (P = 0.70); I² = 0%								
Test for overall effect: Z = 2.10 (P = 0.04)								

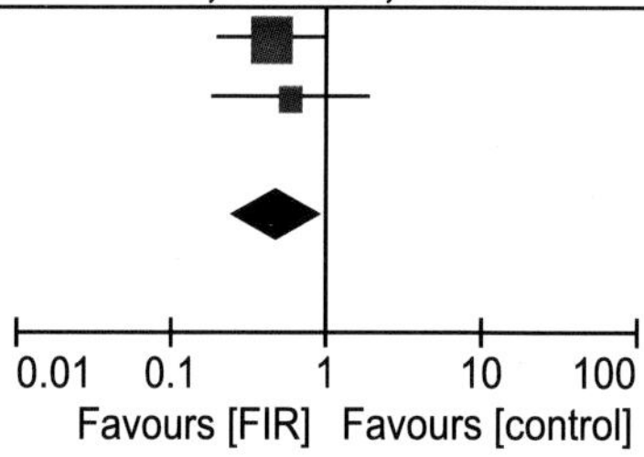

Figure 6. Forest plot showing surgical intervention for AVF malfunction.

control group. Pooled results showed significant difference between the two groups, with those who received FIR showing better primary patency rates compared to control (Pooled risk ratio = 1.23 [1.12, 1.35], 95% CI, p = 0.00001) [Figure 2]. There was no evidence of statistical heterogeneity (Cochran's Q = 0.33; degree of freedom (DF) = 3; p = 0.96; $I^2 = 0\%$). The funnel plot did not suggest bias [Figure 3], and the result was unchanged when fixed effects modelling was used (pooled risk ratio1.24 [1.13–1.37], 95% CI, p<0.0001).

Excluding the RCT by Lin et al on newly formed AVFs in pre-dialysis patients [38] from the analysis for primary patency after 12 months, the remaining studies (490 patients) showed better results in the FIR group with 176/252 AVFs being patent at 12 months compared to 142/238 in the control group [35–37]. This was statistically significant (Pooled risk ratio = 1.23 [1.10, 1.37], 95% CI, p = 0.0001) [Figure 4]. There was no evidence of statistical heterogeneity (Cochran's Q = 0.31; degree of freedom (DF) = 2; p = 0.86; $I^2 = 0\%$).

Secondary - assisted - patency rates

Data could be retrieved from 2 studies (331 patients) for analysis of assisted – secondary – patency rates at 12 months following salvage procedures [36,38]. 160/168 patients in the FIR group had patent AVFs following intervention for dysfunctional fistulas, compared to 140/163 patients in the control arm. Pooled results showed statistically significant difference favouring FIR therapy (Pooled risk ratio = 1.11 [1.04–1.19]; 95% CI, p = 0.003) [Figure 5]. There was no evidence of statistical heterogeneity (Cochran's Q = 0.71; degree of freedom (DF) = 1; p = 0.40; $I^2 = 0\%$).

Intervention

Two studies [35,38] (249 patients) reported the need for intervention to salvage a dysfunctional AVF. Patients who received FIR therapy required less interventions, 11/123 patients compared to 23/126 patients in the control group. The difference was significant (Pooled risk ratio = 0.49 [0.25–0.985; 95% CI; p = 0.04) [Figure 6]. There was no evidence of statistical heterogeneity (Cochran's Q = 0.15; degree of freedom (DF) = 1; p = 0.70; $I^2 = 0\%$).

Discussion

This review identified four studies (666 patients) which evaluated the use of FIR therapy to improve primary and secondary patency rates for AVFs in patients with ESRD. They all reported significant improvement in the outcome measures assessed in this review in favour of FIR therapy. Three of those studies (490 patients) were carried out on patients already started HD sessions, and one study (122 patients) focused on pre-dialysis first time AVF maturation. All four trials following some form of randomisation, and the demographics of patients in included studies did not differ significantly. Pooled analysis showed that primary - unassisted - patency was significantly better in the FIR group (pooled risk ratio of 1.23 [1.12–1.35], p value of 0.0001). Secondary – assisted – patency was reported in two studies (279 patients) and was found to be significantly better in those who received FIR therapy (pooled risk ratio of 1.19 [1.07–1.31], p value of 0.0008).

Post-conditioning using Far Infra-Red therapy has been shown to increase the level of heme oxygenase-1 (HO-1) expression which protects against Ischaemia/reperfusion injury in study by Tu et al [42]. HO-1 is a known vasodilator and at the same time inhibits proliferation of vascular smooth muscle cells, platelet aggregation, and vasospasm leading to favourable conditions for maturation of AVFs. Also, Ikeda et al repeated thermal therapy was shown to up-regulate endothelial nitric oxide synthase expression in Syrian hamsters [24], a finding that was validated by Akasaki et al, who also reported increased angiogenesis via (eNOS) following repeated thermal therapy in mice with hindlimb ischemia. [43]. Kipshidze et al irradiated cultures of rabbit endothelial cells and smooth muscle cells with different doses of non-ablative infrared. They found that non-ablative infrared laser inhibited neointimal hyperplasia after coronary arteries angioplasty in cholesterol-fed rabbits for up to 60 days [44]. FIR therapy is still considered a novel treatment for AVF although the technique has been described since 2007 by Lin et al [35]. This review demonstrated a beneficial use of FIR therapy that improved both primary and secondary patency rates across all studies included. This statistically significant difference was consistent even when one excluded study for having only 3 months of follow-up was added to the sensitivity analysis [39]. Also, excluding the only RCT found by the authors on newly formed AVF did not alter the outcome of the pooled analysis in terms of significance.

FIR therapy was also shown to improve access flow (Qa). The study by Lin et al – which was one of the RCTs included in the review - showed that 40 min of FIR therapy in a single HD session could increase access flow of AVF by about 50 mL/min with a 1-year effect of improving Qa by up to 150 mL/min and increasing unassisted patency of AVF by about 18% in comparison with controls [35].

A serious limiting factor of this systematic review is that the four RCTs came from the same institution (Yang-Ming University in Taiwan), and three of the four were authored by the same two authors (Lin-cc and Yang-wc) [35,36,38]. Dr Lin-cc reported that he was receiving lecture fees from WS Far Infrared Medical Technology, the company that makes the infrared machines used in the studies raising the potential of bias.

Also, all the RCTs were performed in an unblinded fashion, which can impact outcomes as demonstrated by the fact that in one study nine patients opted to join the FIR group despite initially being allocated as controls. Blinding in clinical trials involving FIR therapy would involve additional costs in making machines that resemble the ones used to deliver FIR therapy. Those machines should be convincing to both staff and patients if effective double blinding is to be considered. However, blinding can be attempted by placing a screen between the FIR device and the patient. Also, double-blinding can be achieved by placing a box over the device and then creating simple mock devices that also appear as boxes. This review provides a thorough examination of published evidence supporting the use of FIR therapy to promote AVF access maturation in patients with ESRD in HD, and also for those who are likely to require dialysis in the near future. The meta-analysis showed overwhelming support for regular use of FIR therapy, however there were limitations that need to be considered. Finally, this review may serve to guide future advances in using repeated thermal therapy in postconditioning of AVFs.

Conclusion

Results from four RCTs suggest that regular use of FIR therapy in haemodialysis and pre-haemodialysis patients, in particular those with AVFs, can positively influence AVF function. However, more blinded randomised controlled, multicentre and international clinical trials are required. We also hope to see sub-group analysis in those studies, particularly by age (e.g. using 65 as cut-off), gender and diagnosis of hypertension.

Author Contributions

Conceived and designed the experiments: KB DH EK SRW MCM PB EK MW LB. Performed the experiments: KB DH EK SRW MCM PB EK MW LB. Analyzed the data: KB DH EK SRW MCM PB EK MW. Contributed reagents/materials/analysis tools: KB DH. Contributed to the writing of the manuscript: KB DH EK SRW MCM PB EK MW LB.

References

1. Frankel A (2006) Temporary access and central venous catheters. Eur J Vasc Endovasc Surg 31: 417–422.
2. NKF-KDOQI (2006) 2006 Updates Clinical Practice Guidelines and Recommendations.
3. Hoggard J, Saad T, Schon D, Vesely TM, Royer T (2008) Guidelines for venous access in patients with chronic kidney disease. A Position Statement from the American Society of Diagnostic and Interventional Nephrology, Clinical Practice Committee and the Association for Vascular Access. Semin Dial 21: 186–191.
4. Polkinghorne KR, Chin GK, Macginley RJ, Owen AR, Russell C, et al. (2013) KHA-CARI guideline: Vascular access - central venous catheters, arteriovenous fistulae and arteriovenous grafts. Nephrology (Carlton).
5. Stolic R (2013) Most important chronic complications of arteriovenous fistulas for hemodialysis. Med Princ Pract 22: 220–228.
6. McCann M, Einarsdottir H, Van Waeleghem JP, Murphy F, Sedgewick J (2008) Vascular access management 1: an overview. J Ren Care 34: 77–84.
7. Dixon BS (2006) Why don't fistulas mature? Kidney Int 70: 1413–1422.
8. Allon M, Robbin ML (2002) Increasing arteriovenous fistulas in hemodialysis patients: problems and solutions. Kidney Int 62: 1109–1124.
9. Rayner HC, Pisoni RL, Gillespie BW, Goodkin DA, Akiba T, et al. (2003) Creation, cannulation and survival of arteriovenous fistulae: data from the Dialysis Outcomes and Practice Patterns Study. Kidney Int 63: 323–330.
10. Lok CE, Oliver MJ, Su J, Bhola C, Hannigan N, et al. (2005) Arteriovenous fistula outcomes in the era of the elderly dialysis population. Kidney Int 67: 2462–2469.
11. Allon M, Lockhart ME, Lilly RZ, Gallichio MH, Young CJ, et al. (2001) Effect of preoperative sonographic mapping on vascular access outcomes in hemodialysis patients. Kidney Int 60: 2013–2020.
12. Oliver MJ, McCann RL, Indridason OS, Butterly DW, Schwab SJ (2001) Comparison of transposed brachiobasilic fistulas to upper arm grafts and brachiocephalic fistulas. Kidney Int 60: 1532–1539.
13. Allon M (2007) Current management of vascular access. Clin J Am Soc Nephrol 2: 786–800.
14. Dixon BS, Novak L, Fangman J (2002) Hemodialysis vascular access survival: upper-arm native arteriovenous fistula. Am J Kidney Dis 39: 92–101.
15. Ocak G, Rotmans JI, Vossen CY, Rosendaal FR, Krediet RT, et al. (2013) Type of arteriovenous vascular access and association with patency and mortality. BMC Nephrol 14: 79.
16. Polkinghorne KR, McDonald SP, Atkins RC, Kerr PG (2004) Vascular access and all-cause mortality: a propensity score analysis. J Am Soc Nephrol 15: 477–486.
17. Spergel LM, Ravani P, Roy-Chaudhury P, Asif A, Besarab A (2007) Surgical salvage of the autogenous arteriovenous fistula (AVF). J Nephrol 20: 388–398.
18. Brunori G, Bandera A, Valente F, Laudon A (2008) [Vascular access for dialysis in elderly: AVF versus permanent CVC]. G Ital Nefrol 25: 614–618.
19. McCann M, Einarsdottir H, Van Waeleghem JP, Murphy F, Sedgewick J (2010) Vascular access management III: central venous catheters. J Ren Care 36: 25–33.
20. Ma A, Shroff R, Hothi D, Lopez MM, Veligratli F, et al. (2013) A comparison of arteriovenous fistulas and central venous lines for long-term chronic haemodialysis. Pediatr Nephrol 28: 321–326.
21. Cox JL, Chiasson DA, Gotlieb AI (1991) Stranger in a strange land: the pathogenesis of saphenous vein graft stenosis with emphasis on structural and functional differences between veins and arteries. Prog Cardiovasc Dis 34: 45–68.
22. Davies MG, Hagen PO (1994) Pathobiology of intimal hyperplasia. Br J Surg 81: 1254–1269.
23. Newby AC, Zaltsman AB (2000) Molecular mechanisms in intimal hyperplasia. J Pathol 190: 300–309.
24. Ikeda Y, Biro S, Kamogawa Y, Yoshifuku S, Eto H, et al. (2001) Repeated thermal therapy upregulates arterial endothelial nitric oxide synthase expression in Syrian golden hamsters. Jpn Circ J 65: 434–438.
25. Kawaura A, Tanida N, Kamitani M, Akiyama J, Mizutani M, et al. (2010) The effect of leg hyperthermia using far infrared rays in bedridden subjects with type 2 diabetes mellitus. Acta Med Okayama 64: 143–147.
26. Huang CY, Yang RS, Kuo TS, Hsu KH (2009) Phantom limb pain treated by far infrared ray. Conf Proc IEEE Eng Med Biol Soc 2009: 1589–1591.
27. Toyokawa H, Matsui Y, Uhara J, Tsuchiya H, Teshima S, et al. (2003) Promotive effects of far-infrared ray on full-thickness skin wound healing in rats. Exp Biol Med (Maywood) 228: 724–729.
28. Capon A, Mordon S (2003) Can thermal lasers promote skin wound healing? Am J Clin Dermatol 4: 1–12.
29. Su LH, Wu KD, Lee LS, Wang H, Liu CF (2009) Effects of far infrared acupoint stimulation on autonomic activity and quality of life in hemodialysis patients. Am J Chin Med 37: 215–226.
30. Liberati A, Altman DG, Tetzlaff J, Mulrow C, Gotzsche PC, et al. (2009) The PRISMA statement for reporting systematic reviews and meta-analyses of studies that evaluate health care interventions: explanation and elaboration. PLoS Med 6: e1000100.
31. Higgins JP, Altman DG, Gotzsche PC, Juni P, Moher D, et al. (2011) The Cochrane Collaboration's tool for assessing risk of bias in randomised trials. BMJ 343: d5928.
32. The Nordic Cochrane Centre TCc (2012) Review Manager (RevMan) [Computer Program]. Version 5.2.
33. DerSimonian R, Laird NM (1983) Evaluating the Effect of Coaching on SAT Scores: A Meta-Analysis. Harvard Educational Review 53: 1–15.
34. Sterne JAC EM, Moher D (2011) Chapter 10: Addressing reporting biases. Higgins JPT, Green S (editors) Cochrane Handbook for Systematic Reviews of Intervention Version 5.1.0.
35. Lin CC, Chang CF, Lai MY, Chen TW, Lee PC, et al. (2007) Far-infrared therapy: a novel treatment to improve access blood flow and unassisted patency of arteriovenous fistula in hemodialysis patients. J Am Soc Nephrol 18: 985–992.
36. Lin CC, Chung MY, Yang WC, Lin SJ, Lee PC (2013) Length polymorphisms of heme oxygenase-1 determine the effect of far-infrared therapy on the function of arteriovenous fistula in hemodialysis patients: a novel physicogenomic study. Nephrol Dial Transplant 28: 1284–1293.
37. Lai CC, Fang HC, Mar GY, Liou JC, Tseng CJ, et al. (2013) Post-angioplasty far infrared radiation therapy improves 1-year angioplasty-free hemodialysis access patency of recurrent obstructive lesions. Eur J Vasc Endovasc Surg 46: 726–732.
38. Lin CC, Yang WC, Chen MC, Liu WS, Yang CY, et al. (2013) Effect of Far Infrared Therapy on Arteriovenous Fistula Maturation: An Open-Label Randomized Controlled Trial. Am J Kidney Dis.
39. W.-C LC-CY (2012) Far infrared therapy improves arteriovenous fistula maturation. Nephrology Dialysis Transplantation Conference: 50th ERA-EDTA Congress Istanbul Turkey Conference Start: 20120524 Conference End: 20120527.

40. Shipley T, Adam J, Sweeney D, Fenwick S, Mansy H, et al. (2012) Does far infrared therapy aid av fistula maturation and maintenance?. Nephrology Dialysis Transplantation Conference: 49th ERA-EDTA Congress Paris France Conference Start: 20120524 Conference End: 20120527 Conference Publication: (varpagings) 27 (ii261).
41. Lin CH, Lee LS, Su LH, Huang TC, Liu CF (2011) Thermal therapy in dialysis patients - a randomized trial. Am J Chin Med 39: 839–851.
42. Tu YP, Chen SC, Liu YH, Chen CF, Hour TC (2013) Postconditioning with far-infrared irradiation increases heme oxygenase-1 expression and protects against ischemia/reperfusion injury in rat testis. Life Sci 92: 35–41.
43. Akasaki Y, Miyata M, Eto H, Shirasawa T, Hamada N, et al. (2006) Repeated thermal therapy up-regulates endothelial nitric oxide synthase and augments angiogenesis in a mouse model of hindlimb ischemia. Circ J 70: 463–470.
44. Kipshidze N, Nikolaychik V, Muckerheidi M, Keelan MH, Chekanov V, et al. (2001) Effect of short pulsed nonablative infrared laser irradiation on vascular cells in vitro and neointimal hyperplasia in a rabbit balloon injury model. Circulation 104: 1850–1855.

8

Circulating MiR-133a as a Biomarker Predicts Cardiac Hypertrophy in Chronic Hemodialysis Patients

Ping Wen[1], Dan Song[3], Hong Ye[1], Xiaochun Wu[1], Lei Jiang[1], Bing Tang[1], Yang Zhou[1], Li Fang[1], Hongdi Cao[1], Weichun He[1], Yafang Yang[2], Chunsun Dai[1], Junwei Yang[1]*

1 Center for Kidney Disease, Second Affiliated Hospital, Nanjing Medical University, Nanjing, China, **2** Department of Radiology, Second Affiliated Hospital, Nanjing Medical University, Nanjing, China, **3** Department of Nephrology, Affiliated Wuxi Hospital, Nanjing Medical University, Wuxi, China

Abstract

Background: MicroRNAs (miRNAs) are small ribonucleotides regulating gene expression. MicroRNAs are present in the blood in a remarkably stable form and have emerged as potential diagnostic markers in patients with cardiovascular disease. Our study aimed to assess circulating miR-133a levels in MHD patients and the relation of miR-133a to cardiac hypertrophy.

Methods: We profiled miRNAs using RNA isolated from the plasma of participants. The results were validated in 64 MHD patients and 18 healthy controls.

Results: Levels of plasma miR-133a decreased in MHD patients with LVH compared with those in healthy controls. Plasma miR-133a concentrations were negatively correlated with LVMI and IVS. After single hemodialytic treatment, plasma miR-133a levels remained unchanged. Cardiac Troponin I and T were not associated with LVMI and IVS.

Conclusions: Our observations supplied the possibility that circulating miR-133a could be a surrogate biomarker of cardiac hypertrophy in MHD patients.

Editor: Sakthivel Sadayappan, Loyola University Chicago, United States of America

Funding: This work was supported by National Science Foundation of China Grants 31171093, "973" Science Program of the Ministry of Science and Technology, China (2011CB504005) to Junwei Yang. The author Weichun He was supported by National Science Foundation of China Grants 81170659. Junwei Yang took responsibility of the design of the study and Weichun He was in charge of the preparation of the manuscript. The funders had no role in study design, data collection and analysis, decision to publish, or preparation of the manuscript.

Competing Interests: The authors have declared that no competing interests exist.

* Email: jwyang@njmu.edu.cn

Introduction

Cardiovascular disease (CVD) is the main complication in patients with chronic kidney disease (CKD) and end stage renal disease (ESRD). More importantly, CVD is the leading cause of death in ESRD patients, accounting for 50% of all deaths in renal replacement therapy patients. In ESRD patients, a major pathophysiologic process frequently occurring in uremic hearts is left ventricular hypertrophy (LVH). Even though coronary artery disease and arrhythmia are not uncommon, LVH is the most frequent cardiovascular manifestation in these patients [1,2]. In addition, LVH is a very strong independent predictor of cardiovascular mortality not only among patients with hypertension but also among ESRD patients [3,4].

To date, several imaging modalities such as echocardiography (ECHO), magnetic resonance imaging (MRI) and computerized tomography have been performed to measure LVH [5,6,7]. ECHO is widely available, noninvasive, and has been demonstrated to be of reasonable accuracy in the assessment of LVH. However, ECHO might not be able to detect LVH in all dialysis patients [8]. In addition, there are studies implied serum biomarkers like arterial vasopressin, aldosterone and cardiac Troponin T appear to predict LVH [9,10]. However, stable and accurate serum biomarkers are not found, the present study evaluates whether a new biomarker for LVH can improve detection of LVH.

Recent studies have demonstrated that microRNAs (miRNAs) are present in the human circulation in a cell-free form and can be detected in circulating blood, thus may serve as a new class of blood-based biomarkers [11]. Numerous studies reported altered plasma or serum levels of various miRNAs in patients with cardiovascular diseases, including acute myocardial infarction [12,13], myocarditis [14], acute and chronic heart failure [14,15] and stable coronary artery disease [16]. Previous studies have found that miR-133a level was decreased in hypertrophic heart [17]. In study presented here, we measured plasma miR-133a in MHD patients and healthy controls and analyzed the relationship between miR-133a level and cardiac hypertrophy.

Subjects and Methods

Ethical statement

All of the following details of the study were approval by the responsible ethics committee of Nanjing Medical University

Table 1. Clinical characteristics of the study population.

characteristics	controls	MHD without LVH	MHD with LVH
Number	18	24	40
Men, n(%)	12(66.7)	14(58.3)	26(65)
Median age(range) (yr)	42(27–59)	46(29–69)	54(44–85)
Cardiovascular history, n(%)			
Myocardial infarction	0(0)	1(4.2)	0(0)
PTCA	0(0)	1(4.2)	0(0)
CABG	0(0)	0(0)	0(0)
Pacemaker	0(0)	0(0)	1(4.2)
Hypertension	0(0)	22(91.7)	35(87.5)
Diabetes	0(0)	0(0)	6(15)
Hypercholesterolemia	3(17.6)	2(8.3)	2(5)
Anemia, n(%)	0(0)	21(87.5)	28(70)
Renal failure, n(%)	0(0)	24(100)	40(100)
Hemodialysis, n(%)	0(0)	24(100)	44(100)
Median hemodialysis duration(range) (mo)	-	81(16–165)	94(12–306)
Laboratory examinations			
Hemoglobin (g/L)	-	106.8	100.9
Product of Ca and Pi (mg^2/dl^2)	-	49.4	44.9
iPTH (ng/ml)	-	314.3	210.7
Medication, n(%)			
Aspirin	0(0)	0(0)	1(4.2)
β-blocker	0(0)	8(33.3)	11(27.5)
CCB	0(0)	5(20.8)	18(45)
ACEI	0(0)	3(12.5)	5(12.5)
ARB	0(0)	2(8.3)	4(10)
Statins	0(0)	0(0)	0(0)
Warfarin	0(0)	0(0)	0(0)

PTCA: percutaneous transluminal coronary angioplasty; CABG: coronary artery bypass grafting; β-blocker: β receptor blocker; CCB: calcium-channel blocker; ACEI: angiotensin-converting enzyme inhibitor; ARB: angiotensin II type1 receptor blocker.

(Permit Number: KY2013019). And the written informed consent was supplied by the patients before the study.

Patients

The study population consists of 64 patients with ESRD undergoing regular hemodialysis from one clinical center and 18 healthy controls from one health examination center. Two blood samples of each patient were collected: one before hemodialysis another after hemodialysis, while one blood sample was obtained from each control. All the patients were evaluated with transthoracic echocardiography and 8 of them were measured with cardiac magnetic resonance.

Left ventricular mass index estimated by echocardiography

We measured the following parameters on the M-mode echocardiogram: left ventricular diastolic dimension (LVDd, cm), interventricular septum thickness (IVS, cm), and left ventricular posterior wall thickness (LVPW, cm). LV mass was calculated according to Devereux's formula [18]: left ventricular mass (g) $= 1.04 \times [(LVDd+IVS+LVPW)^3 - (LVDd)]^3 - 13.6$, where 1.04 ($g/cm^3$) is the specific gravity of the myocardium. It is the measurements of the peak value of R wave on the electrocardiograph. The left ventricular mass index (LVMI, g/m^2) was defined as left ventricular mass divided by body surface area (m^2).

Biochemical analyses

Plasma cardiac Troponin I (CA: DRE11443) and Troponin T (CA: DRE11403) were measured using the ELISA kit (fengxiang biotechnology company, Shanghai, China) by sandwich ELISA. The detection range were 10~300 ng/L and 5~220 ng/L respectively.

Plasma microRNA determination

Total RNA was extracted from plasma as previously described [19]. Quantitative RT-PCR was carried out using TaqMan miRNA probes (Applied Biosystems; Foster City, CA) according to the manufacturer's instructions. Real-time PCR was performed using a TaqMan PCR kit on an Applied Biosystems 7300 Sequence Detection System. The primer sequences of miR-133a was UUGGUCCCCUUCAACCAGCUGU. The mixtures of let-7d, let-7g and let-7i were used for our reference gene. To evaluate the change of miR-133a levels before and after hemodialysis, Δct was used, which can be calculated as the following equation: Δct = ct value (miR-133a)- ct value (let-7dgi).

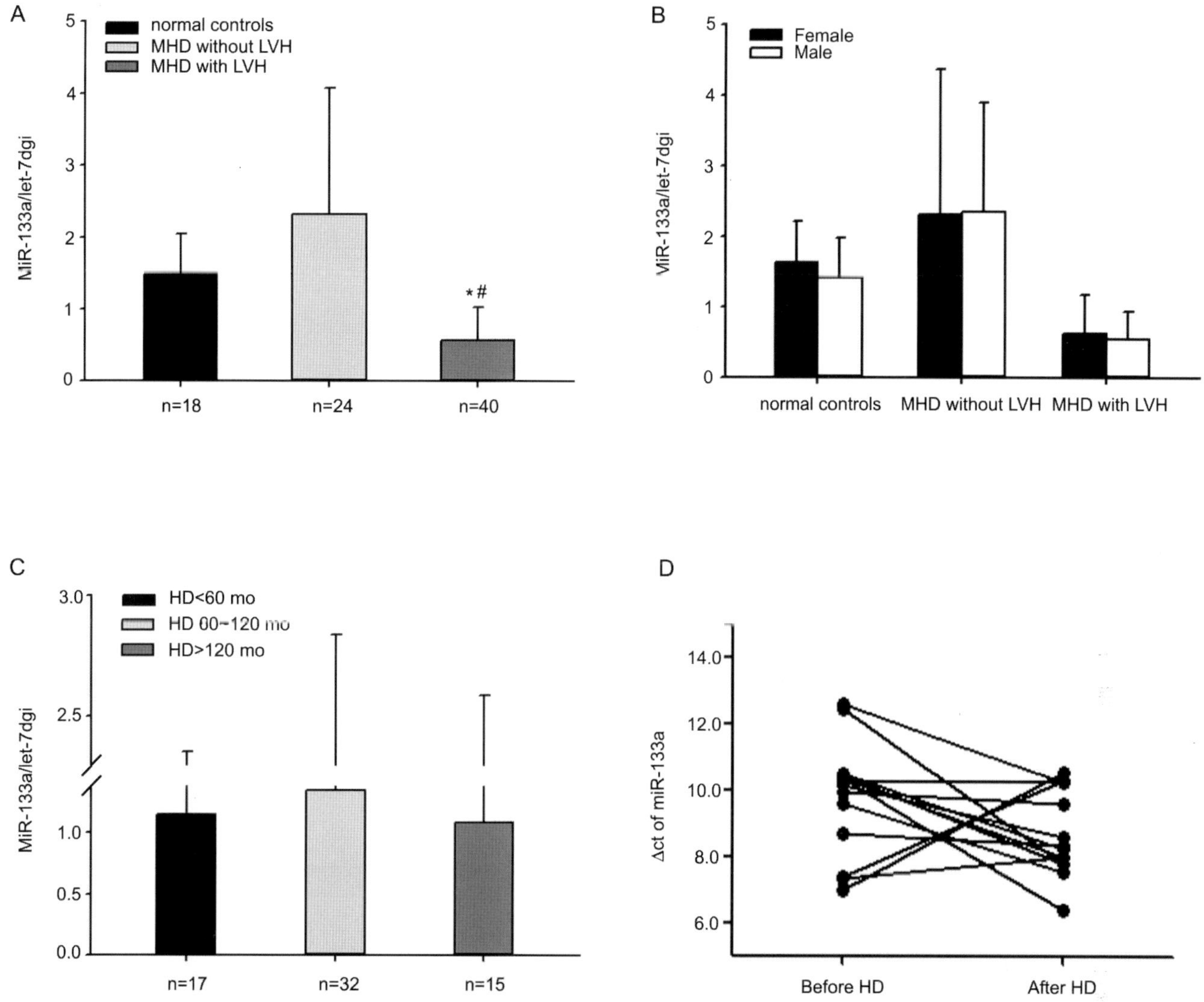

Figure 1. Plasma concentrations of miR-133a in healthy controls and MHD patients. The average miR-133a level of MHD patients with LVH was much lower than that of healthy controls and MHD patients without LVH, (0.57±0.46 *vs* 1.48±0.57, P = 0.000; 0.57±0.46 *vs* 2.33±1.75, P = < 0.001) (A). There were no differences in miR-133a level between male and female in controls (1.40±0.58 *vs* 1.63±0.58, P = 0.457) and MHD patients either with LVH (0.54±0.41 *vs* 0.63±0.55, P = 0.565) or without LVH (2.34±1.56 *vs* 2.31±2.07, P = 0.961) (B). When patients were divided into three groups according to the duration of hemodialysis, there was no significant difference in miR-133a levels between groups (1.15±1.21 *vs* 1.39±1.50 *vs* 1.02±1.48, P = 0.806) (C). Among 14 patients receiving hemodialytic treatment, miR-133a concentration remained unchanged after hemodialysis (D). Δct (ct value of 133a subtract ct value of let-7dgi) was used to evaluate the alteration. If Δct was increased, the level of miR-133a was decreased.

Statistical analyses

Data are presented as mean±SE unless otherwise described. To test the differences of miR-133a between MHD patients and healthy controls, t-test was used. Correlations were assessed using liner regression analysis and univariate logistic regression analysis method. Paired t-test was used to evaluate the change of miR-133a levels, Troponin I/T levels after hemodialysis. PASW statistics, version 18 was used to perform statistical analyses. A probability value <0.05 was considered to indicate statistical significance.

Results

Patient characteristics

A total of 82 subjects were enrolled in this study and 64 of them were ESRD patients receiving maintenance hemodialysis treatment. Clinical characteristics of all patients are shown in Table 1. 18 volunteers without documented kidney or heart diseases were used as healthy controls. Among the 64 patients, 40 had left ventricular hypertrophy which is defined as LVMI>125 g/m^2 in male and LVMI >115 g/m^2 in female. Thereby patients were divided into two groups according to the LVMI value. The traditional risk factors of LVH such as age, hypertension, and anemia were not significantly different between patients with LVH and without LVH. Among patients with LVH, there were 6 patients have diabetes. In contrast, all of the patients without LVH did not suffer the diabetes, suggesting that diabetes is a strong risk factor of LVH. There were no significant differences of laboratory indexes and medications between the two groups.

Plasma levels of miR-133a are decreased in MHD patients with LVH compared with those without LVH.

To investigate plasma miR-133a levels, blood samples were obtained from healthy controls and MHD patients before hemodialysis. The average level of plasma miR-133a was much

Table 2. Left ventricular mass index estimated by echocardiography and cardiac magnetic resonance.

patient	echocardiography			cardiac magnetic resonance		
	LVDd	IVS	LVPW(cm)	LVDd	IVS	LVPW(cm)
1	4.45	0.7	0.68	4.0	0.9	0.6
2	4.77	0.86	0.88	5.1	0.8	0.5
3	4.83	0.95	1.03	5.2	0.9	0.5
4	4.07	0.74	0.63	4.1	0.8	0.6
5	4.58	1.29	1.07	4.7	1.1	0.7
6	4.52	1.2	1.05	4.5	1.5	0.7
7	4.66	1.37	1.22	5.0	1.5	0.5
8	5.66	1.32	1.25	5.1	1.4	0.9

lower in MHD plus left ventricular hypertrophy group compared to MHD group, P = <0.001 (Figure 1A). There were no significant differences in miR-133a level between male and female both in healthy controls and MHD patients with or without LVH (Figure 1B). When patients were divided into three groups according to their duration of hemodialysis, there were no significant differences in plasma miR-133a levels between the groups (Figure 1C). The plasma miR-133a levels after hemodialysis were compared to that before hemodialysis in 14 MHD patients and it was found that miR-133a levels were not changed, P = 0.09 (Figure 1D).

Plasma miR-133a levels are negatively correlated with LVMI and IVS.

Previous study has demonstrated cardiac specific miR-133a control cardiac hypertrophy [17]. Therefore, we estimated the association between plasma miR-133a and cardiac hypertrophy. All of the patients were evaluated with ECHO while 8 of them were measured with MRI. It was confirmed that the findings from echocardiography were consistent with the results of MRI so they were credible (Table 2). To elucidate whether plasma miR-133a concentration were associated with cardiac hypertrophy in MHD patients, the liner regression analysis was used and it indicated that plasma miR-133a level were negatively correlated with IVS and LVMI, $R^2 = 0.319$ and 0.383 respectively, P = <0.001 (Figure 2A, B). To further confirm the correlation between plasma miR-133a level and LVH, univariate logistic regression analysis was used to analyze the association of miR-133a level and IVS/LVMI, other clinical characteristics were also analyzed. Table 3 showed that plasma miR-133a level were only negatively correlated with IVS and LVMI, 95% confidence intervals were 0.084 to 0.677 and 0.043 to 0.396 respectively.

Plasma levels of cardiac Troponin I and Troponin T were not increased in MHD patients before hemodialysis and not correlated with cardiac hypertrophy

Cardiac Troponin I and Troponin T are common biomarkers of cardiac infarction. We assessed plasma levels of cardiac Troponin I and Troponin T in MHD patients and healthy controls. Significant differences were not found in both biomarkers between controls and patients (Figure 3A, B). There was no significant correlations between Troponin I/T levels and LVMI

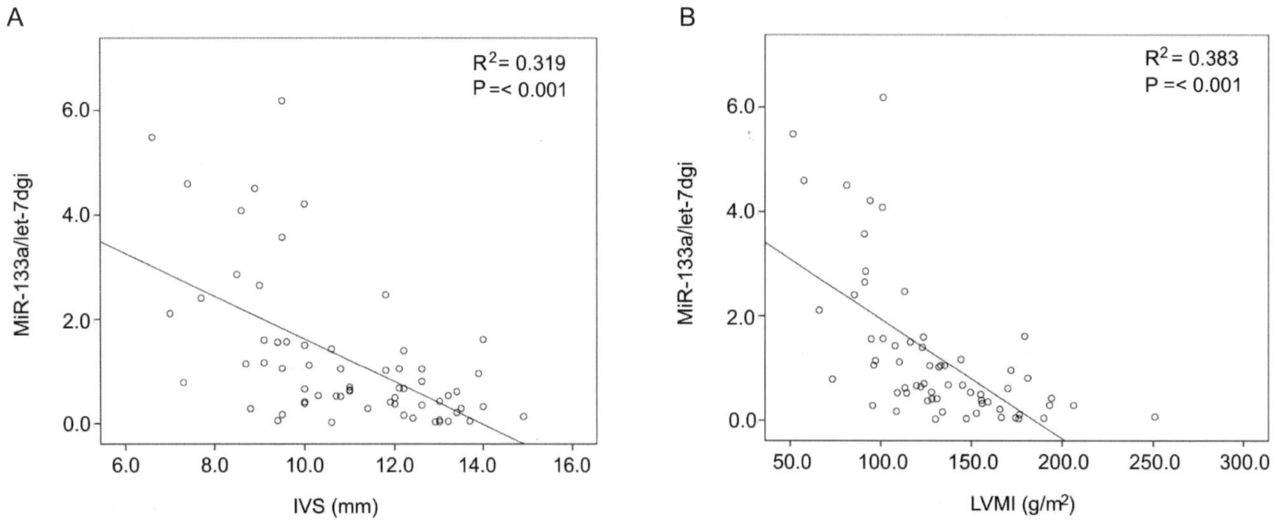

Figure 2. The correlation between plasma miR-133a level and cardiac hypertrophy in ESRD patients receiving maintenance hemodialysis treatment. Liner regression analysis showed that plasma miR-133a concentration was negatively correlated with IVS and LVMI, the correlation coefficient was 0.319 and 0.383 respectively, P = <0.001 (A, B).

Table 3. Univariate logistic regression analysis of plasma miR-133a and clinical characteristics.

Variates	95%CI
Gender	0.402–3.043
Age	0.151–1.129
Cardiovascular history	
Hypertension	0.304–7.226
Diabetes	0.074–2.567
Hypercholesterolemia	0.167–22.482
Left ventricular hypertrophy	0.044–0.461*
Anemia	0.406–7.985
Median hemodialysis duration	0.151–1.129
Medication	
β-blocker	0.269–0.306
CCB	0.215–1.686
ACEI	0.313–2.389
ARB	0.074–2.567
Laboratory index	
Troponin I	0.375–5.437
Troponin T	0.229–3.344
LVMI	0.043–0.396*
IVS	0.084–0.677*

CI: confidence interval.

(Figure 3C, D). Hemodialysis did not change Troponin I levels except that Troponin I decreased dramatically after hemodialysis in one patient (Figure 3E). Also, there was no significant difference between the Troponin T levels before and after hemodialysis, P = 0.289 (Figure 3F).

Discussion

In our study, we demonstrated that circulating miR-133a level was decreased in MHD patients compared with healthy controls. Since the expression of miR-133a in heart is decreased in cardiac hypertrophy animal model [17], we analyzed the correlation between circulating miR-133a levels and cardiac hypertrophy in MHD patients. It was found that the miR-133a level was negatively associated with LVMI, an indicator of left ventricular hypertrophy (LVH), in these patients.

The heart has capable of remodeling in response to various environmental demands and a variety of stimuli can induce it to growth or shrink. In MHD patients, primary or secondary hypertension, volume overload, hemodynamic stress and uremia toxins can alone or together induce cardiac hypertrophy.

MicroRNAs are important regulators of a wide range of cellular processes by modulating gene expression and are estimated to regulate more than 30% of the genes in a cell [20]. Recent studies both in animals and humans have demonstrated that miRNAs are present in the circulation and can be detected and quantified [11,19]. Previous studies have indicated that miR-133a is highly expressed in cardiac and skeletal muscle and is regulated in hypertrophy and failure [17,21]. Circulating miR-133a levels were measured in several studies and were consistently elevated in patients with cardiac infarction and were closely related with high-sensitivity cardiac Troponin [12,22,23,24].

In the present study, we detected circulating miR-133a levels in MHD patients and healthy controls and demonstrated that miR-133a concentrations were decreased in MHD patients with LVH. Among 64 patients enrolled in our study, most of them (89.4%) had hypertension and about half underwent hypertension more than 5 years, but not all of them had decreased miR-133a levels. The significant association between miR-133a level and LVMI indicated that circulating miR-133a may play important role in the process of LVH and could be a biomarker of LVH. In addition, our study showed that plasma miR-133a concentrations were not changed after hemodialysis. There have been some studies investigated the influence of hemodialysis on circulating microRNA levels [25,26,27] and demonstrated different results. Daniel R. and colleagues elucidated miR-499p could be eliminated by hemodialysis [27], however, Thomas Thum [25] and Dai Y [26] indicated that circulating microRNAs could not be cleared by hemodialysis. Although the molecular weight of miRNAs is small enough to permeate the dialysis membrane, it is reported that miRNAs are likely to be transported by larger structures such as proteins and/or microvesicles [28]. Our results implied that miR-133a was not eliminated after hemodialysis. Therefore, we suggest that circulating miR-133a levels before hemodialysis treatment should be used to predict LVH.

Cardiac Troponins are considered the gold standard of biomarkers for the diagnosis of myocardial infarction at present. In our study, no patients suffered from myocardial infarction at the study time. Therefore, the plasma cardiac Troponin-I/T levels were similar to that of healthy controls. Although there was study indicated that cardiac Troponin T concentration positively correlated with left ventricular hypertrophy in hemodialysis patients and predicted lower survival rates [9], we think Troponin-T is more sensitive in cardiac infarction but not hypertrophy.

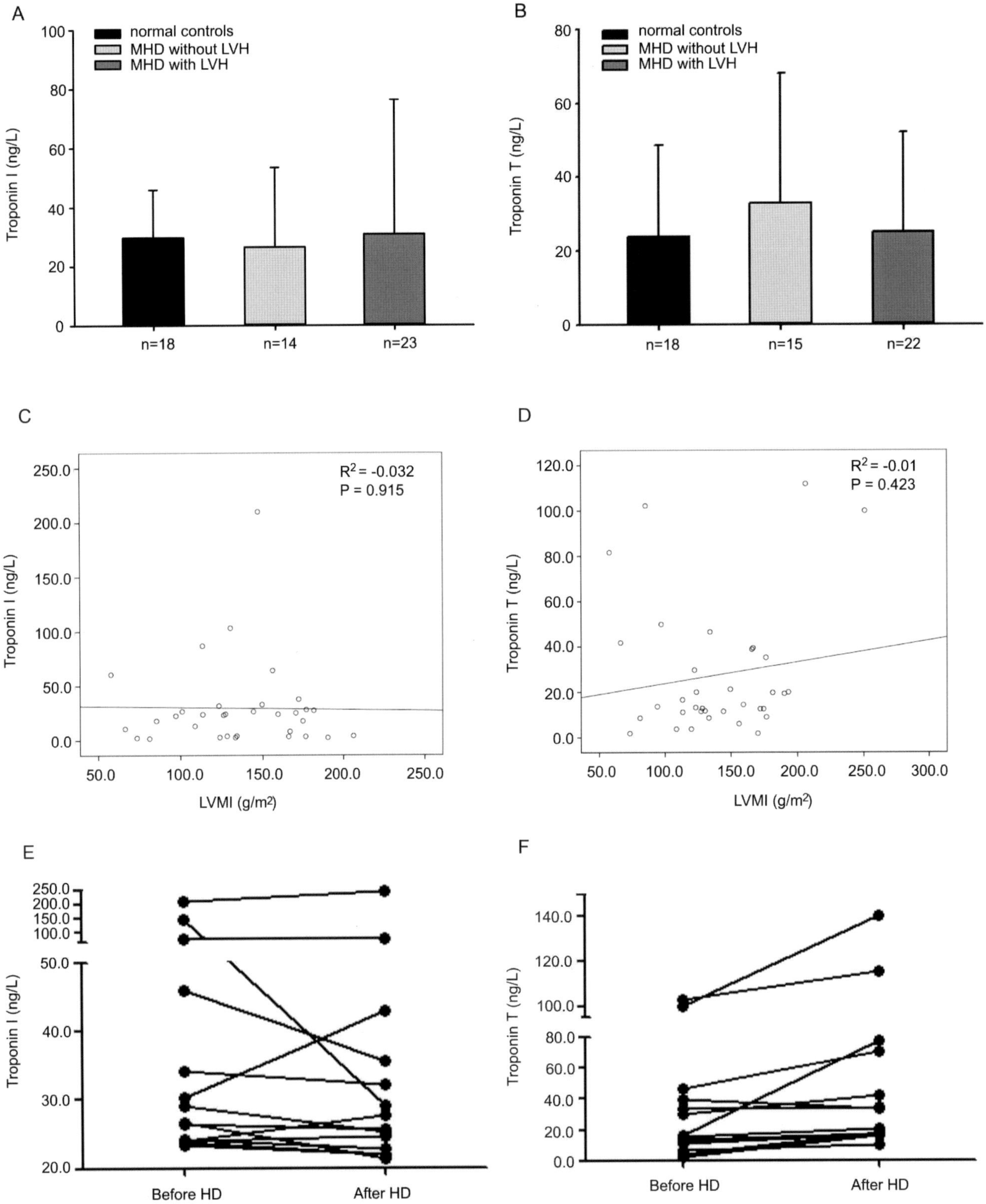

Figure 3. Plasma levels of cardiac Troponin I/T and the correlation between Troponin I/T levels and LVMI/IVS. There were no significant differences between healthy controls and MHD patients in both biomarkers before the hemodialysis treatment (cTnI: 29.72±16.16 *vs* 29.55±40.35, P=0.983; cTnT: 23.85±24.67 *vs* 27.47±29.16, P=0.650) (A, B). No significant differences of Troponin I/T levels were found between MHD patients plus LVH and those without LVH (cTnI: 30.85±45.46 *vs* 26.55±26.85, P=0.784; cTnT: 25.22±26.92 *vs* 33.07±35.07, P=0.480) (A, B). There were no correlation between LVMI and Troponin I/T before hemodialysis treatment (C, D). After hemodialysis, the cardiac Troponin I level remained unchanged in most patients except that it was evident decrease in one patient (E). There were no significant differences of the plasma Troponin T level between before and after hemodialysis (F).

This study is limited by its small size. In addition, MHD patients differed from controls in terms of age, cardiovascular history, and risk factors. More subjects need to be involved in our future study.

In conclusion, plasma miR-133a levels are decreased in MHD patients with LVH. MiR-133a levels are negatively associated with LVMI, indicating that the lower miR-133a level, the more obvious left ventricular hypertrophy. Our observations supplied the possibility that circulating miR-133a can be a blood-based biomarker for cardiac hypertrophy.

Author Contributions

Conceived and designed the experiments: JY. Performed the experiments: PW. Analyzed the data: PW DS. Wrote the paper: PW. Participated in designing the experiment: CD. In charge of the preparation of the manuscript: WH. Made some contributions in the experiments: DS. Collected the information of the patients: HY XW BT. Did part work of the experiment: LJ YZ LF HC. Analysis tools: YY.

References

1. Middleton RJ, Parfrey PS, Foley RN (2001) Left ventricular hypertrophy in the renal patient. J Am Soc Nephrol 12: 1079–1084.
2. Levin A, Djurdjev O, Thompson C, Barrett B, Ethier J, et al. (2005) Canadian randomized trial of hemoglobin maintenance to prevent or delay left ventricular mass growth in patients with CKD. Am J Kidney Dis 46: 799–811.
3. Silberberg JS, Barre PE, Prichard SS, Sniderman AD (1989) Impact of left ventricular hypertrophy on survival in end-stage renal disease. Kidney Int 36: 286–290.
4. Zoccali C, Benedetto FA, Mallamaci F, Tripepi G, Giacone G, et al. (2004) Left ventricular mass monitoring in the follow-up of dialysis patients: prognostic value of left ventricular hypertrophy progression. Kidney Int 65: 1492–1498.
5. Levy D, Garrison RJ, Savage DD, Kannel WB, Castelli WP (1990) Prognostic implications of echocardiographically determined left ventricular mass in the Framingham Heart Study. N Engl J Med 322: 1561–1566.
6. Stewart GA, Foster J, Cowan M, Rooney E, McDonagh T, et al. (1999) Echocardiography overestimates left ventricular mass in hemodialysis patients relative to magnetic resonance imaging. Kidney Int 56: 2248–2253.
7. Truong QA, Ptaszek LM, Charipar EM, Taylor C, Fontes JD, et al. (2010) Performance of electrocardiographic criteria for left ventricular hypertrophy as compared with cardiac computed tomography: from the Rule Out Myocardial Infarction Using Computer Assisted Tomography trial. J Hypertens 28: 1959–1967.
8. Jakubovic BD, Wald R, Goldstein MB, Leong-Poi H, Yuen DA, et al. (2013) Comparative assessment of 2-dimensional echocardiography vs cardiac magnetic resonance imaging in measuring left ventricular mass in patients with and without end-stage renal disease. Can J Cardiol 29: 384–390.
9. Petrovic D, Obrenovic R, Stojimirovic B (2008) Cardiac troponins and left ventricular hypertrophy in hemodialysis patients. Clin Lab 54: 145–152.
10. Strand AH, Gudmundsdottir H, Fossum E, Os I, Bjornerheim R, et al. (2007) Arterial plasma vasopressin and aldosterone predict left ventricular mass in men who develop hypertension over 20 years. J Clin Hypertens (Greenwich) 9: 365–371.
11. Mitchell PS, Parkin RK, Kroh EM, Fritz BR, Wyman SK, et al. (2008) Circulating microRNAs as stable blood-based markers for cancer detection. Proc Natl Acad Sci U S A 105: 10513–10518.
12. D'Alessandra Y, Devanna P, Limana F, Straino S, Di Carlo A, et al. (2010) Circulating microRNAs are new and sensitive biomarkers of myocardial infarction. Eur Heart J 31: 2765–2773.
13. Cheng Y, Tan N, Yang J, Liu X, Cao X, et al. (2010) A translational study of circulating cell-free microRNA-1 in acute myocardial infarction. Clin Sci (Lond) 119: 87–95.
14. Corsten MF, Dennert R, Jochems S, Kuznetsova T, Devaux Y, et al. (2010) Circulating MicroRNA-208b and MicroRNA-499 reflect myocardial damage in cardiovascular disease. Circ Cardiovasc Genet 3: 499–506.
15. Tijsen AJ, Creemers EE, Moerland PD, de Windt LJ, van der Wal AC, et al. (2010) MiR423-5p as a circulating biomarker for heart failure. Circ Res 106: 1035–1039.
16. Fichtlscherer S, De Rosa S, Fox H, Schwietz T, Fischer A, et al. (2010) Circulating microRNAs in patients with coronary artery disease. Circ Res 107: 677–684.
17. Care A, Catalucci D, Felicetti F, Bonci D, Addario A, et al. (2007) MicroRNA-133 controls cardiac hypertrophy. Nat Med 13: 613–618.
18. Devereux RB, Reichek N (1977) Echocardiographic determination of left ventricular mass in man. Anatomic validation of the method. Circulation 55: 613–618.
19. Chen X, Ba Y, Ma L, Cai X, Yin Y, et al. (2008) Characterization of microRNAs in serum: a novel class of biomarkers for diagnosis of cancer and other diseases. Cell Res 18: 997–1006.
20. Lewis BP, Burge CB, Bartel DP (2005) Conserved seed pairing, often flanked by adenosines, indicates that thousands of human genes are microRNA targets. Cell 120: 15–20.
21. Chen JF, Mandel EM, Thomson JM, Wu Q, Callis TE, et al. (2006) The role of microRNA-1 and microRNA-133 in skeletal muscle proliferation and differentiation. Nat Genet 38: 228–233.
22. Wang GK, Zhu JQ, Zhang JT, Li Q, Li Y, et al. (2010) Circulating microRNA: a novel potential biomarker for early diagnosis of acute myocardial infarction in humans. Eur Heart J 31: 659–666.
23. Gidlof O, Andersson P, van der Pals J, Gotberg M, Erlinge D (2011) Cardiospecific microRNA plasma levels correlate with troponin and cardiac function in patients with ST elevation myocardial infarction, are selectively dependent on renal elimination, and can be detected in urine samples. Cardiology 118: 217–226.
24. Eitel I, Adams V, Dieterich P, Fuernau G, de Waha S, et al. (2012) Relation of circulating MicroRNA-133a concentrations with myocardial damage and clinical prognosis in ST-elevation myocardial infarction. Am Heart J 164: 706–714.
25. Martino F, Lorenzen J, Schmidt J, Schmidt M, Broll M, et al. (2012) Circulating microRNAs are not eliminated by hemodialysis. PLoS One 7: e38269.
26. Wang H, Peng W, Ouyang X, Dai Y (2012) Reduced circulating miR-15b is correlated with phosphate metabolism in patients with end-stage renal disease on maintenance hemodialysis. Ren Fail 34: 685–690.
27. Emilian C, Goretti E, Prospert F, Pouthier D, Duhoux P, et al. (2012) MicroRNAs in patients on chronic hemodialysis (MINOS study). Clin J Am Soc Nephrol 7: 619–623.
28. Lorenzen JM, Thum T (2012) Circulating and urinary microRNAs in kidney disease. Clin J Am Soc Nephrol 7: 1528–1533.

Survival after Acute Hemodialysis in Pennsylvania, 2005–2007: A Retrospective Cohort Study

Sarah J. Ramer[1]*, Elan D. Cohen[2], Chung-Chou H. Chang[2,3], Mark L. Unruh[4], Amber E. Barnato[2,5,6,7]

1 Rutgers New Jersey Medical School, Newark, New Jersey, United States of America, **2** Division of General Internal Medicine, Department of Medicine, University of Pittsburgh School of Medicine, Pittsburgh, Pennsylvania, United States of America, **3** Department of Biostatistics, University of Pittsburgh Graduate School of Public Health, Pittsburgh, Pennsylvania, United States of America, **4** Division of Nephrology, Department of Internal Medicine, University of New Mexico School of Medicine, Albuquerque, New Mexico, United States of America, **5** Department of Clinical and Translational Science, University of Pittsburgh School of Medicine, Pittsburgh, Pennsylvania, United States of America, **6** Department of Health Policy and Management, University of Pittsburgh Graduate School of Public Health, Pittsburgh, Pennsylvania, United States of America, **7** The CRISMA Laboratory (Clinical Research, Investigation, and Systems Modeling of Acute Illness), Department of Critical Care Medicine, University of Pittsburgh, Pittsburgh, Pennsylvania, United States of America

Abstract

Background: Little is known about acute hemodialysis in the US. Here we describe predictors of receipt of acute hemodialysis in one state and estimate the marginal impact of acute hemodialysis on survival after accounting for confounding due to illness severity.

Materials and Methods: This is a retrospective cohort study of acute-care hospitalizations in Pennsylvania from October 2005 to December 2007 using data from the Pennsylvania Health Care Cost Containment Council. Exposure variable is acute hemodialysis; dependent variable is survival following acute hemodialysis. We used multivariable logistic regression to determine propensity to receive acute hemodialysis and then, for a Cox proportional hazards model, matched acute hemodialysis and non-acute hemodialysis patients 1:5 on this propensity.

Results: In 2,131,248 admissions of adults without end-stage renal disease, there were 6,657 instances of acute hemodialysis. In analyses adjusted for predicted probability of death upon admission plus other covariates and stratified on age, being male, black, and insured were independent predictors of receipt of acute hemodialysis. One-year post-admission mortality was 43% for those receiving acute hemodialysis, compared to 13% among those not receiving acute hemodialysis. After matching on propensity to receive acute hemodialysis and adjusting for predicted probability of death upon admission, patients who received acute hemodialysis had a higher risk of death than patients who did not over at least 1 year of follow-up (hazard ratio 1·82, 95% confidence interval 1·68–1·97).

Conclusions: In a populous US state, receipt of acute hemodialysis varied by age, sex, race, and insurance status even after adjustment for illness severity. In a comparison of patients with similar propensity to receive acute hemodialysis, those who did receive it were less likely to survive than those who did not. These findings raise questions about reasons for lack of benefit.

Editor: Shree Ram Singh, National Cancer Institute, United States of America

Funding: This work was supported by a Doris Duke Clinical Research Fellowship for Medical Students to SR (http://www.ddcf.org/) and by National Institutes of Health grant R01AG035112 to AB (http://www.nih.gov/). The funders had no role in study design, data collection and analysis, decision to publish, or preparation of the manuscript.

Competing Interests: The authors have declared that no competing interests exist.

* Email: sramer@post.harvard.edu

Introduction

Acute hemodialysis (HD), defined as intermittent or continuous, non-peritoneal renal replacement therapy for patients without end-stage renal disease (ESRD), typically in the context of critical illness, is thought to save lives. Overall, however, the prognosis for patients requiring acute HD is poor, with estimates of in-hospital mortality in the literature ranging from 33% [1]-61% [2]. In a large high-quality clinical trial comparing different intensities of renal support for patients with acute kidney injury (AKI), 60-day mortality was nearly 53% [3]; in another such trial, 90-day mortality approached 45% [4]. Moreover, survivors are at high risk for continued renal failure [5–9] and decreased quality of life [10–12], and acute HD adds to the already substantial cost of care for the critically ill in the US [13,14].

Although the US Renal Data System provides detailed information about patients with ESRD undergoing chronic HD, less is known about the epidemiology of acute HD. Several studies, most notably that of Xue and colleagues [1], have reported on the incidence and mortality of AKI among various populations of

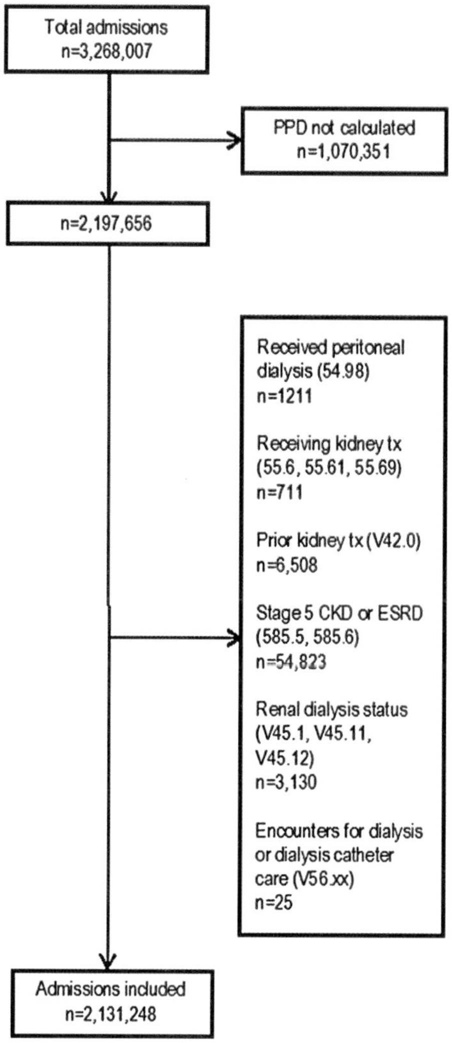

Figure 1. Sample selection process. PPD - predicted probability of death in-hospital, calculated from key clinical findings at admission; tx - transplant; CKD - chronic kidney disease; ESRD - end-stage renal disease.

hospitalized patients in the US [2,6,8]. To our knowledge, however, no study has specifically focused on the predictors of or survival after acute HD.

In the current study, we describe predictors of the receipt of acute HD in a dataset encompassing over 2 million hospital admissions. We then attempt to estimate the marginal impact of acute HD on patient survival after accounting for confounding due to illness severity.

Materials and Methods

Data source

We conducted a retrospective cohort study of adult acute-care hospitalizations in Pennsylvania from October 2005 to December 2007 using data from the Pennsylvania (PA) Health Care Cost Containment Council (PHC4) linked to PA Department of Health death data through December 2008. PHC4 is an independent state agency that collects this data under mandate from the state government. The PHC4 data includes patient demographics, International Classification of Diseases, 9th Revision, Clinical Modification (ICD-9-CM) diagnosis and procedure codes, and the predicted probability of inpatient death at the time of admission for all patients with certain pre-specified diagnosis-related groups (DRGs) and ICD-9-CM codes. (See Text S1. Diagnosis-related groups or International Classification of Diseases, 9th Revision, Clinical Modification principal diagnoses for which the Pennsylvania Health Care Cost Containment Council required predicted probability of inpatient death to be calculated, by year.) The predicted probability of death (PPD) is based upon MediQual mortality models using key clinical findings abstracted from the chart during the first 48 hours of admission. These models significantly out perform those based upon administrative fields alone, with average c-statistics of 0.86 [15]. It is important to note that the PHC4 data does not include any Current Procedural Terminology (CPT) codes; therefore, it is not possible to distinguish between intermittent HD and all other forms of renal replacement therapy in the PHC4 data.

Exposure variable

Our principal exposure variable was acute HD. We defined acute HD as the receipt of HD (ICD-9-CM procedure code 39.95) by patients without ESRD. We excluded from all analyses admissions with ICD-9-CM diagnosis codes that would indicate current ESRD (585.6, V45.1, V45.11, V45.12, V56.xx), imminent ESRD, i.e., stage 5 chronic kidney disease (CKD) (585.5), or prior ESRD treated with kidney transplant (V42.0). We further excluded admissions with ICD-9-CM procedure codes for kidney transplant (55.6, 55.61, 55.69) or peritoneal dialysis (54.98), as these are procedures that only patients with ESRD undergo. For a flowchart depicting the sample selection process, see Figure 1.

Dependent variable

The primary dependent variable is time to death, in days, from hospital admission. The minimum length of follow-up was one year.

Covariates

Patient-level covariates included demographics, insurance status (commercial and/or Medicare, Medicaid with or without Medicare, and uninsured), principal diagnoses (classified into groups from ICD-9-CM codes using Agency for Healthcare Research and Quality Clinical Classification Software), and illness severity, as measured by the MediQual PPD (available for the 67% of admissions with one of the DRGs or ICD-9-CM codes for which PHC4 required that it be calculated). Hospital-level covariates included number of hospital beds, resident-to-bed ratio (a measure of teaching intensity), percent of patients who are black (a measure of racial concentration, correlated with treatment intensity and risk-adjusted mortality), and a Bayesian shrinkage estimator of the observed-to-expected ratio, i.e., standardized rate, of HD among patients at 95th percentile of PPD upon admission ("end-of-life" HD treatment intensity) [16]. (See Figure S1. Standardized [observed-to-expected] hemodialysis use for patients at high probability of dying upon admission, by hospital, Pennsylvania 2001–2007.)

Statistical analyses

We first descriptively summarized the characteristics of admissions in which patients received acute HD and compared them to admissions in which patients did not receive acute HD by employing chi-squared and t-tests. Using multivariable logistic regression with a random effect for hospital, we calculated a propensity score to receive acute HD based on patient- and hospital-level covariates for every admission, stratified by age (less than 65 years old and 65 years or older). We made the decision to stratify after a graphical analysis showed that the proportion of admissions with acute HD peaked at age 65 and declined thereafter.

On the basis of these propensity scores, we matched admissions with acute HD to those without acute HD in a ratio of 1:5. If a patient had more than one admission, we used only the first admission, even if acute HD was not given in the first admission but was given in a subsequent admission. The rationale for this was to avoid bias, as a patient who underwent acute HD on a 2nd, 3rd, or subsequent admission and then died would seem to have a shorter survival if there was "resetting of the survival clock," so to speak, to the time of that 2nd, 3rd, or subsequent admission. In order to improve the closeness of the matches, we employed matching with replacement, meaning that a non-HD admission could be re-used for matching with an HD admission. To gauge the effectiveness of matching, we used inverse probability treatment weighting to check the covariate balance between the acute HD and non-acute HD groups after propensity score matching. This method allowed us to compare pre- and post-matching samples more accurately since it maintained the original sample size. (See Figure S2. Covariate balance before and after inverse probability treatment weighting by propensity score.)

We plotted Kaplan-Meier survival curves of time to death, up to one year from admission, for admissions with and without acute HD. We then used Cox proportional hazards models to assess the effect of acute HD on survival, with covariate adjustment. Covariates included only patient-level variables, as hospital-level variables were not significantly associated with survival. To reduce indication (severity) bias, we calculated hazards of dying among admissions with and without acute HD, matched for propensity to receive acute HD, with covariate adjustment. We accounted for dependence between patients within a hospital by using the Huber-White sandwich estimator for standard errors. We performed all analyses with Stata version 11 (StataCorp, College Station, TX).

Sensitivity analyses

Along with our main analyses, we performed 3 sensitivity analyses. The first only involved the calculation of propensity scores. Due to the possibility that our sample selection process might have incorrectly classified some HD given to ESRD patients as acute HD, we dropped all patients with Medicare, given that ESRD is a Medicare-qualifying condition, as well as all patients 65 years or older, given that most of them have Medicare, and again ran the multivariable logistic regression models.

The next two sensitivity analyses involved both the calculation of propensity scores and the survival modeling. One used the sample selection process depicted in Figure 1 but then further limited the sample to only admissions that included a stay in the intensive care unit (ICU). We then conducted the same statistical procedures as in the main analysis.

The final sensitivity analysis used the sample selection process depicted in Figure 1 but did not exclude admissions for which the MediQual PPD was not calculated. Instead of using the MediQual PPD as the main risk adjustor, we used the Charlson Comorbidity Index [17,18]. Once again, we then carried out the same statistical procedures as in the main analysis.

Ethics statement

We conducted this research under a data use agreement with PHC4, which acted as an honest broker to merge hospital discharge data with PA Department of Health death records. The University of Pittsburgh Institutional Review Board reviewed and approved the study, which met US federal criteria for exemption from written informed consent because data were not connected to any patient identifiers.

Results

The characteristics of the full sample by acute HD status are detailed in Table 1. Patients who received acute HD differed significantly from those who did not in age, sex, race, and insurance status. Men ($P<0.001$), black patients ($P<0.001$), and insured patients ($P<0.001$) were all more likely to receive acute HD. The most common principal diagnoses among those who received acute HD were acute and unspecified renal failure; septicemia; non-hypertensive congestive heart failure; respiratory failure, insufficiency, or arrest; and diabetes mellitus with complications. As would be expected, acute HD patients were sicker, as reflected in their higher PPD on admission ($P<0.001$) and higher mortality at every time point ($P<0.001$ for all).

As shown in Table 2, in multivariable logistic regression, age, sex, race, and PPD were independently associated with receipt of acute HD. For patients less than 65 years old, increasing age predicted higher odds of receiving acute HD ($P=0.001$); for patients 65 years or older, increasing age predicted lower odds of receiving acute HD ($P<0.001$). In both age groups, male and black patients were more likely to receive acute HD ($P<0.001$ for each). In the under-65 age group, being uninsured was associated with lower odds of receiving acute HD ($P<0.001$). In both age groups, admission to a hospital with a larger bed count ($P<0.001$ in under-65, $P=0.005$ in 65 and older, data not shown) and higher standardized rate of HD among patients at a high probability of dying upon admission were associated with receipt of acute HD ($P<0.001$ for both age groups, data not shown).

The characteristics of the matched sample by acute HD status are displayed in Table 1. Of the 6113 patients who received acute HD in the time period covered by the study, only 3483 did so in their first admission and were therefore eligible for matching. After matching, there was no longer a significant difference between the groups in sex ($P=0.615$). A significant difference persisted for age measured continuously ($P=0.004$), but in the matched sample the patients who received acute HD actually had a lower mean age, as opposed to in the full sample, in which they had a higher mean age. Significant differences also persisted for race ($P<0.001$), insurance status ($P<0.001$), and PPD on admission ($P=0.002$), but as Figure S2 in the supplemental digital content demonstrates, these differences were very much attenuated in the matched sample. Patients who did and did not receive acute HD continued to differ significantly in mortality at every time point ($P<0.001$ for all).

Figure 2 shows Kaplan-Meier curves for patients who did and did not receive acute HD. As would be expected based upon their illness severity, the patients who received acute HD were more likely to die throughout the follow-up period. In the fully adjusted Cox model before propensity score matching, the acute HD patients had a higher risk of death (hazard ratio [HR] 1.78, 95% confidence interval [CI] 1.58–2.00). The survival difference persisted essentially unchanged in the fully adjusted Cox model after propensity score matching (HR 1.82, 95% CI 1.68–1.97; Figure 3).

The sensitivity analysis excluding patients insured by Medicare or 65 years or older produced odds ratios qualitatively unchanged from those obtained from the main analysis. The sensitivity analysis restricted to patients admitted to the ICU differed notably from the main analysis in that, for patients younger than 65, increasing age was not significantly associated with higher odds of

Table 1. Characteristics of full and matched samples by acute hemodialysis status, Pennsylvania 2005–2007.

	Full sample			Matched sample		
	No acute HD	Acute HD	P	No acute HD	Acute HD	P
Admissions[a] (n)	2,124,591	6,657		17,415	3,483	
Patients (n)	1,283,053	6,113		16,167	3,483	
Female (%)	1,201,352 (57)	3,043 (46)	<0.001	7,856 (45)	1,555 (45)	0.615
Age (yrs)	65.0±17.9	65.5±15.0	0.024	65.2±15.9	64.4±15.5	0.004
Age (%)[b]			<0.001			0.026
21–49	452,764 (21)	1,034 (16)		2,982 (17)	626 (18)	
50–59	321,349 (15)	1,179 (18)		2,883 (17)	625 (18)	
60–69	358,797 (17)	1,439 (22)		3,863 (22)	746 (21)	
70–79	454,958 (21)	1,697 (25)		4,174 (24)	851 (24)	
80+	536,723 (25)	1,308 (20)		3,513 (20)	635 (18)	
Race (%)[b]			<0.001			<0.001
White	1,792,633 (84)	4,899 (74)		13,065 (75)	2,463 (71)	
Black	218,565 (10)	1,393 (21)		3,496 (20)	816 (23)	
Hispanic	38,395 (1.8)	141 (2.1)		292 (1.7)	80 (2.3)	
Asian/Pacific Islander	7,798 (0.37)	27 (0.41)		84 (0.48)	20 (0.57)	
Other/unknown	67,200 (3.2)	197 (3)		478 (2.7)	104 (3)	
Insurance (%)[b]			<0.001			<0.001
Commercial and/or Medicare	1,688,748 (80)	4,642 (70)		12,646 (73)	2,418 (69)	
Medicaid with/without Medicare	404,928 (19)	1,969 (30)		4,601 (26)	1,037 (30)	
Uninsured	30,142 (1.4)	44 (0.66)		168 (0.96)	28 (0.8)	
Primary diagnosis (%)						
Acute and unspecified renal failure	37,021 (1.7)	1,659 (25)	<0.001	4,087 (23)	816 (23)	0.959
Septicemia (except in labor)	55,833 (2.6)	900 (14)	<0.001	2,041 (12)	460 (13)	0.014
Congestive heart failure, non-hypertensive	121,786 (5.7)	547 (8.2)	<0.001	1,204 (6.9)	234 (6.7)	0.678
Respiratory failure, insufficiency, or arrest	33,132 (1.6)	328 (4.9)	<0.001	820 (4.7)	173 (5)	0.513
Diabetes mellitus with complications	40,435 (1.9)	323 (4.9)	<0.001	912 (5.2)	176 (5.1)	0.656
Predicted probability of death upon admission[c]	0.031±0.084	0.14±0.2	<0.001	0.11±0.21	0.13±0.19	0.002
Mortality (%)						
During admission	50,478 (2.4)	1,258 (19)	<0.001	1,480 (8.5)	589 (17)	<0.001
By 90 d post-admit date	194,257 (9.1)	2,309 (35)	<0.001	3,047 (17)	1,059 (30)	<0.001
By 1 yr post-admit date	271,519 (13)	2,837 (43)	<0.001	3,793 (22)	1,315 (38)	<0.001
By 90 d post-admit date, conditional on surviving to discharge	143,873 (6.9)	1,061 (20)	<0.001	1,571 (9.9)	474 (16)	<0.001
By 1 yr post-admit date, conditional on surviving to discharge	221,041 (11)	1,579 (29)	<0.001	2,313 (15)	726 (25)	<0.001

Continuous variables expressed as mean ± standard deviation; categorical variables expressed as n (%).
T-tests used for continuous variables; chi-squared tests used for categorical variables.
[a]All means and proportions are based on admissions, not individual patients.
[b]Due to rounding, percentages may not add up to 100.
[c]Based upon proprietary MediQual mortality model using key clinical findings abstracted from the chart during the first 48 hours of admission.

receiving acute HD (odds ratio 1.00, 95% CI 1.00–1.01, P = 0.85). In the fully adjusted Cox model after propensity score matching, however, the acute HD patients still had a higher risk of death (HR 1.77, 95% CI 1.64–1.92). In the sensitivity analysis that used the Charlson Comorbidity Index rather than the MediQual PPD as the means of risk adjustment, the sample size increased by almost 50% (2,131,248 to 3,174,283) since the admissions for which PPD was not calculated were included. In this larger sample, the hazard ratio for death after acute HD in the fully adjusted Cox model after propensity score matching increased (HR 2.60, 95% CI 2.41–2.80).

Discussion

This work represents one of the first descriptions of the epidemiology of acute HD not limited to Medicare beneficiaries in a large US population. Receipt of acute HD varied by age, sex, race, and insurance status, even after adjustment for patients' underlying illness severity. Furthermore, in a comparison of patients with similar propensity to receive acute HD and adjusted for predicted probability of death upon admission, those who did receive acute HD had a higher risk of death for at least one year compared to those who did not.

Table 2. Independent predictors of receipt of acute hemodialysis, Pennsylvania 2005–2007.[a]

	Age<65		Age≥65	
	Adjusted odds ratio	95% confidence interval	Adjusted odds ratio	95% confidence interval
Age (per year)	1.01	1.00–1.01	0.95	0.94–0.95
Female	0.79	0.73–0.86	0.85	0.79–0.91
Black	1.37	1.24–1.52	1.54	1.37–1.73
Uninsured (vs. Medicare/commercial)	0.49	0.35–0.68	0.58	0.27–1.25
Uninsured (vs. Medicaid ± Medicare)	0.35	0.25–0.48	0.58	0.27–1.27
Primary diagnoses (top 5 by prevalence over all ages)				
Acute and unspecified renal failure	57.9	51.4–65.2	31.3	28.2–34.6
Septicemia (except in labor)	10.8	9.35–12.6	5.57	4.89–6.36
Congestive heart failure, non-hypertensive	6.30	5.31–7.49	3.80	3.34–4.33
Respiratory failure, insufficiency, or arrest	5.55	4.54–6.77	3.12	2.63–3.71
Diabetes mellitus with complications	7.19	6.06–8.54	8.22	6.85–9.86
Predicted probability of inpatient death (per 1% increase)	49.6	40.0–61.4	39.0	32.9–46.3

[a]Based on the full sample.

Our findings that being male or black are independent predictors of receipt of acute HD are consistent with previous findings that these groups are more likely to receive other intensive interventions such as mechanical ventilation [19–21], pulmonary artery catheters [19,20], and cardiopulmonary resuscitation [22]. Other authors have also previously reported a higher rate of renal replacement therapy among critically ill men [19]. Similarly, our finding that the uninsured are much less likely than those with any type of insurance to receive acute HD is in line with a recent report by Lyon and colleagues, who, also working with the PHC4 data, noted that uninsured patients less than 65 years old had a significantly lower probability of receiving acute HD, tracheostomies, and central venous catheters [23]. It should be noted, however, that Lyon's strategy for differentiating acute from chronic HD relied on older ICD-9-CM codes that didn't allow for separation of CKD and ESRD [24]. As such, their strategy may have unnecessarily eliminated from acute HD analyses some CKD patients whose HD was in fact acute. At first glance, after seeing this kind of disparity between the insured and uninsured, one might attribute it to healthcare providers' reluctance to offer expensive therapies to patients who are unlikely to ever be able to pay for them. As Lyon pointed out, though, the disparity could

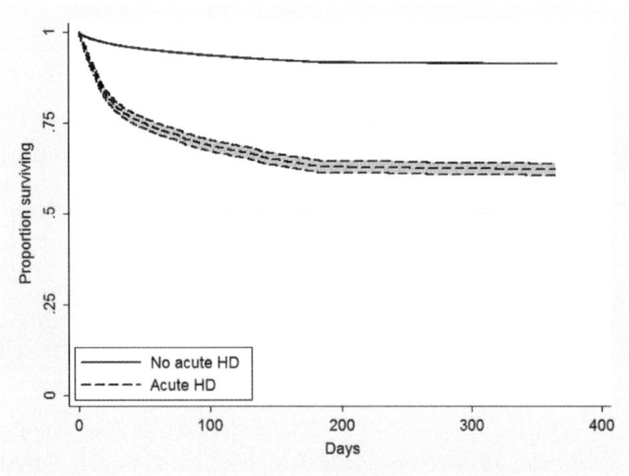

Figure 2. Unadjusted survival among patients with and without acute hemodialysis, Pennsylvania 2005–2007. Kaplan-Meier survival curves for patients who did and did not receive acute hemodialysis, with 95% confidence intervals.

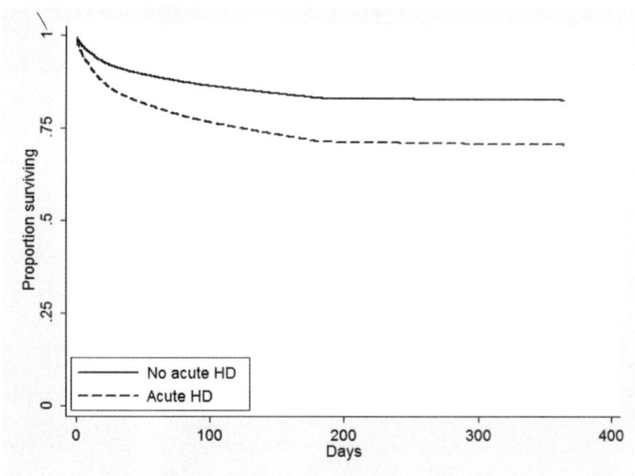

Figure 3. Adjusted survival among propensity-score matched patients with and without acute hemodialysis, Pennsylvania 2005–2007. Cox-adjusted survival curves with covariate adjustment for patients who did and did not receive acute hemodialysis after matching on propensity to receive acute hemodialysis. Variables included in covariate risk adjustment included age; female sex; black race; insurance with Medicare or private insurance vs. no insurance; insurance with Medicaid and/or Medicare vs. no insurance; MediQual predicted probability of death; and the top 25 Clinical Classification Software admission diagnoses for people who received acute hemodialysis, with the exception of hypertension with complications and secondary hypertension (#6) and peripheral and visceral atherosclerosis (#25), which were dropped in the model selection phase.

result more from choices by the uninsured patients and their surrogates than from healthcare providers' decisions—unconscious or otherwise—to forego these interventions in the uninsured. The reasons underlying the observed disparity merit further investigation, perhaps using survey-based or qualitative methods.

Perhaps the most striking finding from our study is the increased mortality risk for patients who received acute HD, even after robust risk-adjustment, including propensity score matching. Even after we limited the sample to the sickest patients, those admitted to the ICU, this increased mortality risk persisted. This finding runs counter to the commonly accepted notion that acute HD decreases mortality for those in whom it is initiated. Certainly, despite our best efforts to match by propensity to receive acute HD patients who did and did not receive it, the possibility of unmeasured confounding by illness severity remains. Though a principal diagnosis of AKI was a covariate in our propensity scoring and survival models, we could not match patients on severity of AKI (e.g., by serum BUN or creatinine or urine output), as our dataset did not include that information.

However, we also cannot rule out the possibility that acute HD is deleterious to patient survival. Elseviers and colleagues reported similar results from a nonrandomized prospective study of 1,303 patients in 9 ICUs [25]. They found that differences in illness severity did not account for the higher in-hospital mortality observed in patients who received acute HD. Intriguingly, they also noted wide variations between ICUs in initiation of acute HD, underscoring the general lack of consensus in nephrology and critical care about the relative indications for this therapy. In our study, we attempted to account for between-institution variations by including each hospital's standardized rate of HD among patients at a high probability of dying in our propensity score calculation and appropriately adjusting Cox model standard errors for clustering of patients within hospitals.

Two even more recent studies, though they did not find higher mortality with acute HD, did find lack of survival benefit. For Clec'h and colleagues, this lack of benefit was in patients who received acute HD versus those who did not after matching on propensity to receive acute HD using detailed clinical information [26]. For Wilson and colleagues, this lack of benefit was in patients who developed severe AKI on days other than Sundays compared to patients who developed severe AKI on Sundays, despite lower frequency of acute HD initiation on Sundays [27]. Moreover, Wilson and colleagues, in their most recent study, observed an association between dialysis for AKI and increased survival when dialysis was initiated in patients with higher serum creatinine but not when it was initiated in patients with lower serum creatinine. In fact, in patients with lower serum creatinine, initiation of dialysis for AKI was associated with increased mortality [28]. Though the reasons that acute HD might exert either no effect or a negative effect on patient survival are far from clear and merit further research, the known risks of HD—episodic hypotension, an indwelling catheter, immune and coagulation disturbances, changes in medication clearance, to name a few—all might play a role.

Our study has several strengths that should be noted. Our sample includes over 2 million observations from a dataset that captured admissions of all adults in almost every hospital in a populous US state, not just Medicare beneficiaries or hospitals within a particular commercial or government healthcare system. Our analyses benefitted from the precise risk adjustment of the MediQual model for predicted probability of death. Furthermore, by restricting our sample to admissions from the last quarter of 2005 onwards, we were able to take advantage of updated ICD-9-CM codes that allow for separation of CKD and ESRD. As such, we can have reasonable confidence in our ability to differentiate between acute and chronic HD using administrative data.

This study is not without weaknesses, however. Though we carefully crafted our strategy to exclude ESRD patients from the sample and backed it up with a sensitivity analysis, without medical records we are unable to fully validate the strategy. Despite adjusting for a wide variety of covariates in our models and propensity-score matching patients who received acute HD with patients who did not, as well as replicating our main results with a sensitivity analysis limited to patients sick enough to be admitted to the ICU, there is still likely to be some degree of unmeasured confounding contributing to the survival difference between the groups. In the most extreme case, if the only patients dialyzed were those who would have definitely died from their illness, then acute HD had to confer a survival benefit, as some patients did survive. While we cannot exclude this possibility using our dataset, we mitigated it to the fullest extent that our dataset would allow. Finally, in order to use the precise risk adjustment of the MediQual model, we excluded all those admissions for which PHC4 did not require calculation of predicted probability of death. Our sample must therefore be considered nonrandom. In fact one of our sensitivity analyses did demonstrate that the inclusion of all admissions in our sample would have altered the results. But the most important finding, the hazard ratio for death in patients who received acute HD versus those who did not, actually became larger in this case.

Taken in the context of previous research, our findings regarding predictors of acute HD suggest factors other than clinical indication at play in determining who receives this therapy; our findings regarding survival after acute HD raise questions about its presumed benefits. Given the extraordinary costs of intensive interventions such as acute HD in the US, and the ever-expanding population of patients who might become ill enough to be viewed as candidates for it, healthcare providers and policy-makers alike must carefully consider why exactly patients receive the therapies they do and whether those reasons impact eventual outcomes.

Supporting Information

Figure S1 Standardized (observed-to-expected) hemodialysis use for patients at high probability of dying upon admission, by hospital, Pennsylvania 2001–2007. Each dot represents 1 hospital.

Figure S2 Covariate balance before and after inverse probability treatment weighting by propensity score. Movement of the open dots towards a Z-value of 0 represents better covariate balance after weighting, with a value of 0 reflecting perfect balance.

Text S1 Diagnosis-related groups or International Classification of Diseases, 9th Revision, Clinical Modification principal diagnoses for which the Pennsylvania Health Care Cost Containment Council required predicted probability of inpatient death to be calculated, by year.

Acknowledgments

The authors wish to thank Khaled Abdel-Kader, MD, MS for his suggestion of the method for one of the sensitivity analyses and his helpful input regarding propensity score matching.

Disclaimer: The Pennsylvania Health Care Cost Containment Council (PHC4) is an independent state agency responsible for addressing the problem of escalating health costs, ensuring the quality of health care, and increasing access to healthcare for all citizens regardless of ability to pay. PHC4 has provided data to this entity in an effort to further PHC4's mission of educating the public and containing health care costs in Pennsylvania. PHC4, its agents, and staff, have made no representation, guarantee, or warranty, express or implied, that the data — financial, patient, payor, and physician specific information — provided to this entity, are error free, or that the use of the data will avoid differences of opinion or interpretation. This analysis was not prepared by PHC4. This analysis was done by the University of Pittsburgh. PHC4, its agents and staff, bear no responsibility or liability for the results of the analysis, which are solely the responsibility of the University of Pittsburgh.

Author Contributions

Conceived and designed the experiments: SR EC CC MU AB. Performed the experiments: SR EC CC AB. Analyzed the data: SR EC CC AB. Contributed reagents/materials/analysis tools: EC CC AB. Contributed to the writing of the manuscript: SR EC MU AB.

References

1. Xue JL, Daniels F, Star RA, Kimmel PL, Eggers PW, et al. (2006) Incidence and mortality of acute renal failure in Medicare beneficiaries, 1992 to 2001. J Am Soc Nephrol 17: 1135–1142.
2. Mehta RL, Pascual MT, Gruta CG, Zhuang S, Chertow GM (2002) Refining predictive models in critically ill patients with acute renal failure. J Am Soc Nephrol 13: 1350–1357.
3. Palevsky PM, Zhang JH, O'Connor TZ, Chertow GM, Crowley ST, et al. (2008) Intensity of renal support in critically ill patients with acute kidney injury. N Engl J Med 359: 7–20.
4. Bellomo R, Cass A, Cole L, Finfer S, Gallagher M, et al. (2009) Intensity of continuous renal-replacement therapy in critically ill patients. N Engl J Med 361: 1627–1638.
5. Mehta RL, Pascual MT, Soroko S, Chertow GM (2002) Diuretics, mortality, and nonrecovery of renal function in acute renal failure. JAMA 288: 2547–2553.
6. Mehta RL, Pascual MT, Soroko S, Savage BR, Himmelfarb J, et al. (2004) Spectrum of acute renal failure in the intensive care unit: the PICARD experience. Kidney Int 66: 1613–1621.
7. Bagshaw SM, Laupland KB, Doig CJ, Mortis G, Fick GH, et al. (2005) Prognosis for long-term survival and renal recovery in critically ill patients with severe acute renal failure: a population-based study. Crit Care 9: R700–709.
8. Hsu CY, Chertow GM, McCulloch CE, Fan D, Ordonez JD, et al. (2009) Nonrecovery of kidney function and death after acute on chronic renal failure. Clin J Am Soc Nephrol 4: 891–898.
9. Wald R, Quinn RR, Luo J, Li P, Scales DC, et al. (2009) Chronic dialysis and death among survivors of acute kidney injury requiring dialysis. JAMA 302: 1179–1185.
10. Gopal I, Bhonagiri S, Ronco C, Bellomo R (1997) Out of hospital outcome and quality of life in survivors of combined acute multiple organ and renal failure treated with continuous venovenous hemofiltration/hemodiafiltration. Intensive Care Med 23: 766–772.
11. Ahlstrom A, Tallgren M, Peltonen S, Rasanen P, Pettila V (2005) Survival and quality of life of patients requiring acute renal replacement therapy. Intensive Care Med 31: 1222–1228.
12. Johansen KL, Smith MW, Unruh ML, Siroka AM, O'Connor TZ, et al. (2010) Predictors of health utility among 60-day survivors of acute kidney injury in the Veterans Affairs/National Institutes of Health Acute Renal Failure Trial Network Study. Clin J Am Soc Nephrol 5: 1366–1372.
13. Hamel MB, Phillips RS, Davis RB, Desbiens N, Connors AF, et al. (1997) Outcomes and cost-effectiveness of initiating dialysis and continuing aggressive care in seriously ill hospitalized adults. SUPPORT Investigators. Study to Understand Prognoses and Preferences for Outcomes and Risks of Treatments. Ann Intern Med 127: 195–202.
14. Rauf AA, Long KH, Gajic O, Anderson SS, Swaminathan L, et al. (2008) Intermittent hemodialysis versus continuous renal replacement therapy for acute renal failure in the intensive care unit: an observational outcomes analysis. J Intensive Care Med 23: 195–203.
15. Pine M, Jordan HS, Elixhauser A, Fry DE, Hoaglin DC, et al. (2007) Enhancement of claims data to improve risk adjustment of hospital mortality. JAMA 297: 71–76.
16. Barnato AE, Farrell MH, Chang CC, Lave JR, Roberts MS, et al. (2009) Development and validation of hospital "end-of-life" treatment intensity measures. Med Care 47: 1098–1105.
17. Charlson ME, Pompei P, Ales KL, MacKenzie CR (1987) A new method of classifying prognostic comorbidity in longitudinal studies: development and validation. J Chronic Dis 40: 373–383.
18. Deyo RA, Cherkin DC, Ciol MA (1992) Adapting a clinical comorbidity index for use with ICD-9-CM administrative databases. J Clin Epidemiol 45: 613–619.
19. Valentin A, Jordan B, Lang T, Hiesmayr M, Metnitz PG (2003) Gender-related differences in intensive care: a multiple-center cohort study of therapeutic interventions and outcome in critically ill patients. Crit Care Med 31: 1901–1907.
20. Fowler RA, Sabur N, Li P, Juurlink DN, Pinto R, et al. (2007) Sex-and age-based differences in the delivery and outcomes of critical care. CMAJ 177: 1513–1519.
21. Pietropaoli AP, Glance LG, Oakes D, Fisher SG (2010) Gender differences in mortality in patients with severe sepsis or septic shock. Gend Med 7: 422–437.
22. Ehlenbach WJ, Barnato AE, Curtis JR, Kreuter W, Koepsell TD, et al. (2009) Epidemiologic study of in-hospital cardiopulmonary resuscitation in the elderly. N Engl J Med 361: 22–31.
23. Lyon SM, Benson NM, Cooke CR, Iwashyna TJ, Ratcliffe SJ, et al. (2011) The effect of insurance status on mortality and procedural use in critically ill patients. Am J Respir Crit Care Med 184: 809–815.
24. Elixhauser A, Steiner C, Harris DR, Coffey RM (1998) Comorbidity measures for use with administrative data. Med Care 36: 8–27.
25. Elseviers MM, Lins RL, Van der Niepen P, Hoste E, Malbrain ML, et al. (2010) Renal replacement therapy is an independent risk factor for mortality in critically ill patients with acute kidney injury. Crit Care 14: R221.
26. Clec'h C, Darmon M, Lautrette A, Chemouni F, Azoulay E, et al. (2012) Efficacy of renal replacement therapy in critically ill patients: a propensity analysis. Crit Care 16: R236.
27. Wilson FP, Yang W, Schrauben S, Machado C, Lin JJ, et al. (2013) Sundays and mortality in patients with AKI. Clin J Am Soc Nephrol 8: 1863–1869.
28. Wilson FP, Yang W, Machado CA, Mariani LH, Borovskiy Y, et al. (2014) Dialysis versus Nondialysis in Patients with AKI: A Propensity-Matched Cohort Study. Clin J Am Soc Nephrol 9: 673–681.

Adventitial Delivery of Lentivirus-shRNA-ADAMTS-1 Reduces Venous Stenosis Formation in Arteriovenous Fistula

Evelyn C. Nieves Torres[1]☯, Binxia Yang[1]☯, Rajiv Janardhanan[1], Akshaar Brahmbhatt[1], Ed Leof[2], Debabrata Mukhopadhyay[2], Sanjay Misra[1,2]*

1 Vascular and Interventional Radiology Translational Laboratory, Department of Radiology, Mayo Clinic, Rochester, Minnesota, United States of America, **2** Department of Biochemistry and Molecular Biology, Mayo Clinic, Rochester, Minnesota, United States of America

Abstract

Hemodialysis vascular access can develop venous neointimal hyperplasia (VNH) causing stenosis. Recent clinical and experimental data has demonstrated that there is increased expression of a disintegrin and metalloproteinase thrombospondin motifs-1 (ADAMTS-1) at site of VNH. The experiments outlined in the present paper were designed to test the hypothesis that targeting of the adventitia of the outflow vein of murine arteriovenous fistula (AVF) using a small hairpin RNA that inhibits ADAMTS-1 expression (LV-shRNA-ADAMTS-1) at the time of fistula creation will decrease VNH. At early time points, ADAMTS-1 expression was significantly decreased associated with a reduction in vascular endothelial growth factor-A (VEGF-A) and matrix metalloproteinase-9 (MMP-9) (LV-shRNA-ADAMTS-1 transduced vessels vs. controls). These changes in gene and protein expression resulted in favorable vascular remodeling with a significant increase in mean lumen vessel area, decrease in media/adventitia area, with a significant increase in TUNEL staining accompanied with a decrease in cellular proliferation accompanied with a reduction in CD68 staining. Collectively, these results demonstrate that ADAMTS-1 transduced vessels of the outflow vein of AVF have positive vascular remodeling.

Editor: Jing-Wei Xiong, Peking University, China

Funding: This work was funded by a R01HL098967 (SM) from the National Heart, Lung, and Blood Institute, Society of Interventional Radiology Foundation (RJ), and Howard Hughes Medical Institute (AB). The funders had no role in study design, data collection and analysis, decision to publish, or preparation of the manuscript.

Competing Interests: The authors have declared that no competing interests exist.

* E-mail: misra.sanjay@mayo.edu

☯ These authors contributed equally to this work.

Introduction

There are more than 400,000 patients in the United States who require hemodialysis because of end-stage renal disease (ESRD) [1]. A well-functioning vascular access is required for optimal hemodialysis to occur. Current recommendations by National Kidney Foundation Kidney Disease Outcomes Quality Initiative (KDOQI) for hemodialysis vascular access are that patients whom require long-term dialysis have an arteriovenous fistula (AVF). However, it is estimated that at one year patency of AVF's is 62%. [2,3]. AVFs fail because of venous stenosis formation which is caused by venous neointimal hyperplasia (VNH) [4]. Consequently, treatment of stenosis to maintain the function of hemodialysis AVFs and grafts costs over one billion dollars annually [1]. Developing therapies that could be used to reduce AVF stenosis would be advantageous to ESRD patients.

A recent study from our laboratory demonstrated that there is increased expression of a disintegrin and metalloproteinase with thrombospondin motif-1 (ADAMTS-1) in specimens removed from patients with failed hemodialysis vascular access and experimental animal models of AVF, but its role in the formation of VNH is unknown [5,6,7]. A disintegrin and metalloproteinase with thrombospondin motif belongs to a new family of matrix metalloproteinases (MMPs) that were initially described from a colon cancer cell line [8]. ADAMTS-1 has been shown to be able to cleave aggrecan and versican that are components of extracellular matrix. Recent studies have shown that there is increased expression of ADAMTS-1 in plaques from patients with acute myocardial infarction which is associated with increased CD68 staining [9].

The experiments outlined using the present manuscript were performed in a murine model of CKD with AVF to test the hypothesis that reduction of ADAMTS-1 gene expression by adventitial delivery to the outflow vein of the AVF at the time of placement would lead to a reduction in VNH. Gene expression for ADAMTS-1 was reduced by adventitial delivery of a small hairpin RNA (shRNA) that inhibits its expression. Gene, protein expression, and histomorphometric analyses were performed at the outflow vein after administration of anti-ADAMTS-1 RNA therapy.

Materials and Methods

Experimental animals

Mayo Clinic Institutional Animal Care and Use Committee approval was obtained prior to performing any procedures. The

Table 1. Q-PCR primers used.

Gene	Sequence
ADAMTS-1	5′ – ACGCCACACTTATCAAACTTCT – 3′ (sense)
	5′ – CTTTTTCGTCTTACAGCCCAAG– 3′ (antisense)
VEGF-A	5′ – ATGAAGTGATCAAGTTCATGG– 3′(sense)
	5′ – GGATCTTGGACAAACAAATGC– 3′ (antisense)
MMP-9	5′ – GTTTTTGATGCTATTGCTGAGATCCA– 3′ (sense)
	5′ – CCCACATTTGACGTCCAGAGAAGAA-3′(antisense)
18S	5′ – GTTCCGACCATAAACGATGCC-3′ (sense)
	5′- TGGTGGTGCCCTTCCGTCAAT- 3′(antisense)

housing and handling of the animals was performed in accordance with the Public Health Service Policy on Humane Care and Use of Laboratory Animals revised in 2000 [10]. We have previously described this animal model and used it extensively [7,11,12,13]. Briefly, male C57BL/6 mice (Jackson Laboratories, Bar Harbor, ME) weighing 25–30 grams were used for the present study. Chronic renal insufficiency was created as described previously [20,] [14]. Four weeks after the nephrectomy, the right carotid artery to the ipsilateral jugular vein was used to create the AVF [11,14]. Five million particle forming units (PFU) of either lentivirus-shRNA-ADAMTS-1 (**LV-shRNA-ADAMTS-1**) or scrambled-shRNA (**control shRNA**) in 5-μL of PBS were injected using a 30-guage needle, into the adventitia of the proximal outflow vein at the time of AVF creation at the time of fistula creation [15]. We have previously shown that in this animal model that venous stenosis forms reproducibly at this location [7,11,12,13]. Animals were sacrificed at day 7 (**D7**), day 14 (**D14**), and day 21 (**D21**) following AV fistula placement. Real time quantitative polymerase chain reaction (qPCR) and histologic analyses were obtained.

Vector constructs

The shRNA for ADAMTS-1 and control shRNA were obtained from Open Biosystems, Huntsville, AL (www.openbiosystems.com, RMM4534-NM_001025250) and the lentivirus was prepared according to the manufacturer's protocol. The shRNA for ADAMTS-1 and controls were tagged to GFP (green fluorescent protein) thus allowing for it to be localized after delivery

Cell culture

We determined the efficacy and efficiency of lentiviral silencing of ADAMTS-1 expression in NIH 3T3 cells which were transduced with either lentivirus-shRNA- ADAMTS-1 (LV-shRNA-VEGF-A) or control shRNA. The gene expression of ADAMTS-1 was determined using RT-PCR [16].

Tissue harvesting

At euthanasia, all mice were anesthetized as described previously and the fistula was dissected free of the surrounding tissue. Animals were euthanized by CO_2 asphyxiation and the outflow veins harvested for qPCR or histologic analyses. For histologic analysis, all vessels were perfusion fixed prior to removal.

Procedures to ensure animal comfort and anesthesia

Mayo strives to ensure that the institutional facilities and procedures adhere in all respects to USDA regulations and NIH guidelines for care and use of laboratory animals. Investigators are required to administer appropriate analgesics to all animals associated with a procedure that would normally require pain medication in humans. The mice undergoing surgery for the creation of the arteriovenous fistula procedure were anesthetized by administering intraperitoneal injection of a mixture of ketamine hydrochloride and xylazine per IACUC recommendations. Surgery was conducted in a disinfected, uncluttered area, which promotes asepsis during surgery. The animals were maintained at a surgical plane of anesthesia throughout the procedure in which the animal is maintained and the vital signs are monitored. The surgical incision was closed using appropriate techniques and materials. After surgery the animal was moved to a warm, dry area and monitored during recovery. Heat lamps or warming pads were used in maintaining or recovering body temperature. All surgical procedures were performed under deep anesthesia with intraperitoneal pentobarbital (20-40 mg/kg). This anesthesia was maintained animal comfort throughout the surgical procedure until recovery or sacrifice.

RNA isolation

The tissue was stored in RNA stabilizing reagent (Qiagen', Gaithersburg, MD) as per the manufactures guidelines. To isolate the RNA, the specimens were homogenized and total RNA isolated using RNeasy mini kit (Qiagen) as described previously [11,14].

Real time polymerase chain reaction (qPCR) analysis

Expression for the gene of interest was determined using qPCR analysis as described previously [11], [17]. Primers used are shown in table 1.

Tissue processing and immunohistochemistry

Each outflow vein from each animal was embedded in paraffin length-wise so that the sections would be orthogonal to the long axis of the vessel as described previously [17]. Four-μm sections from the outflow vein after transduction with either LV-shRNA-ADAMTS-1 or control shRNA were stained with hematoxylin and eosin, Ki-67, α-SMA, CD31, CD68, MMP-9, ADAMTS-1, and VEGF-A using the EnVision (DAKO, Carpinteria, CA) method with a heat-induced antigen retrieval step [18,19]. The following antibodies were used: mouse monoclonal antibody Ki-67 (DAKO, 1:400), CD31 (Abcam, Cambridge, MA; 1:400), rabbit polyclonal antibody to mouse for VEGF-A, ADAMTS-1, CD-68 (assess for macrophage staining), and MMP-9 (Abcam, 1:600), or rabbit polyclonal antibody to mouse for MMP-9 (Novus Biologics, 1:200). IgG antibody staining was performed to serve as controls.

TUNEL staining [17]

TUNEL staining was performed on paraffin-embedded sections from the outflow vein of LV-shRNA-ADAMTS-1 and control shRNA transduced vessels as specified by the manufacturer (DeadEnd Colorimetric tunnel assay system, G7360, Promega). Negative control is shown where the recombinant terminal deoxynucleotidyl transferase enzyme was omitted.

Picrosirius red staining [17]

Picrosirius red staining was performed on unstained sections from the outflow vein of LV-shRNA-ADAMTS-1 and control shRNA transduced vessels as described elsewhere [17].

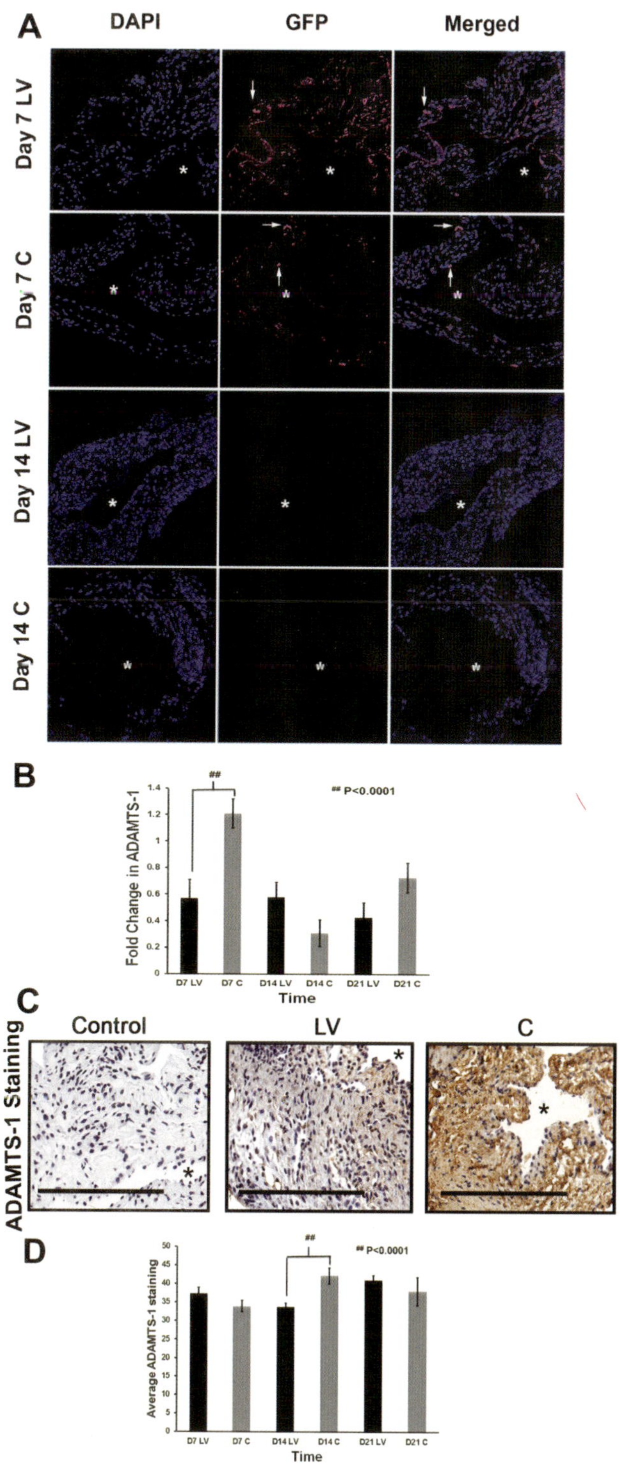

Figure 1. ADAMTS-1 expression is reduced in LV-shRNA-ADAMTS-1 transduced vessels. A) is representative sections using confocal microscopy from the outflow vein after transduction with LV-shRNA-ADAMTS-1 (**LV**) and control shRNA (**C**) at day 7 (**D7**) and 14 (**D14**). Both the **C** and **LV** have a GFP tag. First column shows DAPI intensity indicated by blue staining nuclei. Second column shows GRP intensity. Magenta staining cells are GFP positive. Third column depicts merged images. These sections demonstrate that there is **LV** or **C** delivery to the adventitia and endothelium of the vessel wall. By day 14, the gfp signal decreases and is not detectible. **B**) is the pooled data of the mean gene expression of ADAMTS-1 at the outflow vein after transduction with LV-shRNA-ADAMTS-1 (**LV**) compared to control shRNA (**C**) using qPCR analysis at day 7 (**D7**), 14 (**D14**), and 21 (**D21**). This demonstrates a significant reduction in the mean ADAMTS-1 expression in the **LV** transduced vessels when compared to **C** vessels at **D7** ($P<0.0001$). **C**) is representative sections from ADAMTS-1 staining at the outflow vein of **LV** transduced vessels when compared to **C** vessels at day 14. Cells staining brown are positive for ADAMTS-1. IgG antibody staining was performed to serve as negative control. **D**) is the pooled data of the mean ADAMTS-1 staining at the outflow vein after transduction with **LV** compared to **C** at day 7 (**D7**), 14 (**D14**), and 21 (**D21**). This shows that by **D14**, there is a significant reduction in the mean ADAMTS-1 staining in the **LV** transduced vessels when compared to **C** ($P<0.0001$). All are 40X. Scale bar is 50-μM. * Indicates the lumen. Each bar shows mean ± SEM of 4-6 animals per group (**B, D**). Two-way ANOVA followed by Student *t*-test with post hoc Bonferroni's correction was performed. Significant difference from control value was indicated by $^{\#\#}P<0.0001$.

GFP staining in paraffin tissue

Unstained sections from the outflow vein of LV-shRNA-ADAMTS-1 and control shRNA transduced vessels were deparaffinized in three changes of absolute xylene five minutes each and then with H_20 two times each for three minutes. Slides were stained using Vectashield Dapi stain (Vector Labs, Burlingame, CA) and a cover placed and imaged immediately using a confocal microscope (LSM 510 META, Carl Zeiss; Thornwood, NY) at a 10×/0.3 objective.

Morphometry and image analysis [7,17,21]

Morphometric and image analysis was performed as described previously. Briefly, 4-μm paraffin embedded sections that had been immunostained for hematoxylin and eosin stains were viewed using an Axioplan 2 Microscope (Zeiss, Oberkochen, Germany) equipped with a Neo-Fluor × 20/0.50 objective. Images were captured and digitized to a minimum of 3090×3900 pixels using a Axiocam camera (Zeiss) [18,19]. Only images that covered the entire cross-section from each section of the outflow vein that had been transduced with either LV-shRNA-ADAMTS-1 or control shRNA were acquired and analyzed using KS 400 Image Analysis software (Zeiss). To quantify the lumen vessel area and wall vessel area, we used 3 to 5, 4-um paraffin embedded sections removed from the outflow vein for each animal at each time point. Sections were subsequently viewed with an Axioplan 2 Microscope (Zeiss) equipped with a Neo-Fluor × 20/0.50 objective and digitized to capture at least 1030×1300 pixels and cell density determined along with the vessel wall and luminal vessel areas. The area was measured by tracing the vessel wall using an automated program [19]. Ki-67 (brown), CD68 positive (brown), CD31 positive (brown), α-SMA positive (brown), TUNEL positive (brown), VEGF-A (brown), MMP-9 (brown), and ADAMTS-1 positive (brown) were highlighted, in turn, by selecting the appropriate RGB (red-green-blue) color intensity range and then counted. The color intensity was adjusted for each section to account for decreasing intensity of positive staining over time. This was repeated twice to ensure intra-observer variability was less than 10% [7,13].

Statistical methods

Data are expressed as mean ± SEM. Multiple comparisons were performed with two-way ANOVA followed by Student *t*-test with post hoc Bonferroni's correction. Significant difference from control value was indicated by $^{*}P<0.05$, $^{**}P<0.01$, $^{\#}P<0.001$, or $^{\#\#}P<0.0001$. JMP version 9 (SAS Institute Inc., Cary, N.C.) was used for statistical analyses.

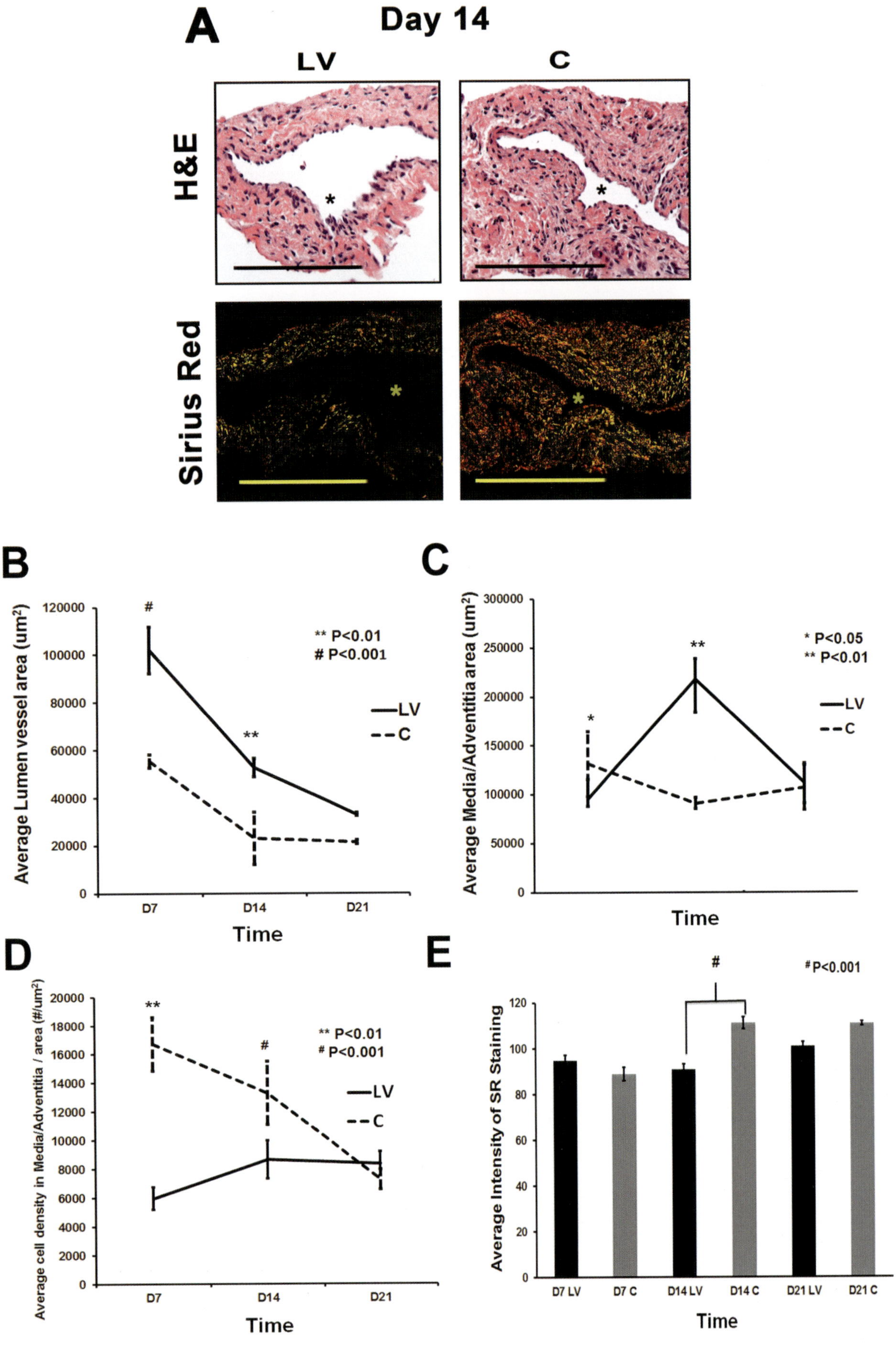
A
Day 14
LV
C
H&E
Sirius Red
B
Average Lumen vessel area (um²)
120000
100000
80000
60000
40000
20000
0
D7
D14
D21
Time
** P<0.01
# P<0.001
LV
C
C
Average Media/Adventitia area (um²)
300000
250000
200000
150000
100000
50000
0
Time
* P<0.05
** P<0.01
LV
C
D
Average cell density in Media/Adventitia / area (#/um²)
20000
18000
16000
14000
12000
10000
8000
6000
4000
2000
0
D7
D14
D21
Time
** P<0.01
# P<0.001
LV
C
E
Average Intensity of SR Staining
120
100
80
60
40
20
0
D7 LV
D7 C
D14 LV
D14 C
D21 LV
D21 C
Time
# P<0.001

Figure 2. Hematoxylin and eosin (H&E) and picrosirius red staining of LV-shRNA-ADAMTS-1 transduced vessels have increased lumen vessel area with decreased collagen expression. A) Upper panel is representative sections after hematoxylin and eosin (H&E) at the venous stenosis of the LV-shRNA-ADAMTS-1 (**LV**) and control shRNA (**C**) transduced vessels at day at day 14 showing increase in lumen vessel area. **A) Lower panel** is representative polarized light microscopy of picrosirius red-stained venous stenosis showing decreased fibrosis (collagen fibers are bright yellow) of the **LV** and **C** transduced vessels. Pooled data for the average lumen vessel area of the **LV** and **C** groups at day 7 (**D7**), 14 (**D14**), and 21 (**D21**) are shown in **B**). There is a significant increase in the average lumen vessel area in the **LV** transduced vessels when compared to **C** vessels for day 7 (P<0.001) and day 14 (P<0.01). Pooled data for average area of the media and adventitia for **LV** and **C** groups at day 7 (**D7**), 14 (**D14**), and 21 (**D21**) are shown in (**C**). By day 7, there is a significant increase in the average area of the media and adventitia in the **LV** transduced vessels when compared to **C** vessels (P<0.05). By day 14, the average area of the media and adventitia is significantly increased in the **LV** transduced vessels when compared to **C** vessels (P<0.01). Pooled data for the average cell density in the media and adventitia in the **LV** and **C** groups at day 7 (**D7**), 14 (**D14**), and 21 (**D21**) are shown in (**D**). There is a significant decrease in average cell density in the media and adventitia in the **LV** transduced vessels when compared to **C** vessels for day 7 (P<0.01) and day 14 (P<0.001). Pooled data for average intensity of picrosirius red staining of the vessel wall for **LV** and **C** groups at day 7 (**D7**), 14 (**D14**), and 21 (**D21**) are shown in (**E**). There is a significant decrease in average intensity of picrosirius red staining of the vessel wall of **LV** transduced vessels when compared to **C** vessels for day 14 (P<0.001). All are 40X. Scale bar is 50-µM. * Indicates the lumen. Each bar shows mean ± SEM of 4-6 animals per group (**B-E**). Two-way ANOVA followed by Student *t*-test with post hoc Bonferroni's correction was performed. $^{*}P<0.05$, $^{**}P<0.01$, or $^{\#}P<0.001$.

Results

Surgical outcomes

One hundred and nineteen male C57BL/6 mice weighing 25-30 grams underwent right nephrectomy and left upper pole occlusion surgery as described previously [17].

Seven mice died after nephrectomy, two after AVF fistula placement, and fifteen had significant arterial thickening and inflammation such that a new AV fistula could not be placed. Ninety five mice underwent placement of an AVF to connect the right carotid artery to the ipsilateral jugular vein [17]. Next, either 1×10^6 PFU of LV-shRNA-ADAMTS-1 (**LV**, n = 48) or control shRNA, scrambled-shRNA, (control, **C**, n = 47) was injected into the adventitia of the outflow vein where the stenosis forms in this model [7,11]. Animals were sacrificed for gene expression, protein, or histologic analyses at 7 (**D7**), 14 (**D14**), and 21 (**D21**) days after AVF placement.

Serum BUN and creatinine after nephrectomy

In this model it is observed that there is an increase in creatinine levels post-nephrectomy when compared to non-nephrectomized animals [12,13].

Adventitial transduction of LV-shRNA-ADAMTS-1 to the outflow vein reduces gene and protein expression of ADAMTS-1 at 7 and 14 days after AVF placement

The efficacy of reducing ADAMTS-1 gene expression *in vitro* was first determined using NIH 3T3 cells that were transduced with either LV-shRNA-ADAMTS-1 or control shRNA. RT-PCR (**Figure S1**) demonstrated greater than two fold decrease in ADAMTS-1 expression in the LV-shRNA-ADAMTS-1 transduced cells when compared to controls.

To determine, if similar findings are present *in vivo*, experiments were conducted to determine the distribution of the lentivirus in the outflow vein after delivery to the vessel wall. GFP staining was used to localize the delivery of the lentivirus to the vessel wall. This demonstrated that GFP positive cells (magenta positive) were present at 7 days after adventitial transduction but not at 14 days (**Fig. 1A**). The amount of reduction of ADAMTS-1 gene expression was determined *in vivo* using qPCR analysis for ADAMTS-1 on sections removed from the outflow vein at days 7, 14, and 21 after lentiviral transduction. By day 7, the mean gene expression of ADAMTS-1 at the LV-shRNA-ADAMTS-1 transduced vessels was significantly lower than the control vessels (0.31±0.1 vs. 1.21±0.11, respectively, P<0.0001, Average reduction: 74%, **Fig. 1B**).

It is well known that the expression of the protein can lag behind the decrease in gene expression. Therefore, the protein expression of ADAMTS-1 was determined using immunohistochemistry on outflow vein specimens removed after transduction with either LV-shRNA-ADAMTS-1 and compared to control shRNA (**Fig. 1C**). Cells staining brown are positive for ADAMTS-1. By day 14, there was a significant reduction in the average ADAMTS-1 staining in the LV-shRNA-ADAMTS-1 transduced vessels when compared to controls (33.7±1.06 vs. 42.1±2.2, respectively, P<0.0001, Average reduction: 44%, **Fig. 1D**). By day 21, there was no difference between the two groups.

Adventitial transduction of LV-shRNA-ADAMTS-1 to the outflow vein promotes positive vascular remodeling with a decrease in constrictive remodeling

We hypothesized that reducing mRNA levels of ADAMTS-1 by adventitial delivery of LV-shRNA-ADAMTS-1 to the outflow vein would result in positive vascular remodeling at the outflow vein (**Fig. 2**). Hematoxylin and eosin staining (H&E) (**Fig. 2A upper row**) and picrosirius red staining (**Fig. 2A lower row**) was used to assess the histomorphometric changes in vascular remodeling. A representative H&E and picrosirius red stains are shown from day 14. There was a significant increase in the average lumen area of the outflow vein of the LV-shRNA-ADAMTS-1 transduced vessels when compared to the control vessels by day 7 (average increase: 184%, P<0.001) and day 14 (average increase: 229%, P<0.01, **Fig. 3B**). Adventitial remodeling has been observed in experimental models of VNH associated with hemodialysis vascular access [18,20,21]. This was assessed by measuring the area of the adventitia and media. By day 7, there was a significant reduction in the average area of the media and adventitia of the LV-shRNA-ADAMTS-1 transduced vessels when compared to controls (average decrease: 27%, P<0.05, **Fig. 2C**). By day 14, there was a significant increase in the average area of the media and adventitia (average increase: 139%, P<0.01) with no differences in the average neointima area between the two groups.

A decrease in cell density can accompany positive vascular remodeling [12,13]. By day 7, there was a significant reduction in the average cell density of the media and adventitia of the LV-shRNA-ADAMTS-1 transduced vessels when compared to controls (average decrease: 55%, P<0.05, **Fig. 2D**). By day 14, there was a significant increase in the average cell density in the LV-shRNA-ADAMTS-1 transduced vessels when compared to controls (average increase: 238%, P<0.01).

Picrosirius staining was used to assess changes in collagen types 1 and 3 content in the LV-shRNA-ADAMTS-1 transduced vessels when compared to controls. Yellow color is positive for collagen

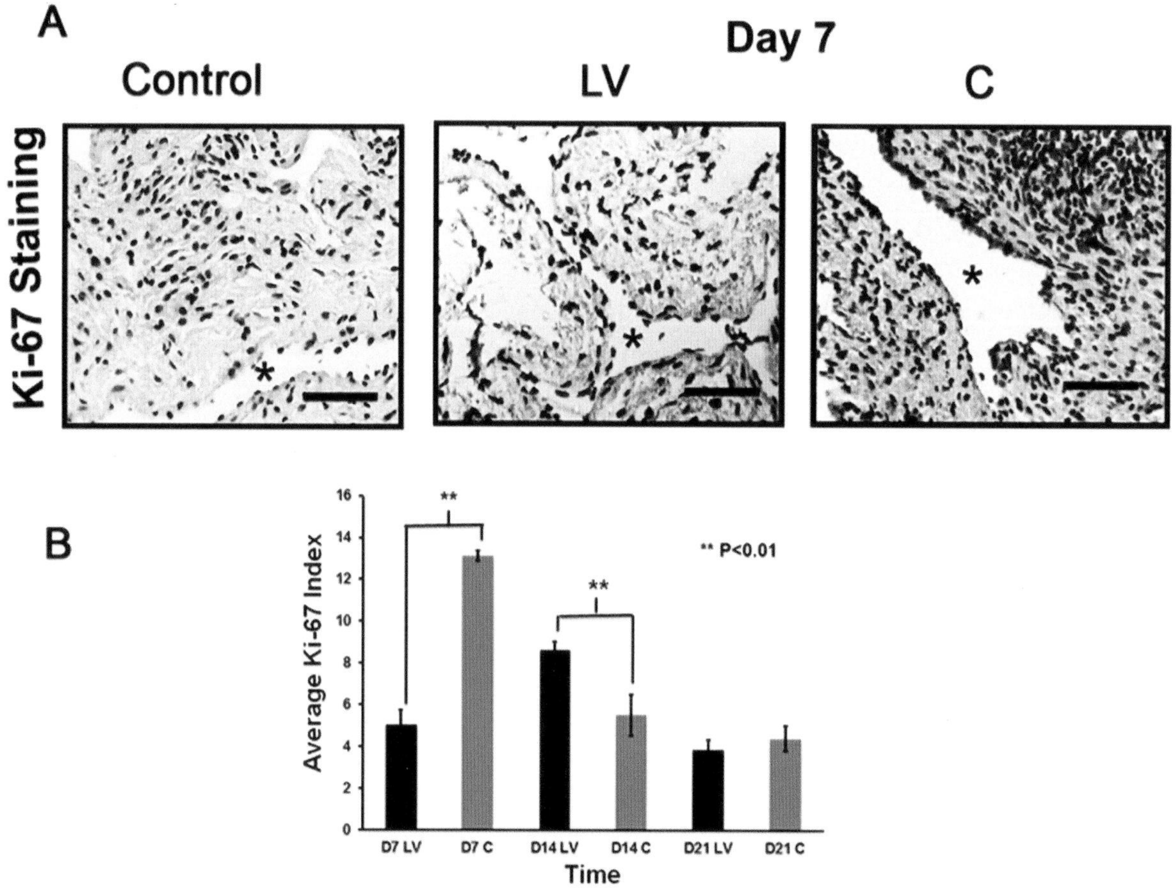

Figure 3. Cellular proliferation is decreased in LV-shRNA-ADAMTS-1 transduced vessels. A) is representative sections after Ki-67 staining at the venous stenosis of the LV-shRNA-ADAMTS-1 (**LV**) and control shRNA (**C**) at day 7. Nuclei staining brown are positive for Ki-67. IgG antibody staining was performed to serve as negative control. All are 40X. Scale bar is 50-μM. * indicates the lumen. Pooled data for Ki-67 index at the outflow vein of the **LV** and **C** transduced vessels at day 7 (**D7**), 14 (**D14**), and 21 (**D21**) is shown in (**B**). By day 7, there is a significant decrease in the mean Ki-67 index in the **LV** transduced vessels when compared to **C** at day 7 (P<0.01). By day 14, the mean Ki-67 index in the **LV** transduced vessels is significantly increased when compared to **C** (P<0.01). Each bar shows mean ± SEM of 4-6 animals per group. Two-way ANOVA followed by Student *t*-test with post hoc Bonferroni's correction was performed. Significant difference from control value was indicated by $^*P<0.01$.

types 1 or 3 staining. By day 14, there was a significant decrease in the average picrosirius staining in the LV-shRNA-ADAMTS-1 transduced vessels when compared to controls (Average reduction: 18%, P<0.001, **Fig. 2E**).

Adventitial transduction of LV-shRNA-ADAMTS-1 to the outflow vein decreases cellular proliferation

Cellular proliferation was determined by performing Ki-67 staining on sections from the outflow vein after transduction with either LV-shRNA-ADAMTS-1 or control shRNA (**Fig. 3A**). By day 7, the average Ki-67 index in the LV-shRNA-ADAMTS-1 group was significantly lower than the control group (5.1±0.7 vs. 9.3±1.7, respectively, average reduction: 45%, P<0.01, **Fig. 3B**). By day 14, a significant increase in the average Ki-67 index in the LV-shRNA-ADAMTS-1 transduced group was observed when compared to control group (8.65±0.4 vs. 5.5±0.98, respectively, average increase: 158%, P<0.01).

Adventitial transduction of LV-shRNA-ADAMTS-1 to the outflow vein increases apoptosis at day 14 and 21

Apoptosis was assessed using TUNEL staining performed on sections removed after transduction with either LV-shRNA-ADAMTS-1 or control shRNA (**Fig. 4A**). The average TUNEL index (number of TUNEL positive cells (brown)/total number of cells ×100) at the outflow vein of the LV-shRNA-ADAMTS-1 group was significantly higher than the control group by day 14 (8.4±1.4 vs. 4.6±0.8, respectively, average increase: 185%, P< 0.01, **Fig. 4B**) and day 21 (6.3±0.9 vs. 2.9±0.9, respectively, average increase: 215%, P<0.05). Overall, these results indicate that adventitial delivery of LV-shRNA-ADAMTS-1 results in a significant increase in TUNEL activity suggesting that there is increased cell death in LV-shRNA-ADAMTS-1 transduced vessels when compared to controls.

Adventitial transduction of LV-shRNA-ADAMTS-1 to the outflow vein decreases CD68 staining at day 7

Studies have demonstrated that ADAMTS-1 expression is associated with CD68 staining [9,22]. CD68 staining was performed to assess the changes after LV-shRNA-ADAMTS-1 transduction at different time points (**Fig. 5A**). This demonstrated that there was a significant decrease in the average CD68 staining at day 7 in the LV-shRNA-ADAMTS-1 transduced vessels when compared to controls (6.29±0.60 vs. 11.9±5.6, respectively, average reduction: 47%, P<0.05, **Fig. 5B**). By day 14, the CD68 staining had increased in the LV-shRNA-ADAMTS-1

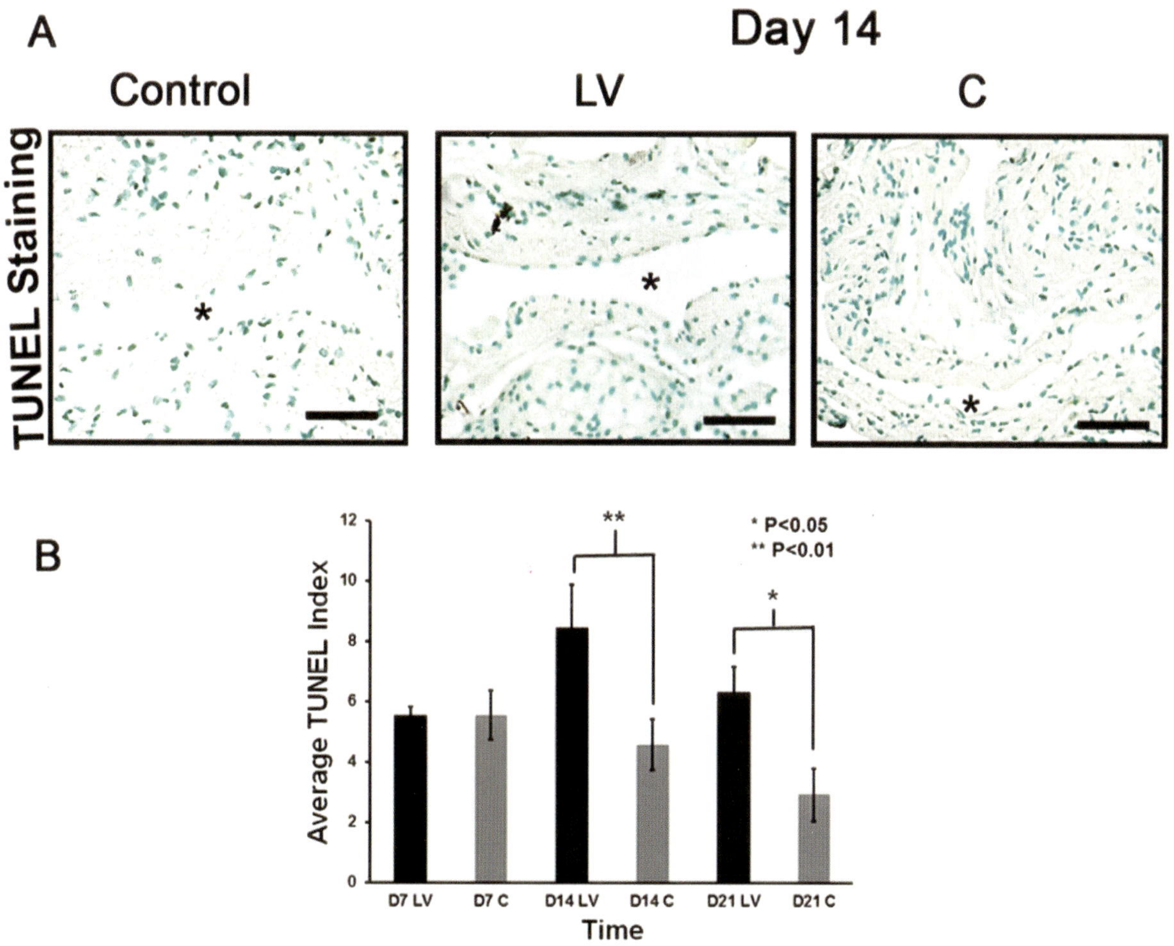

Figure 4. Apoptosis is increased in the LV-shRNA-ADAMTS-1 transduced vessels. A) is a representative section from TUNEL staining at the venous stenosis of the LV-shRNA-ADAMTS-1 (**LV**) and control shRNA(**C**) transduced control vessels at day 14. Nuclei staining brown are positive for TUNEL. Negative control is shown where the recombinant terminal deoxynucleotidyl transferase enzyme was omitted. All are 40X. Scale bar is 50-μM. * Indicates the lumen. Arrow indicates TUNEL positive cells. Pooled data for **LV** and **C** transduced vessels for TUNEL index at the outflow vein of the **LV** and **C** transduced vessels at day 7 (**D7**), 14 (**D14**), and 21 (**D21**) is shown in (**B**). This demonstrates a significant increase in the mean TUNEL index at day 14 ($P<0.01$) and day 21 ($P<0.05$) in the **LV** group when compared to **C**. Each bar shows mean ± SEM of 3–6 animals per group. Two-way ANOVA followed by Student *t*-test with post hoc Bonferroni's correction was performed. Significant difference from control value was indicated by *$P<0.05$ or **$P<0.01$.

transduced vessels when compared to controls however it was not statistically significant.

Adventitial delivery of LV-shRNA-ADAMTS-1 to the outflow vein is associated with a reduction of gene and protein expression of VEGF-A at days 7 and 14

There have been studies that have shown that ADAMTS-1 can modulate the VEGF-A response. This was assessed using qPCR analysis for VEGF-A expression at the outflow vein at days 7, 14, and 21 after lentiviral transduction [23]. The mean gene expression of VEGF-A at the LV-shRNA-ADAMTS-1 transduced vessels was significantly lower than the control vessels by day 7 (0.29±0.17 vs. 1.06±0.17, respectively, $P<0.05$, Average reduction: 73%, **Fig. 6A**) and 14 (0.43±0.21 vs. 2.44±0.17, respectively, $P<0.0001$, Average reduction: 83%). By day 21, the mean VEGF-A expression increased significantly in the LV-shRNA-ADAMTS-1 transduced vessels when compared to controls (1.84±0.17 vs. 1.19±0.17, respectively, $P<0.05$, Average increase: 154%).

To determine the consequence of the reduction in gene expression of VEGF-A, protein expression of VEGF-A was assessed using immunohistochemistry after lentiviral mediated gene silencing of ADAMTS-1 (**Fig. 6B**). Cells staining brown are positive for VEGF-A. There was a significant reduction in the average VEGF-A staining at the LV-shRNA-ADAMTS-1 transduced vessels when compared to controls by day 14 (17.5±0.7 vs. 21±0.7, respectively, $P<0.01$, Average reduction: 17%, **Fig. 6C**) and 21 (16±0.97 vs. 22.8±1.02, respectively, $P<0.001$, Average reduction: 30%).

CD31 staining can be used to assess the formation of new blood vessel formation after anti-angiogenic therapy [12]. Cells staining brown are positive for CD31. The effect of VEGF-A reduction on angiogenesis in LV-shRNA-ADAMTS-1 transduced vessels or control shRNA vessels were assessed using CD31 staining (**Fig. 6D**). By day 14, there was a significant decrease in the average CD31 density in the LV-shRNA-ADAMTS-1 transduced vessels when compared to controls (0.08±0.02 vs. 0.14±0.02, respectively, $P<0.05$, Average reduction: 42%). By day 21, there

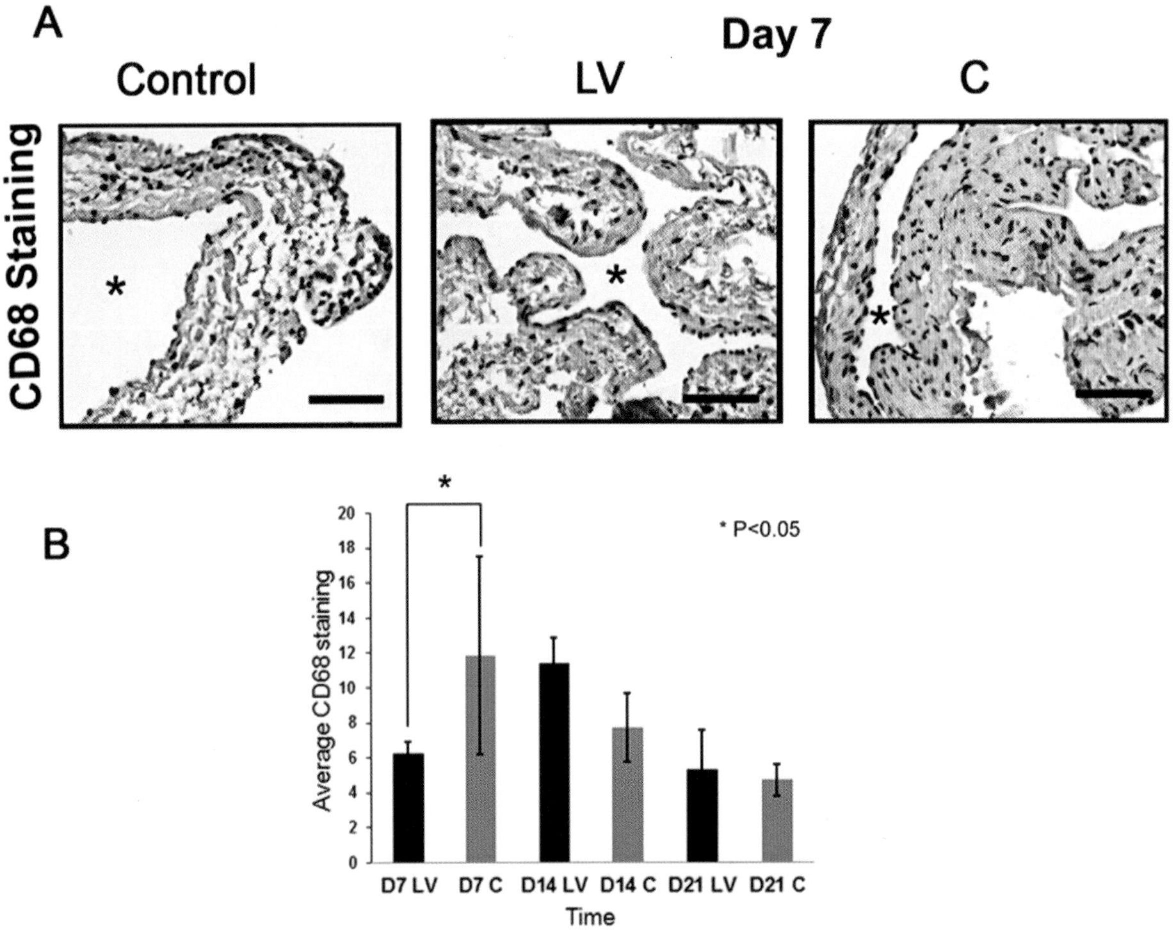

Figure 5. CD68 expression is reduced in LV-shRNA-ADAMTS-1 transduced vessels. A) is a representative section from CD68 staining at the venous stenosis of the LV-shRNA-ADAMTS-1 (**LV**) and control shRNA (**C**) transduced control vessels at day 7. Cells staining brown are positive for CD68. IgG antibody staining was performed to serve as negative control. All are 40X. Scale bar is 50-mM. * Indicates the lumen. Arrow indicates TUNEL positive cells. Pooled data for **LV** and **C** transduced vessels for CD68 index at the outflow vein of the **LV** and **C** transduced vessels at day 7 (**D7**), 14 (**D14**), and 21 (**D21**) is shown in **(B)**. This demonstrates a significant increase in the mean TUNEL index at day 74 ($P<0.05$) in the **LV** group when compared to **C**. Each bar shows mean ± SEM of 3-6 animals per group. Two-way ANOVA followed by Student *t*-test with post hoc Bonferroni's correction was performed. Significant difference from control value was indicated by $^*P<0.05$.

was a reversal of the average CD31 density with an increase in the LV-shRNA-ADAMTS-1 transduced vessels when compared to controls (0.19±0.02 vs. 0.13±0.01, respectively, $P<0.05$, Average increase: 149%, **Fig. 6E**). Collectively, these results indicate that at early time points, ADAMTS-1 silencing is associated with a reduction in the mean gene expression and subsequent protein expression of VEGF-A which is accompanied with a decrease in CD31 density. At later time points, there is an increase in the mean gene expression of VEGF-A expression and CD31 density.

Adventitial transduction of LV-shRNA-ADAMTS-1 to the outflow vein reduces expression of MMP-9 at the outflow vein

Recent study has shown that a decrease in VEGF-A is associated with a decrease in MMP-9 [12]. In addition, several studies have shown that there is increased expression of MMP-9 in animal models of hemodialysis AVF and graft failure as well as clinical samples [14,18,19,24,25]. We determined the gene expression of MMP-9 using qPCR analysis on specimens removed from the outflow vein transduced with either LV-shRNA-ADAMTS-1 or control shRNA. The average gene expression of MMP-9 was significantly lower in the LV-shRNA-ADAMTS-1 transduced vessels when compared to control shRNA by day 7 (0.24±0.06 vs. 1.17±0.21, respectively, average reduction: 80%, $P<0.05$, **Fig. 7A**) and 14 (0.94±0.11 vs. 1.96±0.31, respectively, average reduction: 52%, $P<0.05$). By day 21, there was a significant increase in MMP-9 expression in LV-shRNA-ADAMTS-1 transduced vessels when compared to controls (4.4±0.6 vs. 0.8±0.09, respectively, average increase: 477%, $P<0.001$).

The protein expression of MMP-9 was determined using immunohistochemistry performed on the outflow vein transduced with either LV-shRNA-ADAMTS-1 or control shRNA (**Fig. 7B**). The average MMP-9 staining (brown staining cells) was significantly lower in the LV-shRNA-ADAMTS-1 transduced vessels when compared to control vessels (6.52±1.4 vs. 15.9±1.9, respectively, average reduction: 59%, $P<0.01$, **Fig. 7C**) and by day 14 it remained lower (9±.2 vs. 11.1±.53, respectively, average reduction: 19%, $P<0.05$).

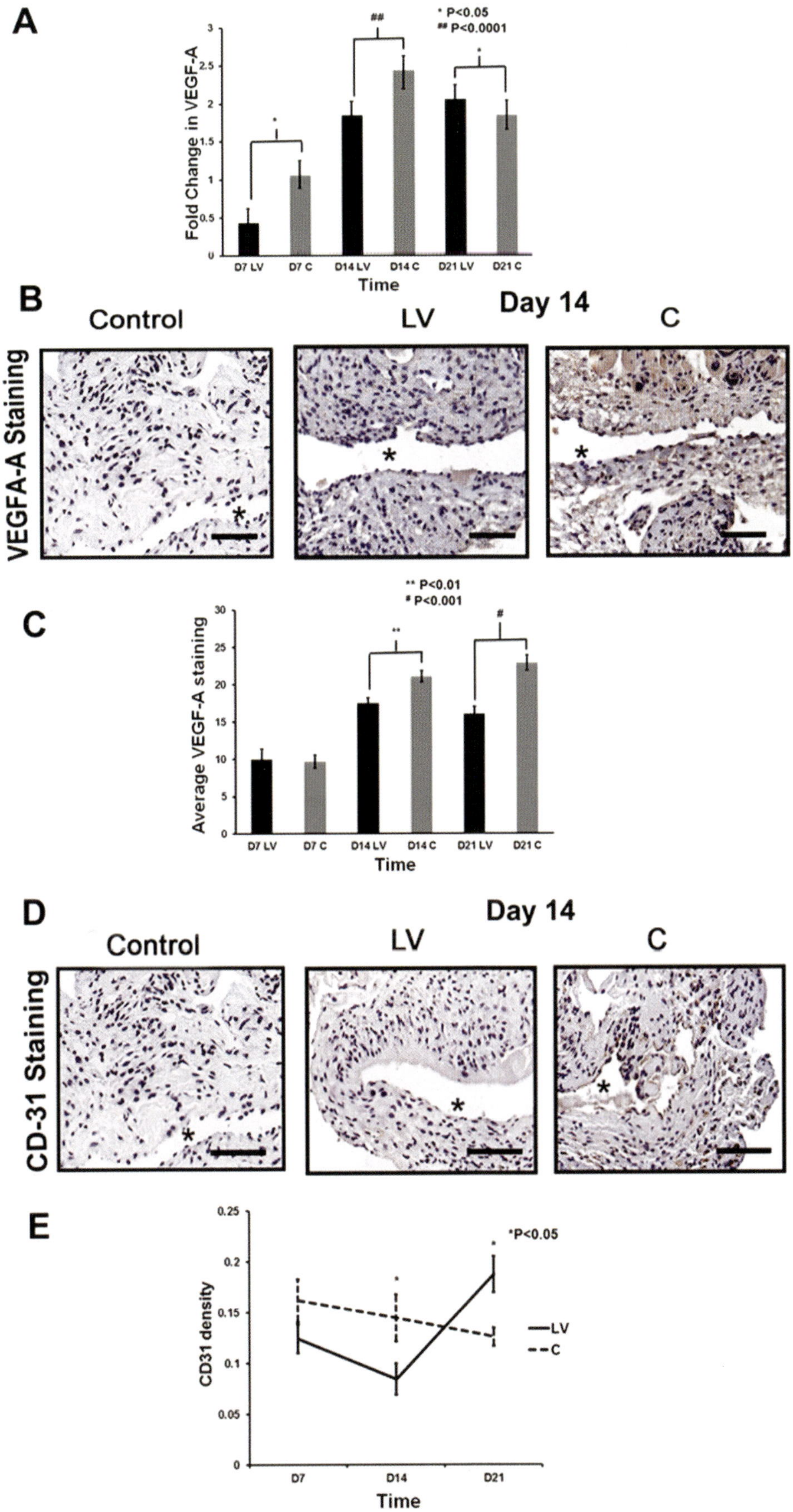
A
* P<0.05
P<0.0001
Fold Change in VEGF-A
D7 LV
D7 C
D14 LV
D14 C
D21 LV
D21 C
Time
B
Control
Day 14
LV
C
VEGFA-A Staining
C
** P<0.01
# P<0.001
Average VEGF-A staining
Time
D
Day 14
Control
LV
C
CD-31 Staining
E
*P<0.05
CD31 density
LV
C
D7
D14
D21
Time

Figure 6. VEGF-A expression is reduced in LV-shRNA-ADAMTS-1 transduced vessels. A) is the pooled data from the mean gene expression of VEGF-A at the outflow vein after transduction with LV-shRNA-ADAMTS-1 (**LV**) compared to control shRNA (**C**) using qPCR analysis at day 7 (**D7**), 14 (**D14**), and 21 (**D21**). This demonstrates that there is significant reduction in the mean VEGF-A expression in the **LV** transduced vessels when compared to **C** vessels at day 7 ($P<0.01$) and day 14 ($P<0.001$). By day 21, there is a significant increase in VEGF-A gene expression in the **LV** treated vessels when compared to **C** vessels (P<0.0.001). **B**) is representative sections from VEGF-A staining at the venous stenosis of the **LV** and **C** transduced vessels at day at day 14. Cells staining brown are positive for VEGF-A. IgG antibody staining serves as negative control. **C**) shows that there is a significant reduction in the mean VEGF-A staining in the **LV** transduced vessels when compared to controls by day 14 ($P<0.01$) and 21 ($P<0.001$). **D**) are representative sections from CD-31 staining at the venous stenosis of the LV-shRNA-ADAMTS-1 (**LV**) and control shRNA (**C**) transduced vessels at day at day 14. Cells staining brown are positive for CD31. IgG antibody staining was performed to serve as negative control. **E**) shows that by day 14, there is a significant reduction in the mean CD31 staining in the **LV** transduced vessels when compared to controls by day 14 ($P<0.05$). By day 21, there is a significant increase in the mean CD31 staining in the **LV** transduced vessels when compared to **C** ($P<0.05$). All are 40X. Scale bar is 50-μM. * Indicates the lumen. Each bar shows mean ± SEM of 4–6 animals per group (**A, C,** and **E**). Two-way ANOVA followed by Student *t*-test with post hoc Bonferroni's correction was performed. Significant difference from control value was indicated by $^{*}P<0.05$ or $^{\#}P<0.001$.

Discussion

Using a proteomic analysis, our laboratory identified ADAMTS-1 as a prominent up-regulated protein in specimens removed from failed hemodialysis grafts, however its role in the formation of VNH remained unknown [6]. In a murine model of AVF with CKD, a significant increase in ADAMTS-1 expression was demonstrated at the outflow vein when compared to controls [7]. In the present study, ADAMTS-1 expression was reduced using a LV-shRNA-ADAMTS-1 administered to the adventitia of the outflow vein at the time of AVF placement. In LV-shRNA-ADAMTS-1 transduced vessels compared to controls, there was a reduction of mRNA for ADAMTS-1 associated with a reduction in mRNA expression of VEGF-A and MMP-9 at days 7 to 14 after adventitial delivery. At day 21, there was a reduction in the protein expression of VEGF-A and MMP-9. Associated with this decrease, the following important histomorphometric changes were observed: 1) significant increase in mean lumen vessel area; 2) significant decrease in average area of the media and adventitia with corresponding cell density; 3) significant decrease in constrictive remodeling; 4) significant decrease in average cellular proliferation; 5) significant increase in TUNEL; and 6) significant decrease in macrophage density. These results suggest that ADAMTS-1 mRNA reduction results in favorable vascular remodeling that is associated with a reduction in VEGF-A (**Fig. 8**).

A disintegrin and metalloproteinase with thrombospondin motif-1 belongs to a new family of matrix metalloproteinases (MMPs) that were initially described from a murine colon cancer cell line [8]. The role of ADAMTS-1 in angiogenesis is controversial [26]. This effect has been demonstrated to occur through the direct binding of ADAMTS-1 to the trans-membrane receptor and thereby inhibiting VEGF-A binding [23,27]. Other studies have demonstrated the opposite effect [28]. These differences in its actions have led some authors to postulate that there may be a feedback inhibition of angiogenesis by ADAMTS-1 on VEGF-A [29]. In fact, a recent study demonstrated that ADAMTS-1 and its fragments have both pro-angiogenic and anti-angiogenic activities [30]. In the present study, reducing mRNA levels of ADAMTS-1 was associated with a decrease in VEGF-A at early time points while at later time points, the levels of VEGF-A were increased. The reduction of VEGF-A was accompanied with a reduction in MMP-9. Previous work from our laboratory and others has shown that decreasing VEGF-A results in a decrease in MMP-9 [12,13].

Since VEGF-A is responsible for angiogenesis, we used CD31, a marker for new blood vessel formation, and found the average CD31 to be decreased at early time points in ADAMTS-1 transduced vessels when compared to controls. These observations are consistent with recent work from our laboratory in which reducing VEGF-A mRNA levels has been shown to decrease CD31 expression [12]. Some investigators have hypothesized that there is a link between microvessel formation as depicted by CD31 staining and stenosis formation [31].

The role of ADAMTS-1 in proliferation is also controversial since there are conflicting reports. Some studies have demonstrated that ADAMTS-1 is associated with increased proliferation while others have shown the opposite [27,29]. In the present study, proliferation was assessed in the vessel wall using Ki-67 staining and found to be decreased in LV-shRNA-ADAMTS-1 transduced vessels when compared to controls. These results are consistent with observations from experimental animal model of vascular injury caused by atherosclerosis involving the carotid artery. In this study, the authors observed a significant increase in mRNA levels of ADAMTS-1 with increase in proliferation and migration [5]. In the present study, the reduction in not only ADAMTS-1 but also VEGF-A and MMP-9 could be responsible for the decrease in proliferation at day 7. Previous studies from our laboratory demonstrated that reducing mRNA for VEGF-A at the outflow vein of AVF decreased cellular proliferation [12]. Other studies have shown that inhibiting MMP activity in a rat and porcine model of arteriovenous hemodialysis graft failure results in a reduction in stenosis formation [32,33]

Accompanied with a decrease in proliferation, an increase in TUNEL staining was observed. In tumor cell lines, ADAMTS-1 over expression has been shown to have no effect on apoptosis [34]. The role of ADAMTS-1 in cell death in vascular injury has not been investigated. TUNEL staining was used to assess changes of cell death in the vessel wall after LV-shRNA-ADAMTS-1 transduction when compared to controls. The increase in TUNEL staining may represent the decrease in VEGF-A expression. It is well known that VEGF-A is needed for cell survival and that reducing VEGF-A expression results in apoptosis and cell death [12,35,36]. Recently, using the same animal model, we observed that reducing VEGF-A mRNA expression using shRNA or statin therapy resulted in an increase in TUNEL staining with increased caspase 3 activity [12,13].

The role of ADAMTS-1 reduction in vascular remodeling with respect to collagen 1 and 3 changes was assessed using picrosirius red staining. This stain is used to assess collagen types 1 and 3. A decrease in collagen types 1 and 3 implies that there is a reduction in constrictive remodeling. There have been no previous studies, which have demonstrated a link between ADAMTS-1 and collagens 1 and 3. The decrease in collagen 1 and 3 staining was observed in the present study in the LV-shRNA-ADAMTS-1 transduced vessels when compared to controls and we speculate that these changes may reflect the reduction in VEGF-A and other cytokines which were not measured.

A recent demonstrated that there is increased expression of ADAMTS-1 which is associated with CD68 staining in patients with acute myocardial infarction [9]. In the present study, we observed a significant decrease in CD68 staining for macrophages

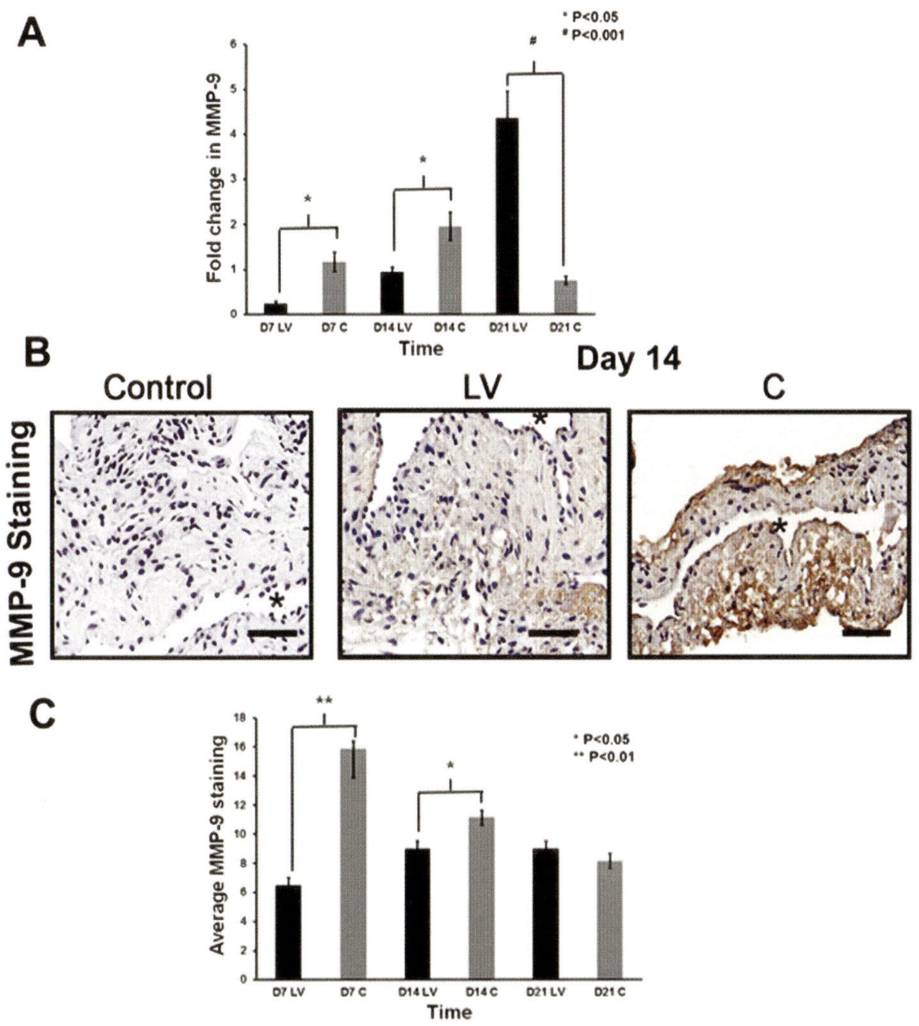

Figure 7. MMP-9 expression is decreased in LV-shRNA-ADAMTS-1 transduced vessels. A) is pooled data for qPCR analysis for MMP-9 expression of the LV-shRNA-ADAMTS-1 (**LV**) and control shRNA (**C**) transduced vessels at day 7 (**D7**), 14 (**D14**), and 21 (**D21**). This demonstrates a significant reduction in the average expression of MMP-9 in the **LV** transduced vessels when compared to **C** at day 7 ($P<0.05$) and 14 ($P<0.05$) with a significant increase in MMP-2 by day 28 ($P<0.001$). **B**) are representative sections from MMP-9 staining at the venous stenosis of the **LV** and **C** transduced vessels at day at day 14. Cells staining brown are positive for MMP-9. IgG antibody staining was performed to serve as negative control. **C**) is pooled data for the average MMP-9 expression at the outflow vein of the **LV** and **C** transduced vessels at day 7 (**D7**), 14 (**D14**), and 21 (**D21**). This shows that there is a significant reduction in the mean MMP-9 staining in the **LV** transduced vessels when compared to controls by day 7 ($P<0.01$) and day 14 ($P<0.05$). All are 40X. Scale bar is 50-μM. * Indicates the lumen. Each bar shows mean ± SEM of 3-6 animals per group (**A, C**). Two-way ANOVA followed by Student *t*-test with post hoc Bonferroni's correction was performed. Significant difference from control value was indicated by $^{*}P<0.05$ or $^{\#}P<0.001$.

at day 7. However, we did not observe a difference in smooth muscle staining at any of the time points. These results imply that ADAMTS-1 reduction results in macrophage density possibly by reducing macrophage infiltration which has been observed in experimental vascular injury [22].

In conclusion, the present study demonstrates that reducing ADAMTS-1 mRNA expression levels at the time of placement of AVF results in a positive vascular associated with a reduction in macrophage staining. There is a decrease in VEGF-A expression as well as a decrease in MMP-9 expression accompanied with a reduction in proliferation, constrictive remodeling, CD31 staining, and an increase in TUNEL. These findings have implications for the development of translational therapies aimed at inhibiting VNH in patients with AVF and ESRD.

Significance

There are more than 400,000 patients in the United States who require hemodialysis because of end-stage renal disease (ESRD). Hemodialysis vascular access can develop venous neointimal hyperplasia (VNH) causing access failure. Recent clinical and experimental data has demonstrated that there is increased expression of a disintegrin and metalloproteinase thrombospondin motifs–1 (ADAMTS-1) at site of VNH. Using a murine model of

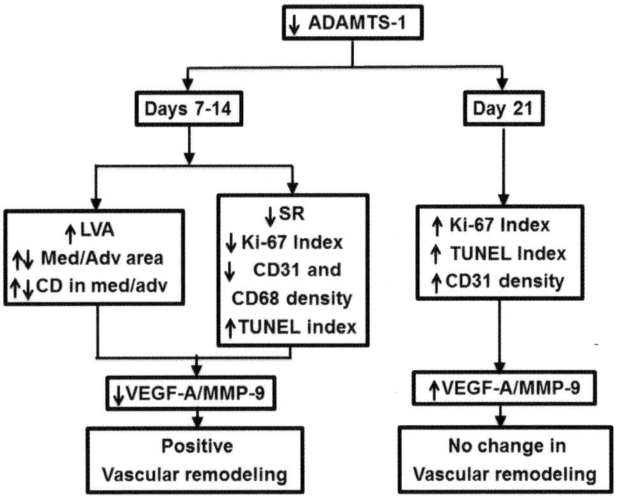

Figure 8. Synopsis of major findings.

AVF with chronic kidney disease, we reduced ADAMTS-1 mRNA expression with a small hairpin RNA that inhibits ADAMTS-1 expression (LV-shRNA-ADAMTS-1) at the time of fistula creation. This resulted in a decrease in VNH accompanied with a decrease in macrophage staining with no change in smooth muscle density. At early time points, ADAMTS-1 expression was significantly decreased accompanied with a decrease in vascular endothelial growth factor-A (VEGF-A) and matrix metalloproteinase-9 (MMP-9). These changes in gene expression resulted in decrease in media/adventitia area, with a significant increase in TUNEL staining accompanied with a decrease in cellular proliferation.

Author Contributions

Conceived and designed the experiments: SM DM ENT BY RJ. Performed the experiments: BY AB RJ ENT. Analyzed the data: BY AB RJ DM EL ENT. Contributed reagents/materials/analysis tools: BY AB RJ ENT. Wrote the paper: BY AB RJ.

References

1. Collins AJ, Kasiske B, Herzog C, Chen SC, Everson S, et al. (2003) Excerpts from the United States Renal Data System 2003 Annual Data Report: atlas of end-stage renal disease in the United States. Am J Kidney Dis 42: A5–7.
2. Rooijens PPGM, Tordoir JHM, Stijnen T, Burgmans JPJ, Smet de AAEA, et al. (2004) Radiocephalic Wrist Arteriovenous Fistula for Hemodialysis: Meta-analysis Indicates a High Primary Failure Rate. European Journal of Vascular and Endovascular Surgery 28: 583–589.
3. (2006) National Kidney Foundation: NKF K/DOQI Guidelines: Clinical Practice Gudelines and Clinical Practice Recommendations.
4. Sullivan KL, Besarab A, Bonn J, Shapiro MJ, Gardiner Jr GA, et al. (1993) Hemodynamics of failing dialysis grafts. Radiology 186: 867–872.
5. Jonsson-Rylander A-C, Nilsson T, Fritsche-Danielson R, Hammarstrom A, Behrendt M, et al. (2005) Role of ADAMTS-1 in Atherosclerosis: Remodeling of Carotid Artery, Immunohistochemistry, and Proteolysis of Versican. 10.1161/01.ATV.0000150045.27127.37. Arterioscler Thromb Vasc Biol 25: 180–185.
6. Misra S, Lee N, Fu AA, Raghavakaimal S, Mandrekar J, et al. (2008) Increased expression of a disintegrin and metalloproteinase thrombospondin 1 in thrombosed hemodialysis grafts. J Vasc Interv Radiol 19: 111–119.
7. Misra S, Shergill U, Yang B, Janardhanan R, Misra KD (2010) Increased expression of HIF-1alpha, VEGF-A and its receptors, MMP-2, TIMP-1, and ADAMTS-1 at the venous stenosis of arteriovenous fistula in a mouse model with renal insufficiency. J Vasc Interv Radiol 21: 1255–1261.
8. Kuno K, Kanada N, Nakashima E, Fujiki F, Ichimura F, et al. (1997) Molecular cloning of a gene encoding a new type of metalloproteinase-disintegrin family protein with thrombospondin motifs as an inflammation associated gene. J Biol Chem 272: 556–562.
9. Lee CW, Hwang I, Park CS, Lee H, Park DW, et al. (2011) Comparison of ADAMTS-1, -4 and -5 expression in culprit plaques between acute myocardial infarction and stable angina. J Clin Pathol 64: 399–404.
10. (1996) Committee on care and use of laboratory animals of the institute of laboratory animal resources. Washington, DC: Government print office.
11. Yang B, Shergill U, Fu AA, Knudsen B, Misra S (2009) The mouse arteriovenous fistula model. J Vasc Interv Radiol 20: 946–950.
12. Yang B, Janardhanan R, Vohra P, Greene EL, Bhattacharya S, et al. (2013) Adventitial Transduction of Lentivirus-shRNA-VEGF-A treatment in Arteriovenous Fistula Reduces Venous Stenosis Formation Kid Int online.
13. Janardhanan R, Yang B, Vohra P, Roy B, Withers S, et al. (2013) Simvastatin reduces venous stenosis formation in a murine hemodialysis vascular access model. Kidney Int.
14. Misra S, Shergill U, Yang B, Janardhanan R, Misra K (2010) Increased expression of HIF-1α, VEGF-A and its receptors, MMP-2, TIMP-1, and ADAMTS-1 at the venous stenosis of arteriovenous fistula in a mouse model with renal insufficiency. J Vasc Interv Radiol in press.
15. Turunen MP, Lehtola T, Heinonen SE, Assefa GS, Korpisalo P, et al. (2009) Efficient regulation of VEGF expression by promoter-targeted lentiviral shRNAs based on epigenetic mechanism: a novel example of epigenetherapy. Circ Res 105: 604–609.
16. Janardhanan R, Yang B, Vohra P, Roy B, Withers S, et al. (2013) Simvastatin Reduces Venous Stenosis Formation in a Murine Hemodialysis Vascular Access Model Kidney International in press.
17. Baboolal K, Evans C, Moore RH (1998) Incidence of end-stage renal disease in medically treated patients with severe bilateral atherosclerotic renovascular disease. Am J Kidney Dis 31: 971–977.
18. Misra S, Doherty MG, Woodrum D, Homburger J, Mandrekar JN, et al. (2005) Adventitial remodeling with increased matrix metalloproteinase-2 activity in a porcine arteriovenous polytetrafluoroethylene grafts. Kidney Int 68: 2890–2900.
19. Misra S, Fu AA, Puggioni A, Karimi KM, Mandrekar JN, et al. (2008) Increased shear stress with up regulation of VEGF-A and its receptors and MMP-2, MMP-9, and TIMP-1 in venous stenosis of hemodialysis grafts Am J Physiol Heart Circ Physiol 294: H2219–2230.
20. Li L, Terry CM, Blumenthal DK, Kuji T, Masaki T, et al. (2007) Cellular and morphological changes during neointimal hyperplasia development in a porcine arteriovenous graft model. Nephrol Dial Transplant 22: 3139–3146.
21. Wang Y, Krishnamoorthy M, Banerjee R, Zhang J, Rudich S, et al. (2007) Venous stenosis in a pig arteriovenous fistula model anatomy, mechanisms and cellular phenotypes. Nephrol Dial Transplant 22: 3139–3146.
22. Ashlin TG, Kwan AP, Ramji DP (2013) Regulation of ADAMTS-1, -4 and -5 expression in human macrophages: differential regulation by key cytokines implicated in atherosclerosis and novel synergism between TL1A and IL-17. Cytokine 64: 234–242.
23. Vazquez F, Hastings G, Ortega M-A, Lane TF, Oikemus S, et al. (1999) METH-1, a Human Ortholog of ADAMTS-1, and METH-2 Are Members of a New Family of Proteins with Angio-inhibitory Activity. 10.1074/jbc.274.33.23349. J Biol Chem 274: 23349–23357.
24. Misra S, Fu A, Rajan D, Juncos L, McKusick M, et al. (2008) Expression of hypoxia inducible factor-1 alpha, macrophage migration inhibition factor, matrix metalloproteinase-2 and -9, and their inhibitors in hemodialysis grafts and arteriovenous fistulas. J Vasc Interv Radiol 19: 252–259.
25. Misra S, Fu A, Anderson J, Glockner J, McKusick M, et al. (2008) The rat femoral arteriovenous fistula model: Increased expression of MMP-2 and MMP-9 at the venous stenosis. J Vasc Interv Radiol 19: 587–594.
26. Luque A, Carpizo DR, Iruela-Arispe ML (2003) ADAMTS1/METH1 inhibits endothelial cell proliferation by direct binding and sequestration of VEGF(165). Journal of Biological Chemistry 278: 23656–23665.
27. Luque A, Carpizo DR, Iruela-Arispe ML (2003) ADAMTS1/METH1 Inhibits Endothelial Cell Proliferation by Direct Binding and Sequestration of VEGF165. 10.1074/jbc.M212964200. J Biol Chem 278: 23656–23665.
28. Fu Y, Nagy JA, Brown LF, Shih SC, Johnson PY, et al. (2011) Proteolytic cleavage of versican and involvement of ADAMTS-1 in VEGF-A/VPF-induced pathological angiogenesis. J Histochem Cytochem 59: 463–473.

29. Xu Z, Yu Y, Duh EJ (2006) Vascular endothelial growth factor upregulates expression of ADAMTS1 in endothelial cells through protein kinase C signaling. Invest Ophthalmol Vis Sci 47: 4059–4066.
30. Liu YJ, Xu Y, Yu Q (2006) Full-length ADAMTS-1 and the ADAMTS-1 fragments display pro- and antimetastatic activity, respectively. Oncogene 25: 2452–2467.
31. Cheema AN, Hong T, Nili N, Segev A, Moffat JG, et al. (2006) Adventitial Microvessel Formation After Coronary Stenting and the Effects of SU11218, a Tyrosine Kinase Inhibitor. Journal of the American College of Cardiology 47: 1067–1075.
32. Rotmans JI, Velema E, Verhagen HJ, Blankensteijn JD, de Kleijn DP, et al. (2004) Matrix metalloproteinase inhibition reduces intimal hyperplasia in a porcine arteriovenous-graft model. J Vasc Surg 39: 432–439.
33. Abbruzzese TA, Guzman RJ, Martin RL, Yee C, Zarins CK, et al. (1998) Matrix metalloproteinase inhibition limits arterial enlargements in a rodent arteriovenous fistula model. Surgery 124: 328–334; discussion 334–325.
34. Rocks N, Paulissen G, El Hour M, Quesada F, Crahay C, et al. (2008) Emerging roles of ADAM and ADAMTS metalloproteinases in cancer. Biochimie 90: 369–379.
35. Katoh O, Takahashi T, Oguri T, Kuramoto K, Mihara K, et al. (1998) Vascular endothelial growth factor inhibits apoptotic death in hematopoietic cells after exposure to chemotherapeutic drugs by inducing MCL1 acting as an antiapoptotic factor. Cancer Res 58: 5565–5569.
36. Katoh O, Tauchi H, Kawaishi K, Kimura A, Satow Y (1995) Expression of the vascular endothelial growth factor (VEGF) receptor gene, KDR, in hematopoietic cells and inhibitory effect of VEGF on apoptotic cell death caused by ionizing radiation. Cancer Res 55: 5687–5692.

11

Short Daily versus Conventional Hemodialysis for Hypertensive Patients

Deborah L. Zimmerman[1]*, Marcel Ruzicka[1], Paul Hebert[2], Dean Fergusson[3], Rhian M. Touyz[4], Kevin D. Burns[5]

1 Associate Professor of Medicine, Division of Nephrology, Ottawa Hospital, Kidney Research Centre of the Ottawa Hospital Research Institute, University of Ottawa, Ottawa, Ontario, Canada, **2** Professor of Medicine, Surgery, Anesthesia and Epidemiology, University of Ottawa; Senior Scientist, Clinical Epidemiology, Ottawa Hospital Research Institute, Ottawa, Ontario, Canada, **3** Associate Professor, Departments of Medicine, Surgery, Epidemiology and Community Medicine, Senior Scientist and Director, Clinical Epidemiology Program, Ottawa Hospital Research Institute, Ottawa, Ontario, Canada, **4** Institute of Cardiovascular and Medical Sciences, BHF Glasgow Cardiovascular Research Centre, University of Glasgow, Glasgow, United Kingdom, **5** Professor of Medicine, Division of Nephrology, Senior Scientist, Kidney Research Centre of the Ottawa Hospital Research Institute, University of Ottawa, Ottawa, Ontario, Canada

Abstract

Background: Treatment of end stage renal disease patients with short daily hemodialysis has been associated with an improvement in blood pressure. It is unclear from these studies if anti-hypertensive management had been optimized prior to starting short daily hemodialysis. Also, the potential mechanism(s) of blood pressure improvement remain to be fully elucidated.

Study Design, Setting and Participants: We undertook a randomized cross-over trial in adult hypertensive patients with ESRD treated with conventional hemodialysis to determine: 1) if short-daily hemodialysis is associated with a reduction in systolic blood pressure after a 3-month blood pressure optimization period and; 2) the potential mechanism(s) of blood pressure reduction. Blood pressure was measured using Canadian Hypertension Education Program guidelines. Extracellular fluid volume (ECFV) was assessed with bioimpedance. Serum catecholamines were used to assess the sympathetic nervous system. Interleukin-6 (IL-6) and thiobarbituric acid reactive substances (T-BARS) were used as markers of inflammation and oxidative stress respectively.

Results: After a 3-month run-in phase in which systolic blood pressure improved, there was no significant difference in pre-dialysis systolic pressure between short-daily and conventional hemodialysis ($p = 0.39$). However, similar blood pressures were achieved on fewer anti-hypertensive medications with short daily hemodialysis compared to conventional hemodialysis ($p = 0.01$). Short daily hemodialysis, compared to conventional hemodialysis, was not associated with a difference in dry weight or ECFV ($p = 0.77$). Sympathetic nervous system activity as assessed by plasma epinephrine ($p = 1.0$) and norepinephrine ($p = 0.52$) was also not different. Markers of inflammation ($p = 0.42$) and oxidative stress ($p = 0.83$) were also similar between the two treatment arms.

Conclusions: Patients treated with short daily, compared to conventional hemodialysis, have similar blood pressure control on fewer anti-hypertensive medications. The mechanism(s) by which short daily hemodialysis allows for decreased anti-hypertensive medication use remains unclear but effects on sodium balance and changes in peripheral vascular resistance require further study.

Editor: Dominique Guerrot, Rouen University Hospital, France

Funding: This study was funded by the Ontario Heart and Stroke Foundation and the Ottawa Hospital Department of Medicine. The funders had no role in study design, data collection and analysis, decison to publish, or preparation of the manuscript.

Competing Interests: The authors have declared no competing interests exist.

* E-mail: dzimmerman@toh.on.ca

Introduction

More than 50% of the patients with end stage renal disease (ESRD) die from cardiovascular disease, a risk 10–20 times greater than the general population [1,2]. Of the potentially modifiable cardiovascular risk factors, greater than 80% of patients with ESRD have hypertension; 70% of whom are poorly controlled using conventional therapy [3]. An expanded extracellular fluid volume (ECFV) and an increase in peripheral vascular resistance (PVR) due to hemodynamic/trophic effects of increased sympathetic nerve activity and inflammation are frequently quoted mechanisms contributing to hypertension in ESRD [4]. Common to these processes is increased bioavailability of reactive oxygen species [5].

The intermittent nature of conventional hemodialysis treatments (4 hours, 3 days/week) results in the majority of patients having a fluctuating ECFV that likely contributes to the activation of neurohormonal pathways [6]. However, daily hemodialysis therapy including short daily (2 hours, 6 days/week) and nocturnal (6–8 hours, 5–6 days/week) improves or even normalizes blood pressure [6–12]. Short daily hemodialysis reportedly improves blood pressure secondary to a reduction in ECFV [6,9] whereas nocturnal hemodialysis appears to be associated with a reduction in PVR [9–11]. This suggests that different mechanisms of blood pressure reduction may vary in different patient groups. In a study by Katzarski et al, patients who were normotensive and dialyzed for 7–8 hours, 3 days/week were compared to normotensive and hypertensive patients whose treatment time was 3–5 hours [13]. There was no overall difference in the ECFV and inferior vena cava diameter between the two normotensive groups, which were lower than the hypertensive patients. However, 24% of the patients treated with long dialysis appeared to have an expanded ECFV such that the authors hypothesized that normotension in these patients might be explained by the removal of a vasoactive hormone. Their results are supported by a small randomized controlled trial of blood pressure control in 21 ESRD patients in which 7 patients had their dialysis time increased by 2 hours, 6 patients had their dialysis time increased by 2 hours and dry weight reduced, and 8 patients only had their dry weight reduced [14]. Despite a decrease in dry weight (and presumably ECFV) in only 2 of the groups, systolic blood pressure and use of anti-hypertensive medication use was reduced in all 3 groups.

In the majority of reported studies it is unclear if the patient's antihypertensive management, including achievement of the appropriate dry weight, had been optimized prior to the introduction of more intensive hemodialysis. A limited number of investigations have been undertaken to determine the mechanisms of blood pressure reduction. For this reason, we undertook a randomized cross-over trial in patients with ESRD treated with hemodialysis. Our primary objective was to determine if short-daily hemodialysis, compared to conventional hemodialysis, is associated with a reduction in systolic blood pressure pre-dialysis after an optimization period. Our secondary objective was to determine the potential mechanism(s) of blood pressure reduction by assessing extracellular fluid volume and the sympathetic nervous system. The potential role of inflammation and oxidative stress were added to the study design because of the increasing evidence suggesting that these mediators may have an etiologic role in hypertension [5,15].

Methods

Study Overview

We undertook a 9-month randomized, crossover trial of adult prevalent hypertensive ESRD patients. Paperwork for the trial was submitted to the Ottawa Hospital Research Institute in June 2007 for registration at clinicaltrials.gov as per protocol at the time but due to administrative delays was not released until September 24, 2008 (NCT00759967). The protocol for this trial and supporting CONSORT checklist is available; see Checklist S1 and Protocol S1. The Ottawa Hospital Research Ethics Board approved the study and all amendments. The study was conducted according to the Declaration of Helsinki.

Run-in Phase

Inclusion criteria included: 1) on hemodialysis for >3 months, 2) any patient on 1 or 2 antihypertensive medications with a pre-dialysis systolic blood pressure of >140 on average over 1 month, 3) any patient on 3 or more antihypertensive medications regardless of pre-dialysis systolic pressure, 4) able to make the time commitment to daily therapy, and 5) able to give informed consent. Patients were excluded if they were expected to switch treatment modality or die within one year or have known dilated cardiomyopathy with an ejection fraction <0.3. Eligible patients provided written informed consent to the study coordinator and then underwent a 3-month run-in phase. All patients were dialyzed with a Fresenius K machine, Optiflux 160 dialyzer, blood pump speed 300–400 mls/min and a dialysate flow of 500 mls/minute. A protocolized blood pressure algorithm was followed to optimize blood pressure control (Figure 1). Briefly, all patients met with the renal dietician. The dietary sodium (<2 grams per day) and fluid restrictions (1L per day) as per unit policy were re-enforced. The dialysate sodium was reduced to 138 mmol/L from 140 mmol/L, the latter being the standard sodium concentration in our Ottawa Hospital hemodialysis units. At each hemodialysis treatment, a pre and post hemodialysis blood pressure was measured using techniques recommended by the Canadian Hypertension Education program. Changes were made to dry weight and/or antihypertensive medications every 2 weeks by the principal investigator if the 2-week average pre-dialysis systolic blood pressure was greater than 140 mmHg. Forty-four hour ambulatory blood pressure was also measured in the last week of the run-in phase. The number, type and strength of antihypertensive medications were recorded at study entry and at the end of each month. Intensity of anti-hypertensive medication use was estimated as multiples of the smallest available dose for that particular medication (eg. amlodipine - smallest available dose 5 mg = 1: 10 mg = 2, 2.5 mg = 0.5). Standard of care monthly laboratory investigations (complete blood count, electrolytes, calcium, phosphate, albumin, creatinine and pre/post hemodialysis urea were collected at baseline and the last month of the run-in phase on a Wednesday or Thursday pre-dialysis.

Randomization

After the 3 month run-in phase, patients were randomized using a computer generated randomization sequence. Each patient completed 3 months of conventional 3 times per week hemodialysis or 6 times per week short daily hemodialysis and then crossed over to the other treatment arm (Fig. 2). The only differences in the short daily dialysis prescription was to increase the frequency from 3 days to 6 days, decrease the hemodialysis session time by 50% and decrease the dialysate bicarbonate concentration to 32 mmol/L from 36 mmol/L to avoid metabolic alkalosis [16]. The assessment of blood pressure with adjustments to weight and anti-hypertensive medications was the same as for the run-in phase. Standard monthly laboratory investigations were also the same except during short daily hemodialysis, blood was collected on Monday (after a day off).

Assessment of Extracellular Fluid Volume

Post treatment extracellular fluid volume was measured with the Xitron Hydra (Xitron Technologies, San Diego, CA) using standard techniques. The Hydra is a multifrequency bioimpedance analyzer that allows for differentiation of ECFV and intracellular fluid volume by detecting differences in the conductive properties of cells by measuring resistance (impedance) to electrical current. The technique is reliable in tracking sequential changes in ECFV with a reported coefficient of variation and intra-observer error of 2.5% [13,17]. All measurements were taken 20 minutes after completion of the hemodialysis treatment, by placing 4 electrodes on the wrist and ankle on the non-fistula side. Yearly calibration of the equipment was performed by the Ottawa Hospital technical department.

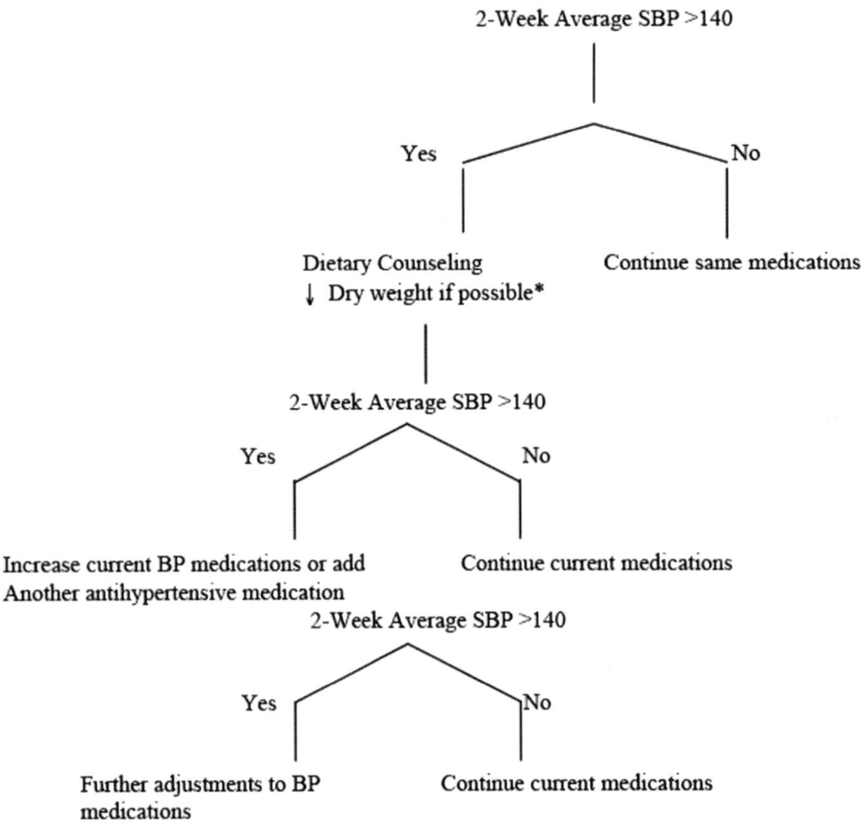

*If SBP is >140, pre-dialysis weight will be decreased by 0.3kg/dialysis session until SBP <140 or the patient develops symptoms such as cramping, headaches, post dialysis fatigue

Figure 1. Protocolized Blood Pressure Management Algorithm.

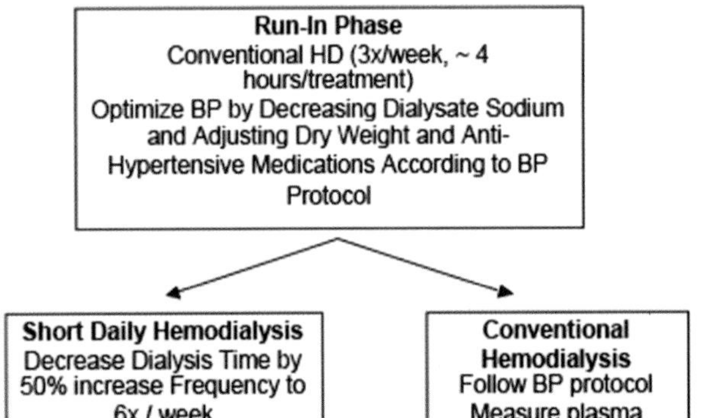

Figure 2. Flow Diagram.

Measurement of Plasma Catecholamines

Blood samples were taken post dialysis with the patient in a quiet dark room prior to the removal of the hemodialysis needles. The plasma samples were prepared immediately and stored at −80C and analyzed within 6 months by high performance liquid chromatography at a commercial laboratory.

Markers of Inflammation and Oxidative Stress

Plasma interleukin-6 (IL-6) and plasma thiobarbituric acid reactive substances (T-BARS) were used as markers of inflammation and oxidative stress respectively. Plasma was prepared from blood collected in EDTA vacutainer tubes pre-dialysis and stored at −80°C. Plasma levels of IL-6 were measured using a solid-phase sandwich ELISA kit from Biosource International according to manufacturer's instructions. Plasma TBARS levels were measured colorimetrically and values were expressed in nmol/ml malondialdehyde (MDA) equivalents as we previously reported [18,19].

Analysis

Based on our previous experience with daily hemofiltration, we calculated that 20 patients would be required to detect a difference of 11 mmHg in systolic blood pressure assuming a standard deviation of 11, a two-sided alpha = 0.05, and a power of 80% [20].

Results are expressed as means and standard deviations or median and interquartile range depending on normality assumptions for continuous data and frequency for categorical data as appropriate. The primary analysis was intention to treat paired t-test of the comparison of the mean pre-dialysis systolic blood pressure values from the last month on conventional hemodialysis and the last month of short daily hemodialysis (last value carried forward for missing blood pressure data). As described by Zoccali et al, this gives an assessment of the pressure load as experienced by the left ventricle [21]. To assess order effect (or period effect) a GEE model with SBP as outcome and treatment and period as predictors, accounting for patient effect in repeated measures was performed.

A paired t-test was also used for weight, ECFV, total ultrafiltration and ultrafiltration rate. Due to the non-normal distribution of the hypertension medication intensity score, serum catecholamines, IL-6 and TBARs, these were compared using the Wilcoxin sign rank test. Linear regression analysis was undertaken to explore the predictors of the intensity of anti-hypertensive medication use after conventional and daily hemodialysis (post-hoc).

Results

Twenty-two patients consented to participate in the study; 3 patients withdrew prior to randomization, 2 patients did not complete the short daily hemodialysis (Figure 3). Therefore data from 19 patients were included in the systolic blood pressure analysis. Patient demographics are depicted in Table 1. The average age of the participating patients was 53 years, 11 patients (58%) had a history of diabetes mellitus and the majority of patients were male.

There was a statistically significant decrease in systolic blood pressure from study entry to the end of the run in phase (151 vs 138 mmHg; $p = 0.004$) without an overall change in dry weight (77.4 vs 77.1 kgs; $p = 0.63$) or intensity of antihypertensive medications (5.46 vs 5.16; $p = 0.57$). Although we did not demonstrate a reduction in average post dialysis body weight at the end of the run-in phase compared to baseline, there was tremendous variability with the weights of some participants being decreased (maximum 8.7 kgs) and the weights of other participants being increased (maximum 5.4 kgs). Similar changes were seen in the anti-hypertensive medication use from baseline to the end of the run-in phase with some patients requiring increased medication while other patients had decreased medication. Overall, there was a decline in the amount of ultrafiltration per treatment from the first month of the run-in phase to the last month of the run-in phase (2.5L vs 2.3L; $p = 0.007$).

Of the standard biochemical tests throughout the study, serum sodium was 138 mmol/L at baseline and 137 mmol/L at the end of the run-in phase. This change was maintained throughout the study. Serum phosphate declined from 1.86 mmol/L at baseline to 1.61 mmol/L at the end of the run-in phase ($p = 0.04$). During conventional hemodialysis and short daily hemodialysis after randomization, serum phosphate was 1.82 mmol/L and 1.58 mmol/L respectively ($p = 0.25$). Weekly Kt/V was similar at the end of the run in phase and 3 months of conventional HD (5.4) but increased (6.6) during short daily HD. No changes were observed in serum potassium, calcium, bicarbonate or albumin throughout the study

Changes in the antihypertensive medication classes are shown in Table 2 at baseline, after the run-in, short daily and conventional hemodialysis phases. After 3 months of short daily, compared to 3 months of conventional hemodialysis, systolic and diastolic blood pressures were not statistically different ($p = 0.39$, $p = 0.56$ respectively; Table 3) and there was no period effect ($p = 0.40$, figure 4). These results are supported by the 44-hour ABPM. However, these similar blood pressures were achieved on a lower intensity of hypertension medication use in the short daily hemodialysis phase compared to conventional hemodialysis phase

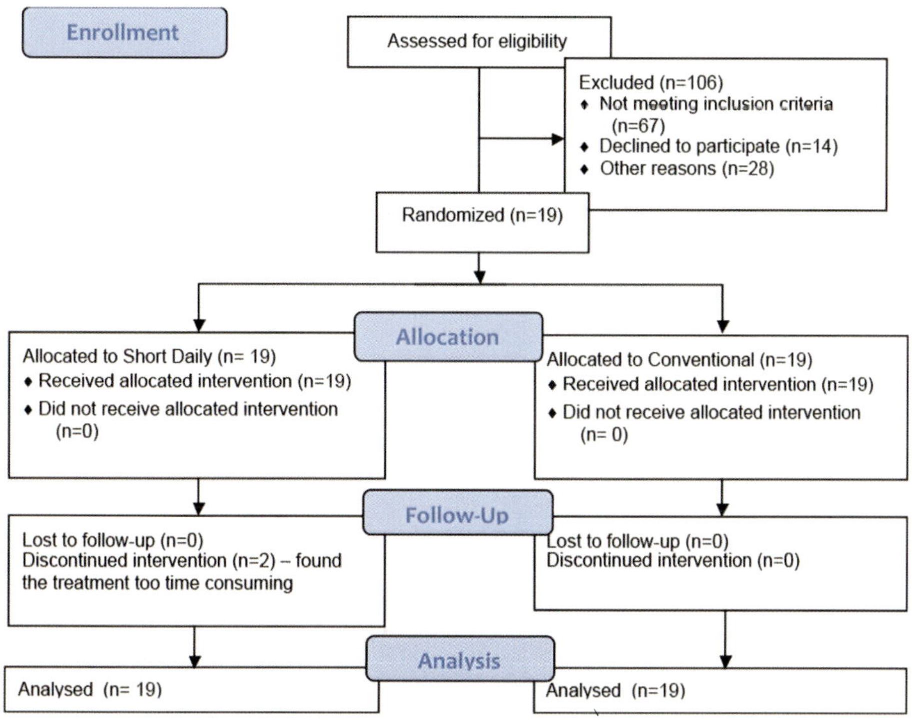

Figure 3. Trial Flow.

Table 1. Baseline Patient Characteristics.

Patient Characteristics	
Age – Years (SD)	53 (13)
Gender (M:F)	13:6
Dialysis Vintage – Day (SD)	1368 (1670)
Charlson Comorbidity Score (SD)	6 (2)
Etiology of ESRD	DM (7), GN (6), HTN (2), Multiple Myeloma (1), Amyloid (1), Other (2)
History of Diabetes Mellitus (Y/N)	11/8
Access Type (AVF/AVG/CVC)	11/2/6
Dry Weight (kgs)	77.4 (14.3)
Baseline BP (SD)	151 (12)/79 (9)
HTN Medication Intensity Score	5.46 (2.94)

SD – standard deviation, M – Male, F – Female, HTN – hypertension, ESRD – end stage renal disease, DM – diabetes mellitus, GN – glomerulonephritis (includes IgA, Goodpasture's, Immunofibrillary), Y/N – yes/no, AVF – arteriovenous fistula, AVG – arteriovenous graft, CVC – central venous catheter, kgs – kilograms.

($p = 0.01$, Table 4). There were no significant differences in dry weight, ECFV, plasma epinephrine or nor-epinephrine levels between conventional hemodialysis and short daily hemodialysis (Table 4). There was no difference between IL-6 and TBARS by treatment modality. Plasma catecholamines, ECFV and serum phosphate were not significantly associated with antihypertensive medication intensity score on conventional ($p = 0.42$, 0.88, 0.09 respectively) or short daily hemodialysis ($p = 0.24$, 0.22, 0.68 respectively).

Serious adverse events were rare during the trial. One patient was hospitalized during the study during the short daily hemodialysis phase with volume overload.

Discussion

Short daily hemodialysis achieves a similar degree of systolic blood pressure control compared to conventional 3 times per week hemodialysis after a blood pressure optimization phase. However, this control is associated with a decreased requirement for antihypertensive medications. Our results highlight the importance of a run-in phase using a protocolized blood pressure algorithm when treatment modalities cannot be blinded.

The decline in blood pressure at the end of the 3 month run-in phase, compared to baseline, was likely multifactorial. Although we did not demonstrate a reduction in average post dialysis weight, there was tremendous variability with some participant's weight being decreased and other participant's weight being increased. Similar changes were seen in the anti-hypertensive medication use. A reduction in dialysate sodium has been associated with a reduction in blood pressure in hypertensive patients without a change in pre-dialysis serum sodium concentration in some [22,23] but not all studies [24]. Post dialysis increases in serum sodium have been demonstrated for patients treated with

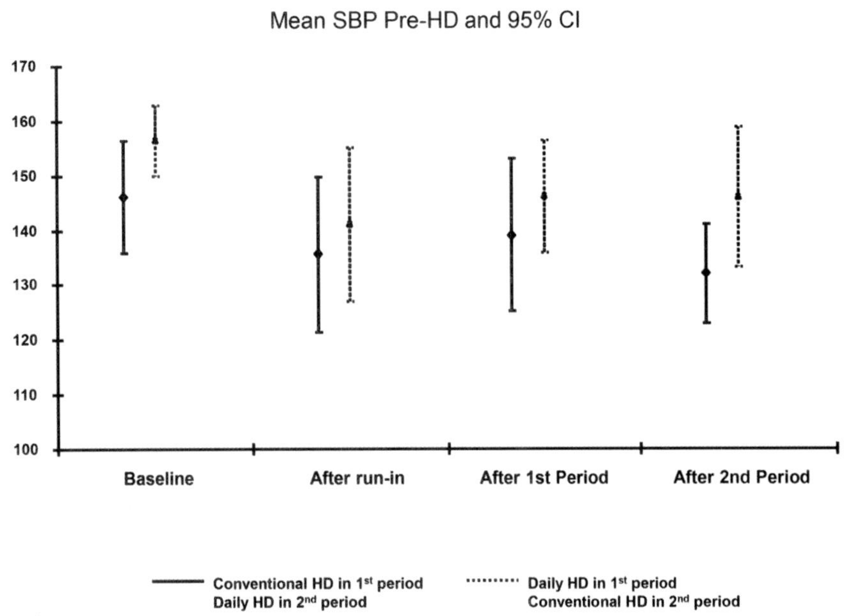

Figure 4. Graph of Period Effects.

Table 2. Changes in Classes of Anti-Hypertensive Medications during the Trial.

	Baseline	Run-In	CHD	DHD
Ace-I	10	9	10	8
ARB	8	5	4	3
β-blocker	11	9	6	6
DHCCB	14	13	11	8
α-blocker	5	2	2	1
Central sympatholytic	1	1	1	1
Diuretic	3	4	3	4
Arterial Vasodilator	2	2	2	2

Ace-I – Angiotensin Converting Enzyme Inhibitor, ARB – angiotensin receptor blocker, DHCCB – dihydropyridine calcium channel blocker.

conventional hemodialysis with dialysate sodium that is higher than the patient's serum sodium with a potential increase in thirst (occurs in 43% when dialysate sodium is 140 mmol/L, 20% when dialysate sodium is 138 mmol/L, [25]). It is unclear if the dietary instruction or the decrease in dialysate sodium in our study caused the small but statistically significant decrease in the total amount of ultrafiltration from the first month of the run in phase to the last month of the run in phase.

The mechanism for the decrease in antihypertensive requirements on short daily hemodialysis, compared to conventional hemodialysis, is unclear. A reduction in ECFV has been demonstrated in some [6,9] but not all [7] studies as a mechanism contributing to the blood pressure lowering effect associated with short daily dialysis. Our study does not support this association for the population. There are a number of potential reasons for the differences in our results compared to other studies. To our knowledge a protocolized blood pressure management algorithm aimed at achieving an optimal dry weight prior to starting short daily hemodialysis has not been followed previously. Even during conventional hemodialysis 'probing dry weight' as was done in the DRIP trial was associated with approximately 7/3 mmHg decline in systolic and diastolic blood pressure respectively [26]. Also, given the inability to blind these modality studies, the possibility of differential patient management is possible.

The activity of the sympathetic nervous system was found to be important in a study that included 11 patients treated with short daily hemodialysis [6]. The investigators demonstrated a reduction in ultrafiltration volumes per session almost identical to those reported in our study. They hypothesized that large volume fluctuations could result in greater sympathetic nervous system stimulation. Greater amounts of ultrafiltration may also lead to increased post dialysis serum sodium which may stimulate the sympathetic nervous system [27]. We were unable demonstrate a difference in serum catecholamines with short daily compared to conventional hemodialysis but this does not rule out increase central sympathetic outflow.

In that last decade there has been an emerging evidence to support importance of oxidative stress in the development of hypertension [28,29]. Hydrogen peroxide production (H_2O_2) was higher in granulocytes of patients with CKD treated with hemodialysis compared to controls [30]. The magnitude of ROS production by granulocytes and monocytes in that study population was significantly related to the plasma concentration of the lipid peroxidation product, malondialdehyde (MDA), which is commonly used as an indirect marker of oxidative stress [30] H_2O_2 levels increased after hemodialysis with a cellulose acetate dialyzer highlighting the potential deleterious effects associated with the dialysis treatment itself [30]. We were unable to show a difference in serum T-BARs (measure of MDA) with short daily

Table 3. Results of the Intervention Phases; Normally Distributed Data.

	3-Months Conventional HD	3-Months Daily HD	Paired-Difference		p-value
			Negative N(%)	Positive N(%)	
SBP pre-HD (mmHg; SD)	142(17)	139(14)	11(58)	8(42)	0.39
DBP pre-HD (mmHg; SD)	79(9)	80(9)	10(53)	9(47)	0.56
SBP post-HD (mmHg; SD)	127(19)	125(14)	8(42)	11(58)	0.40
DBP post-HD (mmHg; SD)	75(11)	76(8)	13(68)	6(32)	0.40
Dry Weight (kgs; SD)	77(14.4)	76.8(15.1)	9(47)	10(53)	0.70
Ultrafiltration/treatment (L; SD)	2.4(0.8)	1.3(0.6)	0(0)	19(100)	<0.001
Ultrafiltration rate (L/hr; SD)	0.60(0.20)	0.65(0.29)	12(63)	7(37)	0.17
ECFV (L; SD)	15.4(2.8)	15.2(3.2)	*11(65)	6(35)	0.77

SBP – systolic blood pressure, HD – hemodialysis, SD – standard deviation, DBP – diastolic blood pressure, kgs – kilograms, L – liter, hr - hour;
*last value not carried forward for the 2 patients who withdrew.

Table 4. Results of the Intervention Phases; Non-Normally Distributed Data.

	'N'	Paired Difference CHD-DHD Median (Quartiles)	Paired-Difference			p-value
			Negative N(%)	No change N(%)	Positive N(%)	
HTN Medication Intensity Score	19	1(0,2)	1(5.3)	7 (36.8)	11 (57.9)	0.01
Epinephrine, umol/L	10*	0(0,0)	1 (10)	8 (80)	1 (10)	1
Nor-Epinephrine, umol/L	15**	−0.2(−0.7, 0.3)	9 (60)	0	6 (40)	0.52
IL_6	12***	−0.35(−1.15, 0.29)	7 (58.3)	0	5 (41.7)	0.42
TBARS	12***	0.15(−0.65, 0.5)	5 (41.7)	0	7 (58.3)	0.83

* 7 samples had chromatographic interference - lab unable to do analysis, 2 patients withdrew from the study;
** 2 patients withdrew from the study, 2 samples were missed,
***started to measure these after the first 5 patients were already enrolled, 2 patients withdrew from the study.

compared to conventional hemodialysis. Interestingly, phosphate has been shown to stimulate endothelial cell apoptosis which was characterized by increased oxidative stress [31]. It is unclear if the effects of an increase in dialysis frequency and exposure to dialysis tubing and membranes is counterbalanced by the improvements in serum phosphate that have been reported with short daily dialysis.

A generalized increase in inflammatory markers including IL-6 may occur via a number of mechanisms including volume overload and oxidative stress. We were unable to show a difference in IL-6 or albumin with short daily compared to conventional hemodialysis. In a prospective cohort study of 26 patients treated with short daily HD in-centre, Ayus et al reported significant improvements in hs-CRP values after 12 months [32]. In a cross-sectional study by Jefferies et al, lower CRP values were only seen for patients who were doing more frequent dialysis at home compared to those patients who were treated in-centre [33]. Post dialysis sodium, ultrafiltration volumes and ultrafiltration rates were much lower for the patients being treated at home compared to the patients being treated in-centre suggesting that post-dialysis increases in serum sodium and/or interdialytic ECFV expansion may explain these differences. They were unable to demonstrate lower IL-6 levels between patients undergoing conventional and short daily dialysis in-centre who had similar post dialysis serum sodium levels and ultrafiltration rates. The impact of more frequent dialysis on markers of oxidative stress and inflammation requires further study.

Our study has a number of limitations including the inability to blind the patients and investigators to the treatment group. We did not measure residual renal function and therefore could not assess the importance of this variable. However, the dialysis vintage of the patients suggests that many of them may have been anuric. Lastly, we did not measure ECFV at baseline and again at the end of the run-in phase; we are therefore unable to comment on the role changes in ECFV in the blood pressure improvement that was seen in the BP optimization phase. Strengths of our study over others that have been published to date include the run-in phase and use of standardized blood pressure algorithm.

In summary after a 3-month run-in phase in which blood pressure was optimized by decreasing dialysate sodium, adjusting dry weight and anti-hypertensive medications,

patients treated with short daily HD compared to conventional HD require fewer anti-hypertensive medications to achieve the same blood pressure. This effect on blood pressure control was not related to a reduction in ECFV, sympathetic nervous system activity, oxidative stress or inflammation. The mechanism(s) by which short daily HD allows for decreased use of anti-hypertensive medication remains unclear but may be related to effects on sodium balance and changes in peripheral vascular resistance that require further study.

Acknowledgments

Elham Sabri provided statistical support for the study. The study would not have been possible without the expertise of the Kidney Research Centre staff. We would like to thank Dr Steven Nadler for retrieving additional data from Nephrocare; our electronic medical record for nephrology patients.

Author Contributions

Conceived and designed the experiments: DLZ MR PH KDB RMT. Performed the experiments: DLZ MR KDB RMT. Analyzed the data: DLZ DF. Contributed reagents/materials/analysis tools: RT DF PH. Wrote the paper: DLZ MR KDB RMT DF PH.

References

1. Laupacis A, Keown P, Pus N, Drueger H, Ferguson B, et al. (1996) A study of the quality of life and const-utility of renal transplant. Kidney Int 50(1):235–42.
2. Foley RN, Parfrey PS, Harnett JD, Kent GM, Murray DC, et al. (1995) The prognositc importance of left ventricular geometry in uremic cardiomyopathy. J Am Soc Nephrol 5(12):2024–31.
3. Agarwal R, Nissenson AR, Batlle D, Coyne DW, Trout JR, et al. (2003) Prevalence, treatment, and control of hypertension in chronic hemodialysis patients in the United States. Am J Med 115:291–297.
4. Horl MP, Horl WH (2002) Hemodialsis-associated hypertension: pathophysiology and therapy. Am J Kidney Dis 39(2):227–244.
5. Montezano AC, Touyez RM (2011) Molecular mechanisms of hypertension: reactive oxygen species and antioxidants: a basic science update for the clinician. Can J Cardiol 28; 288–295.
6. Zilch O, Vos PF, Oey PL, Cramer MJM, Ligtenberg G, et al. (2007) Sympathetic hyperactivity in haemodialysis patients is reduced by short daily haemodialysis. J Hypertension 25:1285–1289.

7. Fagugli RM, Reboldi G, Quintaliani G, Pasini P, Ciao G, et al. (2001) Short daily hemodialysis: blood pressure control and left ventricular mass reduction in hypertensive hemodialysis patients. Am J Kidney Dis 38(2):371–376.
8. FHN Trial Group (2010) In-center hemodialysis six times per week versus three times per week. N Engl J Med 363(24):2287–2300.
9. Nesrallah G, Suri R, Moist L, Kortas C, Lindsay RM (2003) Volume control and blood pressure management in patients undergoing quotidian hemodialysis. Am J Kidney Dis 42(1): S13–17.
10. Chan CT, Floras JS, Miller JA, Richardson MA, Pierratos A (2002) Regression of left ventricular hypertrophy after conversion to nocturnal hemodialysis. Kidney Int 61: 2235–2239.
11. Chan CT, Harvey PJ, Picton P, Pierratos A, Miller JA, et al. (2003) Short-term blood pressure, noradrenergic, and vascular effects of nocturnal home hemodialysis. Hypertension 42: 925–31.
12. Rocco MV, Lockridge RS Jr, Beck GJ, Eggers PW, Gassman JJ, et al. (2011) The effects of frequent nocturnal home hemodialysis: the Frequent Hemodialysis Network Nocturnal Trial. Kidney Int 80(10):1080–1091.
13. Katzarski KS, Charra B, Luik AJ, Nisell J, Divino Filho JC, et al. (1999) Fluid state and blood pressure control in patients treated with long and short haemodialysis. Nephrol Dial Transplant 14(2):369–75.
14. Luik AJ, v d Sande FM, Weideman P, Cheriex E, Kooman JP, et al. (2001) The influence of increasing dialysis treatment and reducing dry weight on blood pressure control in hemodialysis patients: a prospective study. Am J Nephrol 21(6): 471–478.
15. Ponnuchamy B, Khalil RA (2009) Cell mediators in renal vascular dysfunction in hypertension. Am J Physiol Regul Integr Comp Physiol 296: R1001–R1018.
16. Yuen D, Richardson RMA, Chan CT (2005) Improvements in phosphate control with short daily in-center hemodialysis. Clin Nephrol 64: 364–370.
17. Cox-Reijven PL, Looman JP, Soeters PB, van der Sande FM, Leunissen KM (2001) Role of bioimpedance spectroscopy in assessment of body water compartments in hemodialysis patients. Am J Kidney Dis 38:832–838.
18. Virdis A, Neves MF, Amiri F, Viel E, Touyz RM, et al. (2002) Spironolactone improves angiotensin-induced vascular changes and oxidative stress. Hypertension 40: 504–510.
19. White M, Ducharme A, Ibrahim R, Whittom L, Lavoie J, et al. (2006) Increased systemic inflammation and oxidative stress in patients with worsening congestive heart failure: improvement after short-term inotropic support. Clin Sci 110(4):483–9.
20. Zimmerman DL, Swedko PJ, Posen GA, Burns KD (2003) Daily hemofiltration with a simplified method of delivery. ASAIO J 426–429.
21. Zoccali C, Mallamaci F, Tripepi G, Benedetto FA, Cottini E, et al. (1991) Prediction of left ventricular geometry by clinic, pre-dialysis and 24 hour ambulatory BP monitoring in haemodialysis patients. J Hypertens 17:355–360.
22. Song JH, Lee SW, Suh CK, Kim MJ (2002) Time-averaged concentration of dialysate sodium relates with sodium load and interdialytic weight gain during sodium-profiling hemodialysis. Am J Kidney Dis 40(2):291–301.
23. de Paula FM, Peixoto AJ, Pinto LV, Dorigo D, Patricio PJM, et al. (2004) Clinical consequences of an individualized dialysate sodium prescription in hemodialysis patients. Kidney Int 66:1232–1238.
24. Thein H, Haloob I, Marshall MR (2007) Associations of a facility level decrease in dialysate sodium concentration with blood pressure and interdialytic weight gain. Nephrol Dial Transplant 22:2630–2639.
25. Penne EL, Levin NW, Kotanko P (2010) Improving volume status by comprehensive dietary and dialytic sodium management in chronic hemodialysis patients. Blood Purif 30:71–78.
26. Oberleithner H, Riethmuller C, Schillers H, MacGregor GA, de Wardener HE, et al. (2007) Plasma sodium stiffens vascular endothelium and reduced nitric oxide release. PNAS 104(41): 16281–16286.
27. Agarwal R, Alborzi P, Satyan S, Light RP (2009) Dry weight reduction in hypertensive hemodialysis patients (DRIP): a randomized controlled trial. Hypertension 53: 500–507.
28. Hirooka Y, Kishi T, Sakai K, Takeshita A, Sunagawa K (2011) Imbalance of central nitric oxide and reactive oxygen species in the regulation of sympathetic activity and the neural mechanisms of hypertension. Am J Physiol - Regulatory, Integrative and Comparative Physiology 300: R818–R826.
29. Schulz E, Gori T, Munzel T (2011) Oxidative stress and endothelial dysfunction in hypertension. Hypertension Research 34: 665–673.
30. Yoon JW, Pahl MV, Viziri ND (2007) Spontaneous leukocyte activation and oxygen-free radical generation in end-stage renal disease. Kidney Int 71:167–172.
31. Di Marco GS, Hausberg M, Hillebrand U, Rustemeyer P, Wittkowksi W, et al. (2008) Increased inorganic phosphate induces human endothelial cell apoptosis in vitro. Am J Physiol Renal Physiol 294; F1381–F1387.
32. Ayus JC, Mizani MR, Achinger SG, Thadhani R, Go AS, et al. (2005) Effects of short daily versus conventional hemodialysis on left ventricular hypertrophy and inflammatory markers: a prospective controlled study. J Am Soc Nephrol 16: 2778–2788.
33. Jefferies HJ, Virk B, Schiller B, Moran J, McIntyre CW (2011) Frequent hemodialysis schedules are associated with reduced levels of dialysis-induced cardiac injury (myocardial stunning). Clin J Am Soc Nephrol 6: 1326–1332.

Development of Contrast-Induced Acute Kidney Injury after Elective Contrast Media Exposure in Patients with Type 2 Diabetes Mellitus: Effect of Albuminuria

Jun-qing Yang[1,⁋], Peng Ran[1,⁋], Ji-yan Chen[1*], Yi-ting He[2], Li-wen Li[1], Ning Tan[1], Guang Li[1], Shuo Sun[1], Yong Liu[1], Jia-xin Zhan[1], Jian-yi Zheng[1], Ying-ling Zhou[1*]

1 Department of Cardiology, Guangdong Cardiovascular Institute, Guangdong General Hospital, Guangdong Academy of Medical Sciences, Guangzhou, Guangdong, China, **2** Department of Cardiology, Shunde first hospital, Foshan, Guangdong, China

Abstract

Background: The influence of albuminuria and urinary pH on the development of contrast-induced acute kidney disease (CI-AKI) in patients with type 2 diabetes mellitus (T2DM) after elective coronary angiography (CAG) or percutaneous coronary intervention (PCI) is unknown.

Methods: CI-AKI was defined as an increase in serum creatinine >26.4 μmol/L or ≥50% of baseline value within 48 hours after contrast media exposure. Demographics, traditional risk factors, clinical outcomes and CI-AKI incidence were compared between groups. Univariate analysis and multivariate logistic regression were performed to assess risk factors of CI-AKI.

Results: We observed 597 patients with T2DM after CAG or PCI. Patients were divided into 3 groups based on early morning urinary albumin: negative group (urine dipstick negative, n = 483), trace group (urine dipstick trace, n = 60), and positive group (urine dipstick ≥1+, n = 54). CI-AKI occurred in 33 (5.5%) patients, including 19 (3.9%) in the negativealbuminuria group, 4 (6.7%) in the trace group, and 10 (18.5%) in the positive group ($p < 0.001$), respectively. After adjusting for potential confounding risk factors, positive albuminuria (OR = 3.8, 95% CI: 1.5 to 9.2, $p = 0.004$) and urinary pH<6 (OR = 2.4, 95% CI: 1.1 to 5.1, $p = 0.020$) remained significantly associated with CI-AKI.

Conclusion: Preprocedural albuminuria and urinary pH <6 are independent risk factors of CI-AKI in patients with T2DM undergoing elective cardiac catheterization, and may be used to identify patients at high risk of post-procedural CI-AKI.

Editor: Emmanuel A. Burdmann, University of Sao Paulo Medical School, Brazil

Funding: The work was supported by Science and Technology Planning Project of Guangdong Province (grant NO.: 2008A030201002), Guangdong Cardiovascular Institute; and Guangdong Provincial Cardiovascular Clinical Medicine Research Fund (grant NO.: 2009X41), Guangzhou, China. The funders had no role in study design, data collection and analysis, decision to publish, or preparation of the manuscript.

Competing Interests: The authors have declared that no competing interests exist.

* Email: gdphospital@163.com (JYC); gdghospital@163.com (YLZ)

⁋ These authors contributed equally to this work.

Introduction

Contrast-induced acute kidney injury (CI-AKI) is a leading cause of nosocomial acute renal failure [1,2]. It is associated with poor outcomes, including dialysis and in-hospital [3] and 1–2 year mortality [4,5]. Furthermore, it prolongs hospitalization and increases medical costs [6].

Albuminuria is common in patients with type 2 diabetes (T2DM). Previous studies have demonstrated that increased albuminuria and reduced estimated glomerular filtration rate (eGFR) are independent risk factors for acute kidney injury [7], and cardiovascular and renal events [8] in T2DM patients. However, the impact of albuminuria on the prevalence of CI-AKI in T2DM patients is unclear, and few studies have investigated the relationship between urinary albumin levels and CI-AKI. In addition, the pathogenesis of CI-AKI may include free radicals production, which is promoted by the acidic environment in the urinary tubule [9]. Urinary pH may be associated with CI-AKI.

Therefore, we investigated influence of urinary albumin levels and urinary pH on the incidence of CI-AKI in T2DM patients who underwent elective CAG or PCI.

Methods

Study protocol

We conducted an observational study in consecutive patients with T2MD and who underwent elective CAG or PCI at the Guangdong Cardiovascular Institute of Guangdong General Hospital, Guangdong Academy of Medical Sciences, between August 2009 and August 2012. The study protocol was approved by the Guangdong General Hospital ethics committee, and all patients provided a written informed consent.

T2DM patients undergoing CAG or PCI were enrolled. Exclusion criteria were: 1) age <18years; 2) eGFR<15 ml/min/1.73 m^2; 3) dialysis; 4) nephrotic syndrome; 5) nephropyelitis; 6) emergency CAG or PCI; 7) cardiac shock; 8) severe aortic valve disease; 9) multiple myeloma; 10) severe hepatic insufficiency; 11) acute stroke; 12) diabetic ketoacidosis; 13) iodic contrast administration during the preceding 7 days; 14) coronary revascularization surgery; 15) nonsteroidal anti-inflammatory drugs (NSAIDs) use within 48 hours before the procedure; 16) severe sepsis; 17) pregnancy; 18) allergy to contrast medium.

Routine urinalysis of early morning urine samples which involved urinary albumin and pH was performed upon hospital admission and before the procedure. Serum creatinine was measured as part of routine clinical care upon admission, and daily for 2 days after the procedure. Urinary albumin and pH were tested using an Urisys-2400 automatic analyzer (Roche Diagnostics, Basel, Switzerland), a Miditrom Junior analyzer (Roche Diagnostics, Basel, Switzerland), or a COBAS U411 analyzer (Roche Diagnostics, Basel, Switzerland). eGFR was estimated using the abbreviated Modification of Diet in Renal Disease (MDRD) formula [10].

CAG or PCI was performed using standard techniques [11]. The dose and types of contrast medium were left to the discretion of the interventional cardiologist. The use of aspirin, clopidogrel, β-blockers, angiotensin-converting enzyme inhibitors (ACEIs)/angiotensin receptor blockers (ARBs), calcium channel blockers (CCBs), diuretics, intra-aortic balloon pump (IABP) or vascular active drugs was also left to the discretion of the interventional and/or clinical cardiologist. Patients received perioperative hydration for 8–36 hours with normal saline at a rate of 1 ml/kg/hour. The hydration rate was reduced by half in patients with a left ventricular ejection fraction (LVEF) <35% or NYHA class III–IV at admission.

T2DM was defined as fasting plasma glucose ≥126 mg/dl (7.0 mmol/L); or 2-h plasma glucose ≥200 mg/dl (11.1 mmol/L) during an oral glucose tolerance test; or in a patient with classic symptoms of hyperglycemia or hyperglycemic crisis, a random plasma glucose ≥200 mg/dl (11.1 mmol/L) [12], a previous diagnosis or received treatment was also accepted. Anemia was defined as baseline hematocrit <39% for men and <36% for women. Hypotension was defined as systolic blood pressure (SBP) <80 mmHg for at least 1 hour requiring inotropic support with medications or intra-aortic balloon pump (IABP) within 24 hours periprocedurally. Congestive heart failure was defined as New York Heart Association functional classification III/IV and/or history of pulmonary edema [13].

Endpoints

Primary endpoints. The primary endpoint was the occurrence of CI-AKI, was defined as an increase in serum creatinine > 26.4 μmol/L or ≥50% of baseline value within 48 hours after contrast media exposure [14].

Secondary endpoints. Secondary endpoints were absolute change in serum creatinine within 48 hours, in-hospital death and dialysis. The cause of death was ascertained from discharge documents and discussion with attending physician.

Follow-up

Follow-up was performed at an outpatient clinic visit or via telephone interviews. Cardiac death was defined as any death with a demonstrable cardiac cause or any death that was not clearly attributable to a non-cardiac cause [15]. All-cause death, cardiac death, and dialysis were adjudicated by two experienced cardiologists who were blinded to angiographic and biochemical data.

Statistical analysis

SPSS 19.0 was used for statistical analysis. Patients were divided into three groups according to early morning urinary albumin assessment by routine urinalysis: negative group (urine dipstick negative), trace group (urine dipstick trace), and positive group (urine dipstick ≥1+). Data are presented as mean ± standard deviation (SD) for normally distributed data, or medians and interquartile ranges (IQR) for unevenly distributed data. Categorical data are expressed as numbers (%). Demographics, traditional risk factors, clinical outcomes and CI-AKI incidence were compared between groups. Chi-square tests or Fisher exact tests were used for categorical data, as appropriate. Normally distributed variables were compared by one-way ANOVA (with Bonferroni correction for comparisons between groups if the ANOVA p-value was <0.05), or by the Kruskal-Wallis test for unevenly distributed data.Risk factors were initially screened for univariate association with CI-AKI at a p value <0.20, and identified variables were then assessed in a forward stepwise manner using a p-value criterion of <0.05. The final model included the important baseline characteristics. Multivariate logistic regression analysis was performed to identify independent risk factors for CI-AKI. Cumulative event curves were constructed using the Kaplan-Meier survival method, and cumulative event rates were compared using the log-rank test. All p-values were two-tailed, and a p-value <0.05 was considered statistically significant.

Results

A total of 597 patients with T2DM after elective CAG or PCI were included; 173 (29.0%) were female, and the overall patient age was 65.1±10.1 years. Baseline patient eGFR and serum creatinine were were 77.8 ml/min/1.73 m^2 (IQR 61.6–96.7 ml/min/1.73 m^2) and 84.0 μmol/L (IQR 70.5–106.0 μmol/L), respectively. Overall, 33 patients (5.5%) developed CI-AKI

Baseline characteristics

Table 1 shows the baseline characteristics of the study population. There were significant differences among negative, trace and positive groups including: serum creatinine { 82.0(IQR 68.0–101.0)μmol/L vs. 94.4(IQR 75.3–113.5)μmol/L vs. 117.6(IQR 95.3–190.0)μmol/L, p<0.001}, urea nitrogen {4.8(IQR 3.8–6.2) mmol/L vs. 5.4(IQR 4.4–7.0)mmol/L vs.7.4(IQR 5.0–9.8) mmol/L, p<0.001}, eGFR { 80.2 (IQR 64.0–98.9)ml/min/1.73 m^2 vs.72.3(IQR 50.6–97.3)ml/min/1.73 m^2 vs.54.5(IQR 31.1–74.8) ml/min/1.73 m^2, p<0.001}, the proportion of preoperative congestive heart failure (13.0% vs.16.7% vs. 25.9%, p=0.011), anemia (36.5% vs.40.0% vs. 66.7%,p<0.001), hypertension (67.9% vs.75.0% vs. 88.9%, p=0.001), hypoalbuminemia (36.2±4.6 g/L vs. 33.7±4.3 g/L vs. 31.3±4.9 g/L, p<0.001), SBP(133.2±20.0 mmHg vs. 137.6±20.1 mmHg vs. 141.8±27.1 mmHg, p=0.002), HbA1c (7.6±1.5% vs. 8.5±2.2% vs. 7.8±1.6, p=0.014), and use of diuretics (13.9% vs.18.3% vs. 38.9%, p<0.001). There was no difference in age, LVEF, periprocedural hypotension, periprocedural IABP, urinary pH, history of myocardial infarction, or hyperlipidemia.

Procedural characteristics

Table 2 lists the procedural characteristics of the patients. Compared with the negative and trace groups, the patients in the positive urine albumin group were hydrated with higher volumes

Table 1. Baseline Characteristics.

characteristics	Urinary Albumin				*p*			
	All (N = 597)	Negative (N = 483)	Trace (N = 60)	Positive (N = 54)	All	Negative vs. Trace	Trace vs. Positive	Positive vs. Negative
Female, n(%)	173(29.0%)	151(31.3%)	9(15.0%)	13(24.1%)	0.046	-	-	-
Age, years	65.1±10.1	65.0±10.1	64.7±10.0	66.5±9.5	0.541	-	-	-
eGFR,	77.8	80.2	72.3	54.5	<0.001*	-	-	-
ml/min/1.73 m^2	(61.6-96.7)	(64.0-98.9)	(50.6-97.3)	(31.1-74.8)				
SBP, mmHg	134.4±21.0	133.2±20.0	137.6±20.6	141.8±27.1	0.002	0.378#	0.838#	0.012#
DBP, mmHg	77.1±11.9	77.1±11.9	76.6±10.8	78.0±13.5	0.737	-	-	-
HR, bpm	74.7±11.7	74.6±11.3	75.1±11.4	75.7±14.1	0.461	-	-	-
LVEF, %	59.2±12.8	59.7±12.7	57.2±13.4	57.4±12.5	0.120	-	-	-
Hypotension, n(%)	14(2.3%)	12(2.5%)	1(1.7%)	1(1.9%)	0.682	-	-	-
IABP, n(%)	10(1.7%)	7(1.4%)	1(1.7%)	2(3.7%)	0.260	-	-	-
Congestive heart failure, n(%)	87(14.6%)	63(13.0%)	10 (16.7%)	14(25.9%)	0.011	-	-	-
Medical history								
Smoking, n(%)	20(34.3%)	162(33.5%)	28(46.7%)	15(27.8%)	0.965	-	-	-
Hypertension, n(%)	421(70.5%)	328(67. 9%)	45(75.0%)	48(88.9%)	0.001	-	-	-
Dyslipidemia, n(%)	82(13.7%)	69(14.3%)	6(10.0%)	7(13.0%)	0.555	-	-	-
Anemia, n(%)	235(39.6%)	175(36.5%)	24(40.0%)	36(66.7%)	<0.001	-	-	-
MI history, n(%)	87(14.6%)	66(13.7%)	8(13.3%)	13(24.1%)	0.075	-	-	-
CABG history, n(%)	7(1.2%)	6(1.2%)	1(1.7%)	0(0.0%)	0.552	-	-	-
Laboratory measurements								
SCr, μmol/L	84.0 (70.5-106.0)	82.0 (68.0–101.0)	94.4 (75.3–113.5)	117.6 (93.5–190.0)	<0.001*	-	-	-
BUN, mmol/L	5(4.0–6.4)	4.8(3.8–6.2)	5.4(4.4–7.0)	7.4(5.0–9.8)	<0.001*	-	-	-
TC, mmol/L	4.3±1.1	4.2±1.1	4.2±1.0	4.5±1.1	0.211	-	-	-
LDL-C, mmol/L	2.4(1.9–3.0)	2.4(1.9–3.0)	2.3(1.8–3.2)	2.5(2.0–3.1)	0.871*	-	-	-
TG, mmol/L	1.4(1.0–1.9)	1.4(1.0–1.9)	1.5(1.0–1.8)	1.5(1.2–2.6)	0.158*	–	-	-
HbA1c, %	7.7±1.6	7.6±1.5	8.5±2.2	7.8±1.6	0.014	<0.001#	0.029#	1.000#
Urinary PH<6,n(%)	179(30.0%)	140(29.0%)	20(33.3%)	19(35.2%)	0.271	-	-	-
PH<5.5	155	27	13	15				
PH = 5.5	24	13	7	4				
Hematocrit (%)	38.0±4.8	38.0±4.6	39.0±4.4	35.0±6.2	<0.001	1.000#	0.002#	<0.001#
Hemoglobin, g/L	129.2±16.5	130.22±15.4	132.0±16.2	116.8±20.6	<0.001	1.000#	<0.001#	<0.001#
Albumin, g/L	35.5±4.8	36.2±4.6	33.7±4.3	31.3±4.9	<0.001	0.049#	0.097#	<0.001#
Medicine usage								
ACEI/ARB, n (%)	531(88.9%)	434(89.9%)	49(81.7%)	48(88.9%)	0.351	-	-	-

Table 1. Cont.

characteristics	Urinary Albumin				*p*			
	All (N = 597)	Negative (N = 483)	Trace (N = 60)	Positive (N = 54)	All	Negative vs. Trace	Trace vs. Positive	Positive vs. Negative
β-blocker, n (%)	515(86.3%)	421(87.2%)	52(86.7%)	42(77.8%)	0.087	-	-	-
CCB, n (%)	156(26.2%)	116(24.1%)	18(30.0%)	22(40.7%)	0.007	-	-	-
Diuretics, n (%)	99(16.6%)	67(13.9%)	11(18.3%)	21(38.9%)	<0.001	-	-	-
Statin, n (%)	584(97.8%)	473(97.9%)	60(100.0%)	51(94.4%)	0.289	-	-	-
Insulin, n (%)	175 (29.3%)	125 (25.9%)	26 (43.3%)	24(44.4%)	<0.001	-	-	-
α-glycosidase inhibitors, n (%)	341(57.1%)	284(58.8%)	33(55.0%)	24(44.4%)	0.046	-	-	-
Sulfonylureas, n(%)	169(28.3%)	147(30.4%)	17(28.3%)	5(9.3%)	0.003	-	-	-
Repaglinide/Nateglinide, n(%)	80 (13.4%)	67 (13.9%)	8 (13.3%)	5 (9.3%)	0.381	-	-	-
Thiazolidinediones, n(%)	13(2.2%)	11(2.3%)	2 (3.3%)	0 (0%)	0.453	-	-	-

1. Data are expressed as number (%), or mean±SD for normally distributed data, or median (IQR) for unevenly distributed data.
2.* P was tested by Kruskal-Wallis test.
3. # P was tested by Bonferroni correction.
4. Chi-square test or Fisher exact test was used for the frequency of distribution. Means were compared by One-way ANOVA for normally distributed data.
5. SBP: Systolic blood pressure. DBP: diastolic blood pressure. BUN: blood urea nitrogen. LVEF: left ventricular ejection fraction; ACEI/ARB: angiotensin-converting enzyme inhibitor/angiotensin receptor blocker. CABG: coronary artery bypass grafting. CCB: Calcium channel blocker. MI: myocardial infarction. HbA1C: glycosylated hemoglobin A1c. LDL-C: low density lipoprotein-cholesterol. TG: Triglycerides.

Table 2. Procedural Characteristics.

Characteristics	Urinary Albumin				*p*
	All (N = 597)	Negative (N = 483)	Trace (N = 60)	Positive (N = 54)	
Number of lesions (n)	2.1±1.1	2.0±1.1	2.0±1.0	2.3±1.1	0.322
Number of stents (n)	1.6±1.4	1.5±1.4	1.6±1.4	1.6±1.2	0.945
Left main lesion (%)	64(10.7%)	54(11.2%)	5(8.3%)	5(9.3%)	0.520
Left main treated (%)	30(5.0%)	28(5.8%)	1(1.7%)	1(1.9%)	0.100
Total stent length (mm)	38.4±36.6	38.1±37.2	40.3±36.4	38.7±32.4	0.912
Contrast Type					0.263
Iopamidol	328(55.1%)	265(55.0%)	33(55.0%)	30(56.6%)	
Iopromide	238(40.0%)	199(41.3%)	23(38.3%)	16(30.2%)	
Iodixanol	25(4.2%)	16(3.3%)	3 (5.6%)	6 (11.3%)	
Contrast volume, ml	130 (80–170)	130 (80–165)	130 (100–150)	135 (77.5–172.5)	0.901*
Intravenous hydration volume, ml	500 (500–1000)	500 (500–1000)	500 (500–1000)	1000(500–1500)	0.002*

1. Data are expressed as number (%), or mean±SD for normally distributed data, or median (IQR) for unevenly distributed data.
2. *P was tested by Kruskal-Wallis test.
3. PCI: percutaneous coronary intervention.

of fluid (500 ml (IQR 500–1000 ml) and 500 ml (IQR 500–1000 ml) vs. 1000 ml (IQR 500–1500 ml); p = 0.002), presumably because patients with albuminuria presented with reduced baseline renal function and underwent longer hydration. There were no differences in the other procedural characteristics.

CI-AKI incidence and in-hospital outcomes

CI-AKI incidence and in-hospital clinical outcomes are displayed in Table 3. The CI-AKI incidence in positive urine albumin group was higher than the negative and trace groups (negative vs. trace vs. positive: 3.9% vs.6.7% vs. 18.5%, p<0.001). A difference was observed in dialysis frequency (0.2% vs. 1.7% vs. 1.9%, p = 0.005). No difference was observed regarding in-hospital death.

Multivariate analysis

Results of multivariate logistic regression analysis have been displayed in Table 4. After adjusting for potential confounding risk factors (Hosmer-Lemeshow Chi-square: 5.2, p = 0.520), and using the negative group as reference, the odds ratio (OR) of CI-AKI was 3.8 (95% CI: 1.5–9.2, p = 0.004) for the positive urine albumin group, but 1.4 (95%CI: 0.4–4.5, p = 0.562) for the trace urine albumin group. The OR of CI-AKI was 2.4 (95% CI: 1.1–5.1, p = 0.020) for urinary pH <6, and 2.5 (95% CI: 1.1–5.7, p = 0.023) for eGFR <60 ml/min/1.73 m^2. However, age >65 years and congestive heart failure were not associated with CI-AKI in this study.

Follow-up

Median follow-up was 23 months (IQR: 16 to 30 months). Clinical outcomes were available for 572 patients (95.8%). Forty-two (7.5%) patients died. Cardiac death occurred in 11 patients in the positive urine albumin group due to refractory heart failure (n = 6), acute myocardial infarction (n = 1), cardiac arrest (n = 1), or other cardiovascular causes (n = 3). In the trace urine albumin group, 4 cardiac deaths were caused by refractory heart failure (n = 1), acute myocardial infarction (n = 1), cardiac arrest (n = 1), or other cardiovascular causes (n = 1). In the negative urine albumin group, 16 cardiac deaths were attributed to refractory heart failure (n = 6), acute myocardial infarction (n = 6), sudden death (n = 2), or other cardiovascular causes (n = 2).

Table 3. CI-AKI incidence and Clinical outcomes in-hospital.

Outcomes	Urinary Albumin				*p*
	All (N = 597)	Negative (N = 483)	Trace (N = 60)	Positive (N = 54)	
CI-AKI					
SCr increase≥26.4μmol/L or ≥50%, n(%)	33(5.5%)	19(3.9%)	4(6.7%)	10(18.5%)	<0.001
SCr increase≥26.4μmol/L, n(%)	31(5.2%)	18(3.7%)	3(5.0%)	10(18.5%)	<0.001
SCr increase≥50%, n(%)	10(1.7%)	6(1.2%)	2(3.3%)	2 (3.7%)	0.101
Absolute change in SCr, μmol/L	1.3(−5.8–10.0)	0.9(−5.5–9.0)	2.3(−6.0–10.0)	10.1(−7.8–20.1)	0.016*
Death, n(%)	3 (0.5%)	1(0.2%)	2(3.3%)	0(0%)	0.280
Dialysis, n(%)	2(0.5%)	0(0%)	1(1.7%)	1(1.9%)	0.005

CI-AKI: contrast-induced acute kidney injury; SCr: serum creatinine;
* P was tested by Kruskal-Wallis test.

Table 4. Univariate and multivariate analyses of predictors for CI-AKI.

Risk factors	Univariate analysis			Multivariate analysis		
	OR	95%CI	*p*	OR	95%CI	*p*
Urinary Albumin			<0.001			0.015
Negative	-	-	-	-	-	-
Trace (vs. Negative)	1.7	0.6–5.3	0.327	1.4	0.4–4.5	0.562
Positive (vs. Negative)	5.6	2.4–12.7	<0.001	3.8	1.5–9.2	0.004
Urinary PH<6.0	3.0	1.5–6.1	0.002	2.4	1.1–5.1	0.020
eGFR<60 ml/min/1.73 m^2	5.0	2.4–10.3	<0.001	2.5	1.1–5.7	0.023
Age>65 years	2.6	1.2–5.8	0.016	1.8	0.8–4.1	0.191
Congestive heart failure*	3.7	1.8–7.9	0.001	2.1	0.9–4.8	0.074

*Congestive heart failure was defined as New York Heart Association functional classification III/IV and/or history of pulmonary edema.
Hosmer-Lemeshow Chi-square: 5.2, $p = 0.520$.

The cumulative rate of all-cause death (33.4% vs. 7.3%, log rank P<0.001) (Fig.1), cardiac death (30.7% vs. 5.2%, log rank P<0.001) (Fig.2) and dialysis (10.9% vs. 0.7%, log rank P< 0.001)(Fig.3) were higher in patients with CI-AKI compared with those without.

Discussion

The present study suggests that pre-procedural urinary albumin levels, urinary pH <6 and eGFR <60 ml/min/1.73 m^2 were independent predictors for CI-AKI in patients with T2DM undergoing elective cardiac catheterization (CAG or PCI).

The mechanism of CI-AKI/contrast-induced nephropathy (CIN) is not clear. However, it probably involves the direct toxic

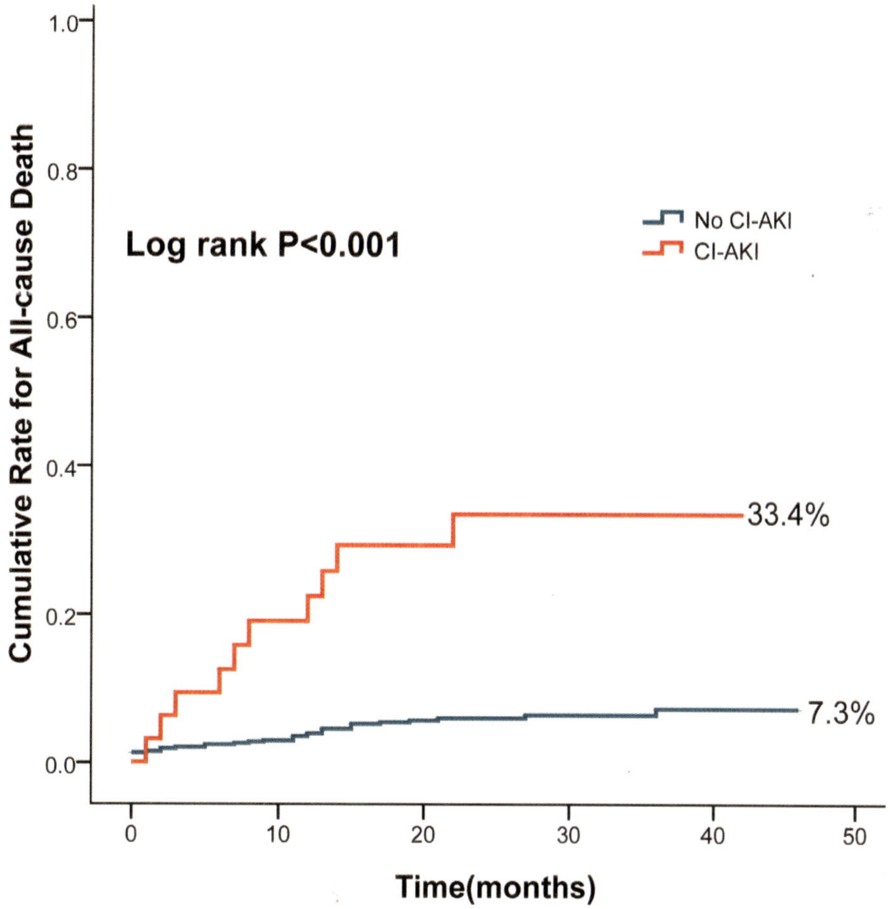

Figure 1. Cumulative rates for all-cause death in patients with CI-AKI and without CI-AKI.

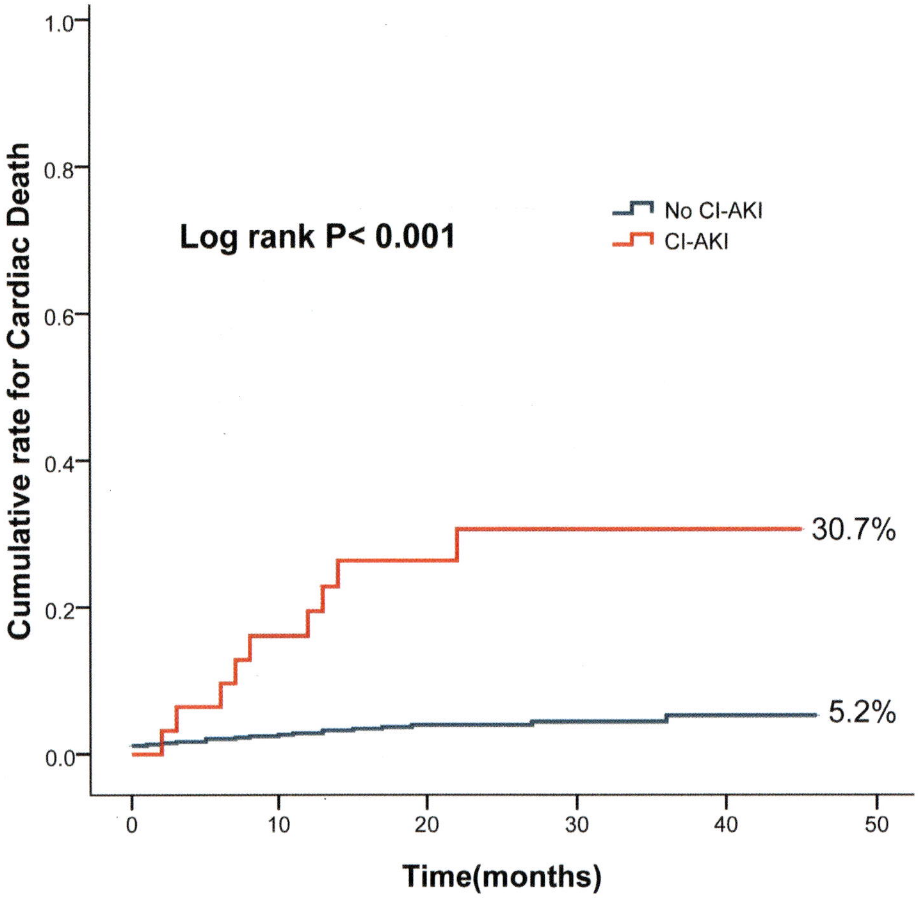

Figure 2. Cumulative rates for cardiac death in patients with CI-AKI and without CI-AKI.

effect of contrast agents and decreased renal medullary blood flow resulting in medullary ischemia that may lead to enhanced ROS formation and oxidative stress.

Many studies have indicated that preexisting renal disease [13,16,17] and T2DM [13,16–20] are risk factors for CI-AKI/CIN. In the Mehran's study, preexisting renal disease including eGFR <60 ml/min/1.73 m^2 or serum creatinine >1.5 mg/dl, is an independent predictor of CIN [13]. European Society of Urogenital Radiology (ESUR) contrast media safety Committee [14] considers that serum creatinine is not an ideal marker for renal function, and support eGFR to identify impaired renal function. In present study, eGFR <60 ml/min/1.73 m^2 was an independent risk factors for CI-AKI (OR = 2.5, 95% CI: 1.1–5.7, P = 0.023). The possible reason is that preexisting renal disease is associated with a decreased vasodilatory response and slower clearance of contrast media compared to normal subjects. Besides, in the Mehran's study [13], T2DM is an independent predictor of CIN. The possible mechanisms are: impaired endothelial function, caused by persistent hyperglycemia [21], leading to impaired renal vasomotor function and renal ischemia; and increased ROS generationas well as preexisting renal failure or metabolic syndrome [17].

Albuminuria may be an additional risk factor for T2DM patients. Albumin is almost totally restricted by the glomerular barrier, filtered albumin is reabsorbed by the proximal tubular cells [22], degraded there, and brings about inflammatory and fibrogenic mediators resulting in inflammation and fibrosis, followed by loss of renal function [22,23]. Albuminuria may contribute to the pathogenesis of CI-AKI/CIN by its toxic effects on the tubular system [24]. Albuminuria could activate Fas-mediated and peroxisome proliferator-activated receptor-γ-dependent apoptosis, and induce proinflammatory molecules, leading to apoptosis and damage of the renal tubular system [25–32]. In addition, albumin overload in proximal tubules could induce ROS formation, which activates NF-κB and consequently evokes NF-κB-dependent inflammatory reactions [33]. Moreover, in animal models of massive proteinuria, excessive oxidative stress induced by oxidized fatty acid was noted in regions with renal tubular damage [34]. Albuminuria and contrast media may share similar effects on kidneys [24], and may coordinate with each other in the pathogenesis of CI-AKI/CIN.

James et al. [7] demonstrated that the incidence of AKI is about 4 times higher in patients with heavy albuminuria (relative risk: 4.4 vs. no albuminuria, 95% CI: 3.7–5.2). Furthermore, long-term outcomes such as dialysis, death and composite renal outcomes are worse in patients with heavy albuminuria. In other studies [8,35–38], similar conclusions were reached, i.e. that albuminuria was an independent risk factor for AKI, renal and cardiovascular events, and all-cause mortality. In addition, albuminuria and eGFR were independently associated with AKI [39]. Chronic kidney disease (CKD) is defined as either kidney damage (proteinuria, hematuria or anatomical abnormality) or eGFR<60 ml/min/1.73 m^2 present on at least 2 occasions for ≥3 months [40]. The diagnosis of proteinuria supports the diagnosis of CKD in T2DM patients, independently of eGFR values [41]. Albuminuria may represent another type of CKD. Albuminuria may be an independent

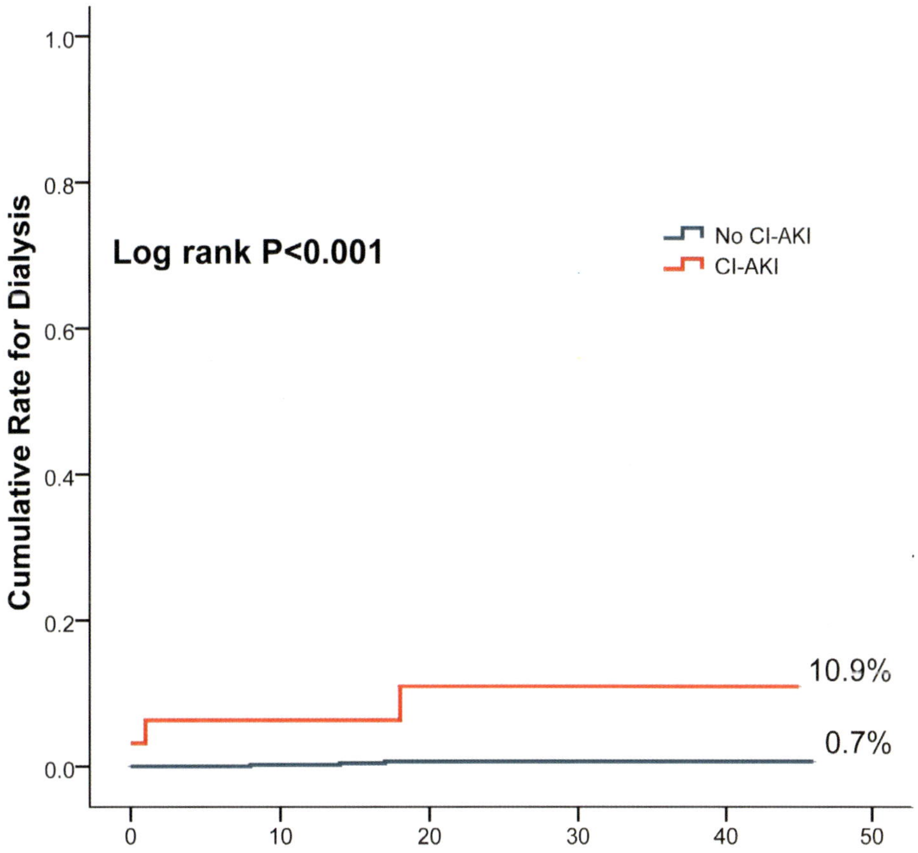

Figure 3. Cumulative rates for dialysis in patients with CI-AKI and without CI-AKI.

predictor for CI-AKI. A recent study [24] concluded that proteinuria may be a new risk factor for CIN in CKD patients; however, the sample size was small. Our data supported the hypothesis that urinary albumin levels were associated with CI-AKI incidence, and that albuminuria was an independent risk factor for CI-AKI in patients with T2DM.

ROS formation plays an important role in the development of CI-AKI/CIN [42] and may be promoted by an acidic urinary environment, but is inhibited by higher pH [22,39], and alkalinizing renal tubular fluid with bicarbonate may reduce injury. As with others, this is the most important mechanism why sodium bicarbonate provided more protection than sodium chloride in animal models for acute ischemic renal failure [43], clinical trials [9,44,45] and meta analyses [46–48] for CIN. Besides, sodium bicarbonate appears capable to scavenge ROS, and increasing urine flow. Additional, sodium bicarbonate avoids the large amounts of chloride which is in isotonic saline that may cause constriction of the renal vasculature. Therefore, guidelines by ESUR contrast media safety Committee considers that sodium bicarbonate seems to provide equal or superior protection to isotonic saline [14]. Actually, urinary pH is used in the diagnosis of renal tubular acidosis (RTA), despite its low specificity. Urinary pH could partly indicate renal tubular fluid pH, and a low urinary pH (<5.5) could be found in various forms of RTA (mostly in types 2 and 4 RTA) [49,50]. In the present study, among patients with urinary pH <6 most (n = 155, 86.59%) were of <5.5, and some may be with RTA. In a recent study[51], CIN incidence was significantly lower in patients with urinary pH >6 (32.8% vs. 2.2% in those with urinary pH >6, P<0.0001). The study by Merten et al. [9] showed that lower post-procedure urinary pH (5.6±0.6 vs.6.5±0.8, P = 0.002) and lower CIN incidence in the group hydrated by sodium bicarbonate compared with sodium chloride. Despite a small sample size (n = 119) and a weak statistical power [52], patients with urinary pH <6 may be a population that could benefit from bicarbonate hydration to prevent CI-AKI/CIN. Another study [53] concluded that daily oral sodium bicarbonate could slow eGFR decline and reduce urinary albumin based on a 5-year follow-up.

Albuminuria and urinary pH <6 are valuable for identifying patients at high risk of CI-AKI. What adds to the value of these parameters is that they are included in the routine test for every patient, and easy to obtain from preoperative urinalysis. Using these existing data, we may assess every patient more accurately and give him/her more precise risk stratification, importantly, with no additional cost and little effort.

Limitations

Our study has several limitations. First, this study was observational, of moderate-scale, and from a single center. Some patients were excluded such as patients with a nephrotic syndrome. The results should be confirmed in a large-scale multicenter clinical trial, including patients excluded from the current analysis. Second, treatment-related details in coronary artery disease were not available. Available information was restricted to cardiovascular drugs used. Finally, the data of some useful biochemical parameters such as cystatin C and urinary albumin/creatinine ratio were lacking in the present study.

Conclusions

Preprocedural albuminuria and urinary pH <6 were independent factors for CI-AKI in T2DM patients undergoing elective cardiac catheterization. Urinary albumin levels and urinary pH may be potential biochemical parameters for screening high-risk patients.

Acknowledgments

We would like to express our deep appreciation to Gary S. Mintz, Cardiovascular Research Foundation, New York, USA, for his insight and editorial assistance.

Author Contributions

Conceived and designed the experiments: JYC YLZ. Performed the experiments: JQY PR. Analyzed the data: JQY PR YTH. Wrote the paper: JQY PR. Contributed to revising manuscript critically for important intellectual content: LWL NT GL YL SS. Contributed to acquisition of data: JXZ JYZ.

References

1. Parfrey P. (2005) The clinical epidemiology of contrast-induced nephropathy. Cardiovasc Intervent Radiol 28 Suppl 2:S3–S11.
2. Mccullough P A, Stacul F, Becker C R, Adam A, Lameire N, et al. (2006) Contrast-Induced Nephropathy (CIN) Consensus Working Panel: executive summary. Rev Cardiovasc Med 7:177–197.
3. Mccullough P A, Wolyn R, Rocher L L, Levin R N, O'Neill WW. (1997) Acute renal failure after coronary intervention: incidence, risk factors, and relationship to mortality. Am J Med 103:368–375.
4. Tublin M E, Murphy M E, Tessler F N. (1998) Current concepts in contrast media-induced nephropathy. AJR Am J Roentgenol 171:933–939.
5. Gupta R, Gurm H S, Bhatt D L, Chew DP, Ellis SG. (2005) Renal failure after percutaneous coronary intervention is associated with high mortality. Catheter Cardiovasc Interv 64:442–448.
6. Weisbord S D, Chen H, Stone R A, Kip K E, Fine M J et al. (2006) Associations of increases in serum creatinine with mortality and length of hospital stay after coronary angiography. J Am Soc Nephrol 17:2871–2877.
7. James M T, Hemmelgarn B R, Wiebe N, Pannu N, Manns BJ et al. (2010) Glomerular filtration rate, proteinuria, and the incidence and consequences of acute kidney injury: a cohort study. Lancet 376:2096–2103.
8. Ninomiya T, Perkovic V, de Galan B E, Zoungas S, Pillai A et al. (2009) Albuminuria and kidney function independently predict cardiovascular and renal outcomes in diabetes. J Am Soc Nephrol, 20:1813–1821.
9. Merten G J, Burgess W P, Gray L V, Holleman J H, Roush T S et al. (2004) Prevention of contrast-induced nephropathy with sodium bicarbonate: a randomized controlled trial. JAMA 291:2328–2334.
10. National Kidney Foundation. (2002) K/DOQI clinical practice guidelines for chronic kidney disease: evaluation, classification, and stratification. Am J Kidney Dis 39:S1–S266.
11. Levine G N, Bates E R, Blankenship J C, Bailey SR, Bittl JA et al. (2011) 2011 ACCF/AHA/SCAI Guideline for Percutaneous Coronary Intervention: executive summary: a report of the American College of Cardiology Foundation/American Heart Association Task Force on Practice Guidelines and the Society for Cardiovascular Angiography and Interventions.Circulation 124:2574–2609.
12. Gavi S, Hensley J. (2009) Diagnosis and management of type 2 diabetes in adults: a review of the ICSI guideline. Geriatrics 64:12–17, 29.
13. Mehran R, Aymong E D, Nikolsky E, Lasic Z, Iakovou I et al. (2004) A simple risk score for prediction of contrast-induced nephropathy after percutaneous coronary intervention: development and initial validation. J Am Coll Cardiol 44:1393–1399.
14. Stacul F, van der Molen A J, Reimer P, Webb J A, Thomsen H S et al. (2011) Contrast induced nephropathy: updated ESUR Contrast Media Safety Committee guidelines. EurRadiol, 21:2527–2541.
15. Yang Z K, Zhang R Y, Hu J, Zhang Q, Ding FH et al. (2013) Impact of successful staged revascularization of a chronic total occlusion in the non-infarct-related artery on long-term outcome in patients with acute ST-segment elevation myocardial infarction. Int J Cardiol 165:76–79.
16. Rihal C S, Textor S C, Grill D E, Berger P B, Ting H H et al. (2002) Incidence and prognostic importance of acute renal failure after percutaneous coronary intervention. Circulation 105:2259–2264.
17. Toprak O, Cirit M, Yesil M, Bayata S, Tanrisev M et al. (2007) Impact of diabetic and pre-diabetic state on development of contrast-induced nephropathy in patients with chronic kidney disease. Nephrol Dial Transplant 22:819–826.
18. Dangas G, Iakovou I, Nikolsky E, Aymong E D, Mintz G S et al. (2005) Contrast-induced nephropathy after percutaneous coronary interventions in relation to chronic kidney disease and hemodynamic variables. Am J Cardiol 95:13–19.
19. Klima T, Christ A, Marana I, Kalbermatter S, Uthoff H et al. (2012) Sodium chloride vs. sodium bicarbonate for the prevention of contrast medium-induced nephropathy: a randomized controlled trial. Eur Heart J 33:2071–2079.
20. Lindsay J, Canos D A, Apple S, Pinnow E, Aggrey G K et al. (2004) Causes of acute renal dysfunction after percutaneous coronary intervention and comparison of late mortality rates with postprocedure rise of creatine kinase-MB versus rise of serum creatinine. Am J Cardiol 94(6):786–789.
21. Kamdar A, Weidmann P, Makoff D L, Massry SG. (1977) Acute renal failure following intravenous use of radiographic contrast dyes in patients with diabetes mellitus. Diabetes 26:643–649.
22. Gorriz J L, Martinez-Castelao A. (2012) Proteinuria: detection and role in native renal disease progression. Transplant Rev (Orlando) 26:3–13.
23. Birn H, Christensen E I. (2006) Renal albumin absorption in physiology and pathology. Kidney Int 69:440–449.
24. Piskinpasa S, Altun B, Akoglu H, Yildirim T, Agbaht K et al. (2013) An uninvestigated risk factor for contrast-induced nephropathy in chronic kidney disease: proteinuria. Ren Fail 35:62–65.
25. Wang Y, Rangan G K, Tay Y C, Wang Y, Harris D C. (1999) Induction of monocyte chemoattractant protein-1 by albumin is mediated by nuclear factor kappaB in proximal tubule cells. J Am Soc Nephrol,10:1204–1213.
26. Erkan E, De Leon M, Devarajan P. (2001) Albumin overload induces apoptosis in LLC-PK(1) cells. Am J Physiol Renal Physiol 280:F1107–F1114.
27. Arici M, Chana R, Lewington A, Brown J, Brunskill N J. (2003) Stimulation of proximal tubular cell apoptosis by albumin-bound fatty acids mediated by peroxisome proliferator activated receptor-gamma. J Am Soc Nephrol 14:17–27.
28. Tang S, Leung J C, Abe K, Chan KW, Chan LY et al. (2003) Albumin stimulates interleukin-8 expression in proximal tubular epithelial cells in vitro and in vivo. J Clin Invest 111:515–527.
29. Zoja C, Morigi M, Figliuzzi M, Bruzzi I, Oldroyd S et al. (1995) Proximal tubular cell synthesis and secretion of endothelin-1 on challenge with albumin and other proteins. Am J Kidney Dis 26:934–941.
30. Cameron J S. (1990) Proteinuria and progression in human glomerular diseases. Am J Nephrol Suppl 1:81–87.
31. Abbate M, Benigni A, Bertani T, Remuzzi G.(1999) Nephrotoxicity of increased glomerular protein traffic. Nephrol Dial Transplant 14:304–312.
32. Ohse T, Inagi R, Tanaka T, Ota T, Miyata T et al. (2006) Albumin induces endoplasmic reticulum stress and apoptosis in renal proximal tubular cells. Kidney Int 70:1447–1455.
33. Morigi M, Macconi D, Zoja C, Donadelli R, Buelli S et al. (2002) Protein overload-induced NF-kappaB activation in proximal tubular cells requires H(2)O(2) through a PKC-dependent pathway. J Am Soc Nephrol 13:1179–1189.
34. Kanaguchi Y, Suzuki Y, Osaki K, Sugaya T, Horikoshi S et al. (2011) Protective effects of L-type fatty acid-binding protein (L-FABP) in proximal tubular cells against glomerular injury in anti-GBM antibody-mediated glomerulonephritis. Nephrol Dial Transplant 26:3465–3473.
35. Grams M E, Astor B C, Bash L D, Matsushita K, Wang Y et al. (2010) Albuminuria and estimated glomerular filtration rate independently associate with acute kidney injury. J Am Soc Nephrol 21:1757–1764.
36. Huang T M, Wu V C, Young G H, Lin YF, Shiao CC et al. (2011) Preoperative proteinuria predicts adverse renal outcomes after coronary artery bypass grafting. J Am Soc Nephrol 22:156–163.
37. Hemmelgarn B R, Manns B J, Lloyd A, James MT, Klarenbach S et al. (2010) Relation between kidney function, proteinuria, and adverse outcomes. JAMA 303:423–429.
38. Hillege H L, Fidler V, Diercks G F, van Gilst WH, de Zeeuw D et al. (2002) Urinary albumin excretion predicts cardiovascular and noncardiovascular mortality in general population. Circulation 106:1777–1782.
39. Hingorani S R, Seidel K, Lindner A, Aneja T, Schoch G et al. (2008) Albuminuria in hematopoietic cell transplantation patients: prevalence, clinical associations, and impact on survival. Biol Blood Marrow Transplant 14:1365–1372.
40. The National Collaborating Centre for Chronic Conditions (UK). (2008) Chronic Kidney Disease: National clinical guideline for early identification andmanagement in adults in primary and secondary care.Royal College of Physicians (UK); Sep.
41. Wijns W, Kolh P, Danchin N, Di Mario C, Falk V et al. (2010) Guidelines on myocardial revascularization. Eur Heart J 31:2501–2555.
42. Heyman S N, Rosen S, Khamaisi M, Idée JM, Rosenberger C et al. (2010) Reactive oxygen species and the pathogenesis of radiocontrast-induced nephropathy. Invest Radiol 45:188–195.

43. Atkins J L.(1986) Effect of sodium bicarbonate preloading on ischemic renal failure. Nephron 44:70–74.
44. Briguori C, Airoldi F, D'Andrea D, Bonizzoni E, Morici N et al. (2007) Renal Insufficiency Following Contrast Media Administration Trial (REMEDIAL): a randomized comparison of 3 preventive strategies. Circulation 115:1211–1217.
45. Recio-Mayoral A, Chaparro M, Prado B, Cózar R, Méndez I et al. (2007) The reno-protective effect of hydration with sodium bicarbonate plus N-acetylcysteine in patients undergoing emergency percutaneous coronary intervention: the RENO Study. J Am Coll Cardiol 49:1283–1288.
46. Meier P, Ko D T, Tamura A, Tamhane U, Gurm HS. (2009) Sodium bicarbonate-based hydration prevents contrast-induced nephropathy: a meta-analysis. BMC Med 7:23.
47. Navaneethan S D, Singh S, Appasamy S, Wing RE, Sehgal AR. (2009) Sodium bicarbonate therapy for prevention of contrast-induced nephropathy: a systematic review and meta-analysis. Am J Kidney Dis 53:617–627.
48. Hogan S E, L'Allier P, Chetcuti S, Grossman PM, Nallamothu BK et al. (2008) Current role of sodium bicarbonate-based preprocedural hydration for the prevention of contrast-induced acute kidney injury: a meta-analysis. Am Heart J 156:414–421.
49. Brown A S. (2010) Renal tubular acidosis. DimensCrit Care Nurs 29:112–119.
50. Smulders Y M, Frissen P H, Slaats E H, Silberbusch J. (1996) Renal tubular acidosis. Pathophysiology and diagnosis. Arch Intern Med 156:1629–1636.
51. Markota D, Markota I, Starcevic B, Tomic M, Prskalo Z et al. (2013) Prevention of contrast-induced nephropathy with Na/K citrate. Eur Heart J 34:2362–2367.
52. Pflueger A, Abramowitz D, Calvin A D. (2009) Role of oxidative stress in contrast-induced acute kidney injury in diabetes mellitus. Med Sci Monit 15:A125–A136.
53. de Brito-Ashurst I, Varagunam M, Raftery M J, Yaqoob MM. (2009)Bicar-Bicarbonate supplementation slows progression of CKD and improves nutritional status. J Am Soc Nephrol 20:2075–2084.

13

Hemodialysis without Systemic Anticoagulation: A Prospective Randomized Trial to Evaluate 3 Strategies in Patients at Risk of Bleeding

Bruno Guéry[1], Corinne Alberti[2], Aude Servais[1], Elarbi Harrami[1], Lynda Bererhi[1], Brigitte Zins[1], Malik Touam[1], Dominique Joly[1,3]*

1 Université Paris-Descartes, Faculté de Médecine, Assistance Publique-Hôpitaux de Paris, Service de Néphrologie, Hôpital Necker-Enfants Malades, Paris, France, **2** Université Denis Diderot, Assistance Publique-Hôpitaux de Paris, Hôpital Robert Debré, Unité d'Epidémiologie Clinique et Institut National de la Santé et de la Recherche Médicale CIE 5, Paris, France, **3** Institut National de la Santé et de la Recherche Médicale U845, Hôpital Necker-Enfants Malades, Paris, France

Abstract

Objective: In this clinical trial, we aimed to compare three means of performing chronic hemodialysis in patients with contra-indication to systemic heparinization.

Methods: This open-label monocentric randomized « n-of-one » trial, conducted in a single tertiary care center, recruited chronic hemodialysis patients with a contra-indication to systemic heparinization for at least 3 consecutive sessions. All patients underwent hemodialysis with an AN69ST dialyzer, and were administered three alternative dialysis procedures in a random sequence: intermittent saline flushes, constant saline infusion, or pre-dialysis heparin coating of the membrane. The primary outcome was the need to interrupt the dialysis session because of clotting events due to either (i) a complete coagulation of the circuit; (ii) a partial coagulation of the circuit; (iii) a>50% rise over baseline in the venous pressure.

Results: At the end of the inclusion period (May, 2007 to December, 2008), the number of patients to include (n = 75) was not reached: only 46 patients were included and underwent randomization. The study was terminated, and statistical analysis took into account 224 hemodialysis sessions performed in 44 patients with analyzable data. Heparin adsorption was associated with a significant reduction of the need to interrupt the dialysis session because of clotting events: odds ratio 0.3 (CI 95% 0.2 to 0.6; p<0.001, versus intermittent saline flushes). Heparin adsorption was also associated with higher odds for performing >3 h dialysis sessions and for having complete blood restitution. There were no significant effects of the dialysis procedure on weight loss, online ionic dialysance, and adverse events.

Conclusion: Heparin-coated AN69ST dialysis membrane is a safe and effective method to avoid or delay per-dialytic clotting events in patients with contra-indication to systemic anticoagulation. However, results are not generalizable safely to patients with active bleeding, since weak heparinemia, not assessed in this study, may occur.

Editor: Hugo ten Cate, Maastricht University Medical Center, Netherlands

Funding: This work was supported by a research grant from the Département à la Recherche Clinique et au Développement, Assistance Publique–Hôpitaux de Paris, which was also the sponsor of the study (CRC 05 032), and AURA (Association pour l'Utilisation du Rein Artificiel). The funders had no role in study design, data collection and analysis, decision to publish, or preparation of the manuscript.

Competing Interests: The authors have declared that no competing interests exist.

* E-mail: doume.joly@gmail.com

Introduction

Heparin, either unfractionated or fractionated, is commonly administered during hemodialysis sessions to prevent clotting events in the extracorporeal circuit [1–6]. This systemic anticoagulation is however contra-indicated in patients at high risk of bleeding. In these challenging cases, a variety of methods have been proposed[7]. Regional heparin/protamine [8], regional citrate/calcium [9–13] and prostacyclin [14,15] are efficient but their use was limited by technical difficulties or clinical complications. Conversely, intermittent saline flushes (ISS) and constant saline infusion (CSI) of the circuit were described as simple and safe techniques to reduce clotting [7,16,17] and are widely used use in daily practice. Finally, the AN69ST membrane (polyacrylonitrile surface, modified by a polyethyleneimine layer) allows stable binding of unfractionated heparin [18]. Heparin coating of the AN69ST membrane produces a local antithrombogenic action which may help perform in some selected patients regular dialysis sessions without systemic heparinization [19,20]. However, the benefits of this technique remained to be established in a comparative trial, especially in patients at risk of bleeding.

In this open-label monocentric randomized prospective study, patients at risk of bleeding that were included underwent hemodialysis without systemic heparinization; all dialysis sessions being performed with AN69ST membrane, we aimed to compare through an individual cross over "n of 1"-type trial the effects of intermittent saline flushes, constant saline infusion, and heparin-coating on clotting events.

Materials and Methods

The protocol for this trial and supporting CONSORT checklist are available as supporting information; see Checklist S1 and Protocol S1.

Patients

We planned to include adult patients on chronic hemodialysis who had a contra-indication to the use of systemic heparinization for at least three consecutive sessions, because of a high bleeding risk (active bleeding, recent surgery or organ biopsy, pericardic effusion), cholesterol emboli, or immunoallergy to heparin. We planned to exclude any patients with either an access blood flow < 250 ml/mn, hemoglobin >13 g/dl, systolic blood pressure < 80 mm Hg, or needing per-dialytic nutritional or blood transfusion support.

The protocol was approved by the local ethics committee (Comité Consultatif de Protection des Personnes en Recherche Biomédicale de l'Ile de France) and written informed consent was obtained from all the patients.

Dialysis Procedures

Dialysis duration was 4 hours, three times per week. Vascular access was either a native arterio-venous fistula (bipuncture) or a double lumen tunneled catheter. Blood flow was wept between 250 and 300 ml/mn. Dialysate prescriptions were as follow: flow 500 ml/mn, sodium conductivity 14.4 mS/cm, bicarbonate conductivity 3.3 mS/cm, temperature 36°C. Ultrafiltration was performed as requested by patient's weight gain and clinical status. All sessions were performed with Nephral 400 ST membranes (AN69ST, hollow-fiber 1.4 m2; Gambro-Hospal, Meyzieu, France).

The three specific procedures to avoid systemic heparinization tested in this study were:

Intermittent saline flushes: every 30 minutes, the blood arterial line was transiently occluded to allow the infusion and quick flush of 125 ml of 0.9% sodium chloride. Constant saline infusion: 0.9% sodium chloride was infused via the arterial line at a constant rate of 250 ml/h during the whole session. Heparin coating was performed according to the manufacturer's recommendations: the AN69ST membrane was primed with 2 liters 0.9% saline containing 10 000 IU of heparin.

Outcomes and Measurements

The primary outcome was defined as the need to interrupt the dialysis session because of clotting events accounting for either (i) a complete coagulation of the circuit; (ii) a partial coagulation of the circuit; (iii) a>50% rise over baseline in the venous pressure. For each dialysis session, we recorded patient's blood pressure and heart rate, initial, dry and final weight, on-line ionic dialysance values (every 30 mn), eventual clinical symptoms and dialysis duration. We also recorded the medical history, treatments. Any adverse events was also recorded; the observation interval was not limited to the duration of the dialysis session, but was extended to the beginning of next dialysis session.

Study Design, Location and Sample Size Calculations

This study was performed at a single tertiary care center (Necker Hospital, Paris). Patients fulfilling all inclusion and exclusion criteria were included in this « N of one » trial in which the three alternative dialysis procedures tested were administered for each patient in a random sequence. The dialysis procedures were used in an open label fashion. The random sequence was generated by computer in an independent center and sent to us by fax. When more than 3 sessions without systemic heparinization had to be performed, order of the three additional sequences was randomly changed. Patients were withdrawn from the study when bleeding risk has disappeared, or after completion of 36 sessions, or if three consecutive complete circuit clotting had occurred with the same specific procedure.

Sample size calculation was based on MacNemar test comparing matched groups for a binary test. Based on our previous unpublished retrospective experience, we hypothesized that the rates of primary outcomes would be 30% with intermittent saline flushes (ISF, standard technique), 20% with constant saline infusion (CSI), and 10% with heparin adsorption (HA). Based on this, with a risk alpha of 5% and a power of 80%, we planned to include 65 pairs of sessions ISF and CSI and 294 pairs of ISF and HA. Thus, 294 triplets of sessions were retained and were inflated to 350 to take into account the clustering of patients (our estimation of a cluster size of 6 and of an intraclass correlation of 0.04 resulted in an inflation factor coefficient of 1.19). Consequently, 75 patients had to be recruited in 18 months time. Based on this calculation, it was decided that the study would be monocentric.

Statistics

Qualitative variables were described as number (percentages) and quantitative variables as median (1st and 3rd quartiles). We built a two levels hierarchical logistic mixed model for qualitative outcomes as interruption of dialysis session and linear mixed model for quantitative outcomes. Level one represented the dialysis sessions as fixed effect and level two the patient as random effect. Results are expressed in Odd Ratio and regression coefficient with their 95% confidence interval (with intermittent saline flushes as the reference method). All tests were bilateral and statistical significance was stated to 5%. Data management was performed with SAS 9.2 (SAS Institute, Cary, NC) and hierarchical models building used MLwiN v2.0.

Results

Patients and Treatment Allocations

At the end of the defined inclusion period (18 months, between May, 2007 and December, 2008), the initially planned number of patients to include (n = 75) had not been reached. During this period, only 48 successive patients on chronic hemodialysis fulfilling all inclusion and exclusion criteria were considered for potential enrolment. One patient declined to be enrolled. Another patient was excluded because his consent form was lost. A total of 46 patients agreed, were included in the study, and underwent randomization. Two additional patients withdrew their consent. The investigators and the sponsor decided to terminate the study and to perform the statistical analysis.

Patient's flow diagram, relevant characteristics and reasons for not performing systemic heparinization are indicated in figure 1 and table 1. This rather unselected group of patients was characterized by a relatively young median age, a reduced dialysis vintage, and a high proportion of patients undergoing urologic surgery (including nephrectomy for 5 patients with autosomal dominant polycystic kidney disease).

Patients underwent a median of 3 sessions (range: 2–36). A total of 224 sessions was performed: 74 with ISS, 74 with CSI, and 76

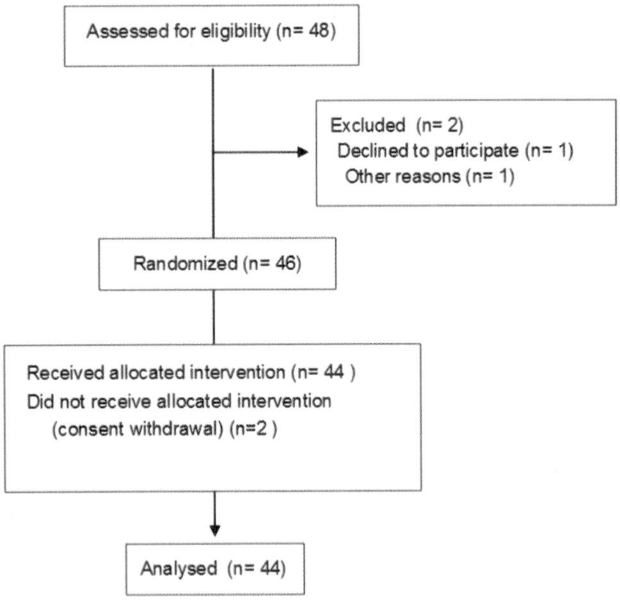

Figure 1. Flow Diagram.

with HA. Overall, the order in the random sequence was comparable for the three dialysis techniques.

Clotting Events

Clotting events leading to premature termination of the dialysis session were observed in 51.4%, 55.4% and 23.7% of dialysis sessions and in 67.4%, 73.8% and 37.2% of patients using ISS, CSI and HA, respectively. Heparin adsorption technique conferred lower odds for premature termination of the dialysis session (OR = 0.3; 95% Confidence Interval, CI (0.2–0.6); $p < 0.001$). HA was also associated with lower rates of, and fewer patients with, complete clotting of the circuit, partial clotting, and with >50% increase in venous pressure (table 2). Finally, complete blood restitution was more frequently reported after HA than with ISS or CSI (respectively 75%, 48.7% and 47.3%, p = 0.001).

Dialysis Duration, Performance and Tolerance

Dialysis sessions performed with the heparin adsorption technique were longer than with other techniques, with a significantly higher probability of lasting more than 3 hours (table 3). Total weight loss was not statistically higher with the heparin adsorption technique. Instantaneous urea nitrogen blood clearances measured after 3 hours of dialysis were not statistically different with the three techniques (table 3). Bleeding of any cause was recorded after 18 of the 224 dialysis sessions (4.5%) performed in this study (the observation period included the dialysis session and the time frame until the beginning of the next dialysis session). Bleeding episodes were never judged as severe, nor required red blood cells transfusion, and were not statistically more frequent after sessions performed with the heparin adsorption technique (p = 0.69 by Fisher's exact test). All dialysis sessions associated with a reported bleeding episode were performed in the 6 patients included in this study because of an active bleeding (see table 1). We did not observe any new or unexpected bleeding during the study.

Perdialytic clinical events including headache, cramps, and hypotension were infrequent in this study (listed table 3). The proportion of sessions and the proportion of patients experiencing these events were similar between the three dialysis techniques.

Discussion

To compare the three dialysis modalities, we performed a n-of-one trial. A n-of-1 trial is a crossover trial conducted in an individual patient. Its results may indicate the best treatment at the individual level. Combining the results of a series of similar n-of-1 trials conducted in different patients may indicate the best treatment at the collective level. The crossover design of n-of-1 trials is particularly appropriate to study of clotting events during hemodialysis sessions: patients have a chronic condition requiring iterative therapeutic interventions; the treatments applied have short-term effects; and finally, measurements in each period are independent [21].

The budget allocated to this study did not allow us to prolong the inclusion period, at the end of which the planned number of patients (n = 75) had not been reached. The number of patients had been calculated based on the assumption that heparin

Table 1. Characteristics of the 44 patients at inclusion.

Variables	median (Q1; Q3) or n (%)
Age (years)	55.3 (42.4; 72.8)
Male gender	22 (48%)
Weight (kg)	63.0 (54.5; 70.5)
Hemoglobin (g/dl)	11.1 (9.2; 12.0)
Diabetes	12 (26%)
Dialysis vintage <12 months	39 (84%)
Native arterio-venous fistula	20 (43%)
Central tunnelized catheters	26 (56%)
Reasons for not using heparin	Recent surgery, n = 29
	Recent organ biopsy/embolization, n = 8
	Current bleeding, n = 6
	Hematologic disorders/thrombopenia, n = 3
	Pericardic effusion, n = 1

Table 2. Clotting events.

Variables		Intermittent Saline flushes	Continuous Saline infusion	Heparin adsorption
Interrupted sessions	n sessions/n patients	74/43	74/42	76/43
	n sessions (%)	38/74 (51%)	41/74 (55%)	18/76 (24%)
	n patients (%)	29/43 (67%)	31/42 (74%)	16/43 (37%)
	OR (95%CI), p	1.0	1.2 (0.6–2.3), p = 0.6	0.3 (0.2–0.6), p = 0.0005
Complete clotting	n sessions (%)	31/74 (42%)	32/74 (43%)	14/76 (18%)
	n patients (%)	25/43 (58%)	24/42 (57%)	13/43 (30%)
	OR (95%CI), p	1.0	1.1 (0.6–2.1), p = 0.8	0.3 (0.2–0.6), p = 0.001
Partial clotting	n sessions (%)	14/74 (19%)	13/74 (18%)	16/76 (21%)
	n patients (%)	11/43 (26%)	10/42 (24%)	14/43 (33%)
	OR (95%CI), p	1.0	0.9 (0.4–2.1), p = 0.9	1.2 (0.5–2.6), p = 0.7
Venous pressure rise >50%	n sessions (%)*	36/73 (49%)	37/74 (50%)	19/76 (25%)
	n patients (%)*	27/42 (64%)	28/42 (67%)	17/43 (40%)
	OR (95%CI), p	1.0	1.0 (0.5–2.0), p = 0.9	0.3 (0.2–0.7), p = 0.002
Incomplete blood restitution	n sessions (%)	38/74 (51.3%)	39/74 (52.7%)	19/76 (25.0%)
	OR (95%CI), p	1.0	1.1 (0.6–2.0), p = 0.9	0.3 (0.2–0.6), p = 0.001

OR: Odd Ratio, CI: Confidence Interval. OR were computed using a two levels hierarchical logistic mixed model.
*data were missing for one patient.

adsorption would reduce the percentage of clotting system by 30%. The decision was made to terminate the study and to perform the statistical analysis, taking the risk of reporting an underpowered study. However, our data clearly indicate that, compared to intermittent saline flushes and continuous saline infusion, heparin-coating significantly reduced the rate of clotting events necessitating the premature termination of the dialysis session.

Clotting in the extracorporeal circuit depends on the anticoagulation procedure, the thrombogenicity of the different circuit components, the patient's thrombophilic potential, and the fluid dynamics. The use of the same membrane in the three modalities strongly suggest that the differences reported in our study are

Table 3. Dialysis efficiency and tolerance.

Variables		Intermittent Saline flushes	Continuous Saline infusion	Heparin adsorption
Dialysis session length (hours)	median (Q1; Q3)	3.5 (2.5; 4.0)	3.6 (2.5; 4.0)	4.0 (3.9; 4.0)
Dialysis >3 hours	n (%)	42/74 (61%)	47/74 (64%)	67/76 (88%)
	OR (95%CI), p	1.0 (ref.)	1.1 (0.6–2.1), 0.8	4.7 (2.2–10.4), <0.001
Weight loss (kgs)**	median (Q1; Q3)	2.0 (1.3; 2.8)	1.8 (1.2; 2.4)	2.4 (1.6; 2.8)
	RC (95%CI), p	0	−0.2 (−0.6; 0.2), 0.3	0.2 (−0.2; 0.6), 0.3
Ionic dialysance (mL/mn)*	median (Q1; Q3)	173 (162; 184)	170 (162; 182)	170 (161; 179)
	RC (95%CI), p	0	−4.3 (−11.6; 2.62), 0.1	−4.9 (−12.0; 2.3), 0.09
Bleeding after dialysis session	n sessions (%)	3/74 (4%)***	5/74 (7%)***	6/76 (8%)***
Headache	n sessions (%)	0/74 (0%)	0/74 (0%)	2/76 (3%)
	n patients (%)	0/43 (0%)	0/42 (0%)	1/43 (2%)
Cramps	n sessions (%)	1/74 (1%)	0/74 (0%)	2/76 (3%)
	n patients (%)	1/43 (2%)	0/42 (0%)	2/43 (5%)
Symptomatic hypotension	n sessions (%)	0/74 (0%)	1/74 (1%)	1/76 (1%)
	n patients (%)	0/43 (0%)	1/42 (2%)	1/43 (2%)
Other symptoms	n sessions (%)	2/74 (3%)	1/74 (1%)	3/76 (4%)
	n patients (%)	2/43 (5%)	1/42 (2%)	3/43 (7%)

CI: confidence interval. OR: Odd Ratio, RC: Regression coefficient, ref: reference OR were computed using a two levels hierarchical logistic mixed model and regression coefficient with a two levels hierarchical linear mixed mode.
*missing data for 48 sessions;
**missing data for 23 sessions.
***p = 0.69 by Fisher's exact test.

mainly due to differences in the membrane thrombogenicity, the latter being reduced by heparin adsorption. The properties and specificities of the AN69 ST membrane have been underscored by many reports [18,19,22]; it should however be stressed here that heparin priming has also been reported with other synthetic membranes, including FX100 polysulphone [23].

Even with the heparin adsorption technique, clotting events occurred quite frequently. However, the rate of complete clotting in our study (18% of sessions) compares favorably to the 38% reported by Evenopol et al. in a study including also patients at risk of bleeding [24]. Part of this difference may be team-dependent; technical experience of the nurses is indeed critical to handle properly heparin-coated AN69 ST membranes, including careful deaeration of the dialyzer and hourly lowering of the blood column in the venous drip chamber, as recommended by the manufacturer. Patient's risk for thrombosis was also probably lower in our study, due to selective inclusion criteria, which required vascular access flow >250 ml/mn and hemoglobin < 13 g/dl. Of note, the incidence of massive clotting with the HA technique could be as low as 1/66 sessions in a different population, made of carefully selected stable hemodialysis patients with no specific risk of bleeding [19].

Two observations may help reduce the rate of clotting events in the future. First, almost all clots observed with heparin-coated AN69ST technique were initially formed in parts of the circuit not coated with heparin (mainly the venous bubble trap). Some authors have reported encouraging results with covalent coating of the whole extracorporeal circuit with low molecular weight heparin [25]. Second, the vast majority of clots observed with heparin-coated AN69ST formed at the very end of the dialysis session, suggesting that a slight reduction of the session length could have dramatically reduced the rate of coagulation events.

In this study, heparin adsorption did not improve membrane permeability to small molecular weight plasma molecules, as measured by online ionic conductance throughout sessions. Other groups have reported that during heparin-free dialysis, small solutes removal could be maintained despite moderate dialyzer clotting, to a possible increase of blood flow through the unclotted fibers [19,26].

Heparin partial desorption from the membrane and incomplete removal of the priming solution before patient's connection to the extracorporeal circuit may occur with the HA protocol, with subsequent systemic anticoagulation due to circulating heparin. Coagulation parameters were not assessed in the present study. However, antiXa activity measurements reported by Lavaud et coll. after 3 hours of dialysis were weakly positive, all values being <0.1 UI/ml [19]. Another study using heparin-coated membranes reported a weak and transient increase in activated partial thromboplastin time [22]. Even if the systemic exposure to heparin is transient and minimal, we consider that heparin-coated membranes should be strictly avoided in patients with heparin-induced allergy. The heparin adsorption protocol should probably also be avoided in patients who suffer from major active bleeding. Only 6 patients with active bleeding were included in our study. Besides patients with active bleeding, our results cannot safely be generalized to patients with acute renal failure, to patients in intensive care units, and to patients with different baseline characteristics, i.e very elderly patients and patients with high dialysis vintage.

In our experience, both ISS and CSI were associated with a very high rate of clotting events, confirming that their efficiency should be questioned [27]. By comparison, the heparin-coated AN69ST membrane technique appeared as a safe and effective method for providing hemodialysis treatments in most (if not all) patients with contra-indication to systemic anticoagulation. Despite its increased cost, this technique has become the preferred anticoagulation strategy in patients at risk of bleeding in our center. However, hemodialysis centers with access to both heparin-coated membranes and sodium citrate regional anticoagulation should be aware that the latter technique may provide an even superior anticoagulation efficacy, at the expense of a higher complexity [24].

Acknowledgments

The authors thank the participating patients, Dr Soraya Soulimane, Mr Patrick Vaillant, Caroline Quintin (Unité de Recherche Clinique, Paris Nord) for their implementation and monitoring of the study, Priscilla Armoogum for statistical analyses, the nurses of Necker dialysis unit for their unvaluable help in this study, Pr Grünfeld and Pr Lesavre for their support.

Author Contributions

Conceived and designed the experiments: DJ, CA, MT, BG. Performed the experiments: BG AS EH LB BZ MT. Analyzed the data: CA, DJ, BG. Wrote the paper: DJ, CA, BG.

References

1. Bartels PC, Schoorl M, Schoorl M, Wiering JG, Nubé MJ (2000) Activation of coagulation during treatment with haemodialysis. Scand. J. Clin. Lab. Invest 60: 283–290.
2. Martin-Malo A, Velasco F, Rojas R, Castillo D, Rodriguez M, et al (1993) Fibrinolytic activity during hemodialysis: a biocompatibility-related phenomenon. Kidney Int. Suppl 41: S213–216.
3. Camici M, Evangelisti L, Balestri P, Cioni L, Rindi P, et al (1997) Coagulation activation in extracorporeal hemodialysis. Int J Artif Organs 20: 163–165.
4. Lim W, Cook DJ, Crowther MA (2004) Safety and efficacy of low molecular weight heparins for hemodialysis in patients with end-stage renal failure: a meta-analysis of randomized trials. J. Am. Soc. Nephrol 15: 3192–3206.
5. Weitz JI: Low-molecular-weight heparins (1997) N. Engl. J. Med 337: 688–698.
6. Nurmohamed MT, Ten Cate J, Stevens P, Hoek JA, Lins RL, et al. (1991) Long-term efficacy and safety of a low molecular weight heparin in chronic hemodialysis patients. A comparison with standard heparin. ASAIO Trans 37: M459–461.
7. Caruana RJ, Raja RM, Bush JV, Kramer MS, Goldstein S (1987) Heparin free dialysis: comparative data and results in high risk patients. Kidney Int 31: 1351–1355.
8. Swartz RD (1981) Hemorrhage during high-risk hemodialysis using controlled heparinization. Nephron 28: 65–69.
9. Pinnick RV, Wiegmann TB, Diederich DA (1983) Regional citrate anticoagulation for hemodialysis in the patient at high risk for bleeding. N. Engl. J. Med 308: 258–261.
10. Flanigan MJ, Von Brecht J, Freeman RM, Lim VS (1987) Reducing the hemorrhagic complications of hemodialysis: a controlled comparison of low-dose heparin and citrate anticoagulation. Am. J. Kidney Dis 9: 147–153.
11. Kelleher SP, Schulman G (1987) Severe metabolic alkalosis complicating regional citrate hemodialysis. Am. J. Kidney Dis 9: 235–236.
12. Apsner R, Buchmayer H, Lang T, Unver B, Speiser W, et al. (2001) Simplified citrate anticoagulation for high-flux hemodialysis. Am. J. Kidney Dis 38: 979–987.
13. Janssen MJ, Huijgens PC, Bouman AA, Oe PL, Donker AJ, et al. (1993) Citrate versus heparin anticoagulation in chronic haemodialysis patients. Nephrol. Dial. Transplant 8: 1228–1233.
14. Caruana RJ, Smith MC, Clyne D, Crow JW, Zinn JM, et al. (1991) Controlled study of heparin versus epoprostenol sodium (prostacyclin) as the sole anticoagulant for chronic hemodialysis. Blood Purif 9: 296–304.

15. Swartz RD, Flamenbaum W, Dubrow A, Hall JC, Crow JW, et al. (1988) Epoprostenol (PGI2, prostacyclin) during high-risk hemodialysis: preventing further bleeding complications. J Clin Pharmacol 28: 818–825.
16. Schwab SJ, Onorato JJ, Sharar LR, Dennis PA (1987) Hemodialysis without anticoagulation. One-year prospective trial in hospitalized patients at risk for bleeding. Am. J. Med 83: 405–410.
17. Preuschof L, Keller F, Seemann J, Offermann G (1988) Heparin-free hemodialysis with prophylactic change of dialyser and blood lines. Int J Artif Organs 11: 255–258.
18. Chanard J, Lavaud S, Paris B, Toure F, Rieu P, et al. (2005) Assessment of heparin binding to the AN69 ST hemodialysis membrane: I. Preclinical studies. ASAIO J 51: 342–347.
19. Lavaud S, Canivet E, Wuillai A, Maheut H, Randoux C, et al. (2005) Optimal anticoagulation strategy in haemodialysis with heparin-coated polyacrylonitrile membrane. Nephrol. Dial. Transplant 18: 2097–2104.
20. Lavaud S, Paris B, Maheut H, Randoux C, Renaux J, et al. (2005) Assessment of the heparin-binding AN69 ST hemodialysis membrane: II. Clinical studies without heparin administration. ASAIO J 51: 348–351.
21. Zucker DR, Deo A, Schmid CH (2010) Dialysis research and N-of-1 trials: made for each other? Am. J. Kidney Dis 55: 635–638.
22. Richtrova P, Opatrny K, Vit L, Sefrna F, Perlik R (2007) The AN69 ST haemodialysis membrane under conditions of two different extracorporeal circuit rinse protocols a comparison of thrombogenicity parameters. Nephrol. Dial. Transplant 22: 2978–2984.
23. Kodras K, Benesch T, Neumann I, Haas M (2008): Comparison of two dialysers (AN69ST vs. FX100) for heparin-free dialysis in patients with oral anticoagulation. Blood Purif 26: 226–230.
24. Evenepoel P, Dejagere T, Verhamme P, Claes K, Kuypers D, et al. (2008) Heparin-coated polyacrylonitrile membrane versus regional citrate anticoagulation: a prospective randomized study of 2 anticoagulation strategies in patients at risk of bleeding. Am. J. Kidney Dis 49: 642–649.
25. Frank RD, Müller U, Lanzmich R, Groeger C, Floege J (2006) Anticoagulant-free Genius haemodialysis using low molecular weight heparin-coated circuits. Nephrol. Dial. Transplant 21: 1013–1018.
26. Romão JE, Fadil MA, Sabbaga E, Marcondes M (1997) Haemodialysis without anticoagulant: haemostasis parameters, fibrinogen kinetic, and dialysis efficiency. Nephrol. Dial. Transplant 12: 106–110.
27. Sagedal S, Hartmann A, Osnes K, Bjørnsen S, Torremocha J, et al. (2006) Intermittent saline flushes during haemodialysis do not alleviate coagulation and clot formation in stable patients receiving reduced doses of dalteparin. Nephrol. Dial. Transplant 21: 444–449.

14

Prognostic Value and Link to Atrial Fibrillation of Soluble Klotho and FGF23 in Hemodialysis Patients

Albina Nowak[1]*⁹, Björn Friedrich[2,3]⁹, Ferruh Artunc[2], Andreas L. Serra[4], Tobias Breidthardt[5], Raphael Twerenbold[6], Myriam Peter[6], Christian Mueller[6]

1 Division of Internal Medicine, University Hospital Zürich, Zürich, Switzerland, **2** Department of Internal Medicine, Division of Endocrinology, Diabetology, Vascular Disease, Nephrology and Clinical Chemistry, University of Tübingen, Tübingen, Germany, **3** Dialysis center Leonberg, Leonberg, Germany, **4** Division of Nephrology, University Hospital Zürich, Zürich, Switzerland, **5** Division of Nephrology, University Hospital Basel, Basel, Switzerland, **6** Division of Cardiology, University Hospital Basel, Basel, Switzerland

Abstract

Deranged calcium-phosphate metabolism contributes to the burden of morbidity and mortality in dialysis patients. This study aimed to assess the association of the phosphaturic hormone fibroblast growth factor 23 (FGF23) and soluble Klotho with all-cause mortality. We measured soluble Klotho and FGF23 levels at enrolment and two weeks later in 239 prevalent hemodialysis patients. The primary hypothesis was that low Klotho and high FGF23 are associated with increased mortality. The association between Klotho and atrial fibrillation (AF) at baseline was explored as secondary outcome. AF was defined as presence of paroxysmal, persistent or permanent AF. During a median follow-up of 924 days, 59 (25%) patients died from any cause. Lower Klotho levels were not associated with mortality in a multivariable adjusted analysis when examined either on a continuous scale (HR 1.25 per SD increase, 95% CI 0.84–1.86) or in tertiles, with tertile 1 as the reference category (HR for tertile two 0.65, 95% CI 0.26–1.64; HR for tertile three 2.18, 95% CI 0.91–2.23). Higher Klotho levels were associated with the absence of AF in a multivariable logistic regression analysis (OR 0.66 per SD increase, 95% CI 0.41–1.00). Higher FGF23 levels were associated with mortality risk in a multivariable adjusted analysis when examined either on a continuous scale (HR 1.45 per SD increase, 95% CI 1.05–1.99) or in tertiles, with the tertile 1 as the reference category (HR for tertile two 1.63, 95% CI 0.64–4.14; HR for tertile three 3.91, 95% CI 1.28–12.20). FGF23 but not Klotho levels are associated with mortality in hemodialysis patients. Klotho may be protective against AF.

Editor: Christos Chatziantoniou, Institut National de la Santé et de la Recherche Médicale, France

Funding: The authors thank TECOmedical AG, Switzerland for measurements of soluble Klotho and FGF23 levels. The funders had no role in study design, data collection and analysis, decision to publish, or preparation of the manuscript. In addition to the above, there was no other funding for this study. The authors' organisations had no other external or internal funding.

Competing Interests: The authors declare that TECOmedical AG, Switzerland measured the soluble Klotho and FGF23 levels in their hemodialysis cohort for this study. The authors of this manuscript have no commercial or professional association with TECOmedical AG. They have nothing to declare concerning employment, consultancy, patents, products in development, marketed products, etc.

* Email: albina.nowak@usz.ch

⁹ These authors contributed equally to this work.

Introduction

Cardiovascular mortality in hemodialysis patients is 55% higher than in patients with normal kidney function [1]. Vascular calcification has been linked to deranged calcium-phosphate metabolism. Fibroblast growth factor 23 (FGF23) regulates phosphate metabolism by inhibiting renal phosphate reabsorption [2,3].

The transmembrane form of Klotho functions as co-receptor of FGF23 increasing the affinity of FGF23 to the FGF-receptor. Klotho is a 130-kDa single-pass transmembrane protein that is mainly expressed in the kidney [4]. The extracellular Klotho domain is cleaved into the circulation [5]. Klotho protects against arterial calcification [6] reduces arterial stiffness in chronic kidney disease (CKD) [7], increases endothelial survival [8]. Klotho expression decreases early in the course of CKD [9,10] possibly causing FGF23 resistance [11].

High FGF23 levels were associated with an increased all-cause mortality in hemodialysis patients [12], increased risk for end stage renal disease (ESRD), cardiovascular events and mortality in CKD patients [13,14]. An excess of FGF23 in CKD may be caused by low Klotho levels triggering FGFR's peripheral resistance to FGF23 and thus linking FGF23-associated mortality to Klotho. To test this hypothesis, we assessed the association of soluble Klotho (sKlotho) with all-cause mortality as the primary outcome in a large cohort of hemodialysis patients.

Atrial fibrillation (AF) is one of the important cardiac comorbidities in hemodialysis patients. High FGF23 levels were associated with AF in a recent study [15]. Little is known of the association between low Klotho levels and AF. Experimental data demonstrated that sKlotho is important for the function of ion channels by regulating their cell-surface abundance through enzymatic activation [16–18]. This can influence the peacemaker activity of the channels in the sinoatrial node. Klotho's expression in the sinoatrial node has been demonstrated in animal studies,

Klotho-deficient animals develop sinoatrial dysfunction under stress conditions [19]. Thus, we tested a possible association between low Klotho level and AF.

Subjects and Methods

This study was approved by the ethics committee of medical faculty Eberhard-Karls-university Tübingen (project 191/2009BO2). All study participants provided a written informed consent, both for taking of blood samples and for their clinical records to be used in the study. The research was done in accordance with the Helsinki declaration.

Patients and control group

The study population consists of 239 prevalent maintenance hemodialysis patients from four dialysis centers in Southwest Germany participating in a prospective multicenter study. All the patients received bicarbonate hemodialysis. This cohort was established between September 2009 and September 2012 and investigate the associations between novel biochemical risk parameters and all-cause mortality [20,21].

Patients were eligible if they had given written informed consent, initiation of hemodialysis was more than three months previously and there was no evidence of acute life-threatening illness, cardiac event, cardiac amyloidosis or cardiac procedure within the previous two months. Clinical data were collected at baseline from the patients' medical records. The follow-up was complete in all patients.

Endpoint evaluation

We defined all-cause mortality as the primary endpoint. The primary exposure variables were plasma Klotho and FGF23 levels, measured at study enrolment. Mortality was prospectively recorded and coded. The follow-up was conducted by the primary physicians of the cohort. Patients received status "survived" if they continued attending their regular thrice-weekly hemodialysis facility on 31.08.2012. No patient recovered kidney function. To ascertain the survival status of 18 patients who moved to another dialysis center, the new responsible primary physician was contacted. The follow-up of 14 transplanted patients was censored at the transplantation date.

The association between sKlotho and the prevalence of AF at baseline was explored as a secondary outcome in a cross-sectional manner. The diagnosis of AF was extracted from patient records. In this cohort, 12-lead ECGs were routinely performed every 6 months and additionally if patients complained of palpitations or chestpain. If no AF was seen on the 12-lead ECG, a 24-hour ECG was recorded promptly. AF was defined as the presence of paroxysmal, persistent or permanent AF.

Control group

The Klotho control group consisted of 80 healthy blood donors who permitted use of their samples for research purposes (age 45±13 years). Blinded to Klotho, we generated age-adjusted groups by excluding hemodialysis patients older than 70 and controls younger than 50 years. The age-adjusted groups included 109 hemodialysis patients aged 56±11 and 32 controls aged 56±4 years.

The FGF23 control group consisted of 55 healthy blood donors who permitted use of their samples for research purposes. Blinded to FGF23, we generated age-adjusted groups by including all dialysis patients in the cohort and controls older than 60 years. The age-adjusted groups included 239 hemodialysis patients aged 68±14 and 19 controls aged 69±8 years.

Laboratory assays

Blood was drawn prior to the dialysis session at enrolment and two weeks later, collected in EDTA, cooled to 4°C, centrifuged within 4 hours, the plasma samples were stored at −80°C for further batched analysis. Klotho and FGF23 levels were measured in a blinded fashion.

Human soluble α-Klotho levels were measured by Enzyme Linked Immunosorbent Assay (ELISA) (Immuno-Biologic Laboratories Co., Ltd. Japan). This novel method detects sKlotho using a monoclonal antibody with high affinity to the human α-Klotho protein. According to the manufacturer's manual, the intra assay variation coefficients (VC) are 2.7% and 3.1% at 757 pg/ml and 2969 pg/ml, the interassay VC are 6.5% and 2.9% at 706 pg/mL and 2903 pg/mL, respectively; the analytic sensitivity is ≥ 6.15 pg/mL. Plasma FGF23 concentrations were measured using the two-site second generation Human FGF23 (C-Term) ELISA Kit (Immutopics, San Clemente, CA) with mean intra-assay VC < 3%, as specified by the manufacturer. We additionally measured FGF23 levels in 36 patients using Millipore human FGF23 (intact) ELISA Kit (Billerica, MA, USA) and in 32 patients using Kainos (Tokyo, Japan) murine FGF23 (intact) ELISA Kit. To verify the capability of the chosen FGF23 and Klotho assays, we performed dilution experiments in 11 random samples. We tested sample: diluent ratios 1:2 and 1:4. The correlation between measured and expected Klotho and FGF23 levels in the diluted samples was very high: R = 0.97, P>0.001 for Klotho and R = 0.99, P<0.001 for FGF23 (Figure S1 in File S1).

Due to low sample volume in some patients, we first measured FGF23 as it required a lower sample volume, then measuring Klotho if enough volume remained.

Laboratory values of PTH, hemoglobin, albumin, C-reactive protein (CRP), calcium, phosphate and alkaline phosphatase were extracted from the patient medical records and averaged from the available values of the previous year (4–12 values). 25(OH)vitamin D levels were measured between 3 months before and 3 months after study enrolment and were available in 223 patients Body Mass Index (BMI) was calculated as postdialytic dry weight at study enrolment in kilograms divided by the square of the height in meters.

Clinical data

All clinical evaluation of the patients was performed at the time the prospective cohort was established. Data on residual diuresis (measured by 24 h urine collection and quantified in milliliters per day), single pool Kt/V (mean of the last 4 values), interdialytic weight gain, predialytic blood pressure (means from the last 12 values), dialysis access and membrane, time on dialysis, blood pump, arterio-venous fistula flow (measured with a Transonic system, Ithaca, NY, USA), presence of pulmonary hypertension (using echocardiography or right heart catheter as indicated) were extracted from the medical records. Transthoracic echocardiography (TTE) was performed as clinically indicated. The results of TTE performed within one year before and one year after the study enrolment were extracted from the medical records and analysed for the presence of left ventricular hypertrophy (LVH) and left atrium dilation (LAD). These results were available in166 patients for LVH and in 177 for LAD.

Statistical analysis

We used descriptive statistics to compare baseline characteristics and laboratory parameters according to the baseline Klotho tertiles. Categorical variables were expressed as proportions, continuous variables as means with standard deviations and medians with interquartile ranges [IQR]. Normal distribution was assessed by Kolmogorov-Smirnov-Test. Comparisons of groups were made using one-way analysis of variance (ANOVA) for continuous and the chi-squared test for categorical variables.

Kaplan-Meier analysis was performed and log-rank test of survival distributions equality for the Klotho and FGF23 tertiles was calculated.

Cox regression analysis was used to examine the mortality risk associated with baseline Klotho and FGF23 levels. Similarly to previous studies examining FGF23 and mortality risk in CKD [13,14] and hemodialysis [12], multivariable models were applied to adjust for potential confounders, using prior knowledge of variables that have been associated with mortality risk in patients undergoing hemodialysis in previous studies. We hierarchically adjusted for demographics (age, gender, dialysis center) in model 1, dialysis-specific risk factors and comorbid conditions (dialysis vintage, blood pressure, BMI, vascular access at study enrolment, diabetes mellitus, coronary and valvular heart disease, AF, ICD carriage, peripheral and cerebrovascular disease, COPD, malignancy, cause of renal failure, medication and pooled Kt/V) in model 2, and mineral metabolism levels (PTH, 25(OH)vitamin D, phosphate and calcium), albumin, hemoglobin, CRP, cholesterol in model 3.

We used logistic regression analysis to explore the association between baseline Klotho levels and AF. Multivariable models were applied to adjust for potential confounders, using variables that have been associated with AF in previous studies. We hierarchically adjusted for demographics (age, gender, dialysis center) in model 1, cardiovascular comorbidities (diabetes mellitus, coronary artery and valvular heart disease, peripheral artery and cerebrovascular disease), anuria in model 2, and mineral metabolism levels (FGF23, PTH, phosphate, calcium), calcium dialysate, potassium serum and dialysate, albumin, hemoglobin, CRP, cholesterol, thyroid stimulating hormone in model 3. Regression analysis for Klotho tertiles at baseline with the absence of AF as dependent variable was performed using the same models.

The statistical analyses were performed using the SPSS/PC (version 19.0; SPSS Inc., Chicago, IL, USA) software package. Numbers at risk were calculated using SAS 9.3 (SAS Institute, Cary, NC, USA). All statistical tests were two-sided, and P values <0.05 were considered significant.

Results

Baseline characteristics and outcome

From a total of 250 eligible patients, 239 (96%) were enrolled in our study. The exclusion reasons were: six declined to participate, two died within two weeks after enrolment, two suffered from cardiac amyloidosis and one had initiated hemodialysis less than three months before. The follow-up was complete in all patients. Fifty-nine patients (25%) died within the median follow-up period of 924 [735–996] days.

Klotho at enrolment was measured in 55 (93%) non-survivors and 172 (96%) survivors, FGF23 in 57 (97%) non-survivors and 177 (98%) survivors. Both, Klotho and FGF23 levels at baseline were measured in 226 (95%) patients. The baseline characteristics and laboratory results for the full cohort and according to the Klotho level tertiles are given in Table 1.

All-cause mortality

Median Klotho levels were similar in non-survivors and survivors (351 [264–454] vs 338 [255–420] pg/ml, P = 0.85). Median FGF23 levels tended to be higher in non-survivors than in survivors (394 [111–1147] vs 201 [83–707] RU/ml, P = 0.07).

In Cox regression analysis, higher Klotho levels were not associated with mortality in crude model and after multiple adjustments when examined either on a continuous scale or in tertiles, with tertile 1 as the reference category. In contrast, higher FGF23 levels were associated with mortality after the same adjustments (Table 2). Similar results were obtained analysing the second blood sample (Table S1 in File S1).

Following adjustment for demographics and markers of bone metabolism, haemoglobin, albumin and cholesterol, Klotho remained not associated with mortality (HR 1.21 per SD increase, 95% CI 0.87–1.68, P = 0.25), in contrast to FGF23 (HR 1.56 per SD increase, 95% CI 1.21–2.01, P = 0.001).

Cumulative survival among the three groups, stratified according to the baseline Klotho tertiles, was similar in a Kaplan-Meier analysis (P = 0.42) (Figure 1). For FGF23, the poorest cumulative survival was observed among patients with levels within the top tertile, with a log-rank test approaching significance (P = 0.05) (Figure 2).

There was no correlation between FGF23 and Klotho levels (R = −0.03, P = 0.64).

The ratio between FGF23 (RU/ml) per SD increase and Klotho (pg/ml) per SD increase did not substantially improve the association with mortality (HR 1.59 95% CI 1.16–2.19, P = 0.004) compared to FGF23 per SD increase alone in a crude Cox regression model.

Atrial fibrillation

In 54 (23%) of 239 patients, AF had been diagnosed. The baseline characteristics and laboratory results according to presence or absence of AF are presented in Table S2 in File S1.

Both low Klotho and high FGF23 levels were associated with AF (Figure 3). In logistic regression analysis, low Klotho levels remained associated with AF in crude model, in model 1, model 2, this association was slightly attenuated in model 3 (Table 3).

This association was similar if we adjusted only for demographics and markers of bone metabolism, haemoglobin, albumin and cholesterol (HR 0.66 per SD increase, 95% CI 0.43–1.00, P = 0.05).

Patients with Klotho levels within the third tertile were more frequently free of AF (Table 4). This effect remained significant after multiple adjustments. A similar association was observed analysing the results of the second blood sample (Tables S3 and S4 in File S1).

The presence of AF tended to be associated with mortality in a crude Cox regression model (HR 1.67; 95%CI 0.97–2.89; P = 0.07).

Klotho and FGF23 levels in control group versus hemodialysis patients

The median Klotho level in controls was higher than in hemodialysis patients before (Figure 4A) and after age adjustment (647 [381–974], versus 344 [116–752] pg/ml, P<0.001). Klotho levels correlated with age in controls ($R^2 = -0.293$, P = 0.008) but not in haemodialysis patients (P = 0.78).

The mean FGF23 level in controls was lower than in haemodialysis patients before (Figure 4B) and after age adjustment (93±25, versus 883±1940 RU/ml, P = 0.001). FGF23 levels did not correlate with age in controls (P = 0.11) and in hemodialysis patients (P = 0.17).

FGF23 levels measured with different kits

The mean FGF23 level measured using the Millipore assay was 1028±2119 pg/ml, using Immutopics assay in the same samples

Table 1. Baseline characteristics and laboratory parameters according to Klotho tertiles.

	Full Cohort	Klotho Tertile 1	Klotho Tertile 2	Klotho Tertile 3	P value
	339 [260–427] N = 239	(<286 pg/ml) N = 75	(286–392 pg/ml) N = 75	(>392 pg/ml) N = 77	
Age (yr)	68±14	67±15	69±12	66±15	0.42
Male gender n (%)	153 (64)	55 (73)	41 (55)	49 (64)	0.06
Body-mass index*	26 [23–30]	27 [24–30]	26 [23–29]	26 [22–30]	0.41
Blood pressure (mmHg)					
Systolic	134 [122–144]	137 [128–147]	134 [124–144]	127 [117–140]	0.005
Diastolic	69 [63–74]	69 [63–76]	68 [64–74]	69 [61–73]	0.55
Cause of renal failure n (%)					
Diabetes mellitus	63 (26)	24 (36)	19 (25)	18 (23)	0.48
Hypertension	19 (8)	5 (7)	8 (11)	3 (4)	0.26
Glomerulonephritis	71 (30)	24 (32)	23 (31)	22 (29)	0.90
PKD	11 (5)	2 (3)	5 (7)	4 (5)	0.51
Others/unknown	75 (31)	20 (27)	20 (27)	30 (39)	0.17
Cardiac comorbidities n (%)					
Coronary artery disease	73 (31)	24 (32)	24 (32)	19 (25)	0.52
PCI/CABG	45 (19)	16 (21)	19 (25)	17 (22)	0.78
Valvular heart disease	61 (26)	13 (17)	20 (27)	22 (29)	0.27
Atrial fibrillation	54 (23)	19 (25)	20 (27)	10 (13)	0.08
ICD implantation	4 (2)	1 (1)	0 (0)	2 (3)	0.37
LVH†	101 (61)	36 (62)	34 (62)	28 (52)	0.18
Pulmonary hypertension	16 (7)	3 (4)	6 (8)	5 (6)	0.59
Other comorbidities n (%)					
Diabetes mellitus	90 (38)	29 (39)	24 (32)	32 (43)	0.46
PVD	80 (33)	28 (37)	23 (31)	23 (31)	0.56
Stroke	38 (16)	8 (11)	18 (24)	9 (12)	0.04
Vasculitis	8 (3)	3 (4)	2 (3)	2 (3)	0.85
Malignoma	34 (14)	14 (19)	7 (9)	11 (14)	0.26
COPD	19 (8)	3 (4)	8 (11)	7 (9)	0.29
Dialysis vintage (months)	59±53	49±40	67±56	62±60	0.10
Duration of dialysis session (hours)	4.2±0.4	4.3±0.5	4.1±0.3	4.2±0.42	0.24
Dialysis access at baseline n (%)					
Arteriovenous fistula	169 (71)	49 (65)	54 (72)	56 (73)	0.51
PTFE graft	31 (13)	11 (15)	7 (9)	11 (14)	0.57
Tunnelled catheter	38 (16)	15 (20)	13 (17)	10 (13)	0.50
Dialysis membrane n (%)					
High-flux	228 (95)	73 (97)	70 (93)	73 (95)	0.51
Low-flux	11 (5)	2 (3)	5 (7)	4 (5)	
Dialysis modality					
Hemodiafiltration	54 (23)	18	17	15	0.79
Hemodialysis only	185 (77)	57	58	62	
Anuric patients n (%)	93 (39)	28 (37)	30 (40)	32 (42)	0.86
Residual diuresis (ml/24 hours)	250 [0–1005]	300 [0–1100]	200 [0–1025]	200 [0–900]	0.75
Interdialytic weight gain (kg)	1.9 [1.3–2.5]	1.9 [1.4–2.7]	1.82 [1.22–2.43]	1.86 [1.17–2.48]	0.52
Shunt flow (ml/min)	1177±638	1099±512	1287±670	1160±694	0.28
Singe pool Kt/V	1.6 [1.4–1.7]	1.52 [1.33–1.65]	1.60 [1.40–1.77]	1.53 [1.39–1.71]	0.24
Ca, dialysate	1.4±0.2	1.4±0.2	1.4±0.2	1.4±0.2	0.98
K, dialysate	2.4±0.6	2.3±0.6	2.3±0.6	2.5±0.6	0.40
FGF23 (RU/ml)	883±1940	1117±2866	609±1025	761±1370	0.25
PTH (pg/ml)	249±177	282±184	240±188	234±152	0.20

Table 1. Cont.

	Full Cohort 339 [260–427] N = 239	Klotho Tertile 1 (<286 pg/ml) N = 75	Klotho Tertile 2 (286–392 pg/ml) N = 75	Klotho Tertile 3 (>392 pg/ml) N = 77	P value
25(OH)vitamin D (ng/ml)	28 [21–35]	28 [20–35]	27 [21–34]	29 [20–36]	0.52
Phosphate (mmol/l)	1.6 [1.4–1.9]	1.6 [1.3–1.9]	1.6 [1.3–1.8]	1.6 [1.4–1.9]	0.70
Ca, serum (mmol/l)	2.3 [2.2–2.4]	2.3 [2.2–2.4]	2.3 [2.2–2.4]	2.3 [2.2–2.4]	0.40
AP (U/l)	91±42	85±41	91±43	97±45	0.14
K, serum (mmol/l)	5.0±0.6	5.1±0.6	5.1±0.6	5.0±0.6	0.37
Albumin (g/l)	37±4	37±5	37±4	37±4	0.82
Hemoglobin (g/dL)	11.5 [11.1–12.0]	11.5 [11.2–11.8]	11.6 [11.2–12.0]	11.5 [11.2–12.0]	0.9
C-reactive protein (mg/l)	12±12	13±14	12±11	12±11	0.80
Cholsterol (mg/dl)	167 [141–196]	171 [147–200]	172 [143–199]	156 [141–193]	0.52
Medication use n (%)					
Phosphate binders	205 (86)	64 (85)	64 (85)	67 (87)	0.88
Vitamin d replacement	233 (97)	72 (96)	74 (99)	75 (97)	0.76
ACE-I or ARB	126 (53)	48 (64)	39 (52)	33 (43)	0.04
β-Blockers	153 (64)	56 (75)	45 (60)	42 (55)	0.03
Statin	101 (42)	41 (55)	28 (37)	26 (34)	0.02

Plus-minus values are means ± SD. Numbers with ranges in square brackets are medians and interquartile ranges. P values are for the comparisons between the three Klotho tertiles. To convert the values for calcium to milligrams per deciliter, multiply by 4.000. To convert the values for phosphate to milligrams per deciliter, multiply by 3.0969.
*The body-mass index is the weight in kilograms divided by the square of the height in meters.
†Based on 166 available clinically indicated transthoracic echocardiography results.
Abbreviations: ACE-I, angiotensin-converting enzyme inhibitors; AF, atrial fibrillation; AP, alkaline phosphatase; ARB, angiotensin receptor blocker; COPD, chronic obstructive pulmonary disease; FGF23, fibroblast growth factor 23; ICD, implantable cardioverter defibrillator; IQR, interquartile range; PTFE, Polytetrafluorethylen; PTH, parathyroid hormone; PKD, polycystic kidney disease; PVD Peripheral vascular disease; T, Tertile; U, unit.

1001±1627 RU/ml. The mean FGF23 level measured using Kainos assay was 690±1001 pg/ml, using the Immutopics assay in the same samples 723±1279 RU/ml.

FGF23 levels measured using the Immunotopic assay correlated with the levels measured using the Millipore (R = 0.73, P<0.001) and Kainos assay (R = 0.66, P<0.001). FGF23 levels measured using Millipore assay correlated with the levels measured using Kainos assay (R = 0.97, P<0.001).

Discussion

In this cohort of ESRD patients with long-term follow-up, we report three major findings. First, FGF23 but not Klotho levels were predictive for all-cause mortality. This association remained significant after multivariate adjustments and was confirmed analysing the results of the second blood sample drawn two weeks after study enrolment. Second, high Klotho levels may exert a protective effect against AF. Interestingly, Klotho was more strongly associated with AF than the presence of traditional cardiovascular risk factors such as complete loss of kidney function, age, gender, arteriosclerosis and valvular heart disease. Even the fully adjusted model, additionally including levels of other mineral metabolites known as risk factors for structural heart disease, approached statistical significance. Third, Klotho levels in healthy controls were higher than in hemodialysis patients.

Assays for Klotho have been lacking until now, and data on the regulatory mechanism, function and expression of Klotho has been scant. Only very recently, a sandwich enzyme-linked immunosorbent assay (ELISA) has been developed for the soluble form of Klotho [22]. Using this, we determined Klotho and FGF23 blood levels in a large multicentre cohort of hemodialysis patients and tested the hypothesis that low blood Klotho levels could be associated with all-cause mortality. To our knowledge, this is the first study exploring an association of Klotho with all-cause mortality in hemodialysis patients.

Although Klotho has been shown to exert direct vasculoprotective effects, our data extend recent observations by Seiler et al in patients with stage 2–4 chronic kidney disease which showed Klotho levels not to be associated with mortality. As Seiler and authors excluded ESRD patients, the need for a study with ESRD-patients has been highlighted [23].

Moreover, recent experimental and clinical studies have challenged previous views on Klotho. Anour et al. failed to prove a physiological role for soluble and transmembrane Klotho in mineral metabolism and glucose homeostasis [24]. A study by Komaba et al. found no association between Klotho and the major players in arterial calcification in CKD-related mineral bone disorder PTH and FGF23 [25]. Furthermore, calcimimetic therapy in a hemodialysis patients was followed by very modest effects on Klotho levels, raising the question of whether these effects are biologically meaningful [25]. Levels of Klotho did not appear to correlate with residual renal function in a prevalent cohort of peritoneal dialysis patients [26], findings that were also seen in our cohort. No association between Klotho gene variants and the presence of valvular or vascular calcification was observed in the Framingham Offspring Cohort [27]. Taken together, the current data allow the conclusion that soluble Klotho levels do not reflect clinical outcome in patients with CKD.

FGF23 rather than Klotho more appropriately reflects cardiovascular risk. FGF23 is the earliest marker of deranged phosphate

Table 2. Hazard Ratios (and 95% CIs) for Death per Standard Deviation of FGF23 and Klotho levels and according to the level tertiles.

Parameter	Crude			Model 1*			Model 2†			Model 3‡		
	HR	95%CI	P value	HR	95%CI	P value	HR	95%CI	P value	HR	95%CI	P value
Klotho (N = 227)	1.03	0.77–1.34	0.85	1.03	0.78–1.36	0.83	1.10	0.76–1.60	0.62	1.30	0.86–1.96	0.22
Klotho§												
Tertile 1 (N = 75)	R			R			R			R		
Tertile 2 (N = 75)	0.79	0.40–1.57	0.50	0.67	0.33–1.33	0.25	0.55	0.23–1.31	0.18	0.68	0.27–1.74	0.42
Tertile 3 (N = 77)	1.22	0.66–2.28	0.53	1.19	0.63–2.22	0.59	1.70	0.74–3.88	0.21	2.42	1.00–5.87	0.05
FGF23 (N = 234)	1.36	1.09–1.70	0.006	1.39	1.12–1.74	0.003	1.40	1.04–1.89	0.03	1.59	1.13–2.22	0.007
FGF23‖												
Tertile 1 (N = 77)	R			R			R			R		
Tertile 2 (N = 78)	0.93	0.46–1.91	0.85	0.98	0.48–2.01	0.95	1.61	0.67–3.89	0.29	1.75	0.69–4.44	0.24
Tertile 3 (N = 79)	1.82	0.97–3.43	0.06	2.17	1.15–4.09	0.02	2.65	1.09–6.44	0.03	3.73	1.15–12.11	0.03

*Model 1 = demographics: adjusted for age, gender (male) and by dialysis center clustering.

†Model 2 = dialysis specific risk factors and comorbid conditions: adjusted for covariates in Model 1 plus dialysis vintage, systolic and diastolic blood pressure, body-mass index, vascular access on study enrolment (fistula, graft, catheter), coexisting conditions listed in Table 1 (coronary artery disease, valvular heart disease, atrial fibrillation, pulmonary hypertension, implantable cardioverter defibrillator carrier; diabetes mellitus, peripheral vascular disease, stroke, vasculitis, malignoma, chronic obstructive pulmonary disease), cause of renal failure (diabetic nephropathy, hypertensive nephropathy glomerulonephritis, polycystic kidney disease, others/unknown), medication use listed in Table 1 (phosphate binders, vitamin D replacement, angiotensin converting enzyme inhibitors or angiotensin receptor blockers, beta blockers, aspirin, anticoagulant or clopidogrel, statin), pooled Kt/V.

‡Model 3 = fully adjusted model: adjusted for covariates in Model 2 plus parathyroid hormone, 25(OH)vitamin D, phosphate, calcium, albumin, hemoglobin, C-reactive protein, cholesterol.

§Patients were categorized according to Klotho level tertiles at enrolment (1st tertile <286 pg/ml, 2nd tertile 286–392 pg/ml, 3rd tertile >392 pg/ml).

‖Patients were categorized according to FGF23 level tertiles at enrolment (1st tertile <118 RU/ml, 2nd tertile 118–468 RU/ml, 3rd tertile >468 RU/ml).

Abbreviations: FGF23, fibroblast growth factor 23; HR, hazard ratio; R, reference.

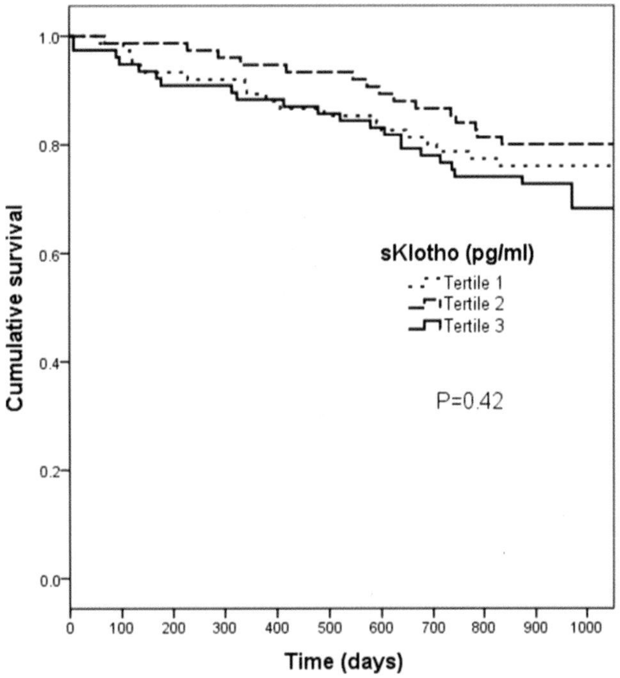

Figure 1. Cumulative survival by tertiles of secreted Klotho. Patients were stratified by their baseline Klotho levels according to the tertiles. Kaplan-Meier analysis with long-rank test did not reveal a significant difference between groups (P = 0.42).

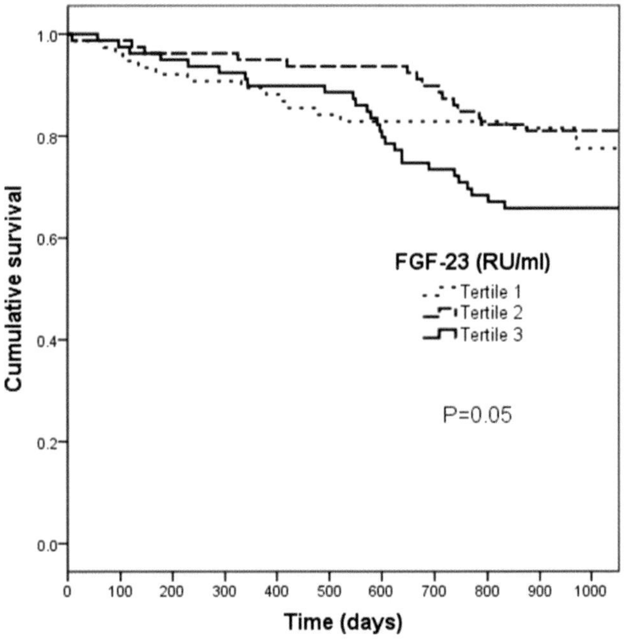

Figure 2. Cumulative survival by tertiles of Fibroblast growth factor 23 (FGF23). Patients were stratified by their FGF23 levels according to the tertiles. Kaplan-Meier analysis with long-rank test approached a significant difference between groups (P = 0.05).

metabolism, increasing before PTH and phosphate levels and before vitamin D levels decrease [14]. Studies found FGF23 to be independently associated with mortality in hemodialysis patients [12], with ESRD development, cardiovascular events and mortality in CKD patients [13,14]. In accordance with those previous studies, our study highlighted FGF23 as a valuable biomarker for assessment of cardiovascular risk in hemodialysis patients.

The FGF23 levels in this cohort appear lower compared to previous studies measuring C-terminal FGF23 in hemodialysis patients [12]. The cause is not completely clear. First, despite a good recovery in the dilution experiments using our samples, we cannot exclude some assay differences. Second, as FGF23 increases in the circulation with increasing phosphate load and vice versa [28], a further contributor could be differences in phosphate load. In our cohort, we may have had a high phosphate-clearance due to relatively long dialysis duration [29], a high percentages of high-flux dialysis membrane and hemodiafiltration (HDF) usage. All three modalities enhance phosphate clearance and possibly FGF23 removal itself. Previous studies showed that more intensive dialysis treatment can substantially lower FGF23 levels. Zaritzky et al achieved a median of 823 RU/ml in daily hemodialysis versus 2521 RU/ml in conventional hemodialysis patients [30]. Using HDF, Patrier et al achieved a 20% higher FGF23 clearance over high-flux hemodialysis only. Hemodialysis studies with FGF23 mostly do not give the exact information about dialysis treatment details hindering a direct comparison between studies. Importantly, although the FGF23 levels are lower in this study, its association with mortality is in accordance with previous work [12,14].

Interestingly, the analytical concordance between Kainos and Millipore assays was in much closer agreement than between each of them and the Immutopics assay. A similar lack of agreement was found by Smith et al in a smaller group of hemodialysis patients [31]. The authors suggest that this might be due to differences in calibration. As the sample number where FGF23 levels were determined using different assays was not high in our study, further studies are warranted and careful interpretation of our results is recommended. Harmonisation of available assays would facilitate interpretation of studies where different assays are used.

Of note, patients with AF had lower Klotho levels than patients without AF. This effect remained significant even after the adjustment for cardiovascular comorbidities and approached significance in the fully adjusted model. Thus, high Klotho levels seem to exert a protective effect against AF. The absolute differences in Klotho levels between the patients groups with and without AF was small albeit significant. Small differences in sKlotho levels may be physiologically relevant. Relatively small increases in sKlotho levels were for example shown to induce overt changes in vascular tone of animal and human blood vessels in an experimental study by Six et al [32]. These dose dependent effects were shown to be due to sKlotho mediated intracellular reactive oxygen species (ROS) and nitric oxide (NO) production. We found no studies examining dose-dependent influence of ion channels by sKlotho. The physiological relevance of this relatively small difference in our study needs to be confirmed by further studies and must be regarded as a pilot hypothesis.

Concomitantly, patients with AF had higher FGF23 levels than patients without AF. The latter finding is in agreement with data from Seiler et al who found higher FGF23 levels in patients with AF in 885 subjects with normal and reduced kidney function undergoing elective coronary angiography [15].

A mechanistic explanation for the sinoatrial dysfunction might be arteriosclerotic changes caused by Klotho deficiency. But an even more plausible hypothesis is that Klotho might be essential for the function of ion channels which are responsible for the peacemaking activity in the sinoatrial node. In fact, a study by

Table 3. Association of Klotho levels with the presence of atrial fibrillation.

Parameter	Crude			Model 1*			Model 2†			Model 3‡		
	OR	95%CI	P value	OR	95%CI	P value	OR	95%CI	P value	OR	95%CI	P value
Klotho§ (pg/mL)	0.60	0.52–0.68	<0.001	0.45	0.31–0.65	<0.001	0.43	0.29–0.64	<0.001	0.60	0.38–0.95	0.03
Age (years)				1.01	1.01–1.04	0.08	1.00	0.98–1.01	0.59	1.07	1.03–1.11	0.002
Gender (male)				0.83	0.44–1.59	0.58	0.76	0.36–1.61	0.48	1.26	0.48–3.27	0.64
DM							0.85	0.36–2.01	0.71	0.08	0.41–2.84	0.88
CAD							2.96	1.37–6.37	0.006	2.37	1.00–5.63	0.05
VHD							4.05	1.82–9.02	0.001	3.85	1.51–9.62	0.004
PAD							1.80	0.78–4.14	0.17	1.43	0.57–3.63	0.45
Stroke							1.14	0.45–2.89	0.78	1.11	0.38–3.26	0.84
Anuria							2.07	1.02–4.22	0.04	2.38	1.37–8.32	0.008
PTH (pg/ml)										1.00	1.00–1.00	0.79
FGF23§ (RU/ml)										1.65	0.86–3.17	0.13
Phosphate (mmol/l)										0.40	0.12–1.48	0.17
Ca, serum (mmol/l)										0.28	0.02–4.07	0.35
Ca, dialysate (mmol/l)										0.90	0.01–1.14	0.06
K, serum (mmol/l)										1.22	0.62–2.40	0.56
K, dialysate (mmol/l)										1.44	0.70–2.93	0.32
Albumin (g/l)										1.03	0.91–1.17	0.67
Hb (g/dl)										0.88	0.51–1.51	0.67
CRP (mg/l)										1.02	0.98–1.05	0.32
Cholesterol (mg/dl)										1.00	0.99–1.01	0.61
TSH (mU/l)										1.15	0.86–1.53	0.35

*Model 1: adjusted for age and gender (male).
†Model 2: adjusted for covariates in Model 1 plus cardiovascular comorbidities and anuria.
‡Model 3: adjusted for covariates in Model 2 plus laboratory results for mineral metabolism, calcium dialysate, potassium serum and dialysate, inflammation, cholesterol, hemoglobin and TSH.
§per standard deviation.
Abbreviations: Ca, Calcium; CAD, coronary artery disease; CI, confidence interval; CRP, C-reactive protein; DM, diabetes mellitus; FGF23, fibroblast growth factor 23; Hb, hemoglobin; K, potassium; PAD, peripheral artery disease; TSH, thyroid stimulating hormone.
OR, odds ratio; VHD, valvular heart disease.

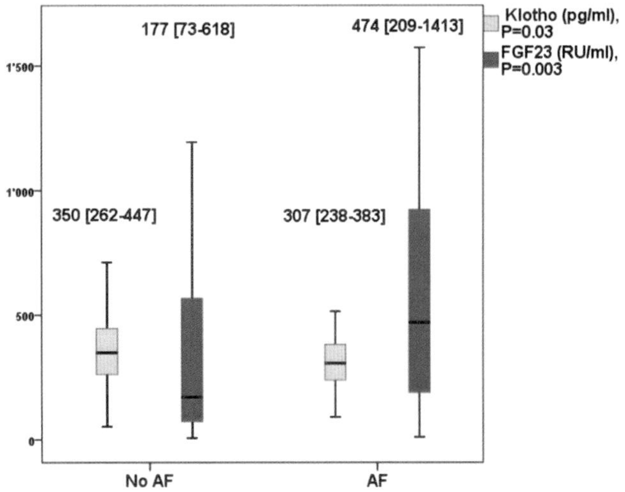

Figure 3. Klotho and FGF23 levels in patients with and without atrial fibrillation.

Takeshita et al. demonstrated specific expression of Klotho in the sinoatrial node peacemaker cells [19]. Furthermore, electrophysiological studies revealed significant sinus node dysfunction in Klotho knock-out mice [19]. Recent experimental research demonstrates that sKlotho can regulate the cell-surface abundance of ion channels such as Ca2+ and K+ channels [16]. The stimulation of the Ca2+ channel TRPV5, promoting the renal Ca2+ reabsorption by sKlotho was demonstrated in an animal study by Alexander et al [33]. Klotho has been shown to exhibit cardioprotective effects by downregulation of TRPC6 channels in the heart. But, these studies were performed only on isolated cardiac myocytes using supraphysiologic soluble Klotho concentrations. [17,18,34]. Low Klotho levels may therefore have led to sinoatrial dysfunction secondary to disturbed ion channels regulation in the cardiac peacemaker cells. Through protecting against AF, which is mostly attributed to senescence processes, Klotho appears to have anti-aging properties. With decreasing Klotho tertiles and therefore increasing AF prevalance, the treating physicians prescribed beta-, renin-angiotensin-aldosteron-blockers and statins more frequently (Table 1).

Klotho mainly derives from the renal tubular cells [4] both declining early in the CKD course [9,35]. Correspondingly, Klotho levels in our healthy control group were higher than in CKD patients in the Study by Seiler et al [23] and the latter higher than in our hemodialysis patients (respective medians 690, 538 and 349 pg/ml). All levels measured using the same assay. But, Klotho levels were neither associated with CKD stages 2–4 [23] nor with residual kidney function in our patients. A possible explanation could be a reduced renal clearance in CKD. The fact that Klotho levels are maintained even with complete loss of kidney function suggests that sKlotho may be important for physiologic functions such as ion channels. The lack of association with mortality remains to be elucidated. One possibility is that Klotho level does not reflect membrane-bound Klotho function, the latter only being measurable by invasive methods.

Several limitations merit consideration. Firstly, the study was not designed to establish the exact cause of death. This limitation is common and may partly be due to the relatively low autopsy rate [14]. Due to this, we defined all-cause mortality rather than myocardial infarction (MI) as the primary end-point of the study with the knowledge that cardiovascular disease is the main contributor to mortality in ESRD [1]. Secondly, we did not define non-fatal MI as an end-point. Non-fatal MI rarely occurs in hemodialysis patients [36], the competing risk of cardiac death is observed to be several-fold greater than that of non-fatal MI [37] corresponding to the finding that coronary media calcifications rather than arterial plaques have a greater impact on mortality in dialysis patients [38,39] and are the main autopsy finding [40]. We also did not record smoking and alcohol consumption habits at study enrolment. Thirdly, we cannot comment on unreported, asymptomatic or still undetected AF episodes. Furthermore, the association between low Klotho levels and AF was analysed in a cross-sectional manner and we have no data on AF incidence during the observational period. Nevertheless our hypothesis is supported, as the association between low Klotho levels and AF remained significant during analysis of the second independent blood sample, even after multiple adjustments. This hypothesis needs to be confirmed by further prospective studies. Experimental studies with systemic Klotho delivery in Klotho-deficient animals with AF could provide valuable information for understanding the mechanism underlying sinoatrial dysfunction and possibly lead to new therapeutic approaches in patients with AF. Another potential problem is that the three commercially available assays for the Klotho measurement differ in quality, as recently demonstrated by Heijboer et al [41]. However, we used the so far best validated assay with the lowest within- and between-run variation among the commercially available assays [41].

In conclusion, FGF23, but not Klotho levels, are associated with long-term mortality in ESRD-patients.

Table 4. Regression analysis for Klotho tertiles with the absence of atrial fibrillation.

	Klotho Tertile 1, N=75 (<286 pg/ml)	Klotho Tertile 2, N=75 (286–392 pg/ml)		Klotho Tertile 3, N=77 (>392 pg/ml)	
		OR (95%CI)	P value	OR (95%CI)	P value
Crude	Reference	2.75 (1.65–4.59)	<0.001	6.70 (3.45–13.02)	<0.001
Model 1*	Reference	1.09 (0.52–2.27)	0.83	2.90 (1.27–6.64)	0.01
Model 2†	Reference	1.23 (0.54–2.78)	0.63	3.71 (1.49–9.25)	0.005
Model 3‡	Reference	1.00 (0.40–2.59)	1.00	3.02 (1.03.89–8.82)	0.04

*Model 1: adjusted for age and gender.
†Model 2: adjusted for covariates in Model 1 plus diabetes mellitus, coronary artery disease, valvular heart disease, peripheral vascular disease, stroke and anuria.
‡Model 3: adjusted for covariates in Model 2 plus parathyroid hormone, fibroblast growth factor 23, calcium, phosphate, albumin, calcium dialysate, potassium serum and dialysate, hemoglobin C-reactive protein, cholesterol and thyroid stimulating hormone.
Abbreviations: CI, confidence interval; OR, odds ratio.

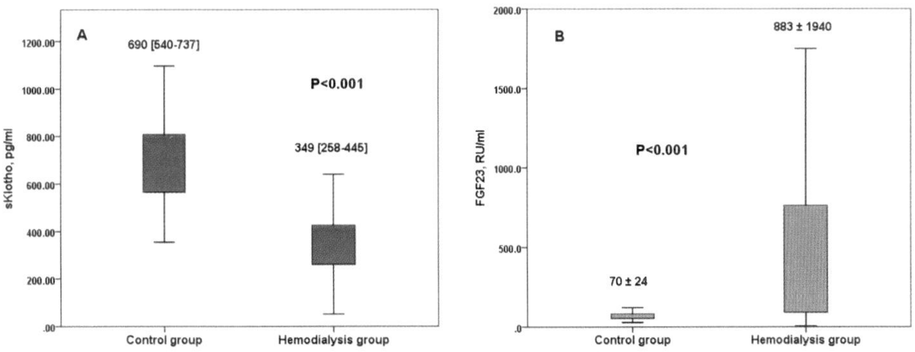

Figure 4. Klotho (A) and FGF23 (B) levels in controls versus hemodialysis patients.

Acknowledgments

We thank Emily Pollock for careful proofreading of the manuscript.

Author Contributions

Conceived and designed the experiments: AN BF FA CM. Performed the experiments: BF FA. Analyzed the data: AN AS. Contributed reagents/materials/analysis tools: AN BF FA TB RT MP. Wrote the paper: AN.

References

1. Shroff GR, Frederick PD, Herzog CA (2012) Renal failure and acute myocardial infarction: clinical characteristics in patients with advanced chronic kidney disease, on dialysis, and without chronic kidney disease. A collaborative project of the United States Renal Data System/National Institutes of Health and the National Registry of Myocardial Infarction. Am Heart J 163: 399–406.
2. Quarles LD (2008) Endocrine functions of bone in mineral metabolism regulation. J Clin Invest 118: 3820–3828.
3. Drueke TB (2010) Klotho, FGF23, and FGF receptors in chronic kidney disease: a yin-yang situation? Kidney Int 78: 1057–1060.
4. Urakawa I, Yamazaki Y, Shimada T, Iijima K, Hasegawa H, et al. (2006) Klotho converts canonical FGF receptor into a specific receptor for FGF23. Nature 444: 770–774.
5. Imura A, Iwano A, Tohyama O, Tsuji Y, Nozaki K, et al. (2004) Secreted Klotho protein in sera and CSF: implication for post-translational cleavage in release of Klotho protein from cell membrane. FEBS Lett 565: 143–147.
6. Lim K, Lu TS, Molostvov G, Lee C, Lam FT, et al. (2012) Vascular klotho deficiency potentiates the development of human artery calcification and mediates resistance to fibroblast growth factor 23. Circulation 125: 2243–2255.
7. Kitagawa M, Sugiyama H, Morinaga H, Inoue T, Takiue K, et al. (2013) A decreased level of serum soluble Klotho is an independent biomarker associated with arterial stiffness in patients with chronic kidney disease. PLoS One 8: e56695.
8. Maekawa Y, Ishikawa K, Yasuda O, Oguro R, Hanasaki H, et al. (2009) Klotho suppresses TNF-alpha-induced expression of adhesion molecules in the endothelium and attenuates NF-kappaB activation. Endocrine 35: 341–346.
9. Moe SM, Radcliffe JS, White KE, Gattone VH, 2nd, Seifert MF, et al. (2011) The pathophysiology of early-stage chronic kidney disease-mineral bone disorder (CKD-MBD) and response to phosphate binders in the rat. J Bone Miner Res 26: 2672–2681.
10. Pavik I, Jaeger P, Ebner L, Wagner CA, Petzold K, et al. (2012) Secreted Klotho and FGF23 in chronic kidney disease Stage 1 to 5: a sequence suggested from a cross-sectional study. Nephrol Dial Transplant.
11. Kuro-o M, Matsumura Y, Aizawa H, Kawaguchi H, Suga T, et al. (1997) Mutation of the mouse klotho gene leads to a syndrome resembling ageing. Nature 390: 45–51.
12. Gutierrez OM, Mannstadt M, Isakova T, Rauh-Hain JA, Tamez H, et al. (2008) Fibroblast growth factor 23 and mortality among patients undergoing hemodialysis. N Engl J Med 359: 584–592.
13. Kendrick J, Cheung AK, Kaufman JS, Greene T, Roberts WL, et al. (2011) FGF-23 associates with death, cardiovascular events, and initiation of chronic dialysis. J Am Soc Nephrol 22: 1913–1922.
14. Isakova T, Xie H, Yang W, Xie D, Anderson AH, et al. (2011) Fibroblast growth factor 23 and risks of mortality and end-stage renal disease in patients with chronic kidney disease. JAMA 305: 2432–2439.
15. Seiler S, Cremers B, Rebling NM, Hornof F, Jeken J, et al. (2011) The phosphatonin fibroblast growth factor 23 links calcium-phosphate metabolism with left-ventricular dysfunction and atrial fibrillation. Eur Heart J 32: 2688–2696.
16. Huang CL (2010) Regulation of ion channels by secreted Klotho: mechanisms and implications. Kidney Int 77: 855–860.
17. Kuwahara K, Wang Y, McAnally J, Richardson JA, Bassel-Duby R, et al. (2006) TRPC6 fulfills a calcineurin signaling circuit during pathologic cardiac remodeling. J Clin Invest 116: 3114–3126.
18. Xie J, Cha SK, An SW, Kuro OM, Birnbaumer L, et al. (2012) Cardioprotection by Klotho through downregulation of TRPC6 channels in the mouse heart. Nat Commun 3: 1238.
19. Takeshita K, Fujimori T, Kurotaki Y, Honjo H, Tsujikawa H, et al. (2004) Sinoatrial node dysfunction and early unexpected death of mice with a defect of klotho gene expression. Circulation 109: 1776–1782.
20. Artunc F, Mueller C, Breidthardt T, Twerenbold R, Peter A, et al. (2012) Sensitive troponins–which suits better for hemodialysis patients? Associated factors and prediction of mortality. PLoS One 7: e47610.
21. Artunc F, Mueller C, Breidthardt T, Twerenbold R, Rettig I, et al. (2012) Comparison of the diagnostic performance of three natriuretic peptides in hemodialysis patients: which is the appropriate biomarker? Kidney Blood Press Res 36: 172–181.
22. Yamazaki Y, Imura A, Urakawa I, Shimada T, Murakami J, et al. (2010) Establishment of sandwich ELISA for soluble alpha-Klotho measurement: Age-dependent change of soluble alpha-Klotho levels in healthy subjects. Biochem Biophys Res Commun 398: 513–518.
23. Seiler S, Wen M, Roth HJ, Fehrenz M, Flugge F, et al. (2013) Plasma Klotho is not related to kidney function and does not predict adverse outcome in patients with chronic kidney disease. Kidney Int 83: 121–128.
24. Anour R, Andrukhova O, Ritter E, Zeitz U, Erben RG (2012) Klotho lacks a vitamin D independent physiological role in glucose homeostasis, bone turnover, and steady-state PTH secretion in vivo. PLoS One 7: e31376.
25. Komaba H, Koizumi M, Tanaka H, Takahashi H, Sawada K, et al. (2012) Effects of cinacalcet treatment on serum soluble Klotho levels in haemodialysis patients with secondary hyperparathyroidism. Nephrol Dial Transplant 27: 1967–1969.
26. Akimoto T, Shiizaki K, Sugase T, Watanabe Y, Yoshizawa H, et al. (2012) The relationship between the soluble Klotho protein and the residual renal function among peritoneal dialysis patients. Clin Exp Nephrol 16: 442–447.

27. Tangri N, Alam A, Wooten EC, Huggins GS (2011) Lack of association of Klotho gene variants with valvular and vascular calcification in Caucasians: a candidate gene study of the Framingham Offspring Cohort. Nephrol Dial Transplant 26: 3998–4002.
28. Gutierrez OM, Wolf M, Taylor EN (2011) Fibroblast growth factor 23, cardiovascular disease risk factors, and phosphorus intake in the health professionals follow-up study. Clin J Am Soc Nephrol 6: 2871–2878.
29. Tandon T, Sinha AD, Agarwal R (2013) Shorter delivered dialysis times associate with a higher and more difficult to treat blood pressure. Nephrol Dial Transplant 28: 1562–1568.
30. Zaritsky J, Rastogi A, Fischmann G, Yan J, Kleinman K, et al. (2013) Short daily hemodialysis is associated with lower plasma FGF23 levels when compared with conventional hemodialysis. Nephrol Dial Transplant.
31. Smith ER, McMahon LP, Holt SG (2013) Method-specific differences in plasma fibroblast growth factor 23 measurement using four commercial ELISAs. Clin Chem Lab Med 51: 1971–1981.
32. Six I, Okazaki H, Gross P, Cagnard J, Boudot C, et al. (2014) Direct, Acute Effects of Klotho and FGF23 on Vascular Smooth Muscle and Endothelium. PLoS One 9: e93423.
33. Alexander RT, Woudenberg-Vrenken TE, Buurman J, Dijkman H, van der Eerden BC, et al. (2009) Klotho prevents renal calcium loss. J Am Soc Nephrol 20: 2371–2379.
34. Winn MP, Conlon PJ, Lynn KL, Farrington MK, Creazzo T, et al. (2005) A mutation in the TRPC6 cation channel causes familial focal segmental glomerulosclerosis. Science 308: 1801–1804.
35. Pavik I, Jaeger P, Ebner L, Wagner CA, Petzold K, et al. (2013) Secreted Klotho and FGF23 in chronic kidney disease Stage 1 to 5: a sequence suggested from a cross-sectional study. Nephrol Dial Transplant 28: 352–359.
36. Etter C, Straub Y, Hersberger M, Raz HR, Kistler T, et al. (2010) Pregnancy-associated plasma protein-A is an independent short-time predictor of mortality in patients on maintenance haemodialysis. Eur Heart J 31: 354–359.
37. Trivedi H, Xiang Q, Klein JP (2009) Risk factors for non-fatal myocardial infarction and cardiac death in incident dialysis patients. Nephrol Dial Transplant 24: 258–266.
38. London GM, Guerin AP, Marchais SJ, Metivier F, Pannier B, et al. (2003) Arterial media calcification in end-stage renal disease: impact on all-cause and cardiovascular mortality. Nephrol Dial Transplant 18: 1731–1740.
39. Tong LL, Mehrotra R, Shavelle DM, Budoff M, Adler S (2008) Poor correlation between coronary artery calcification and obstructive coronary artery disease in an end-stage renal disease patient. Hemodial Int 12: 16–22.
40. Yoshida H, Yokoyama K, Yaginuma T, Ohkido I, Yamamoto H, et al. (2011) Difference in coronary artery intima and media calcification in autopsied patients with chronic kidney disease. Clin Nephrol 75: 1–7.
41. Heijboer AC, Blankenstein MA, Hoenderop J, de Borst MH, Vervloet MG (2013) Laboratory aspects of circulating alpha-Klotho. Nephrol Dial Transplant.

Long-Term Outcome of Anti-Glomerular Basement Membrane Antibody Disease Treated with Immunoadsorption

Peter Biesenbach[1]*, Renate Kain[2], Kurt Derfler[1], Thomas Perkmann[3], Afschin Soleiman[2], Alexandra Benharkou[2], Wilfred Druml[1], Andrew Rees[2], Marcus D. Säemann[1]

1 Internal Medicine III/Clinical Division of Nephrology & Dialysis, Medical University of Vienna, Vienna, Austria, **2** Clinical Institute of Pathology, Medical University of Vienna, Vienna, Austria, **3** Department of Laboratory Medicine, Medical University of Vienna, Vienna, Austria

Abstract

Background: Anti-glomerular basement membrane (GBM) antibody disease may lead to acute crescentic glomerulonephritis with poor renal prognosis. Current therapy favours plasma exchange (PE) for removal of pathogenic antibodies. Immunoadsorption (IAS) is superior to PE regarding efficiency of antibody-removal and safety. Apart from anecdotal data, there is no systemic analysis of the long-term effects of IAS on anti-GBM-disease and antibody kinetics.

Objective: To examine the long-term effect of high-frequency IAS combined with standard immunosuppression on patient and renal survival in patients with anti-GBM-disease and to quantify antibody removal and kinetics through IAS.

Design: Retrospective review of patients treated with IAS for anti-GBM-antibody disease confirmed by biopsy and/or anti-GBM-antibodies.

Setting: University Hospital of Vienna, Austria.

Participants: 10 patients with anti-GBM-disease treated with IAS.

Measurements: Patient and renal survival, renal histology, anti-GBM-antibodies.

Results: Anti-GBM-antibodies were reduced by the first 9 IAS treatments (mean number of 23) to negative levels in all patients. Renal survival was 40% at diagnosis, 70% after the end of IAS, 63% after one year and 50% at the end of observation (mean 84 months, range 9 to 186). Dialysis dependency was successfully reversed in three of six patients. Patient survival was 90% at the end of observation.

Conclusion: IAS efficiently eliminates anti-GBM-antibodies suggesting non-inferiority to PE with regard to renal and patient survival. Hence IAS should be considered as a valuable treatment option for anti-GBM-disease, especially in patients presenting with a high percentage of crescents and dialysis dependency due to an unusual high proportion of responders.

Editor: Effie C. Tsilibary, National Center for Scientific Research Demokritos, Greece

Funding: The authors have no support or funding to report.

Competing Interests: The authors have declared that no competing interests exist.

* Email: Peter.biesenbach@meduniwien.ac.at

Introduction

Anti-glomerular basement membrane (GBM) disease is defined by circulating autoantibodies specific for the alpha-3 chain of type IV collagen [1] and characterised by focal necrotizing glomerulonephritis with linear deposition of IgG along the GBM. Those affected present with acute renal failure often accompanied by pulmonary haemorrhage because the anti-GBM-antibodies also bind to the alveolar basement membrane. Although rare with an incidence of two per million population per year, anti-GBM-disease accounts for approximately 10 to 20 percent of crescentic nephritis [2–4]. Untreated, it rapidly destroys the kidney emphasizing the need for rapid diagnosis and therapy [2,5,6].

The treatment aims at limiting further renal injury by rapidly reducing circulating anti-GBM-antibodies. The current standard treatment consists of plasma exchange (PE) combined with cyclophosphamide and corticosteroids. Although never submitted to randomised controlled clinical trials, there is compelling evidence that morbidity and mortality have improved markedly since PE was introduced [2,6–11].

Immunoadsorption (IAS) with high-affinity matrices selectively binding human IgG and IgM provides an alternative way of removing antibodies and immune complexes [12]. Theoretically it is more efficient than PE because unlimited volumes of plasma can be processed at each treatment [13] whereas PE is usually restricted to a single plasma volume, resulting in higher antibody reduction of more than 85% in IAS [14] compared to up to 70% in PE [15]. IAS is successfully employed in sensitized allograft recipients and in autoimmune disorders including hemophilia A, pemphigus, thrombocytopenic purpura and lupus [13,16–20], whereas only isolated case reports describe IAS against anti-GBM-disease [21–23], including a dialysis-dependant patient who recovered renal function despite 100% crescents in the renal biopsy [24]. Here we describe our results of high intensity IAS in 10 consecutive patients with anti-GBM-disease. Examining the effectiveness, safety and costs of IAS in anti-GBM-disease, we show that IAS is at least as effective as PE and may control anti-GBM-antibodies more rapidly.

Patients, Materials and Methods

Patients

The study group consisted of patients presenting with anti-GBM-disease to the University Hospital of Vienna, Austria, between 1997 and 2012. Diagnosis was based on the presence of anti-GBM-antibodies in serum by indirect immunofluorescence and ELISA (mean concentration at start of treatment 73.6 U/ml: range 6.6–207.1), and in glomeruli in patients with renal biopsies. The mean age was 29 years and five were male and five female. Eight of the patients displayed pulmonary haemorrhage. Patient details are described in the individual case reports and are summarized (Table 1).

Treatment

Immunosuppressive regimen (Table 2) consisted of pulse corticosteroids followed by tapering doses of oral prednisolone and cyclophosphamide, given either as intravenous boli or daily oral doses of 2–3 mg/kg body weight. Additionally, all patients received a course of high intensity IAS whose frequency and duration was determined by clinical course and anti-GBM-antibody levels. Five patients were converted to IAS after 2 to 4 PE treatments after anti-GBM-antibody levels had remained refractory. IAS was performed using our standard previously published protocol [14,19,25]. Up to 80 ml/min of blood was taken from a central or peripheral vein and anti-coagulated with citrate and/or heparin before separation on a plasmaseparator (COBE Spectra Apheresis system, Terumo). The plasma fraction was forwarded into the Adsorption-Desorption-Automated system (ADAsorb, Medicap Ulrichstadt, Germany) prepared with either TheraSorb (Milteny Biotec, Bergisch Gladbach, Germany) or Immunosorba (Fresenius Medical Care, Bad Homburg, Germany) adsorbers selectively binding IgG, IgM and immune complexes in human plasma; the procedure was continued until 2.5 to 3 times the plasma volume had been processed.

Clinical assessment and laboratory studies

Clinical data were recorded at diagnosis and then monthly for six months and yearly thereafter. Anti-GBM-antibodies were re-assayed in all sera using a commercial ELISA (Wieslab, Malmö, Sweden) according to the manufacturer's instructions. Sera were batched with those from an individual patient run of the same ELISA.

Ethics statement

The study was approved by the ethics committee of the Medical University of Vienna (EK1819/2013). Participants did not provide written or verbal consent as the retrospective design did not allow obtaining consent. Patient records were anonymized prior to analysis.

Table 1. Baseline characteristics of patients treated.

			Renal function	Glomerula in biopsy, n (%)		Lung	
	Age (years)	Sex (male)	serum-creatinine	with crescents	with necrosis	confirmed in HR-CT	Follow-up (months)
Pat 1	44	No	Dialysis	3/4 (75)	0/4 (0)	None	144
Pat 2	19	No	Dialysis	25/25 (100)	19/25 (76)	Confirmed	186
Pat 3	35	Yes	1.82 mg/dl	2/7 (28)	2/7 (28)	Confirmed	5
Pat 4	19	Yes	0.96 mg/dl	No biopsy		Confirmed	49
Pat 5	18	No	1.07 mg/dl	No biopsy		Confirmed	123
Pat 6	25	No	3.7 mg/dl	5/27 (19)	2/27 (7)	Confirmed	153
Pat 7	19	Yes	Dialysis	27/27 (100)	21/27 (78)	Confirmed	51
Pat 8	25	Yes	Dialysis	24/25 (96)	9/25 (36)	Confirmed	49
Pat 9	19	Yes	Dialysis	15/16 (94)	8/16 (50)	None	72
Pat 10	66	No	Dialysis	5/8 (63)	2/8 (25)	None	9

Table 2. Extracorporal treatment and concomitant immunosuppression.

Immunoadsorption			Plasma exchange	Cyclophosphamide		Steroids
# of treatments	Duration	volume	# of treatments	Oral	Pulse	
22.7±12.1	85±112 days	7660 ml	1.5±1.7	60%	60%	100%

Results

Case reports

Patient 1 presented with a serum-creatinine of 7.4 mg/dl necessitating hemodialysis. Anti-GBM-antibody titer was 1:80 and renal biopsy showed necrotising glomerulonephritis with 75% crescents and linear deposition of IgG. She was treated with three dexamethasone pulses (50 mg) and prednisolone for six months. Oral cyclophosphamide was given for two months. After two PEs and refractory anti-GBM-antibodies, she was converted to IAS and received 12 sessions over 27 days resulting in negative anti-GBM-antibodies after 2 treatments but renal function did not recover. Four years later, she received a renal allograft and remains well with excellent graft function and without recurrence of anti-GBM-disease.

Patient 2 presented anuric with hemoptysis and a serum-creatinine of 5.5 mg/dl necessitating dialysis. Renal biopsy showed necrotizing glomerulonephritis with 100% crescents and linear IgG deposition. Anti-GBM-antibody concentration was 43.8 U/ml. She was treated with six boli of cyclophosphamide (total dose of 6 g) and methylprednisolone (650 mg for three days, subsequently tapered). IAS was performed 25 times over 171 days and assays for anti-GBM-antibodies were negative after 4 weeks. Renal function recovered and she was discharged with a serum-creatinine of 2 mg/dl. After three years maintenance immunosuppression (mycophenolate mofetil 1 g/day and prednisolone 5 mg/day) was stopped while serum-creatinine was 2.5 mg/dl. However, her renal function deteriorated despite negative anti-GBM-antibodies testing. Renal biopsy showed chronic scarring without active glomerulonephritis or linear deposition of IgG. She restarted dialysis 64 months after diagnosis and received four years later a renal transplant with excellent graft function and no recurrence of anti-GBM-disease. The initial course of the patient has previously been reported [24].

Patient 3 presented with macroscopic hematuria, a serum-creatinine of 1.8 mg/dl and proteinuria (5.5 g/day) without pulmonary involvement. Anti-GBM-antibody concentration was 24.5 U/ml. Renal biopsy showed necrotizing glomerulonephritis with 28% crescents and linear deposition of IgG. He was treated with three 250 mg pulses of prednisolone (followed by 3 months of oral prednisolone), cyclophosphamide (150 mg daily) and IAS, 16 sessions over four weeks. After 1 week anti-GBM-antibodies tested negative and serum-creatinine initially stabilized at 1.75 mg/dl before rising to 3.8 mg/dl after three months despite continuing immunosuppression. He developed severe hemoptysis and a second renal biopsy revealed necrotising glomerulonephritis with fibrocellular crescents in two thirds of glomeruli. Three further pulses of methylprednisolone (250 mg) were given and he received ten PE sessions but did not respond. IAS was re-instituted for 23 sessions together with empiric intravenous immunoglobulin therapy. Renal function stabilized but after two weeks the patient was readmitted with sepsis and died three weeks later with multi-organ failure.

Patient 4 presented with haemoptysis and respiratory distress together with macroscopic haematuria and proteinuria (5 g/day): serum-creatinine was normal and anti-GBM-antibody titer was 1:160. The patient was treated with three daily pulses of methylprednisolone, intravenous cyclophosphamide (5 times 200 mg) and IAS. Symptoms resolved and anti-GBM-antibodies became undetectable but IAS was continued at lower intensity (45 treatments over one year) because treatment with cyclophosphamide had to be stopped due to anaemia. Anti-GBM-antibodies remained undetectable and proteinuria returned to normal being stable for four years along with serum-creatinine.

Patient 5 presented with respiratory distress, macroscopic hematuria and proteinuria (0.6 g/day) and an initial serum-creatinine of 1.21 mg/dl. Anti-GBM-antibody titer was 1:80 and she was treated with prednisolone (50 mg daily) and 18 sessions of IAS over 10 weeks. The symptoms resolved and the serum-creatinine fell to 0.8 mg/dl. One month later, the patient had a second episode of acute respiratory distress and was treated with a short course of cyclophosphamide despite negative assays for anti-GBM-antibodies. There has been no recurrence of symptoms over 10 years of follow-up and the patient currently has a serum-creatinine of 0.58 mg/dl.

Patient 6 was admitted with pulmonary haemorrhage and respiratory failure requiring mechanical ventilation. Serum-creatinine was 1.83 mg/dl and anti-GBM-antibody titer was 1:40. A renal biopsy showed a focal necrotizing glomerulonephritis with 19% crescents and linear IgG deposition along the GBM. She was treated with dexamethasone (initially 100 mg over three days), cyclophosphamide (five boluses of 750 mg cyclophosphamide) and 13 sessions of IAS over one month. Respiratory failure resolved rapidly and serum-creatinine, after increasing to a maximum of 3.7 mg/dl on day 3 normalized within a month. For eight years she remained well but then presented with a recurrence of anti-GBM-disease with hemoptysis, dyspnoea and positive anti-GBM-antibodies. The symptoms resolved after a course of six boli of cyclophosphamide and she has since enjoyed excellent renal function.

Patient 7 presented with acute renal failure and dyspnoea. Serum-creatinine was 14.5 mg/dl and anti-GBM-antibody concentration was 207.8 U/ml. Renal biopsy showed necrotizing glomerulonephritis (100% crescents with linear IgG deposition). Hemodialysis was started and he was treated with pulse methylprednisolone (1 g daily for three doses) followed by tapering doses of prednisolone and oral cyclophosphamide. He received PE twice before institution of 15 IAS sessions over three weeks. Pulmonary disease resolved but the patient remained dialysis-dependent. After eight months the patient received a kidney transplant with a stable serum-creatinine of 1.5 mg/dl and no anti-GBM-antibody recurrence.

Patient 8 presented with dialysis-dependent acute renal failure, haemoptysis and dyspnoea. Serum-creatinine was 6.1 mg/dl and anti-GBM-antibody concentration was 58.5 U/ml. Renal biopsy showed necrotizing glomerulonephritis (96% crescents and linear

IgG deposits). He was treated with three 1 g pulses of methyl-prednisolone followed by oral prednisolone and cyclophosphamide. He received four PEs but anti-GBM-antibodies remained positive. After conversion to IAS (15 sessions over three weeks) pulmonary haemorrhage resolved swiftly and renal function recovered after 2 weeks with a final serum-creatinine of 2.5 mg/dl. After 10 months serum-creatinine increased to 3.75 mg/dl. He was given a second course of steroids and 17 IAS sessions, although assays for anti-GBM-antibodies were negative; renal biopsy showed severe sclerosis. Two years after presentation he restarted dialysis currently awaiting renal transplantion.

Patient 9 presented with serum-creatinine of 4.99 mg/dl necessitating hemodialysis. A renal biopsy showed necrotising glomerulonephritis (94% crescents and segmental scars affecting half of the glomeruli and linear IgG deposition along the GBM) and serum anti-GBM-antibodies were 122.6 U/ml. He was treated with prednisolone (100 mg/day tapering), pulse cyclophosphamide and PE. Anti-GBM-antibodies remained positive and his condition deteriorated despite three PE cycles and IAS was substituted (10 sessions over two weeks). He remained on hemodialysis until receiving a renal graft 18 months later. Due to incompliance he required a second allograft but is now well with stable renal function and no recurrence of anti-GBM-disease.

Patient 10 presented with acute dialysis-dependent renal failure one year after a nephrectomy due to arterial rupture. Anti-GBM-antibody concentration was 51.4 U/ml. Biopsy showed necrotizing glomerulonephritis (63% crescents and linear IgG deposition). The nephrectomy specimen confirmed vasculitis accompanied by a mild focal proliferative glomerulonephritis without detectable IgG deposits, ANCA were negative. She was treated with prednisolone and pulse cyclophosphamide. Anti-GBM-antibodies were reduced by 86% with one IAS treatment and remained negative after 5 treatments. She regained independent renal function after one month and is currently well with a serum-creatinine of 2.96 mg/dl and no detectable anti-GBM-antibodies.

Anti-GBM-antibody removal

IAS was highly effective at removing anti-GBM-antibodies with a reduction of 71.1 to 86.4% per treatment, and in controlling anti-GBM-antibody concentrations. Combined with immunosuppression, anti-GBM-antibodies became undetectable (<10 U/ml) in all patients within 2 to 9 IAS treatments (Figure 1). Autoantibody concentrations decreased from a mean of 73.6 U/ml (range 6.6 to 207.1) at IAS start to 7.8 U/ml after one month and remained undetectable thereafter. The mean value was 6.2 U/ml after a year and 6.6 U/ml at latest follow up (mean 29 months after presentation, Table 3). An exception was patient 6 who had a pulmonary relapse of anti-GBM-disease after eight years which resolved quickly with cyclophosphamide but otherwise enjoyed excellent renal function.

We studied the kinetics of anti-GBM-antibody removal and resynthesis in one patient more detail (Figure 2). Anti-GBM-antibody concentrations fell from 49.2 to 6.7 U/ml (86.4%) during the first IAS session and were consistently less than 10 U/ml after 5 IAS sessions. Anti-GBM-antibodies were measured before and after each IAS and at the midpoint between treatments after equilibration between intra- and extravascular was complete. Consequently the difference between the mid-point and pre-IAS values provides an estimate of the rate of anti-GBM-antibody synthesis indicating that anti-GBM-antibody synthesis was substantially reduced after four IAS, being negligible after five. IAS was equally efficient at removing IgG1, IgG2 and IgG4 (85%, 81% and 85% respectively) whereas IgG3 was removed with about half the efficiency (44%, Figure S1).

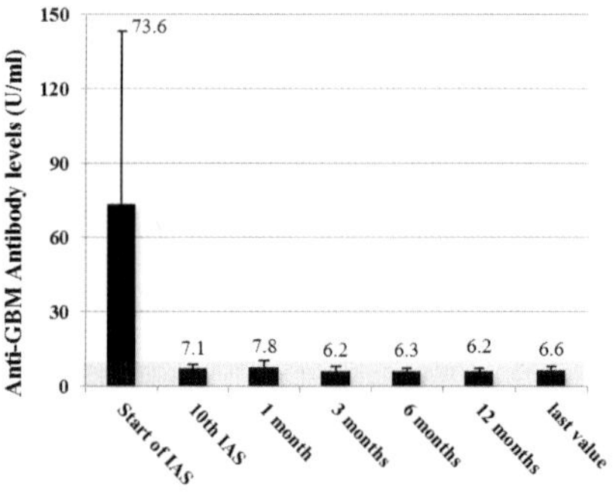

Figure 1. Anti-GBM antibody levels from start of immunoadsorption until end of observation. Mean values ± standard deviation of all patients measured with ELISA depicted. Grey area denotes negativity of the assay.

Renal function and patient survival

Pulmonary haemorrhage resolved rapidly after starting immunosuppression and IAS enabling discontinuation of artificial ventilation in the two patients who had previously needed it. Renal function improved in 4 of 8 patients with increased serum-creatinine, including three of six who where initially dialysis dependent with 100%, 96% and 63% crescents on their renal biopsies (Figure 3). Consequently renal survival increased from 40% at presentation to 70% at the end of IAS (mean 3 months) and decreased to 63% after 1 year and 50% at last follow-up (mean 84 months, range 9–186), respectively (Table 3).

One patient died of fungal infection including septic renal failure after control of his anti-GBM-disease whilst the remaining 9 patients were alive at last follow-up (mean 84 months).

Adverse events

No anaphylactic adverse events were observed during or after IAS. Infections were rare with only one infection requiring hospitalization. There was no reported case of malignancy over a combined follow-up of 70 patient years.

Cost analysis

The per-treatment cost of IAS varies depends on the type of adsorber and on the number of treatments performed as the absorber can be reused. In our study, the mean number of IAS per patient was 23, resulting in the cost of 896 € per single Immunosorba IAS treatment including all disposables and personnel time. The costs for 23 Therasorb treatments were 1035 € per treatment, PE with 4 liters of human albumin including personnel and disposables costs 1194 € at our center (Figure 4).

Discussion

Our study provides the largest evaluation of a series of patients with anti-GBM-disease treated with IAS whose use has only previously been reported in case studies [21–24]. Our results demonstrate that a) the IAS protocol presented enables rapid removal of anti-GBM-antibodies, with efficiency exceeding that of PE; b) that IAS and immunosuppression led to rapid clinical improvement both of pulmonary haemorrhage and of renal function and c) that IAS is an economical choice in anti-GBM-disease. As always in conditions as rare as anti-GBM-disease, the

Table 3. Renal function and patient survival.

Patients	Follow-Up	Patient survival		Independent renal function			
		1 year	Last FU	Start of IAS	End of IAS	1 year	Last FU
(n)	mean, range	n (%)	n (%)	n (%)	n (%)	n (%)	n (%)
10	84, 9–186	9 (90%)	9 (90)	4 (40)	7 (70)	5 (63)	5 (50)

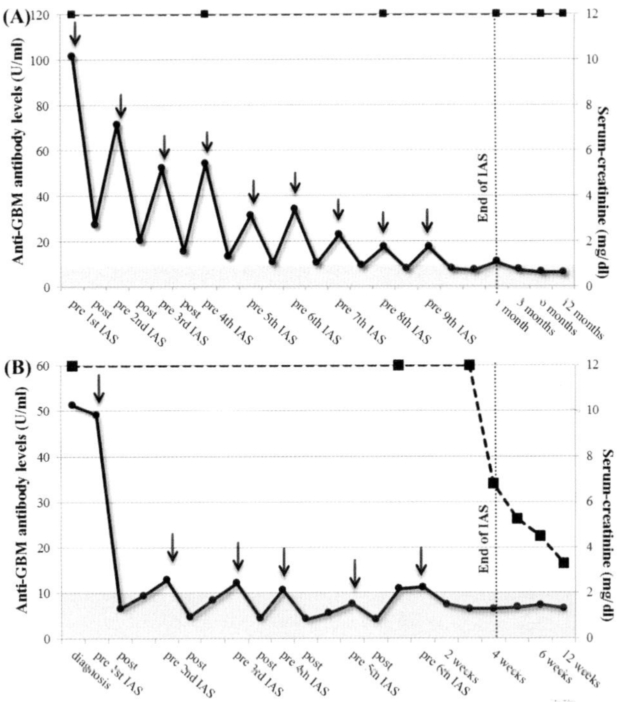

Figure 2. Anti-GBM antibody kinetics and renal function in patient #7 (2a) and patient #10 (2b). Antibody values at diagnosis, before and after IAS, 12 hours in between sessions and up to 6 weeks; arrows depict daily IAS sessions. Grey area depicts negativity of the assay.

conclusions need to be qualified because of the number of patients studied and retrospective design. Nonetheless, the consistency of the patient responses suggests that IAS is a safe and cost-effective alternative to PE for the management of anti-GBM-disease.

IAS was effective at removing all IgG subclasses and anti-GBM-antibodies were 71 to 84% lower after the first IAS and in normal range after 2 to 9 treatments. Anti-GBM-antibody synthesis may

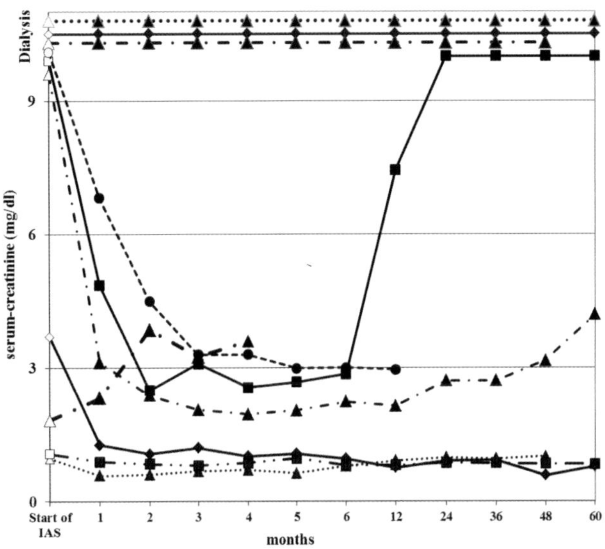

Figure 3. Dynamics of serum-creatinine of individual patients. Observation period from start of IAS until 5 years. White coloured time points depict positive anti-GBM antibody testing.

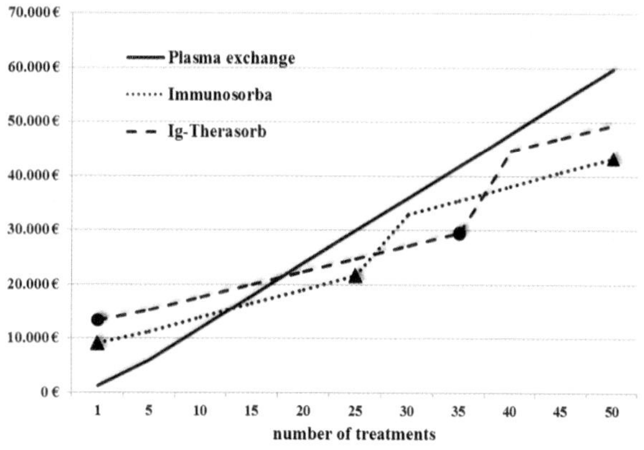

Figure 4. Cumulative costs of immunoadsorption and plasma exchange. Circles and triangles depict earliest timepoints of adsorber change due to reduced adsorption capacity (every 25 treatments for Immunosorba, every 35 treatments for Globaffin).

have already ceased by this time as demonstrated in patient 10 in whom we analyzed autoantibody kinetics.

These results are consistent with previous studies by Peters et al. [26] who showed that the combination of anti-GBM-antibody removal with PE and immunosuppression with cyclophosphamide shortened the duration of autoantibody synthesis compared to either treatment. However, both the rapidity of anti-GBM-antibody reduction and duration of synthesis were shorter in our patients treated with IAS than in patients treated with PE [26]. The rate of antibody removal was greater in our patients than in the four patients treated by IAS reported by Hu et al [21] but they processed one plasma volume (3L) at each session whereas we processed 2.5–3 plasma volumes (8L) at each session.

Clinical studies have consistently demonstrated the need for rapid control of anti-GBM-antibody concentration if renal function is to improve and have emphasised the poor prognosis for those with compromised renal function before this is achieved [7,8,11,27]. For example, only two of 39 dialysis-dependent patients treated with PE and cyclophosphamide were alive with renal function after 1 year in the cohort studies by Levy et al., and accordingly Cui et al. reported 63 patients with serum-creatinine ≥6.8 mg/dl of which only 2 were alive and had intact renal function after one year [11]. Against this background, the recovery of renal function in three of the six dialysis dependent patients in our group was unexpected, especially as renal biopsies showed fulminant crescents. Recovered patients remained free of dialysis for 64, 23 and 9 months (still free so far). These excellent results may be attributable to the intensive anti-GBM-antibody removal and more rapid control of circulating autoantibody concentrations achieved by our protocol.

Long-term patient and renal survival in our study were 90% and 50% respectively at the last follow-up (mean of 84 months) compared to 54% and 35% at a median of 90 months (71 patients) reported by Levy et al [8].

Treatment with IAS is commonly considered prohibitively expensive compared to PE but this is not the case for those needing intensive apheresis therapy as is usual in anti-GBM-disease. Costs for IAS gradually decreased due to reusable adsorbers resulting in lower total treatment costs than PE (exchange against 4 liters human albumin 5%) for those receiving 15 or more treatments. Furthermore, IAS-adsorbers can be stored for up to two years and are potentially available to treat early relapses (Table S1).

The safety profile of IAS was highly acceptable and there were no major procedure-related adverse events. One patient died with sepsis after renal function had been improved. The excellent safety profile when used with cyclophosphamide and high dose steroids is consistent with reports in other autoimmune diseases [28,29].

In conclusion, we have shown that IAS is a highly efficient, safe and cost-effective technique to remove autoantibodies in anti-GBM-disease compared to PE. We also demonstrate the feasibility of increasing the volume of plasma processed at each session from one plasma volume as is normal with PE to 3 plasma volumes. With this regimen, anti-GBM-antibodies consistently became undetectable more rapidly than has been reported with PE, which could translate into a major clinical benefit. Further studies are necessary to determine the clinical value of IAS as potential standard management of anti-GBM disease.

Author Contributions

Conceived and designed the experiments: PB AR RK MS KD. Performed the experiments: AB TP AS RK. Analyzed the data: WD PB AR MS KD. Contributed reagents/materials/analysis tools: TP AB AS. Wrote the paper: PB AR MS.

References

1. Turner N, Mason PJ, Brown R, Fox M, Povey S, et al. (1992) Molecular cloning of the human Goodpasture antigen demonstrates it to be the alpha 3 chain of type IV collagen. J Clin Invest 89: 592–601.
2. Couser WG (1988) Rapidly progressive glomerulonephritis: classification, pathogenetic mechanisms, and therapy. Am J Kidney Dis 11: 449–464.
3. Andrassy K, Küster S, Waldherr R, Ritz E (1991) Rapidly progressive glomerulonephritis: analysis of prevalence and clinical course. Nephron 59: 206–212.
4. Heaf J, Løkkegaard H, Larsen S (1999) The epidemiology and prognosis of glomerulonephritis in Denmark 1985–1997. Nephrol Dial Transplant 14: 1889–1897.
5. Bolton WK (1996) Goodpasture's syndrome. Kidney Int 50: 1753–1766.
6. Madore F, Lazarus JM, Brady HR (1996) Therapeutic plasma exchange in renal diseases. J Am Soc Nephrol 7: 367–386.
7. Savage CO, Pusey CD, Bowman C, Rees AJ, Lockwood CM (1986) Antiglomerular basement membrane antibody mediated disease in the British Isles 1980–4. Br Med J (Clin Res Ed) 292: 301–304.
8. Levy JB, Turner AN, Rees AJ, Pusey CD (2001) Long-term outcome of anti-glomerular basement membrane antibody disease treated with plasma exchange and immunosuppression. Ann Intern Med 134: 1033–1042.
9. Jindal KK (1999) Management of idiopathic crescentic and diffuse proliferative glomerulonephritis: evidence-based recommendations. Kidney Int Suppl 70: S33–40.
10. Kaplan AA (2003) The use of apheresis in immune renal disorders. Ther Apher Dial 7: 165–172.
11. Cui Z, Zhao J, Jia XY, Zhu SN, Jin QZ, et al. (2011) Anti-glomerular basement membrane disease: outcomes of different therapeutic regimens in a large single-center Chinese cohort study. Medicine (Baltimore) 90: 303–311.
12. Biesenbach P, Schmaldienst S, Smolen JS, Hörl WH, Derfler K, et al. (2009) Immunoadsorption in SLE: three different high affinity columns are adequately effective in removing autoantibodies and controlling disease activity. Atheroscler Suppl 10: 114–121.

13. Knöbl P, Derfler K, Korninger L, Kapiotis S, Jäger U, et al. (1995) Elimination of acquired factor VIII antibodies by extracorporal antibody-based immunoadsorption (Ig-Therasorb). Thromb Haemost 74: 1035–1038.
14. Schmaldienst S, Müllner M, Goldammer A, Spitzauer S, Banyai S, et al. (2001) Intravenous immunoglobulin application following immunoadsorption: benefit or risk in patients with autoimmune diseases? Rheumatology (Oxford) 40: 513–521.
15. Pusey CD, Levy JB (2012) Plasmapheresis in immunologic renal disease. Blood Purif 33: 190–198.
16. Snyder HW Jr, Cochran SK, Balint JP Jr, Bertram JH, Mittelman A, et al. (1992) Experience with protein A-immunoadsorption in treatment-resistant adult immune thrombocytopenic purpura. Blood 79: 2237–2245.
17. Kasperkiewicz M, Schmidt E, Zillikens D (2012) Current therapy of the pemphigus group. Clinics in dermatology 30: 84–94
18. Dantal J, Godfrin Y, Koll R, Perretto S, Naulet J, et al. (1998) Antihuman immunoglobulin affinity immunoadsorption strongly decreases proteinuria in patients with relapsing nephrotic syndrome. J Am Soc Nephrol 9: 1709–1715.
19. Schmaldienst S, Jansen M, Hollenstein U, Graninger W, Regele H, et al. (2002) Treatment of systemic lupus erythematosus by immunoadsorption in a patient suffering from tuberculosis. Am J Kidney Dis 39: 415–418.
20. Stummvoll GH, Schmaldienst S, Smolen JS, Derfler K, Biesenbach P (2012) Lupus nephritis: prolonged immunoadsorption (IAS) reduces proteinuria and stabilizes global disease activity. Nephrol Dial Transplant 27: 618–626.
21. Hu W, Liu Z, Ji D, Xie H, Gong D, et al. (2006) Staphylococcal protein A immunoadsorption for Goodpasture's syndrome in four Chinese patients. J Nephrol 19: 312–317.
22. Stegmayr BG, Almroth G, Berlin G, Fehrman I, Kurkus J, et al. (1999) Plasma exchange or immunoadsorption in patients with rapidly progressive crescentic glomerulonephritis. A Swedish multi-center study. Int J Artif Organs 22: 81–87.
23. Moreso F, Poveda R, Gil-Vernet S, Carreras L, Garcia-Osuna R, et al. (1995) [Therapeutic immunoadsorption in Goodpasture disease]. Med Clin (Barc) 105: 59–61.
24. Laczika K, Knapp S, Derfler K, Soleiman A, Hörl WH, et al. (2000) Immunoadsorption in Goodpasture's syndrome. Am J Kidney Dis 36: 392–395.
25. Schmaldienst S, Goldammer A, Spitzauer S, Derfler K, Hörl WH, et al. (2000) Local anticoagulation of the extracorporeal circuit with heparin and subsequent neutralization with protamine during immunoadsorption. Am J Kidney Dis 36: 490–497.
26. Peters DK, Rees AJ, Lockwood CM, Pusey CD (1982) Treatment and prognosis in antibasement membrane antibody-mediated nephritis. Transplant Proc 14: 513–521.
27. Pusey CD (2003) Anti-glomerular basement membrane disease. Kidney Int 64: 1535–1550.
28. Stummvoll GH, Aringer M, Jansen M, Smolen JS, Derfler K, et al. (2004) Immunoadsorption (IAS) as a rescue therapy in SLE: considerations on safety and efficacy. Wien Klin Wochenschr 116: 716–724.
29. Aringer M, Smolen JS, Graninger WB (1998) Severe infections in plasmapheresis-treated systemic lupus erythematosus. Arthritis Rheum 41: 414–420.

16

The Impact of Endothelial Progenitor Cells on Restenosis after Percutaneous Angioplasty of Hemodialysis Vascular Access

Chih-Cheng Wu[1,5,8], Po-Hsun Huang[2,6,7,8,9]*, Chao-Lun Lai[1,5], Hsin-Bang Leu[1,4,9], Jaw-Wen Chen[2,3,9,10], Shing-Jong Lin[2,3,6,7,8,9]

1 Cardiovascular center, National Taiwan University Hospital, Hsinchu Branch, Hsinchu, Taiwan, **2** Division of Cardiology, Taipei Veterans General Hospital, Taipei, Taiwan, **3** Department of Medical Research and Education, Taipei Veterans General Hospital, Taipei, Taiwan, **4** Healthcare and Management Center, Taipei Veterans General Hospital, Taipei, Taiwan, **5** School of Medicine, National Taiwan University, Taipei, Taiwan, **6** Department of Medicine, National Yang-Ming University, Taipei, Taiwan, **7** Institute of Clinical Medicine, National Yang-Ming University, Taipei, Taiwan, **8** School of Medicine, National Yang-Ming University, Taipei, Taiwan, **9** Cardiovascular Research Center, National Yang-Ming University, Taipei, Taiwan, **10** Institute and Department of Pharmacology, National Yang-Ming University, Taipei, Taiwan

Abstract

Objective: We prospectively investigate the relation between baseline circulating endothelial progenitor cells and the subsequent development of restenosis after angioplasty of hemodialysis vascular access.

Background: Effect of angioplasty for hemodialysis vascular access is greatly attenuated by early and frequent restenosis. Circulating endothelial progenitor cells (EPCs) play a key role in vascular repair but are deficient in hemodialysis patients.

Method: After excluding 14 patients due to arterial stenosis, central vein stenosis, and failed angioplasty, 130 patients undergoing angioplasty for dysfunctional vascular access were prospectively enrolled. Flow cytometry with quantification of EPC markers (defined as $CD34^+$, $CD34^+KDR^+$, $CD34^+KDR^+CD133^+$) in peripheral blood immediately before angioplasty procedures was used to assess circulating EPC numbers. Patients were followed clinically for up to one year after angioplasty.

Results: During the one-year follow-up, 95 patients (73%) received interventions for recurrent access dysfunction. Patients in the lower tertile of $CD34^+KDR^+$ cell count had the highest restenosis rates (46%) at three month (early restenosis), compared with patients in the medium and upper tertiles of $CD34^+KDR^+$ cell count (27% and 12% respectively, $p = 0.002$). Patients in the lower tertile of $CD34^+KDR^+$ cell count received more re-interventions during one year. Patients with early restenosis had impaired EPC adhesive function and increased senescence and apoptosis. In multivariate analysis, the $CD34^+KDR^+$ and $CD34^+KDR^+CD133^+$ cell counts were independent predictors of target-lesion early restenosis.

Conclusion: Our results suggest that the deficiency of circulating EPCs is associated with early and frequent restenosis after angioplasty of hemodialysis vascular access.

Editor: Alberico Catapano, University of Milan, Italy

Funding: This study was supported by grants from the National Taiwan University Hospital, Hsinchu Branch (HCH100-4, HCH101-13), and the UST-UCSD International Centre of Excellence in Advanced Bio-engineering NSC-100-2911-I-009-101-A2. The funders had no role in study design, data collection and analysis, decision to publish, or preparation of the manuscript.

Competing Interests: The authors have declared that no competing interests exist.

* Email: huangbs@vghtpe.gov.tw

Introduction

A functioning vascular access greatly influences the survival and quality of life of patients undergoing hemodialysis. Vascular accesses are subject to failure and the underlying pathology is usually a stenosis due to venous intimal hyperplasia. [1] Endovascular interventions are useful in restoring the function of vascular access. [2] Nonetheless, their benefits are attenuated by a high restenosis rate, far more aggressive than that of arterial lesions in non-uremic patients. Physiological and anatomical differences between arteries and veins, continuous hemodynamic stress, repeated puncture, uremia and endothelial dysfunction have all been proposed as possible causes. [1] However, in all patients, it is not precisely known how much the listed factors contribute to the high restenosis rates.

Maintenance of the integrity and function of the endothelium has been shown to play a pivotal role in the prevention of restenosis after angioplasty. [3] Accumulating evidence suggests that circulating endothelial progenitor cells (EPCs) incorporate into sites of endothelial denudation. [4] The circulating EPCs reflect not only repair capacity but also the health of the endothelium. [5] Clinical studies have shown that circulating EPC numbers are decreased and associated with vascular events in hemodialysis patients. [6,7] However, limited data are available about the role of EPCs for venous intimal hyperplasia in hemodialysis patients.

Accordingly, we conducted this prospective study to evaluate the impact of circulating EPC number and function on the outcome of vascular access.

Methods

Ethical statements

The study was based on the Declaration of Helsinki (edition 6, revised 2000). Written informed consent was obtained from all study participants, and the study was approved by the Institutional Review Board of our hospital (Hsinchu General Hospital Institutional Review Board, No. HCGH99G005 and National Taiwan University Hospital Hsinchu Branch Institutional Review Board, No. HCGH100G003).

Study participants

From January 2010 to July 2011, a series of patients with dysfunctional hemodialysis vascular access scheduled for percutaneous intervention were prospectively enrolled. Patients were referred based on one or more of the following criteria: clinical signs suggesting fistula dysfunction, reduction of flow rate and increased venous pressure during dialysis. Participants had to have received regular dialysis treatment for at least 6 months without clinical evidence of acute or chronic inflammation, recent myocardial infarction, unstable angina, or circulatory congestion. According to the same criteria, 26 patients who had normal functioning vascular access for at least two years were invited as the uremic control group. Another 30 non-uremic patients who received cardiac catheterization examination with patent coronary arteries were invited as the non-uremic control group.

Study protocol

Patients eligible for this study were scheduled for diagnostic fistulography and angioplasty on a mid-week non-dialysis day. Baseline characteristics and blood samples were collected on the morning of fistulography. After diagnostic fistulography or angioplasty, patients with insignificant stenosis (less than 50% diameter stenosis), thrombosed fistulas, arterial side stenosis, central vein lesions, or those who failed to obtain anatomic success after angioplasty were excluded. Diagnostic fistulography and angiograms of the angioplasty procedures were independently reviewed by another expert angiographer who was unaware of the patients' clinical and analytic data. The degree of stenosis was evaluated by two orthogonal planes and the greatest degree of stenosis was used for subsequent anatomical measurements. Anatomic measurements were made with use of a calibrated reference maker or computer-assisted edge detection software within the angiographic imaging system. The reference vessel was defined as an adjacent segment of normal vein located upstream from the target lesion. The degree of stenosis was reported as the maximum diameter reduction compared to the reference vessel diameter.

Laboratory methods

Blood samples were drawn after a 12 hour overnight fast and cessation of medications before diagnostic procedures. Plasma biochemical parameters were analyzed by standard laboratory methods. Assessment of the circulating EPCs by flow cytometry was performed by researchers blinded to clinical data. [8–10] A volume of 1000-μL peripheral blood was incubated for 30 minutes in the dark with Allophycocyanin (APC)-conjugated monoclonal antibody against human KDR (R&D, Minneapolis, MN, USA), Phycoerythrin (PE)-conjugated monoclonal antibody against human CD133 (Miltenyi Biotec, Germany), and Fluorescein isothiocyanate (FITC)-conjugated monoclonal antibodies against human CD34 (Becton Dickinson Pharmingen, USA). After incubation, cells were lysed, washed with phosphate-buffered saline (PBS), and fixed in 2% paraformaldehyde before analysis. Each analysis included 150,000 events. The number of cells was normalized and expressed as a percentage (%) of cells and cells per 1×10^5 mononuclear cells (MNC). To assess the reproducibility of EPC measurements, circulating EPCs were measured from 2 separate blood samples in 10 subjects, and there was a strong correlation between the two measurements ($r = 0.90$, $P<0.001$).

Human EPC culture and functional studies

Peripheral blood samples for EPC culture were obtained from twenty of the study participants, ten from the early restenosis group (restenosis developed within three months after angioplasty) and ten from the late restenosis group (restenosis within 4–12 months after angioplasty), matched by age and types of vascular access. These samples were collected retrospectively while vascular accesses were functioning well after angioplasty. Total MNCs were isolated by density gradient centrifugation with Histopaque-1077 (Sigma, St. Louis, MO, USA). [11] Briefly, MNCs (5×10^6) were plated in 2 ml endothelial growth medium (EGM-2 MV Cambrex, East Rutherford, NJ, USA) on fibronectin-coated 6-well plates. After 4 days of culturing, the medium was changed and non-adherent cells were removed; attached EPCs appeared elongated with a spindle shape. EPCs were collected and used for the functional assays in this study.

Fibronectin adhesion test were assessed as previous described. [12] Cellular aging was determined with a Senescence Cell Staining kit (Sigma). TUNEL assay (Terminal deoxynucleotidyl transferase mediated deoxyuridine triphosphate nick-end labeling) was performed using the In Situ Cell Death Detection kit (Roche Diagnostics, Basel, Switzerland) according to the instructions of the manufacturers (**Methods S1**).

Follow-up and definitions

After the angioplasty procedure, all the participants of this study were prospectively followed for one year under the same protocol at respective hemodialysis centers. Medications of the participants were continued or adjusted according to their original indications but not for the maintenance of their vascular accesses. Follow-up surveillance included physical examination and dynamic venous pressure monitoring at each hemodialysis session, and transonic examination of access blood flow rate immediately after the intervention followed by monthly examinations. The referring nephrologists were blinded to the EPC levels of their patients. When abnormal clinical or hemodynamic parameters fulfilling the original referral criteria were detected, patients were referred for repeat fistulography and angioplasty as appropriate.

Anatomic success was defined as less than 30% residual stenosis. Clinical success was defined as an improvement from baseline in clinical or hemodynamic parameters indicative of access dysfunction. Success of the procedure was defined as the combination of anatomic and clinical success. Target-lesion restenosis was defined as more than 50% diameter reduction of the original target lesion. Primary patency of vascular access was defined as time until the next intervention on the access of any kind; secondary patency of vascular access was defined as time from the intervention until surgical revision or abandonment of the access.

Statistical analysis

All data are presented as means ± standard deviations or percentages. Categorical data were compared using the Chi-square test with Yates' correction and Fisher's exact test as appropriate. Continuous variables were tested for a normal distribution by the Kolmogorov-Smirnov test. For normally distributed data, means between categories were compared by one-way analysis-of-variance. For non-normally distributed data, the Kruskal-Wallis test was used for comparison between categories. We made the assumption of three times relative risk of restenosis according to a previous study about the role of $CD34^+$ cell counts on cardiovascular events in hemodialysis patients. [7] There were 39 restenosis events in the 130 patients enrolled in our study. With the assumption of a hazard ratio for restenosis = 3.0, alpha level = 0.05, and power = 80%, each group needs 16 restenosis events by the log rank test. Thus, we stratified our patients into tertiles to compare the relative risk or restenosis between tertiles of $CD34^+KDR^+$ cell counts. The primary patency of the whole access in each group was estimated by the Kaplan-Meier method and differences were assessed using the log-rank test. Proportions of patients with early restenosis, late restenosis, and no restenosis were compared by Chi-square test. Cox regression analysis was used for estimating the relative hazard of vascular access events by tertile of $CD34^+KDR^+$ cell count with subjects in the lower tertile of $CD34^+KDR^+$ cell count as the reference group. All variables with $P<0.2$ in the univariate analysis (including use of calcium channel blocker, side of access, location of access, nature of access, diameter of access and post-dilatation stenosis) and traditional cardiovascular risk factors (including age, hypertension, diabetes mellitus, dyslipidemia, and smoking) were entered into a multivariate analysis to determine independent predictors. A P value of less than 0.05 was considered to be statistically significant. Statistical analysis was performed with the use of SPSS software, version 20.0 for Windows.

Results

Baseline characteristics of study participants

One hundred and forty-four patients with dysfunctional vascular access were enrolled prior to the diagnostic procedures. After diagnostic fistulography and angioplasty, fourteen patients were excluded: five due to central vein lesions; two due to arterial lesions, five due to thrombosed lesions, and two due to a failed angioplasty procedure. Therefore, the study group consisted of 130 patients. All patients underwent one-year clinical follow-up after the angioplasty procedure apart from six patients who died before the end of one-year.

As shown in **Figure 1**, the circulating EPCs were gated with monocytes and defined as $CD34^+$, $CD34^+KDR^+$, and $CD34^+KDR^+CD133^+$, respectively. Compared to the non-uremic control group, patient with dysfunctional vascular access had significantly lower $CD34^+$ cells (50 ± 60 vs. 83 ± 54 cells/10^5 MNCs, p = 0.014), $CD34^+KDR^+$ cells (9 ± 9 vs. 20 ± 15 cells/10^5 MNCs, $p<0.001$), and $CD34^+KDR^+CD133^+$ cells (6 ± 6 vs. 15 ± 15, $p<0.001$). Compared to the uremic control group, patients with dysfunction vascular access had a trend of lower $CD34^+$ cell counts (50 ± 60 vs. 61 ± 31 cells/10^5 MNCs, p = 0.66), $CD34^+KDR^+$ cell counts (9 ± 9 vs. 10 ± 5 cells/10^5 MNCs, p = 0.88), and $CD34^+KDR^+CD133^+$ cell counts (6 ± 6 vs. 10 ± 5, p = 0.08) but the difference didn't reach statistical significance (**Figure 2**).

Endothelial progenitor cell counts and baseline variables

Participants with abnormal vascular access function were stratified into tertiles according to their baseline $CD34^+KDR^+$ cell count (lower, <4.0; medium, 4.0 to 9.0; upper, >9.0 cells/10^6 MNCs). The baseline characteristics of study participants and vascular accesses were shown in **Table 1**. In terms of baseline characteristics, only albumin level and white cell count were associated with tertile of baseline $CD34^+KDR^+$ cell count. In addition to $CD34^+KDR^+$ cells, we also estimated surface marker $CD133^+$ cells, which were expressed as a subfraction of immature EPCs. Increased age and white cell count were associated with a higher $CD34^+KDR^+CD133^+$ cell count.

Incidence of vascular and clinical events (Table 2)

At the end of one year follow-up, 95 patients underwent a re-intervention; 94 of whom had a restenosis at the same location. All the patients with target lesion restenosis received re-interventions and were included in the re-intervention group as well. Nine patients lost their vascular access and six patients died during the follow-up period: three patients due to cardiovascular causes (myocardial infarction or sudden cardiac death) and the others due to non-cardiovascular causes.

Because the majority of patients had target-lesion restenosis at the end of one-year follow-up, the vascular access events were further stratified according the presence and timing of target-lesion restenosis: early restenosis (within 3 months), late restenosis (between 4–12 months) and no restenosis (within 12 months). The same time frame was applied in the stratification of vascular access re-intervention. Patients in the lower tertile of $CD34^+KDR^+$ cell count had the highest rate of early restenosis and re-intervention. In contrast, patients in the highest tertile of $CD34^+KDR^+$ cell count possessed the highest proportions of late or no restenosis compared to the other two tertiles, although they did not achieve statistical significance. The discrepancy in cumulative primary patency rates between EPC groups was largest at three months and then declined as the follow-up period extended (**Table 2 and Figure 3**).

As shown in Figure 3, patients in the lower tertile of EPC received an average of 3.4 ± 2.8 interventions in one year, which was higher than those in the medium tertile (2.6 ± 2.5, P = 0.15) and the upper tertile (1.5 ± 1.5, P = 0.004). As presented in **Table 3**, patients with target-lesion early restenosis had significantly lower $CD34^+KDR^+$ and $CD34^+KDR^+CD133^+$ cell counts, but not $CD34^+$ cell counts, than those with late restenosis.

Characterization of human EPC and function

The peripheral blood mononuclear cells (MNCs) that were initially seeded on fibronectin-coated wells were round in shape. After the medium was changed on day 4, attached EPCs had an elongated and spindle shape. The EPCs were characterized as adherent cells positive for acetylated low-density lipoprotein (AcLDL) uptake and lectin binding by direct fluorescent staining and immunohistochemical staining. Most of the EPCs expressed endothelial and hematopoietic stem cell markers, CD34, VE-cadherin, CD133, Kinase insert domain receptor (KDR), and CD31 (**Figure 4A**), which are considered critical markers of EPCs.

There were no significant differences in clinical or access characteristics between the two groups of patients, except for lower $CD34^+KDR^+$ and $CD34^+KDR^+CD133^+$ cell counts in the early restenosis group. (**Table S1**) Patients with early restenosis had attenuated EPC adhesive function compared to those with late restenosis (9.7 ± 2.3 vs. 17.7 ± 3.3 cells/HPF, $P<0.001$; **Figure 4B**). Patients with early restenosis also had higher

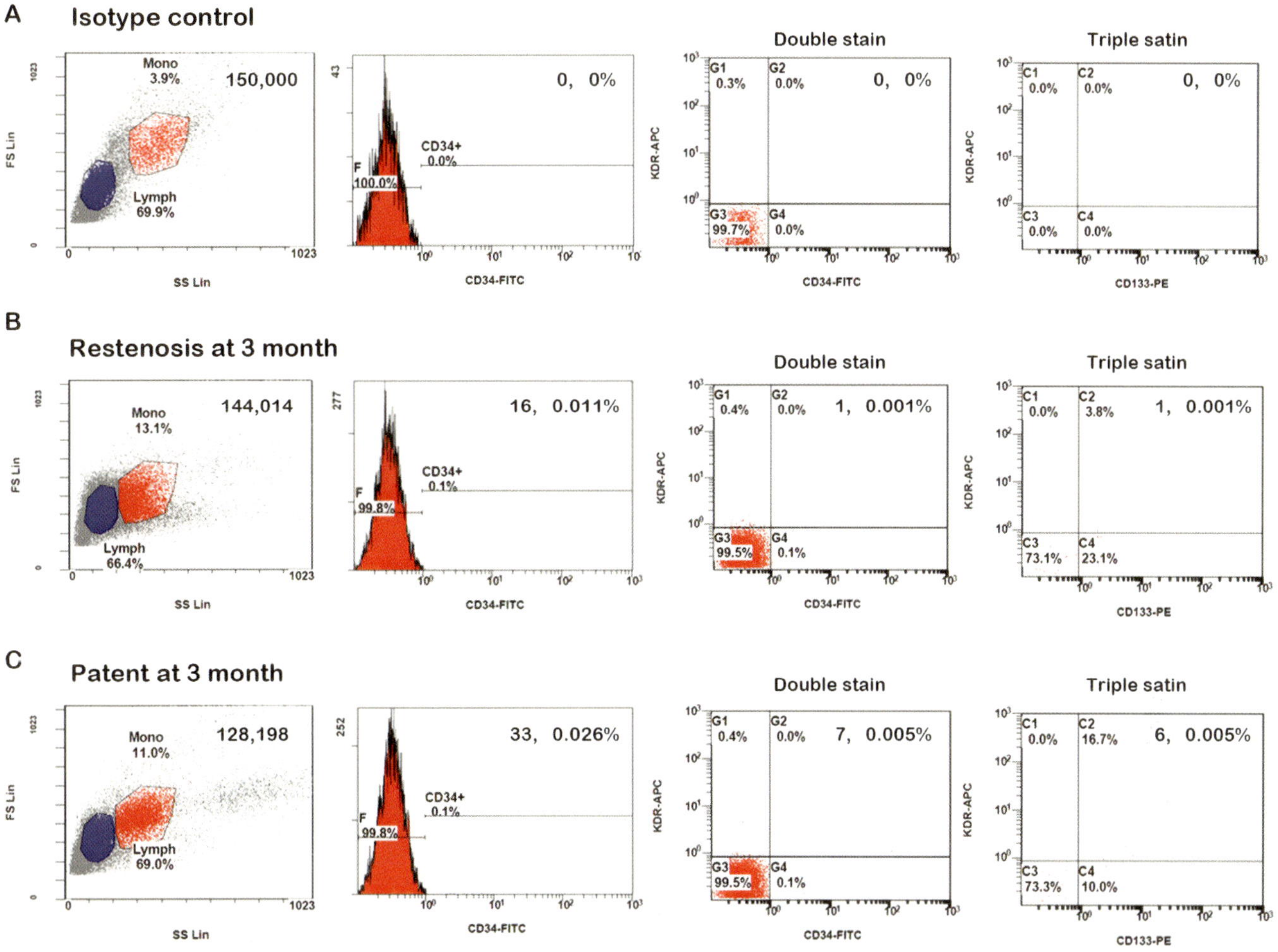

Figure 1. Representative flow cytometry analysis. Panels show mononuclear cells (MNCs) that were gated by forward/sideward scatter (FSC/SSC) in isotype controls (A), patients with restenosis (B), and patients without (C) restenosis at 3 months. The numbers of circulating endogenous progenitor cells (EPCs) were defined as $CD34^+$, $CD34^+KDR^+$, and $CD34^+KDR^+CD133^+$, respectively.

percentage of senescence-associated β-galactosidase-positive EPCs (65.5±18.0% vs. 37.6±10.7, P<0.001, **Figure 4C**) and TUNEL-positive EPCs (29.7±8.2% vs. 12.7±5.5, P<0.001; **Figure 4D**) that that with late restenosis.

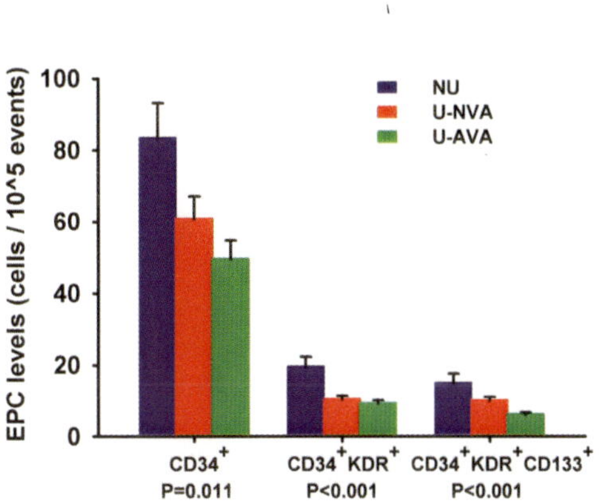

Figure 2. Circulating EPC counts between different groups. Comparisons of EPCs counts between the non-uremic controls (NU), uremic controls (normal vascular access function without interventions in previous two years, U-NVA), and uremic patients with abnormal vascular access function referred for interventions (U-AVA). (Values presented as mean ± standard error).

Univariate analysis for factors associated with target-lesion early restenosis

In univariate Cox regression analysis, the incidence of target-lesion early restenosis was not associated with demographic factors, cardiovascular risk factors, medications, or biochemical profiles; but significantly associated with access factors, including upper-arm access (hazard ratio [HR], 2.31, 95% confidence interval [CI], 1.09–4.92, p = 0.030), right-sided access (HR, 2.94; CI, 1.03–4.34, p = 0.043), graft access (HR, 2.22; CI, 1.03–4.34, p = 0.020), post-dilatation stenosis (HR, 1.01; 95% CI, 1.00–1.01, p = 0.032), and baseline level of circulating EPCs, including $CD34^+KDR^+$ cell count (HR, 0.91; CI, 0.85–0.98, p = 0.013) or tertiles (high vs. low, HR, 0.20; 95% CI, 0.08–0.53, p = 0.001) and $CD34^+KDR^+CD133^+$ cell count (HR, 0.89; CI, 0.80–0.98, p = 0.024) or tertiles (high vs. low, HR, 0.25; CI, 0.11–0.59, p = 0.002) (**Table S2**).

Table 1. Baseline characteristics of patients and vascular accesses.

		Tertiles of $CD34^+KDR^+$ Cell Count			
Characteristic	**Total (N = 130)**	**Lower (N = 43)**	**Medium (N = 44)**	**Upper (N = 43)**	**P value**
Age (yr)	66±13	71±12	65±12	63±14	0.06
Gender (men/women)	47/83	14/29	20/24	13/30	0.31
Risk factors					
Hypertension (%)	76(58%)	24(56%)	26(59%)	26(60%)	0.90
Diabetes (%)	48(37%)	15(35%)	17(39%)	16(37%)	0.94
Dyslipidemia (%)	23(18%)	11(26%)	4(9%)	8(19%)	0.13
Current smoker (%)	15(11%)	5(11%)	6(14%)	4(9%)	0.71
Cardiovascular disease (%)	26(20%)	12(28%)	8(18%)	6(14%)	0.25
Biochemical data					
Cholesterol (mg/dl)	166±40	170±38	164±48	163±33	0.71
Triglycerides (mg/dl)	161±108	177±106	147±99	159±117	0.51
Albumin (g/dl)	3.9±0.5	3.8±0.5	3.8±0.4	4.1±0.4	0.004
Hemoglobin (g/dl)	10.8±1.4	10.7±1.7	10.8±1.3	10.9±1.2	0.88
WBC (10^3/μL)	6.7±2.0	7.2±2.7	5.8±1.4	7.1±1.5	0.01
Calcium (mg/dl)	9.4±1.2	9.1±1.7	9.6±0.9	9.6±0.9	0.16
Phosphate (mg/dl)	4.4±1.3	4.3±1.3	4.4±1.5	4.6±1.1	0.53
Kt/V	1.46±0.30	1.28±0.30	1.62±0.30	1.63±0.27	0.07
Medications					
Anti-platelet	50(43%)	15(38%)	17(47%)	18(46%)	0.64
Nitrates	22(19%)	9(23%)	7(19%)	6(15%)	0.72
β-blocker	23(50%)	7(18%)	7(19.4%)	9(23%)	0.82
Calcium blocker	34(30%)	11(28%)	12(33%)	11(28%)	0.83
ACEI/ARB	23(20%)	6(15%)	8(22.2%)	9(23%)	0.62
Lipid-lowering agents	18(16%)	5(13%)	5(14%)	8(21%)	0.58
Erythropoietin (U/kg/week)	80±36	78±40	79±37	82±34	0.94
Access/lesion					
Shunt age (month)	48±44	42±31	58±57	45±40	0.30
Prosthetic graft	70(54%)	20(47%)	22(50%)	28(65%)	0.18
Upper arm access	19(15%)	7(16%)	8(18%)	4(9%)	0.50
Right arm access	32(25%)	13(30%)	10(23%)	9(21%)	0.60
Diameter (mm)	7.2±1.3	7.1±1.2	7.3±1.4	7.2±1.2	0.76
Pre-stenosis (%)	73±15	71±15	75±15	72±14	0.47
Post-stenosis (%)	22±17	24±17	23±16	21±19	0.78
$CD34^+KDR^+$ cells/10^5MNCs	9.2±9.4	2.3±1.2	6.3±1.3	19.1±10.4	<0.001

ACEI, angiotensin converting enzyme inhibitor; ARB, angiotensin receptor blocker; Kt/V, urea clearance; MNC, mononuclear cell; WBC, white blood cell.
P for ANOVA or Kruskal-Wallis test in continuous variables and p for Chi-square test in categorical variables.

Multivariate analysis for factors associated with target-lesion early restenosis

A multivariate Cox regression analysis with adjustment for covariates confirmed a significant association of $CD34^+KDR^+$ cell tertile (high vs. low, HR, 0.24, CI, 0.08–0.76, $p = 0.016$) and $CD34^+KDR^+CD133^+$ cell tertile (high vs. low, HR, 0.23, CI, 0.08–0.64, $p = 0.005$) with the development of target-lesion early restenosis. In addition, use of calcium channel blockers, side of access and nature of access were identified as independent predictors of early restenosis as well (**Table 4**).

Discussion

Main findings

Our study showed the impact of circulating EPCs on restenosis of hemodialysis vascular access. Deficiency of $CD34^+KDR^+$ cells was significantly associated with an increased risk of early restenosis. Patients in the lower $CD34^+KDR^+$ cell tertile were four times as likely to experience restenosis compared to those in the upper tertile. In addition, patients with early restenosis were more likely to have impaired EPC adhesive function, and increased cellular apoptosis and senescence. In the clinical setting, uremic patients usually have a cluster of cardiovascular risk factors, which significantly influence the number and function of

Table 2. Vascular access and clinical events during follow-up period.

		Tertiles of CD34⁺KDR⁺ Cell Count			
Event	**Total (N = 130)**	**Low (N = 43)**	**Medium (N = 44)**	**High (N = 43)**	**P value**
Vascular access event					
Target-lesion restenosis					
Early restenosis	37(28%)	20(46%)	12(27%)	5(12%)	0.002
Late restenosis	57(44%)	14(33%)	19(43%)	24(56%)	0.09
No restenosis	36(28%)	9(21%)	13(30%)	14(33%)	0.46
Access re-intervention					
Early re-intervention	39(30%)	20(46%)	13(30%)	6(14%)	0.004
Late re-intervention	56(43%)	14(33%)	18(41%)	24(56%)	0.09
No re-intervention	35(27%)	9(21%)	13(29%)	13(30%)	0.56
Access primary patency rate					
At 3 months	70%	53%	70%	86%	0.004
At 6 months	41%	30%	39%	56%	0.009
At 12 months	27%	21%	29%	30%	0.50
Access secondary patency rate					
At 12 months	93%	94%	86%	98%	0.09
Clinical event					
Death (any cause)	6(5%)	1(2%)	3(7%)	2(5%)	0.61
Death (cardiac cause)	3(2%)	1(2%)	2(5%)	0(0%)	0.37
Hospitalization (any cause)	21(16%)	8(19%)	10(23%)	3(7%)	0.12
Hospitalization (cardiac cause)	11(9%)	5(12%)	5(11%)	1(2%)	0.21

Timing of restenosis or re-intervention: early, within 3 months; late, within 4–12 months; P for Chi-square test.

EPCs. [6] Our study has demonstrated for the first time that there is an association between circulating EPCs and the aggressive venous intimal hyperplasia of hemodialysis vascular access, independent of traditional risk factors.

Possible mechanisms from animal studies

Angioplasty is associated with mechanical vascular injury, followed by an intensive local inflammatory response, platelet activation, thrombus formation, and intimal hyperplasia. [13] Endothelial disruption is considered to be the primary event in the initiation of restenosis after balloon angioplasty. [14] Besides acting as a mechanical barrier protecting smooth cell migration, a functional endothelium modulates local hemostasis and thrombolysis, and regulates smooth muscle cell proliferation. [14] The importance of endothelial integrity has been demonstrated in animal studies, suggesting that a functionally intact endothelium is

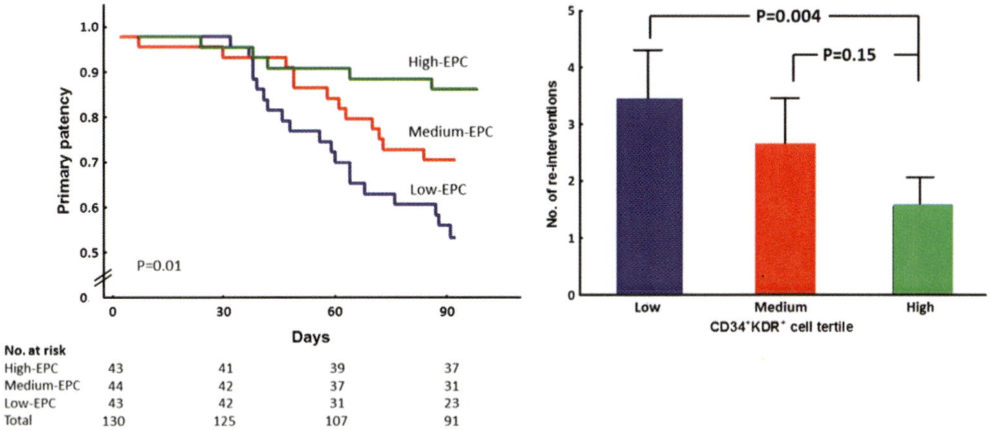

Figure 3. Kaplan-Meier analyses at three months and frequency of re-intervention at one year stratified by EPC tertiles. Left: The figure demonstrates the proportion of patients without target-lesion early restenosis according to their baseline circulating CD34⁺KDR⁺ cell count. Patients are divided into tertiles (low, medium, high) according to their baseline circulating CD34⁺KDR⁺ cell count. Right: Frequency of re-interventions at one year after angioplasty stratified by baseline circulating CD34⁺KDR⁺ cell count. (Values presented as mean ± standard error).

Table 3. Comparisons of EPC levels according to the presence and timing of target-lesion restenosis at one year.

	All patients (N = 130)			Restenosis patients (N = 94)		
EPC	Patent (N = 36)	Restenosis (N = 94)	P value	Late (N = 57)	Early (N = 37)	P value
EPC (%)						
$CD34^+$	0.062±0.082	0.044±0.047	0.12	0.043±0.038	0.046±0.057	0.77
$CD34^+KDR^+$	0.012±0.017	0.009±0.010	0.33	0.012±0.012	0.005±0.005	<0.001
$CD34^+KDR^+CD133^+$	0.009±0.017	0.007±0.007	0.27	0.008±0.008	0.004±0.003	<0.001
EPC (cells/10^5MNCs)						
$CD34^+$	63±83	45±47	0.13	44±39	46±57	0.89
$CD34^+KDR^+$	9±7	9±10	0.90	12±12	5±5	<0.001
$CD34^+KDR^+CD133^+$	6±5	6±6	0.85	8±7	4±3	<0.001

EPC, endothelial progenitor cell; MNCs: mononuclear cells.
Timing of restenosis: early restenosis, within 3 months; late, restenosis within 4–12 months.

requisite for the inhibition of intimal hyperplasia. [14,15] Accordingly, it is believed that faster re-endothelialization may inhibit the formation of intimal hyperplasia. [16] The traditional paradigm of re-endothelialization is based on the proliferation and migration of pre-existing mature adjacent endothelial cells. Increasing evidence suggests that the injured endothelium is regenerated by circulating EPCs and that the levels of EPCs reflect vascular repair capacity. These cells are derived from the bone marrow and can be mobilized into the peripheral circulation in response to many stimuli, including tissue ischemia and vascular damage, through the release of growth factors and cytokines. [4,15,16] In animal studies, Werner et al demonstrated that bone marrow-derived progenitor cells home in to areas of endothelial denudation. [17] Furthermore, intravenous injection of these EPCs can accelerate re-endothelialization and decrease neo-intimal hyperplasia. [18] These animal studies provided mechan-

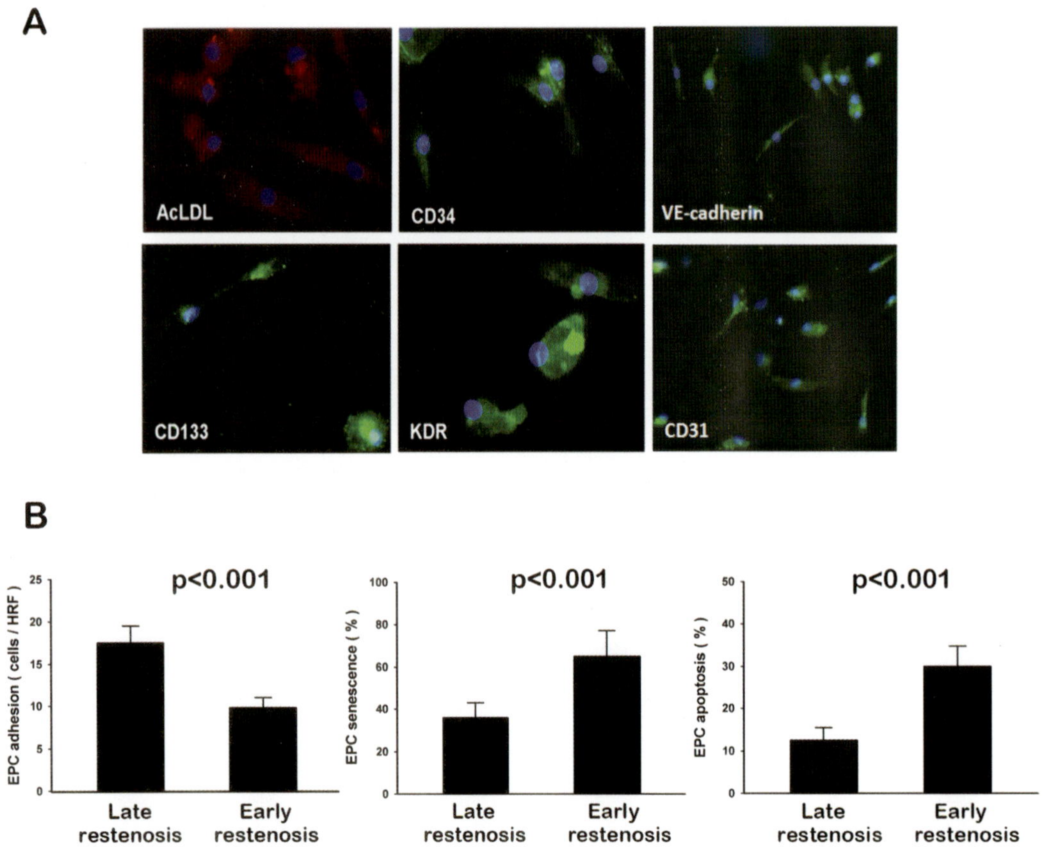

Figure 4. Morphology and functional study. Morphological characterization of human endothelial progenitor cells (EPCs) from peripheral blood (A) and comparisons of the EPC adhesive function (B), senescence assay (C), and apoptosis assay (D) in participants stratified by early (within 3 months) or late (within 4–12 months) restenosis. Values presented as mean ± standard deviation.

Table 4. Multivariate Cox regression analysis for factors predicting target-lesion early restenosis.

Factors	Unit of increase	Hazard Ratio	95% CI	P value
$CD34^+KDR^+$ cells entered as a continuous variable				
Use of CCB	Yes vs. no	0.31	0.11–0.87	0.025
Side of access	Left vs. right	0.23	0.07–0.79	0.020
Nature of access	Native vs. graft	0.40	0.18–0.92	0.030
$CD34^+KDR^+$ cells	1 cell/10^5 MNCs	0.89	0.81–0.97	0.011
$CD34^+KDR^+$ cells entered as a categorical variable				
Use of CCB	Yes vs. no	0.33	0.12–0.88	0.027
Side of access	Left vs. right	0.26	0.08–0.88	0.031
Nature of access	Native vs. graft	0.38	0.16–0.86	0.020
$CD34^+KDR^+$ cells	High vs. low	0.24	0.08–0.76	0.016
$CD34^+KDR^+CD133^+$cells entered as a continuous variable				
Use of CCB	Yes vs. no	0.37	0.14–0.99	0.049
Side of access	Left vs. right	0.21	0.06–0.74	0.015
Nature of access	Native vs. graft	0.37	0.16–0.84	0.018
$CD34^+KDR^+CD133^+$cells	1 cell/10^5 MNCs	0.82	0.72–0.94	0.003
$CD34^+KDR^+CD133^+$cells entered as a categorical variable				
Use of CCB	Yes vs. no	0.35	0.13–0.94	0.037
Side of access	Left vs. right	0.22	0.06–0.76	0.017
Nature of access	Native vs. graft	0.37	0.16–0.84	0.017
Post-stenosis (%)	1%	1.02	1.00–1.05	0.047
$CD34^+KDR^+CD133^+$cells	High vs. low	0.23	0.08–0.64	0.005

CCB, calcium channel blocker; CI, confidence interval; MNC, mononuclear cell.
Age, hypertension, diabetes, smoking, dyslipidemia, use of calcium channel blocker, side of access, nature of access, diameter of access, post-angioplasty stenosis were entered as covariates.

ical basis for the association between the circulating EPCs and intimal hyperplasia.

Evidence from clinical studies

In retrospective studies, George et al demonstrated a reduced number and adhesive function of EPCs in patients with proliferative type in-stent restenosis; Matsuo et al also showed reduced EPC numbers and senescence function in patients with in-stent restenosis. [19,20] In addition, some studies have demonstrated mobilization of EPCs after angioplasty, providing indirect evidence that EPCs may participate in the response to vascular injury. [17] Despite this, conflicting results exist in regards to the relationship between EPC mobilization and subsequent restenosis. [21] Using baseline EPC levels, our study demonstrated that a reduced number of baseline EPCs is an aggravating factor for venous intimal hyperplasia in uremic patients.

Besides being a marker of vascular repair capacity, circulating EPCs are also a surrogate marker for endothelial dysfunction and vascular health. [5] Accordingly, it is possible that deficiency of circulating EPCs may be just a marker of cumulative cardiovascular risk, rather than a direct mediator of intimal hyperplasia. This distinction is important because modulation of EPCs will be beneficial only if it is a 'disease maker'. Our data favors that EPC deficiency may not only be a marker of intimal hyperplasia for the following reasons. First, most of the cardiovascular risk factors were not correlated with the number of EPCs in our hemodialysis patients. Second, our data is consistent with previous studies demonstrating that cardiovascular risk factors do not predict venous intimal hyperplasia of hemodialysis vascular accesses [22–24].

Early vs. late restenosis

Compared to the 30% restenosis rate after coronary angioplasty [4], the 72% target-lesion restenosis rate in our study confirms the aggressive nature of venous intimal hyperplasia. Although the group with high EPC levels had a better patency rate initially, this difference vanished rapidly within one year. This late catch-up phenomenon suggests that rapid re-endothelialization only delays but does not stop the development of intimal hyperplasia. This is further supported by our observation that no difference in EPC counts between patients with late or no restenosis. Our explanation is biologically plausible as the inflammatory activation and intimal hyperplasia develop earlier than re-endothelialization. According to the animal models of restenosis, the inflammation and cellular proliferation phase occur rapidly after balloon injury, usually within days to weeks. [25] In contrast, the regeneration of the endothelium usually takes weeks to months to complete. [14] In consequence, EPCs seem to play a more significant role in the early stage after angioplasty. After the critical point of re-endothelialization, uremia or hemodialysis-related factors may dominate the development of restenosis, such as endothelial dysfunction, systemic inflammation, repeated punctures of vascular access and less well-defined elastic lamina of veins.

Comparisons of EPCs of uremic patients between different studies

It is difficult to compare studies because different surface markers or units have been used to measure EPCs. EPC counts in our study were expressed as a fraction of the number of events, rather than events per microliter. We believe this unit is more appropriate for hemodialysis patients because of the substantial variation in fluid status. Although low circulating $CD34^+$ cells have been found to be associated with all-cause and cardiovascular mortality in uremic patients [7], we didn't find a similar association in our study. Furthermore, $CD34^+$ cells were not associated with the presence or timing of restenosis in our study as well. This marker is common to a variety of progenitor cells, including smooth muscle progenitor cells, not only endothelial progenitor cells. [26] In a recent animal study using $CD34^+$ antibodies to accelerate endothelialization of synthetic grafts, intimal hyperplasia was also stimulated. [27] The dichotomy implies that $CD34^+$ antibodies may attract cells with potential transforming into smooth muscle cell or myofibroblasts as well. EPCs represent only a minor cell population in whole blood, and the choice of markers is very important. Because CD34 and KDR are also expressed on circulating mature endothelial cells, surface marker CD133 was used to ensure the identity of EPCs. Despite the rarity of these cells in the circulation, a significant correlation was still observed between counts of these cells and restenosis. There is still confusion about the cell markers used for EPC. The putative EPCs identified by surface marker CD34, KDR, and CD133 in this study are not certainly EPC but also various amounts of hematopoietic stem cells and circulating endothelial cells. These cells could only be discriminated by extensive gene expression analysis or use of a variety of functional assays. [28,29] Nonetheless, these meticulous methods are not often applied and no simple universal definition exists at the present time. [30,31] Therefore, putative EPCs in the study were still identified by the panel of CD34, KDR, and CD133 markers, which have been widely used in publications and consistently used as a surrogate marker for cells displaying regenerative properties in human study.

Limitations

Our study has several limitations that should be considered when interpreting our results. Only pre-procedure EPC levels were measured and the effect of EPC activation, migration, and homing was not evaluated. Second, we were not able to demonstrate increased EPC homing and migration to the injured endothelium, as has been demonstrated in animal studies. Third, there is still no universal definition of EPCs. KDR is not exclusively a marker of EPC but also expressed on hematopoietic stem cells and circulating mature endothelial cells. [29] Various methods to more specifically identify EPCs are emerging but they were not applicable when the study was conducted. [30,31] Forth, the number of EPCs per 150,000 events analyzed in peripheral blood is relatively low in hemodialysis patients and analysis of more blood amount may be helpful to improve the yield rate. Finally and most importantly, despite our observation of association between EPCs and early restenosis, this is not a sufficient evidence for their causal relationship. Further study to evaluate the effect of EPC manipulation and explore the underlying pathway was needed to prove the mechanical link.

Clinical implications and conclusion

Although the contribution of EPC deficiency to restenosis remains to be proven, EPC-capturing stents are undergoing clinical evaluation as a coronary intervention. [32] The most relevant clinical implication of our study is that deficiency of certain circulating EPCs is possibly pathogenic for the rapid venous intimal hyperplasia observed in hemodialysis patients. Based on this putative mechanism, methods of modifying EPC number or function, including physical exercise, pharmacological modulation (statin, GSF), infusion of autologous EPCs, capturing EPC to the denudated endothelium, may have the potential to delay the development of restenosis. [13] Studies aimed at modulating the number or function of more specific EPCs is warranted not only to clarify the causal role of EPCs but also as a potential strategy to decrease the frequency. In addition, $CD34^+KDR^+$ cells may serve as a biomarker for patients vulnerable to restenosis. It will be helpful in therapeutic planning, such as aggressive monitoring, EPC-modulating intervention, or early surgical revision. Finally, EPCs seems to play a significant role only in the development of early restenosis. In consequence, therapeutic approach to modulating EPC may focus on this critical period of re-endothelialization.

In conclusion, this study demonstrated for the first time that deficiency of circulating EPCs predicts early restenosis of hemodialysis vascular access. Our observation supports a significant role of circulating EPCs on intimal hyperplasia in human, as that was demonstrated in previous animal models. Further studies to clarify their pathogenic role in human by therapeutic approach are warranted.

Acknowledgments

We would like to thank the following hemodialysis centers for the referral and follow-up of patients: Hemodialysis center of Nanmen Hospital and Zen-Tz hospital; Hung-Zen Hemodialysis clinic, and Ansn Hemodialysis Clinic.

Author Contributions

Conceived and designed the experiments: CCW PHH. Performed the experiments: CCW PHH. Analyzed the data: CCW CLL. Contributed reagents/materials/analysis tools: HBL JWC SJL. Wrote the paper: CCW.

References

1. Roy-Chaudhury P, Sukhatme VP, Cheung AK (2006) Hemodialysis vascular access dysfunction: a cellular and molecular viewpoint. J Am Soc Nephrol 17: 1112–1127.
2. Bittl JA (2010) Catheter interventions for hemodialysis fistulas and grafts. J Am Coll Cardiol Intv 3: 1–11.
3. Inoue T, Croce K, Morooka T, Sakuma M, Node K, et al. (2011) Vascular Inflammation and Repair Implications for Re-Endothelialization, Restenosis, and Stent Thrombosis. J Am Coll Cardiol Intv 4: 1057–1066.
4. Werner N, Priller J, Laufs U, Endres M, Böhm M, et al. (2002) Bone Marrow–Derived Progenitor Cells Modulate Vascular Reendothelialization and Neointimal Formation. Arterioscler Thromb Vasc Biol 22: 1567–1572.

5. Hill JM, Zalos G, Halcox JPJ, Schenke WH, Waclawiw MA, et al. (2003) Circulating Endothelial Progenitor Cells, Vascular Function, and Cardiovascular Risk. N Engl J Med 348: 593–600.
6. de Groot K, Bahlmann FH, Sowa J, Koenig J, Menne J, et al. (2004) Uremia causes endothelial progenitor cell deficiency. Kidney Int 66: 641–646.
7. Maruyama S, Taguchi A, Iwashima S, Ozaki T, Yasuda K, et al. (2008) Low circulating CD34+ cell count is associated with poor prognosis in chronic hemodialysis patients. Kidney Int 74: 1603–1609.
8. Vasa M, Fichtlscherer S, Aicher A, Adler K, Urbich C, et al. (2001) Number and Migratory Activity of Circulating Endothelial Progenitor Cells Inversely Correlate With Risk Factors for Coronary Artery Disease. Circ Res 89: e1–e7.
9. Chiang CH, Huang PH, Chung FP, Chen ZY, Leu HB, et al. (2012) Decreased circulating endothelial progenitor cell levels and function in patients with nonalcoholic fatty liver disease. PLoS One 7: e31799.
10. Chiang CH, Huang PH, Chiu CC, Hsu CY, Leu HB, et al. (2014) Reduction of circulating endothelial progenitor cell level is associated with contrast-induced nephropathy in patients undergoing percutaneous coronary and peripheral interventions. PLoS One 9: e89942.
11. Huang PH, Chen YH, Tsai HY, Chen JS, Wu TC, et al. (2010) Intake of red wine increases the number and functional capacity of circulating endothelial progenitor cells by enhancing nitric oxide bioavailability. Arterioscler Thromb Vasc Biol 30: 869–877.
12. Fadini GP, Baesso I, Albiero M, Sartore S, Agostini C, et al. (2008) Technical notes on endothelial progenitor cells: ways to escape from the knowledge plateau. Atherosclerosis 197: 496–503.
13. Padfield GJ, Newby DE, Mills NL (2010) Understanding the role of endothelial progenitor cells in percutaneous coronary intervention. J Am Coll Cardiol 55: 1553–1565.
14. Kipshidze N, Dangas G, Tsapenko M, Moses J, Leon MB, et al. (2004) Role of the endothelium in modulating neointimal formation: vasculoprotective approaches to attenuate restenosis after percutaneous coronary interventions. J Am Coll Cardiol 44: 733–739.
15. Marboeuf P, Corseaux D, Mouquet F, Van Belle E, Jude B, et al. (2008) Inflammation triggers colony forming endothelial cell mobilization after angioplasty in chronic lower limb ischemia. J Thromb Haemost 6: 195–197.
16. Asahara T, Murohara T, Sullivan A, Silver M, van der Zee R, et al. (1997) Isolation of putative progenitor endothelial cells for angiogenesis. Science 275: 964–967.
17. Banerjee S, Brilakis E, Zhang S, Roesle M, Lindsey J, et al. (2006) Endothelial progenitor cell mobilization after percutaneous coronary intervention. Atherosclerosis 189: 70–75.
18. Mills NL, Tura O, Padfield GJ, Millar C, Lang NN, et al. (2009) Dissociation of phenotypic and functional endothelial progenitor cells in patients undergoing percutaneous coronary intervention. Heart 95: 2003–2008.
19. George J, Herz I, Goldstein E, Abashidze S, Deutch V, et al. (2003) Number and adhesive properties of circulating endothelial progenitor cells in patients with in-stent restenosis. Arterioscler Thromb Vasc Biol 23: e57–60.
20. Matsuo Y, Imanishi T, Hayashi Y, Tomobuchi Y, Kubo T, et al. (2006) The Effect of Senescence of Endothelial Progenitor Cells on In-stent Restenosis in Patients Undergoing Coronary Stenting. Intern Med 45: 581–587.
21. Pelliccia F, Cianfrocca C, Rosano G, Mercuro G, Speciale G, et al. (2010) Role of endothelial progenitor cells in restenosis and progression of coronary atherosclerosis after percutaneous coronary intervention: a prospective study. J Am Coll Cardiol Intv 3: 78–86.
22. Wu CC, Wen SC, Yang CW, Pu SY, Tsai KC, et al. (2009) Plasma ADMA predicts restenosis of arteriovenous fistula. J Am Soc Nephrol 20: 213–222.
23. Rajan DK, Bunston S, Misra S, Pinto R, Lok CE (2004) Dysfunctional autogenous hemodialysis fistulas: outcomes after angioplasty–are there clinical predictors of patency? Radiology 232: 508–515.
24. Wu C-C, Wen S-C, Yang C-W, Pu S-Y, Tsai K-C, et al. (2010) Baseline plasma glycemic profiles but not inflammatory biomarkers predict symptomatic restenosis after angioplasty of arteriovenous fistulas in patients with hemodialysis. Atherosclerosis 209: 598–600.
25. Otsuka F, Finn AV, Yazdani SK, Nakano M, Kolodgie FD, et al. (2012) The importance of the endothelium in atherothrombosis and coronary stenting. Nat Rev Cardiol 9: 439–453.
26. Stam F, van Guldener C, Becker A, Dekker JM, Heine RJ, et al. (2006) Endothelial Dysfunction Contributes to Renal Function–Associated Cardiovascular Mortality in a Population with Mild Renal Insufficiency: The Hoorn Study. J Am Soc Nephrol 17: 537–545.
27. Rotmans JI, Heyligers JM, Verhagen HJ, Velema E, Nagtegaal MM, et al. (2005) In vivo cell seeding with anti-CD34 antibodies successfully accelerates endothelialization but stimulates intimal hyperplasia in porcine arteriovenous expanded polytetrafluoroethylene grafts. Circulation 112: 12–18.
28. Kraan J, Sleijfer S, Foekens JA, Gratama JW (2012) Clinical value of circulating endothelial cell detection in oncology. Drug Discov Today 17: 710–717.
29. Yoder MC (2012) Human endothelial progenitor cells. Cold Spring Harb Perspect Med 2: a006692.
30. Lanuti P, Santilli F, Marchisio M, Pierdomenico L, Vitacolonna E, et al. (2012) A novel flow cytometric approach to distinguish circulating endothelial cells from endothelial microparticles: relevance for the evaluation of endothelial dysfunction. J Immunol Methods 380: 16–22.
31. Kraan J, Strijbos MH, Sieuwerts AM, Foekens JA, den Bakker MA, et al. (2012) A new approach for rapid and reliable enumeration of circulating endothelial cells in patients. J Thromb Haemost 10: 931–939.
32. Nakazawa G, Granada JF, Alviar CL, Tellez A, Kaluza GL, et al. (2010) Anti-CD34 Antibodies Immobilized on the Surface of Sirolimus-Eluting Stents Enhance Stent Endothelialization. J Am Coll Cardiol Intv 3: 68–75.

The Montreal Cognitive Assessment (MoCA) - A Sensitive Screening Instrument for Detecting Cognitive Impairment in Chronic Hemodialysis Patients

Frances E. Tiffin-Richards[1,2], Ana S. Costa[1,2], Bernhard Holschbach[3], Rolf D. Frank[4], Athina Vassiliadou[5], Thilo Krüger[6], Karl Kuckuck[1,2], Theresa Gross[6,7], Frank Eitner[6,8], Jürgen Floege[6], Jörg B. Schulz[1,2], Kathrin Reetz[1,2,9]*

1 Department of Neurology, RWTH Aachen University Hospital, Aachen, Germany, **2** Jülich Aachen Research Alliance (JARA) – Translational Brain Medicine, Aachen and Jülich, Germany, **3** KfH Curatorship for Dialysis and Kidney Transplant e.V., KfH-Nephrology Center, Stolberg, Germany, **4** Department of Internal Medicine, St.-Antonius-Hospital Eschweiler, Eschweiler, Germany, **5** Dialysis Center Aachen, Dialysis Center, Aachen, Germany, **6** Division of Nephrology and Clinical Immunology, RWTH Aachen University, Aachen, Germany, **7** Department of Internal Medicine, Dresden-Friedreichstadt Hospital, Dresden, Germany, **8** Bayer Pharma AG, Global Drug Development, Kidney Diseases Research, Wuppertal, Germany, **9** Institute of Neuroscience and Medicine (INM-4), Research Center Jülich GmbH, Jülich, Germany

Abstract

Background: Chronic kidney disease (CKD) patients undergoing hemodialysis (HD) therapy have an increased risk of developing cognitive impairment and dementia, which are known relevant factors in disease prognosis and therapeutic success, but still lack adequate screening in clinical routine. We evaluated the Montreal Cognitive Assessment (MoCA) for suitability in assessing cognitive performance in HD patients in comparison to the commonly used Mini-Mental State Examination (MMSE) and a detailed neuropsychological test battery, used as gold standard.

Methods: 43 HD patients and 42 healthy controls with an average age of 58 years, were assessed with the MoCA, the MMSE and a detailed neuropsychological test battery, covering the domains of memory, attention, language, visuospatial and executive functions. Composite scores were created for comparison of cognitive domains and test results were analyzed using Spearman's correlation and linear regression. Cognitive dysfunction was defined using z-score values and predictive values were calculated. Sensitivity and specificity of the MoCA were determined using receiver operating characteristic (ROC) analysis.

Results: HD patients performed worse in all cognitive domains, especially in memory recall and executive functions. The MoCA correlated well with the detailed test battery and identified patients with cognitive impairment with a sensitivity of 76.7% and specificity of 78.6% for a cut-off value of ≤24 out of 30 points. In the detailed assessment executive functions accounted significantly for performance in the MoCA. The MMSE only discriminated weakly between groups.

Conclusions: The MoCA represents a suitable cognitive screening tool for hemodialysis patients, demonstrating good sensitivity and specificity levels, and covering executive functions, which appear to play an important role in cognitive performance of HD patients.

Editor: Karl Herholz, University of Manchester, United Kingdom

Funding: Ana S. Costa was supported by a PhD fellowship (SFRH/BD/65743/2009) from Fundação para a Ciência e Tecnologia (FCT, Portugal) and financed by the POPH – QREN Program. Kathrin Reetz was funded by the Excellence Initiative of the German federal and state governments (DFG ZUK32/1). Jörg B. Schulz was in part funded by the Helmholtz Alliance ICEMED - Imaging and Curing Environmental Metabolic Diseases, through the Initiative and Network Fund of the Helmholtz Association. The funders had no role in study design, data collection and analysis, decision to publish, or preparation of the manuscript.

Competing Interests: The authors have declared that no competing interests exist.

* Email: kreetz@ukaachen.de

Introduction

The association of cognitive impairment and a higher incidence of dementia in patients with chronic kidney disease (CKD) has been increasingly acknowledged over the last few years [1–3] and represents an important issue in an already vulnerable population. The prevalence of cognitive impairment in chronic hemodialysis (HD) patients has been estimated at 30–80% [4–7]. In addition to being associated with cerebrovascular disease and potentially other types of brain injury [8], cognitive impairment may jeopardize treatment adherence by affecting the efficiency of every-day tasks, including correct medication and dietary rules [9]. Moreover, cognitive impairment is a significant predictor of mortality in HD patients [5].

The call for early detection of cognitive impairment in patients with CKD has yet to be translated to every-day clinical practice. The necessity has, however, been voiced in earlier studies and the use of short and easy-to-apply cognitive screening tools has been suggested [5,10]. The Montreal Cognitive Assessment (MoCA) [11] is a screening test for cognitive impairment that covers major cognitive domains including episodic memory, language, attention, orientation, visuospatial ability and executive functions, while remaining brief and easy to administer. It is generally considered superior to the well-established Mini-Mental State Examination (MMSE) screening test [12,13], since the MoCA not only assesses executive functioning, which may be particularly important in the CKD population [14,15], but also presents a higher sensitivity for mild cognitive impairment. Accordingly, the MoCA has been evaluated and found to be an adequate screening tool in various clinical populations, e.g. Alzheimer's dementia (AD) [16], cerebral small vessel disease [17], and other medical conditions such as cardiovascular disease [18], as well as being able to discriminate between mild cognitive impairment and elderly controls [19]. Recently, the MoCA was also recommended as a standardized approach to cognitive assessment in patients undergoing HD [20]. Therefore our primary goal was to further evaluate the MoCA as a brief screening tool for cognitive impairment in HD patients in comparison to a comprehensive cognitive testing. To achieve this, the ability to distinguish between HD patients with and without cognitive impairment, the sensitivity, specificity and predictive values of the MoCA were assessed. Additionally, psychometric criteria such as concurrent and criterion validity of performance on the MoCA, a comprehensive neuropsychological test battery and the standard brief cognitive screening test MMSE were evaluated.

Subjects and Methods

Ethics Statement

The research project was carried out in accordance with the latest version of the Declaration of Helsinki and approved by the ethics committee of the Medical Faculty of the RWTH Aachen University in Germany (EK 179/11). All participants gave informed, written consent before participating.

Study population

Between February 2012 and March 2013, forty-eight patients on hemodialysis treatment were recruited from the Division of Nephrology of the RWTH Aachen University Hospital in Germany and three community based dialysis centers in the Aachen region. Forty-two matching healthy controls of varied intellectual and educational level, but without specific experience in neuropsychology, were recruited from the community and staff of the RWTH Aachen University. All participants with a history of neurological or psychiatric disease were excluded. In two cases of severe visual or motor impairment, specific tasks were not administered and therefore considered missing values. These cases included one patient with residual eye sight of 30% due to diabetic retinopathy and glaucoma and one patient with a disabilitating hand tremor.

Clinical and demographic data

Medical history and demographic data were gained *via* self-report and/or from medical records. Patients' clinical data included medical history, current medication, CKD etiology, dialysis vintage, serum values of sodium, potassium, hemoglobin, hematocrit, creatinine, pH value and blood sugar and were obtained from routine clinical blood samples taken at the beginning of each dialysis treatment. The duration of dialysis treatment, ultrafiltration volume, pre-dialysis blood pressure values and intradialytic hypotensive episodes, defined as systolic blood pressure $<$ 90 mmHg and/or diastolic blood pressure $<$ 50 mmHg, were collected from the dialysis protocols. Cardiovascular risk factors, including nicotine consumption, body mass index (BMI), serum cholesterol and high blood pressure were rated using the SCORE risk charts of the European Society of Cardiology [21] using the low risk chart for the German population. Hypertension was defined as the prescription of antihypertensive medication. Comorbidities were quantified using the Charlson Comorbidity Index (CCI) [22] corrected for dialysis [23], or age in the healthy control group [22].

Neuropsychological testing

The neuropsychological test battery was administered to all subjects on a dialysis-free day by a psychologist or trained assistants. It consisted of two cognitive screening tests, the MoCA and the MMSE, as well as a detailed cognitive test battery that evaluated memory, language, attention, visuospatial ability and executive functions. As participants were partaking in a cross-sectional observational study with a repeated-measures design [24], previously validated alternate versions of the MoCA [25], as well as from other tests, were used to avoid practice effects. For all patients and controls the same order of test administration was used. The alternate versions of tests were contra-balanced in a pseudo-randomized order. Although all patients and controls underwent two rounds of testing, only the data of the first assessment was used in the current analyses and therefore not all participants completed the exact same version of all tests. Testing was performed in a quiet room with a low distraction level, but in cases of reduced mobility, testing was also performed in patients' hospital rooms. For the order of test administration, view List S1 in File S1.

The MoCA [11] is a brief screening tool assessing visuospatial and executive functions, attention, short-term memory, language and orientation, has been translated and adapted into several languages and is available freely on the Internet (http://www.mocatest.org). It includes tasks such as trail making test – part B, cube copying, clock drawing, naming, digit span backwards and forwards, serial subtraction, selective attention, sentence repetition, phonemic word fluency, verbal abstraction, a 5-word learning and delayed recall task, and spatial and temporal orientation. Completion time is approximately 10 to 15 minutes and a maximum of 30 points can be obtained.

The ability of the MoCA to screen for cognitive impairment in HD patients was to be evaluated through the comparison to a well-known screening test, the MMSE, and a detailed neuropsychological test battery. Given that our emphasis lay on the evaluation of the MoCA, detailed group analyses, such as correlation analysis, were not performed with the MMSE and the detailed neuropsychological battery.

The MMSE is a ten-minute screening test including questions to spatial and temporal orientation, immediate and delayed recall, language ability and oral command comprehension, serial subtraction and tasks to visuospatial ability. Here the German adaptation was used for all participants [12].

A more detailed analysis of the cognitive domains and psychometric characteristics, such as sensitivity, specificity and concurrent validity, of the MoCA was achieved by comparison to a detailed neuropsychological test battery. In the detailed neuropsychological test battery, verbal memory was examined using the California Verbal Learning Test (CVLT) [26], a word list recall task, and non-verbal memory was assessed with the Medical College of Georgia Complex Figures (MCGCF) test [27]. Attention was evaluated through a computer-based cued and non-cued reaction time (phasic and intrinsic alertness) task [28] and digit span forwards. Processing speed and executive functions were assessed using the Trail Making Task (TMT) forms A and B [29], phonemic and semantic word fluency [30], digit span backwards

[31], and the interference task of the Stroop test [32]. The Boston Naming Test [33] gave information on overall language processing ability. Visuospatial abilities were tested with the copying task of the MCGCF and the Incomplete Letters subtest of the Visual Object and Space Perception (VOSP) test [34], which also served to identify individuals with visual impediments that could hinder further testing. We also included the Epworth Sleepiness Scale (ESS) [35] to measure daytime sleepiness. Subjective fatigue level was evaluated through a 10-point scale (0 = no fatigue to 10 = worst imaginable fatigue) adapted from the Brief Fatigue Inventory [36]. Depression and anxiety were quantified with the Hospital Anxiety and Depression Scale (HADS) [37]. For further detail on individual tests, see Table S1 in File S1.

Statistical analysis

Data analysis was performed using Microsoft Excel 2010, IBM SPSS Statistics 20 for Windows and MedCalc Software Version 12.5.0. The distribution of the collected data was determined using the Kolmogorov-Smirnov test. Due to heterogeneous normal and non-normal distribution of data, non-parametric tests were used and all test results are presented with median and interquartile ranges for better comparability. Demographic data is presented according to the distribution of the respective data. Differences, and respective effect sizes (r), between patients and controls regarding demographic and clinical data, as well as the neuropsychological test scores, were computed using the non-parametric Mann-Whitney-U test with Bonferroni correction for multiple testing. The interpretation of effect sizes followed Cohen's proposal for r as small at 0.10–0.29, medium at 0.30–0.49 and large at >0.50 [38]. Correlation analyses were carried out using Spearman's rank correlation coefficient rho (r_s). We calculated standard z-scores for each cognitive test, using the healthy control group as the reference group and without replacing missing values. Based on the median of z-scores of the individual tests, we calculated composite scores for each cognitive domain – memory, attention, language, visuospatial, executive functions – as well as two overall composite scores. The overall composite scores were an executive composite score, including the executive functions and attention tasks, and a non-executive composite score comprising of the language, visuospatial and memory tasks. The same procedure was used to create composite scores of the cognitive domains of the MoCA. For further analysis, cognitive dysfunction was defined using z-score values. Mild cognitive impairment was classified as z-scores one to two standard deviation (SD) below the norm and severe cognitive impairment as more than two SD below the norm in ≥2 neuropsychological tests [5,9]. To examine concurrent validity between the MoCA total scores and the test battery overall composite scores, a bivariate linear regression model with the MoCA as the dependent variable and the composite scores as the independent variables was calculated. The raw total scores of the MoCA were used without education correction [16], and age, years of education, depression and fatigue levels were added as covariates [2]. To establish the discriminative validity of the MoCA in identifying patients with and without cognitive impairment, sensitivity and specificity levels were evaluated using the receiver operating curve (ROC) analysis and the criteria for cognitive impairment as described above. The cut-off score was determined based on maximal sensitivity and specificity. Positive and Negative Predictive Values (PPV/NPV) were calculated for the optimal cut-off value identified by the ROC analysis.

Results

Characterization of the HD patient sample

Forty-three HD patients completed testing and were included in the current analyses. Details of clinical and demographic data are presented in Table 1. In comparison to the control group, HD patients had a significantly higher rate of hypertension, diabetes type 2, hypercholesterolemia and nicotine consumption, yet no significant difference concerning BMI. Levels of fatigue and sleepiness, as well as scores on the depression scale were higher in the patient group. On average, patients had been on dialysis treatment for 50 months and spent four hours on dialysis, three times per week, with an average ultrafiltration volume of 1.2 liters. The 10-year risk of a fatal cardiovascular disease lay at 3–4% [21] while the CCI scoring system for HD patients presented a mean 10-year survival rate of 25% [23].

Performance on the MoCA and association with demographic and clinical variables

HD patients achieved lower mean total scores in the MoCA than the control group. The deficits were especially prominent in the areas of executive functions, language ability and short-term memory capacity (Figure 1). The most difficult tasks appeared to be digit span backwards and forwards, phonemic word fluency, sentence repetition, verbal abstraction and immediate and delayed word recall (see Table S2 in File S1). No significant differences could be identified between groups in respect to visuospatial tasks, naming, level of attention (as tested in the letter cancellation and number subtraction tasks) or temporal and spatial orientation.

In the patient group there was a negative association between the MoCA total score and age ($r_s = -.38$, $p<.05$), which was not found in the control group. There was a positive association ($r_s = .28$, $p<.01$) between the MoCA and education. From the association analysis between clinical variables and performance on the MoCA, only the CCI score for dialysis patients correlated negatively with the MoCA total scores ($r_s = -.53$, $p<.001$), indicating that patients with a higher comorbidity score achieved lower results in the MoCA.

Performance on the detailed neuropsychological test battery

In the detailed neuropsychological testing, patients performed worse than the control group in all cognitive domains (Table 2). Patient performance was worse in tasks such as immediate and delayed verbal and visual memory, semantic and phonemic word fluency, as well as performance on the TMT, reaction-timed alertness and the Stroop interference task. Cognitive dysfunction was identified in 29 patients (70%), whereby for 10 patients (24%) cognitive dysfunction could be classified as mild cognitive impairment and for 19 patients (46%) as severe cognitive impairment.

Correlation analysis showed that the composite scores of the MoCA and the test battery correlated in the domains of executive functions ($r_s = .60$, $p<.001$) and memory ($r_s = .53$, $p<.001$), whereas the attention, language and visuospatial composites revealed no significant association. The MoCA and the MMSE total scores showed a moderate positive correlation ($r_s = .54$, $p<.001$).

Association between the MoCA and the detailed neuropsychological assessment

Linear regression analysis revealed that the composite score including executive functions tasks explained 39% ($\beta = 0.62$,

Table 1. Demographic and health characteristics.

Demographics	**Patients**	**Controls**	p[e]
Age	58.3±13.9	57.9±11.8	.96
Gender	Male 52.1% (25)	Male 47.6% (20)	.67
Education (years)	12.0 (2.0)	13.0 (3.3)	.01
Comorbidities			
BMI	24.4 (6.7)	25.2±3.8	.71
Hypertension	83.3% (40)	33.3% (14)	<.001
Diabetes	45.8% (22)	4.8% (2)	<.001
Nicotine consumption	25.0% (12)	7.1% (3)	.02
Hypercholesterolemia	31.3% (15)	0%	<.001
Cardiovascular Score (ESC - SCORE)	1.0 (4.0)	-	-
Charlson Comorbidity Index (CCI)[a]	4.0 (3.0)	-	-
Hemodialysis			
Dialysis Vintage (months)	36.0 (47.0)	-	-
Time on dialysis (hours)	4.0 (0.0)	-	-
Ultrafiltration volume (l)	1.2 (2.1)	-	-
Etiology of renal disease			
Diabetic nephropathy	27.1% (13)	-	-
Glomerulonephritis and systemic diseases	27.1% (13)	-	-
Vascular (hypertensive) kidney disease	14.6% (7)	-	-
Other causes[b]	12.5% (6)	-	-
Polycystic kidney disease	10.4% (5)	-	-
Unknown	8.3% (4)	-	-
Secondary diseases			
Renal anemia	38.5% (20)	-	-
Secondary hyperparathyroidism	34.6% (18)	-	-
Renovascular hypertension	19.2% (10)	-	-
Kidney transplant in medical history	13.5% (7)	-	-
Medication			
Antihypertensive Medication (total number)	3.0 (4.0)	0.0 (0.0)	<.001
ACE* inhibitors	37.2% (16)	7.1% (3)	<.001
Beta blockers	67.4% (29)	16.7% (7)	<.001
Calcium channel blockers	48.8% (21)	7.1% (3)	<.001
Angiotensin receptor blockers	20.9% (9)	4.8% (2)	.03
Alpha-1 blockers	25.6% (11)	0%	<.001
Adrenergic alpha agonists	23.3% (10)	0%	<.001
Direct vasodilators	9.3% (4)	0%	.04
Diuretics	46.5% (20)	4.8% (2)	<.001
Antidiabetics[c]	37.2% (16)	2.4% (1)	<.001
Thyroid drugs	30.2% (13)	7.1% (3)	.01
Psychoactive drugs[d]	23.3% (10)	0%	.02
Analgesics	16.3% (7)	2.4% (1)	.01
Glucocorticoids	25.6% (11)	0%	<.001

Notes. Values are presented as mean ± SD for normally distributed continuous variables, median (interquartile range) for non-normally distributed continuous variables and % (N) for percentages.

[a] History of cerebral disease found in two cases;

[b] Other causes include progression of acute kidney disease due to post-operative infections, urologic reflux diseases, analgesic medication;

[c] Including oral antidiabetics and insuline therapie;

[d] Psychoactive drugs include antipsychotics, antidepressants, anticonvulsives and drugs containing L-DOPA;

[e] p-value of nonparametric Mann-Whitney-U test for independent samples;

* ACE = Angiotensin Converting Enzyme.

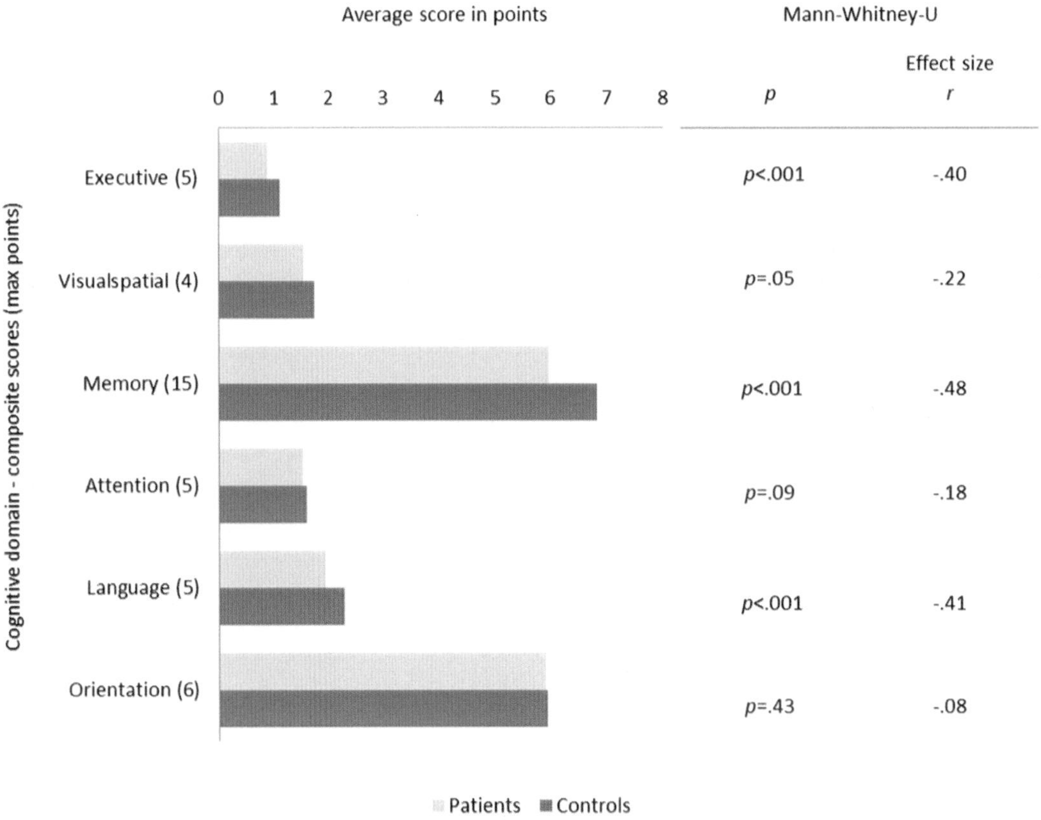

Figure 1. Group differences in cognitive domain composite scores of the Montreal Cognitive Assessment. The bar chart in figure 1 displays the average points scored by the patient and control group for each of the cognitive domains of the Montreal Cognitive Assessment (MoCA). The group differences were assessed using the non-parametric Mann-Whitney-U test with respective p-values showing a significantly ($p \leq .001$) poorer performance of the patient group in the domains of executive functions, episodic memory and language. Notes. *Executive: Trail Making Test (TMT) B, verbal abstraction, digit span backwards, phonemic word fluency; Visuospatial: cube copying, clock drawing; Memory: immediate and delayed word recall; Attention: digit span forwards, letter cancelation, number subtraction; Language: sentence repetition, animal naming; Orientation: temporal and spatial orientation. Group differences were assessed using the Mann-Whitney-U test with a significance level of $p \leq .001$.

$R^2 = .39$, $p < .001$) of the variance in the MoCA and the non-executive functions composite score explained 34% ($\beta = 0.58$, $R^2 = .34$, $p < .001$). Together, executive and non-executive functions accounted significantly for overall performance on the MoCA ($\beta = 0.42$, $R^2 = .44$, $p < .001$), while the covariates age ($\beta = 0.26$, $R^2 = .07$, $p < .05$) and education ($\beta = 0.23$, $R^2 = .05$, $p < .05$) only marginally affected variance in performance. Sleepiness and fatigue did not show a significant effect on cognitive performance, yet high scores on the depression scale had a mild effect ($\beta = -0.36$, $R^2 = .13$, $p < .001$).

ROC analysis and predictive values

The ROC analysis disclosed an optimal cut-off for the MoCA at ≤24 points (Table 3), with a sensitivity of 76.7%, specificity of 78.6% and an area under the curve (AUC) of 0.755 (95% CI, 0.602–0.872). In comparison, the MMSE only achieved a sensitivity of 55.2%, and a specificity of 75.0%, and AUC of 0.701 (95% CI, 0.538 to 0.834) for an optimal cut-off of ≤ 28 points (Figure 2). Using a cut-off value of ≤24 for MoCA results, a total of 26 patients (59%) scored 24 points or lower, while 18 patients achieved a higher score. Respectively, a PPV of 0.88 and NPV of 0.61 could be calculated for the patient cohort. We identified 19 patients (46.3%) with a MMSE score of ≤ 28 points.

Discussion

Here we demonstrate that the MoCA is a valid and well-suited screening tool for cognitive impairment in HD patients. The MoCA was capable of discriminating between HD patients with and without cognitive impairment, as defined by performance on a comprehensive neuropsychological test battery, presenting good sensitivity and specificity levels, as well as a good concurrent validity. In contrast, the MMSE revealed only a weak group discriminative power.

Our main results confirm that the MoCA is able to reliably identify cognitive impairment in CKD patients undergoing hemodialysis. We could establish an optimal cut-off of ≤24 points out of a 30 points maximum, which is lower than the cut-off value of ≤26 described in the original data collected in a population of patients with AD and mild cognitive impairment (MCI) [11]. Given that cut-off values are population specific [39], several other studies have determined lower values in different populations, e.g. a cut-off of 23.5 in a population with MCI [19] and of 21/22 in a population with cerebral small vessel disease [17]. With a good sensitivity (76.67) and specificity (78.57) our findings are consistent with previous research, where the MoCA's sensitivity in detecting cognitive impairment ranged from 56% to 100%, while specificity varied between 29% and 87%, depending on the study population [11,18,40]. More specifically, in the detection of vascular cognitive impairment the MoCA presented a specificity of 68% and lower sensitivity of 56% in a population with silent cerebral infarction [40].

Table 2. Neuropsychological test results.

Neuropsychological domain/test	Test results				Mann-Whitney-U	
	N	Patients	N	Controls	*p*	Effect size *r*
Screening tests						
Montreal Cognitive Assessment (MoCA)	43	24.0 (4.0)	42	28.0 (3.0)	<.001*	−.573
Mini Mental State Examination (MMSE)	41	29.0 (2.0)	41	29.0 (2.0)	.03	−.247
Attention						
Test of attentional performance (TAP)						
TAP Phasic Alertness	35	276.0 (73.0)	39	243.0 (60.0)	.03	−.262
TAP Intrinsic Alertness	35	273.0 (51.0)	39	255.0 (64.0)	.01	−.301
Digit span forwards	41	7.0 (2.0)	42	8.0 (4.0)	.002	−.338
Verbal Memory						
California Verbal Learning Test (CVLT)						
CVLT Total learned	37	50.0 (16.0)	42	61.0 (15.0)	<.001*	−.415
CVLT Interference	37	5.0 (4.0)	42	6.0 (3.0)	.04	−.232
CVLT Immediate Recall	37	9.0 (6.0)	42	12.5 (6.0)	.002	−.327
CVLT Delayed Recall	37	11.0 (6.0)	42	12.5 (4.0)	.002	−.341
CVLT Recognition (correct)	37	16.0 (2.0)	42	16.0 (1.0)	.60	−.059
Non-verbal Memory						
Medical College of Georgia Complex Figures (MCGCF)						
MCGCF Immediate Recall	36	17.8 (12.4)	42	28.0 (13.5)	.004	−.325
MCGCF Delayed Recall	36	16.5 (12.6)	41	28.0 (13.5)	.008	−.266
Visuospatial						
MCGCF Copy	36	31.5 (8.5)	42	34.0 (2.0)	.02	−.264
Visual Object Space Perception (VOSP) Incomplete letters	40	20.0 (1.0)	42	20.0 (1.0)	.39	−.095
Language						
Boston Naming Test	39	15.0 (0.0)	42	15.0 (0.0)	.06	−.207
Executive						
Semantic word fluency	39	28.0 (17.0)	42	39.5 (12)	<.001*	−.409
Phonemic word fluency	39	14.0 (9.0)	42	21.0 (10.0)	<.001*	−.492
Digit span backwards	41	6.0 (2.0)	42	6.0 (1.0)	.25	−.126
Stroop Test						
Colour reading	33	35.0 (14.0)	41	32.0 (6.0)	.01	−.288
Colour naming	33	54.0 (17.0)	41	47.0 (12.0)	.01	−.285
Inteference	33	96.0 (49.0)	41	86.0 (28.0)	.02	−.269
Trail Making Test (TMT) Part A	39	51.0 (38.0)	42	32.5 (15.0)	<.001*	−.512
Trail Making Test (TMT) Part B	38	110.5 (96.0)	42	73.5 (37.0)	<.001*	−.427
Depression						
Hospital Anxiety and Depression Scale (HADS)						
Total score	42	11.0 (9.0)	42	4.5 (7.0)	<.001*	−.373
Anxiety	42	6.0 (5.0)	42	3.0 (5.0)	.02	−.266
Depression	42	4.5 (5.0)	42	1.0 (4.0)	<.001*	−.428
Fatigue						
Epworth Sleepiness Scale (ESS)	42	6.5 (5.0)	42	5.5 (5.0)	.05	−.217
Fatigue	21	5.0 (5.0)	34	2.0 (4.0)	.02	−.318

Notes. Test results presented as median (IQR).
**p*-values with Bonferroni correction for multiple comparisons.
Significant difference at $p<.001$. Effect sizes, *r*: small (0.10–0.29), medium (0.30–0.49), large (>0.50).

The detailed cognitive assessment showed a distinct difference in achievement between groups. This tendency was equally present in the MoCA results, whereas performance did not differ between groups for the MMSE. The prevalence of cognitive impairment of 70% in this cohort, as classified by the testing battery, corresponds to the levels of cognitive dysfunction stated in

Table 3. Criterion (cut-off) values and coordinates of the ROC curves of MoCA and MMSE.

Screening test	Criterion	Sensitivity	95% CI	Specificity	95% CI
MoCA	≤22	46.67	28.3–65.7	78.57	49.2–95.3
	≤24*	76.67	57.7–90.1	78.57	49.2–95.3
	≤25	86.67	69.3–96.2	57.14	28.9–82.3
	≤26	90.00	73.5–97.9	35.71	12.8–64.9
MMSE	≤27	37.93	20.7–57.7	83.33	51.6–97.9
	≤28*	55.17	35.7–73.6	75.00	42.8–94.5
	≤29	89.66	72.6–97.8	33.33	9.9–65.1

Note:
*optimal cut-off score based on maximal sensitivity and specificity using the receiver operating characteristic (ROC) analysis.

previous studies with larger cohorts of dialysis patients [5,7]. The results presented by the MMSE equally match previous characterizations of CKD patient cohorts, where the level of cognitive dysfunction was measured at 30% when only using the MMSE as a diagnostic measure [4,6]. The prevalence of cognitive dysfunction in this patient cohort appears, therefore, to be similar to previous findings and allows the assumption that it is representative for this population. Correlation analysis showed a strong relationship between MoCA results and the detailed neuropsychological testing, especially for memory and executive functions, which may suggest good diagnostic ability in these areas. There remains, nevertheless, a limitation for interpretation of correlation between tests, due to a partial overlap between tasks that may affect association analysis.

The profile of cognitive deficits found in our patient population, including significant impairment in executive functions, processing speed, word fluency and short-term verbal and non-verbal memory capacity, stands in accordance to previous findings [3,41] and similar results have been associated with vascular disease as a potential cause of cognitive impairment in HD patients [15,42]. Given the high prevalence of executive dysfunction in CKD patients and our findings that performance in the MoCA was predominantly dependent on executive ability (as has been described before [43]), we believe that this is one of the strengths of the MoCA in comparison to other generally used cognitive screening instruments. In this regard, the focus of the MoCA on executive functions is believed to be a reason why it is far superior to the MMSE in particular clinical populations, given that the MMSE lacks the assessment of such cognitive domains and has a tendency to produce ceiling effects [43,44].

This may be particularly important considering that the majority of previous studies with CKD patients have included the MMSE as the preferred cognitive screening test [42] or even the only cognitive instrument [45,46]. Methodologically, the fact that the MoCA and the MMSE subtests partially overlap may limit considerations of their differential discriminant validity, but it should be noted that the original rationale behind MoCA, through the inclusion of a wider range of cognitive domains than the MMSE, especially considering the executive functions, already entails some advantage in terms of sensitivity and specificity.

Based on our current results, and as others have suggested [8], the MMSE may be inadequate for this population and may underestimate the extent of cognitive impairment. Nevertheless, a recent study showed that the MMSE was able to detect progression of cognitive impairment in HD patients [47], but may be less suited for early detection of mild cognitive deficits in other populations [48]. In a similar fashion, another screening test, the Kidney Disease Quality of Life Cognitive Function (KDQOL-CF), was found to be inadequate for assessing cognitive function in HD patients, due particularly to the lack of executive tasks [49].

A procedural advantage of the MoCA over the MMSE may also be the availability of alternative versions [25], which enables longitudinal testing while avoiding practice effects. Longitudinal testing is especially interesting in HD patients, as fluctuations in cognitive performance during the hemodialysis cycle have been identified [20,50].

Concerning predictive clinical variables, we were able to show that high comorbidity rates were associated with lower performance on the MoCA, which opens the question of the etiological

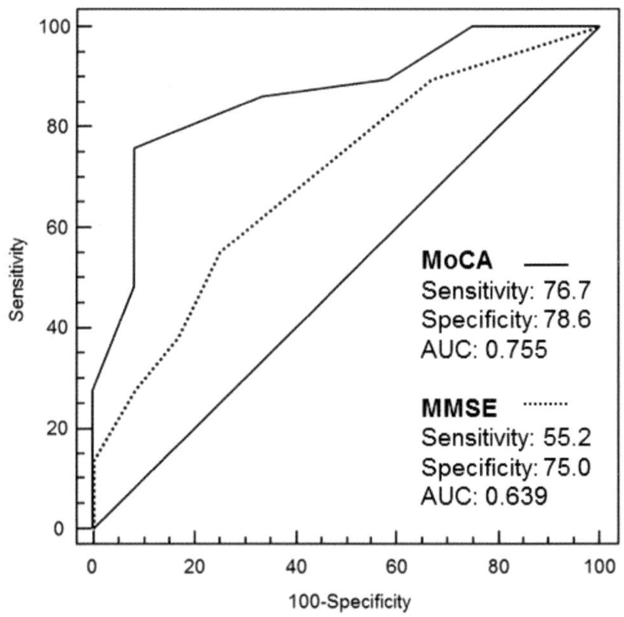

Figure 2. ROC curves for the cognitive screening tests Montreal Cognitive Assessment and Mini-Mental State Examination. The receiver operating characteristics curves for the Montreal Cognitive Assessment (MoCA) and the Mini-Mental State Examination (MMSE) illustrate the discriminative capacity of each of the screening tests, displaying their individual sensitivity, specificity and area under the curve (AUC). The MoCA shows good levels of sensitivity and specificity, as well as an overall greater AUC than the MMSE, while the MMSE presents a high specificity and relatively low sensitivity. Notes. MoCA = Montreal Cognitive Assessment; MMSE = Mini-Mental State Examination; AUC = Area under the curve.

or mediator role that different comorbidities play in cognitive impairment in such a heterogeneous group.

Other interesting findings were that although levels of fatigue and sleepiness were higher in the patient group, which is in line with statements from earlier studies that fatigue is a common problem in HD patients [3,51], we did not find fatigue or sleepiness to influence cognitive performance. It is possible that conducting the assessment on a dialysis-free day avoided post-dialytic fatigue and enabled a more objective assessment of cognitive performance. In contrast, a significant association was found between lower performance and higher levels of depressive symptoms, which supports assumptions that depression may be a relevant co-factor for poor cognitive performance and should also be screened for in CKD patients [52–54]. This is especially important when taking into account the prevalence of depression of up to 25% in HD patients [51] and the number of associated problems, including lower quality of life and higher hospitalization and mortality rates [54].

Further strengths of our study include the detailed neuropsychological testing, which enabled a comprehensive evaluation of cognition and the interpretation of concurrent validity, as well as the inclusion of a healthy control group that served as reference for cognitive performance. The MoCA has recently been suggested for cognitive screening in a small cohort of HD patients showing similar results for MoCA with an average of 24 points before dialysis [20], yet the emphasis was put on testing environment and variation in performance during the HD cycle and only the MMSE was used as a reference. This is therefore a valuable addition, as there is no precedent data on the psychometric characteristics of MoCA in comparison to detailed cognitive analysis and clinical characterization of a moderate size sample of HD patients. Limitations are, nevertheless, the relatively small sample size, which makes it difficult to generalize our findings. Although our results allow the assumption of cognitive impairment in HD patients below the cut-off value of 24 points in the MoCA, a clear distinction between MCI and dementia cannot be made in this study, due to the exclusion of patients with dementia. Equally, one must mention again the concordance of tests used in the screening tests and the detailed test battery that may influence correlation analyses in form of a positive bias. Our decision to enter education as a covariate rather than using the education correction for MoCA values, for which there is no normative data for a German population, may be seen as inadequate as there is a slight difference in educational levels between groups. Furthermore, data on subjective cognitive impairment, and clinical data were limited, the latter especially for the control sample, reducing our ability to assess variables, such as cardiovascular risk factors and hemodialysis parameters, in more detail. Further research is warranted to confirm these findings in a larger patient sample, possibly including non-dialysis CKD patients to further define indications for cognitive screening with the MoCA.

Cognitive impairment is a highly relevant clinical factor for disease progression in HD patients, possibly also affecting daily-life activities, thereby impeding adherence to therapeutic regimes and compromising quality of life. With the aims of improvement of individual outcome and optimizing the utilization of medical care resources, a brief cognitive screening test for HD patients is an essential addition to clinical practice. We presume that the MoCA, granted its validity and psychometric characteristics, is very suitable for this purpose, as it represents a multi-dimensional screening test that not only includes relevant tasks for the assessment of the HD population, but also offers the possibility of longitudinal measurements with available alternate versions.

In conclusion, the MoCA is an adequate screening tool for a brief bedside evaluation of global cognitive performance in HD patients and has the potential to assist in the daily clinical care of HD patients.

Acknowledgments

We sincerely thank all our patients and control participants for their enduring collaboration and interest in this research.

Author Contributions

Conceived and designed the experiments: FT-R AC KK TG FE JF JBS KR. Performed the experiments: FT-R AC BH RF AV TK KK TG FE JF KR. Analyzed the data: FT-R AC KK KR. Contributed reagents/materials/analysis tools: FT-R AC BH RF AV TK KK TG FE JF JBS KR. Wrote the paper: FT-R AC KR.

References

1. Kurella Tamura M, Wadley V, Yaffe K, McClure LA, Howard G, et al. (2008) Kidney function and cognitive impairment in US adults: the Reasons for Geographic and Racial Differences in Stroke (REGARDS) Study. Am J Kidney Dis 52: 227–234.
2. Elias MF, Elias PK, Seliger SL, Narsipur SS, Dore GA, et al. (2009) Chronic kidney disease, creatinine and cognitive functioning. Nephrol Dial Transplant 24: 2446–2452.
3. Sánchez-Román S, Ostrosky-Solís F, Morales-Buenrostro LE, Nogués-Vizcaíno MG, Alberú J, et al. (2011) Neurocognitive profile of an adult sample with chronic kidney disease. J Int Neuropsychol Soc 17: 80–90.
4. Sehgal AR, Grey SF, DeOreo PB, Whitehouse PJ (1997) Prevalence, recognition, and implications of mental impairment among hemodialysis patients. Am J Kidney Dis 30: 41–49.
5. Griva K, Stygall J, Hankins M, Davenport A, Harrison M, et al. (2010) Cognitive impairment and 7-year mortality in dialysis patients. Am J Kidney Dis 56: 693–703.
6. Kurella M, Chertow GM, Luan J, Yaffe K (2004) Cognitive impairment in chronic kidney disease. J Am Geriatr Soc 52: 1863–1869.
7. Murray AM, Tupper DE, Knopman DS, Gilbertson DT, Pederson SL, et al. (2006) Cognitive impairment in hemodialysis patients is common. Neurology 67: 216–223.
8. Bugnicourt J-M, Godefroy O, Chillon J-M, Choukroun G, Massy ZA (2013) Cognitive disorders and dementia in CKD: the neglected kidney-brain axis. J Am Soc Nephrol 24: 353–363.
9. Murray AM, Knopman DS (2010) Cognitive impairment in CKD: no longer an occult burden. Am J Kidney Dis 56: 615–618.
10. Kurella Tamura M, Yaffe K (2011) Dementia and cognitive impairment in ESRD: diagnostic and therapeutic strategies. Kidney Int 79: 14–22.
11. Nasreddine ZS, Phillips NA, Bédirian V, Charbonneau S, Whitehead V, et al. (2005) The Montreal Cognitive Assessment, MoCA: a brief screening tool for mild cognitive impairment. J Am Geriatr Soc 53: 695–699.
12. Kessler J, Markowitsch HJ, Denzler P (2000) Mini-Mental-Status-Test (MMST) German Adaptation. Göttingen: Beltz Test GMBH.
13. Folstein MF, Folstein SE, McHugh PR (1975) "Mini-mental state". A practical method for grading the cognitive state of patients for the clinician. J Psychiatr Res 12: 189–19.
14. Pereira AA, Weiner DE, Scott T, Chandra P, Bluestein R, et al. (2007) Subcortical cognitive impairment in dialysis patients. Hemodial Int 11: 309–314.
15. Post JB, Jegede AB, Morin K, Spungen AM, Langhoff E, et al. (2010) Cognitive profile of chronic kidney disease and hemodialysis patients without dementia. Nephron Clin Pract 116: c247–55.
16. Freitas S, Simões MR, Alves L, Santana I (2011) Montreal Cognitive Assessment: Validation Study for Mild Cognitive Impairment and Alzheimer Disease. Alzheimer Dis Assoc Disord 00: 1–7.
17. Wong A, Xiong YY, Kwan PWL, Chan AYY, Lam WWM, et al. (2009) The validity, reliability and clinical utility of the Hong Kong Montreal Cognitive Assessment (HK-MoCA) in patients with cerebral small vessel disease. Dement Geriatr Cogn Disord 28: 81–87.

18. McLennan SN, Mathias JL, Brennan LC, Stewart S (2011) Validity of the montreal cognitive assessment (MoCA) as a screening test for mild cognitive impairment (MCI) in a cardiovascular population. J Geriatr Psychiatry Neurol 24: 33–38.
19. Ahmed S, de Jager C, Wilcock G (2011) A comparison of screening tools for the assessment of Mild Cognitive Impairment: Preliminary findings. Neurocase.
20. Tholen S, Schmaderer C, Kusmenkov E, Chmielewski S, Förstl H, et al. (2014) Variability of Cognitive Performance during Hemodialysis: Standardization of Cognitive Assessment. Dement Geriatr Cogn Disord 38: 31–38.
21. Perk J, De Backer G, Gohlke H, Graham I, Reiner Z, et al. (2012) "European Guidelines on cardiovascular disease prevention in clinical practice (version 2012)" The Fifth Joint Task Force of the European Society of Cardiology and Other Societies on Cardiovascular Disease Prevention in Clinical Practice. Eur Hear J 33: 2126–2126.
22. Charlson ME, Pompei P, Ales KL, MacKenzie CR (1987) A new method of classifying prognostic comorbidity in longitudinal studies: development and validation. J Chronic Dis 40: 373–383.
23. Beddhu S, Bruns FJ, Saul M, Seddon P, Zeidel M (2000) A simple comorbidity scale predicts clinical outcomes and costs in dialysis patients. Am J Med 108: 609–613.
24. Costa AS, Tiffin-Richards FE, Holschbach B, Frank RD, Vassiliadou A, et al. (2014) Clinical Predictors of Individual Cognitive Fluctuations in Patients Undergoing Hemodialysis. Am J Kidney Dis pii: S0272.
25. Costa AS, Fimm B, Friesen P, Soundjock H, Rottschy C, et al. (2012) Alternate-form reliability of the montreal cognitive assessment screening test in a clinical setting. Dement Geriatr Cogn Disord 33: 379–384.
26. Niemann H, Sturm W, Thöne-Otto A, Willmes-von-Hinkeldey K (2008) California Verbal Learning Test - German adaptation. Pearson As. Frankfurt.
27. Ingram F, Soukoup VM, Ingram PTF (1997) The Medical College of Georgia Complex Figures: reliability and preliminary normative data using an intentional learning paradigm in older adults. Neuropsychiatry, Neuropsychol Behav Neurol 10: 144–146.
28. Zimmermann P, Fimm B (2012) Testbatterie zur Aufmerksamkeitsprüfung. Version 2.3. Herzogenrath: Psytest.
29. Wagner S, Helmreich I, Dahmen N, Lieb K, Tadic A (2011) Reliability of three alternate forms of the trail making tests a and B. Arch Clin Neuropsychol 26: 314–321.
30. Aschenbrenner S, Tucha O, Lange KW (2000) Regensburg Word Fluency Test [Regensburger Wortflüssigkeits-Test (RWT)]. Göttingen: Hogrefe.
31. Von Aste M, Neubauer A, Horn R (2006) Wechsler Intelligenztest für Erwachsene (WIE). Deutschsprachige Bearbeitung und Adaptation des WAIS-III von David Wechsler. Frankfurt: Harcourt Test Services.
32. Bäumler G (1985) Farbe-Wort-Interferenztest. Göttingen: Hogrefe.
33. Aebi C (2002) Valiedirung der neuropsychologischen Testbatterie CERAD-NP: eine Multi-Center Studie [Validation of the CERAD-NP neuropsychological test batery: a multi-center study Basel University.
34. Warrington E, James M (1992) Testbatterie für Visuelle Objekt- und Raumwahrnehmung (VOSP). Frankfurt: Harcourt Test Services.
35. Johns M (1991) A new method for measuring daytime sleepiness: the Epworth sleepiness scale. Sleep.
36. Radbruch L, Sabatowski R, Elsner F, Everts J, Mendoza T, et al. (2003) Validation of the German Version of the Brief Fatigue Inventory. J Pain Symptom Manage 25: 449–45.
37. Herrmann-Lingen C, Buss U, Snaith RP (1995) Hospital Anxiety and Depression Scale - deutsche Version (HADS-D). Bern: Verlag Hans-Huber.
38. Cohen J (1988) Statistical power analysis for the behavioral sciences (2nd ed.). Hillsdale, NJ, England: Lawrence Erlbaum Associates, Inc.
39. Luis CA, Keegan AP, Mullan M (2009) Cross validation of the Montreal Cognitive Assessment in community dwelling older adults residing in the Southeastern US. Int J Geriatr Psychiatry.
40. Zhao J, Tang H, Sun J, Wang B, Chen S, et al. (2012) Analysis of cognitive dysfunction with silent cerebral infarction: a prospective study in Chinese patients. Metab Brain Dis 27: 17–22.
41. Yaffe K, Ackerson L, Kurella Tamura M, Le Blanc P, Kusek JW, et al. (2010) Chronic kidney disease and cognitive function in older adults: findings from the chronic renal insufficiency cohort cognitive study. J Am Geriatr Soc 58: 338–345.
42. Sarnak MJ, Tighiouart H, Scott TM, Lou KV, Sorensen EP, et al. (2013) Frequency of and risk factors for poor cognitive performance in hemodialysis patients. Neurology 80: 471–480.
43. Zadikoff C, Fox SH, Tang-Wai DF, Thomsen T, de Bie RM, et al. (2008) A comparison of the mini mental state exam to the Montreal cognitive assessment in identifying cognitive deficits in Parkinson's disease. Mov Disord 23: 297–299.
44. Gill DJ, Freshman A, Blender JA, Ravina B (2008) The Montreal cognitive assessment as a screening tool for cognitive impairment in Parkinson's disease. Mov Disord 23: 1043–1046.
45. Wang F, Zhang L, Liu L, Wang H (2010) Level of kidney function correlates with cognitive decline. Am J Nephrol 32: 117–121.
46. Helmer C, Stengel B, Metzger M, Froissart M, Massy Z-A, et al. (2011) Chronic kidney disease, cognitive decline, and incident dementia: The 3C Study. Neurology 77: 2043–2051.
47. Bossola M, Antocicco M, Di Stasio E, Ciciarelli C, Luciani G, et al. (2011) Mini Mental State Examination over time in chronic hemodialysis patients. J Psychosom Res 71: 50–54. doi:10.1016/j.jpsychores.2011.01.001.
48. Lessig S, Nie D, Xu R, Corey-Bloom J (2012) Changes on brief cognitive instruments over time in Parkinson's disease. Mov Disord 27: 1125–1128.
49. Sorensen EP, Sarnak MJ, Tighiouart H, Scott T, Giang LM, et al. (2012) The Kidney Disease Quality of Life Cognitive Function Subscale and Cognitive Performance in Maintenance Hemodialysis Patients. Am J Kidney Dis: 1–10.
50. Williams MA, Sklar AH, Burright RG, Donovick PJ (2004) Temporal effects of dialysis on cognitive functioning in patients with ESRD. Am J Kidney Dis 43: 705–711.
51. Bossola M, Luciani G, Tazza L (2009) Fatigue and its correlates in chronic hemodialysis patients. Blood Purif 28: 245–252.
52. Madero M, Gul A, Sarnak MJ (n.d.) Cognitive function in chronic kidney disease. Semin Dial 21: 29–37.
53. Watnick S, Kirwin P, Mahnensmith R, Concato J (2003) The prevalence and treatment of depression among patients starting dialysis. Am J Kidney Dis 41: 105–110.
54. Agganis BT, Weiner DE, Giang LM, Scott T, Tighiouart H, et al. (2010) Depression and cognitive function in maintenance hemodialysis patients. Am J Kidney Dis 56: 704–712.

18

Efficacy and Safety of Dipeptidyl Peptidase-4 Inhibitors in Type 2 Diabetes Mellitus Patients with Moderate to Severe Renal Impairment

Dongsheng Cheng, Yang Fei, Yumei Liu, Junhui Li, Yuqiang Chen, Xiaoxia Wang, Niansong Wang*

Department of Nephrology and Rheumatology, Shanghai Jiaotong University Affiliated Sixth People's Hospital, Shanghai, P.R. China

Abstract

Objective: To perform a systematic review and meta-analysis regarding the efficacy and safety of dipeptidyl peptidase-4 (DDP-4) inhibitors ("gliptins") for the treatment of type 2 diabetes mellitus (T2DM) patients with moderate to severe renal impairment.

Methods: All available randomized-controlled trials (RCTs) that assessed the efficacy and safety of DDP-4 inhibitors compared with placebo, no treatment, or active drugs were identified using PubMed, EMBASE, Cochrane CENTRAL, conference abstracts, clinical trials.gov, pharmaceutical company websites, the FDA, and the EMA (up to June 2014). Two independent reviewers extracted the data, and a random-effects model was applied to estimate summary effects.

Results: Thirteen reports of ten studies with a total of 1,915 participants were included in the final analysis. Compared with placebo or no treatment, DPP-4 inhibitors reduced HbA1c significantly (−0.52%, 95%CI −0.64 to −0.39) and had no increased risk of hypoglycemia (RR 1.10, 95%CI 0.92 to 1.32) or weight gain. In contrast to glipizide monotherapy, DPP-4 inhibitors showed no difference in HbA1c lowering effect (−0.08%, 95% CI −0.40 to 0.25) but had a lower incidence of hypoglycemia (RR 0.40, 95%CI 0.23 to 0.69). Furthermore, DPP-4 inhibitors were well-tolerated, without any additional mortality and adverse events. However, the quality of evidence was mostly as low, as assessed using the GRADE system for each outcome.

Conclusions: DPP-4 inhibitors are effective at lowering HbA1c in T2DM patients with moderate to severe renal impairment. DPP-4 inhibitors also have a potential advantage in lowering the risk of adverse events. Regarding the low quality of the evidence according to GRADE, additional well-designed randomized trials that focus on the safety and efficacy of DPP-4 inhibitors in various CKD stages are needed urgently.

Editor: Jaap A. Joles, University Medical Center Utrecht, Netherlands

Funding: This research is supported by grant from the Project of National Nature Science Foundation of China (81270824), Shanghai Science and Technology Project (11DZ1921904 and 11410708500). The funders played no role in the study design, data collection and analysis, decision to publish, and preparation of the manuscript.

Competing Interests: The authors have declared that no competing interests exist.

* Email: wangniansong2012@163.com

Introduction

The prevalence of type 2 diabetes mellitus (T2DM) and chronic kidney disease (CKD) is increasing steadily. Diabetes is the leading cause of CKD, which might progress to end-stage renal disease and increase the risk of death [1]. It is known that good glycemic control might delay the deterioration in kidney function [2]. However, antihyperglycemic therapy, including the use of metformin, sulfonylureas, thiazolidinediones, and insulin, in T2DM patients with renal impairment remains controversial regarding its tolerability and safety. Metformin might no longer be the first choice for CKD patients because of the risk of lactic acidosis. The KDIGO recommended that metformin could be continued in individuals with a glomerular filtration rate (GFR)> 45 ml/min/1.73 m^2, should be reviewed in those with a GFR 30–44 ml/min/1.73 m^2, and should be discontinued in patients with a GFR<30 ml/min/1.73 m^2 [3]. Selected sulfonylureas are associated with a higher risk of hypoglycemia, which can be worse in CKD patients [4]. For thiazolidinediones, although there is no higher risk of hypoglycemia or dose adjustment in renal failure patients, they might cause fluid retention and edema, which are common manifestations of kidney disease [5]. Although insulin is used widely, its dose has to be adjusted occasionally based on blood glucose to avoid hypoglycemia because it is partially metabolized by the kidney [6].

Dipeptidyl peptidase-4 (DPP-4) inhibitors are a novel type of oral glucose-lowering agents that modulate fasting plasma glucose, postprandial glucose, and HbAlc levels by decreasing the inactivation of incretins such as glucagon-like peptide 1 and glucose-dependent insulinotropic polypeptide to stimulate the release of insulin in a glucose-dependent manner [7–8]. Since most DPP-4 inhibitors are eliminated by the kidney, a dose reduction is required for patients with moderate to severe renal impairment, except for linagliptin because of its relatively reduced renal metabolism [9–10]. Giorda et al [9] conducted a systematic review on the pharmacokinetics, safety, and efficacy of DPP-4 inhibitors in patients with both T2DM and renal impairment, and suggested that DDP-4 inhibitors could be appropriate drugs for patients with renal impairment. However, their study lacked sufficient randomized trials; therefore, a further meta-analysis is needed.

The aim of the current study was to perform a systematic review and meta-analysis of the safety and efficacy of DPP-4 inhibitors for the treatment of T2DM patients with moderate to severe renal impairment.

Methods

This review was conducted and reported according to PRISMA (Preferred Reporting Items for Systematic Reviews and Meta-Analysis; Table S1) [11].

Search Strategy

Literature searches were performed using PubMed, EMBASE, and Cochrane CENTRAL to identify studies published before June 20, 2014, with no language restrictions. The main search term was a combination of MESH terms and text words for DPP-4 inhibitors and renal impairment. The details of the search are presented in File S1. To find additional relevant studies, a full search was conducted of the references lists of the identified studies and abstracts from the 2011 to 2013 annual meetings of the American Diabetes Association and the European Association for the Study of Diabetes. Additional unpublished trials were searched from clinicaltrials.gov (www.clinicaltrials.gov) and relevant pharmaceutical company websites. Finally, the Food and Drug Administration (FDA; www.fda.gov) and European Medicines Agency (EMA; www.ema.europa.eu) websites were searched for medical reviews of DPP-4 inhibitors (alogliptin, linagliptin, saxagliptin, and sitagliptin in the FDA, and vildaligptin in the EMA).

Eligibility criteria for the inclusion in the meta-analysis

The inclusion criteria were as follows: (1) randomized controlled trials, (2) duration ≥12 weeks, (3) studies assessing T2DM patients with moderate or severe renal insufficiency, including dialysis patients, and (4) a comparison of DPP-4 inhibitors with placebo, no treatment, or other active drugs.

The degree of renal impairment was classified as non-dialysis patients including moderate renal insufficiency (estimated glomerular filtration rate [eGFR] 30–60 ml/min or ml/min/1.73 m^2), severe renal insufficiency (eGFR<30 ml/min or ml/min/1.73 m^2, not on dialysis), and persons receiving dialysis.

Study selection

The titles, abstracts, and/or full-text were assessed independently by DC and YL using the abovementioned inclusion criteria. Discrepancies were resolved by consensus, and the reasons for exclusion were recorded. Endnote X4 was used for literature management and selection.

Data extraction

Data were extracted independently by DC and YL using electronic extraction forms. The extracted data included the authors, study title, publication year, study design, number of participants, mean age of the participants, follow-up duration, completeness, inclusion criteria, baseline HbA1C, intervention type, intervention dose, sponsor information, and pre-specified outcomes. The main outcome for efficacy was the mean change in HbA1c from baseline. Other efficacy outcomes included the mean changes in glycated albumin, fasting blood glucose (FPG), 2-h postprandial glucose, and the proportion of participants that achieved the goal of an HbA1c<7%. The parameters used to assess safety included the incidence of hypoglycemia, the mean change in body weight and renal function, the incidence of cardiovascular disease events, mortality, the incidence of any adverse events (AE), serious adverse events (SAE), drug-related AE, drug-related SAE, and the discontinuation rate. In the current meta-analysis, data from the longest follow-up report were extracted. For studies that contained a 12-week placebo treatment as the initial control and an extended 40–42-week sulfonylurea treatment, only the data from the first period were extracted.

Risk of bias assessment and grading the quality of the evidence

The risk of bias was evaluated using the Cochrane Collaboration's "risk of bias" tool [12]. The overall risk of bias was classified into three grades: low risk of bias if all bias domains were low, high risk if any bias domain was high, and the remaining cases were judged as unclear. The quality of evidence for each outcome was assessed using Grading of Recommendations Assessment, Development, and Evaluation (GRADE) [13], and GRADEprofiler was used to create a GRADE evidence profile (Version 3.6.1, GRADE Working Group).

Data analysis and synthesis

The mean difference (MD) and its 95% confidence interval (CI) were applied for continuous variables, whereas the risk ratio (RR) and its 95%CI were used for dichotomous outcomes. All analyses were based on a random-effects model. Statistical heterogeneity across trials was analyzed using χ^2 tests ($p<0.10$) and I^2 tests [14]. I^2 values of 25%, 50%, and 75% corresponded to low, medium, and high levels of heterogeneity, respectively [15]. Subgroup analyses were performed to investigate potential sources of heterogeneity (such as participants, interventions, and study quality). Sensitivity analyses were performed to assess changes in HbA1c by excluding reports at high risk of bias, eliminating unpublished reports, removing open label studies, and using fixed effects models. Publication bias for the main outcome was assessed primarily using funnel plots. Egger's and Begg's tests were applied to provide statistical evidence of funnel graph symmetry. In addition, the trim and fill method was applied to evaluate the influence of missing studies. Meta analyses were performed using Review Manager Software (Version 5.1. The Cochrane Collaboration, 2011). Funnel plots, Egger's and Begg's tests, and the trim and fill method were performed using Stata software (Version 11, College Station, TX).

Results

Search results and study characteristics

Figure 1 shows the flow diagram of trial selection. From the initial 607 records in the electronic databases, a total of 28 articles were examined in full, among which nine reports on seven studies (seven primary reports and two extensions) [16–24] were finally selected. Furthermore, four additional unpublished reports (three primary reports and one extension) [25–28] obtained from conference abstracts, ClinicalTrials.gov and company website were selected, yet one trial on gemigliptin conducted in October 2013 identified in ClinicalTrials.gov was excluded [29]. Ultimately, thirteen reports on ten RCT studies were included in this systematic review.

The characteristics of the included trials are presented in Table 1. With the exception of one open label study, all trials were designed as double-blinded parallel studies and included a total of 1,915 participants, the enrollment sizes ranged from 51 369 individuals. The reports were published between 2008 and 2013, with durations of 12–54 weeks. The mean baseline HbA1c varied from 6.7% to 8.5%.

Among the enrolled articles, six studies (or eight reports) focused mainly on non-dialysis patients, two assessed dialysis patients, and two (or three reports) analyzed both types of patients. The study by Kothny et al. [21], which contained only two hemodialysis subjects, was included in the non-dialysis group. The studies also differed in the type of DPP-4 inhibitors used: five (or six reports) on sitagliptin, three (or four reports) on vildagliptin, two on linagliptin, and one (or two reports) on saxagliptin.

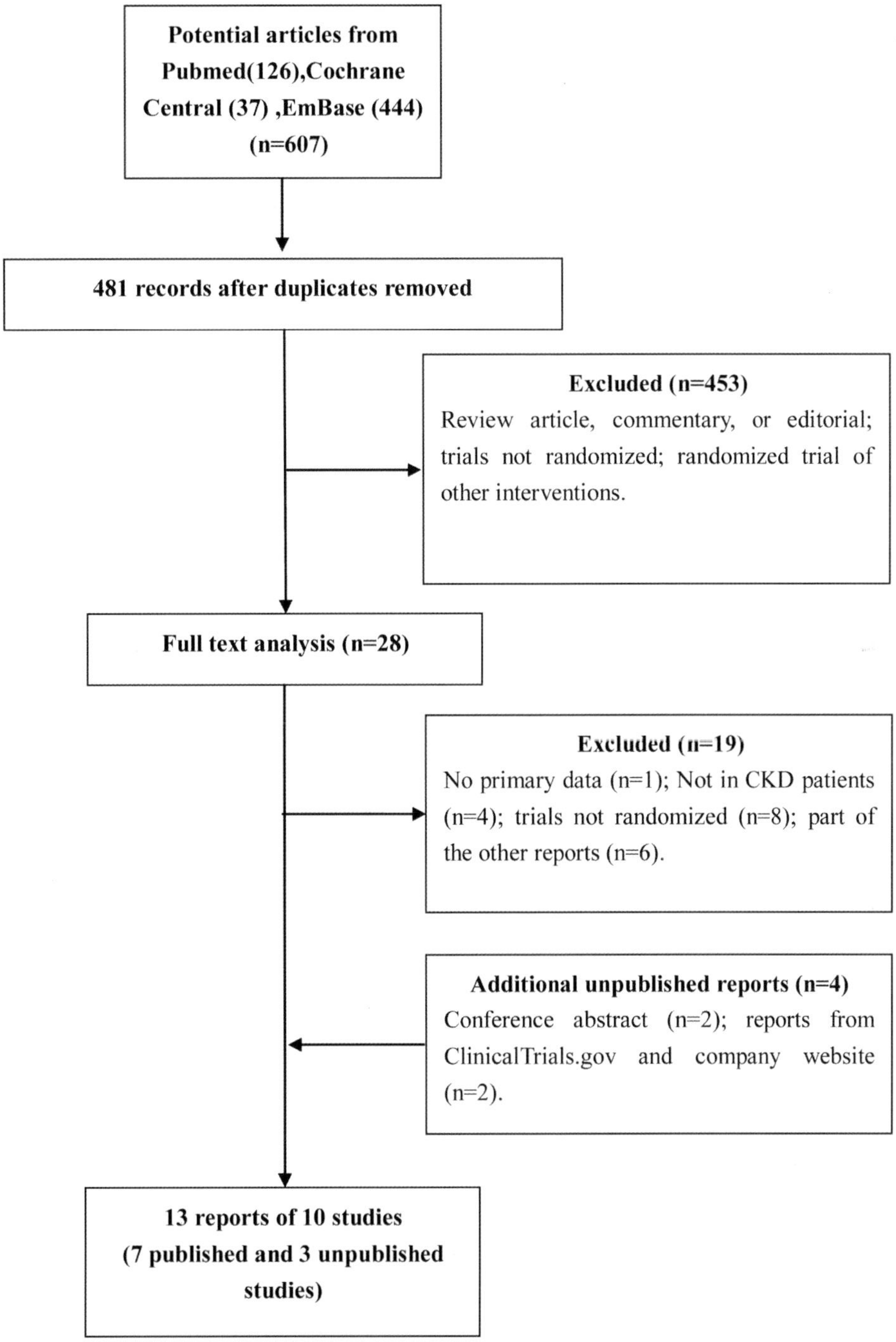

Figure 1. Study flow diagram for trial selection and exclusion.

Table 1. Characteristics of the randomized controlled clinical trials included in this analysis.

Trial	Design	Extension periods	Participant details			Type of prevention		Follow-up details	
			Total number	Baseline HbA1C	Renal status	I	C	Duration	Completeness
DPP-4 inhibitor vs. placebo or no treatment									
Chan, 2008 [16]*	Double blinded RCT	NA	91	I, 7.6% vs. C, 7.8%	eGFR<50 ml/min, including HD and PD patients	Sitagliptin (25–50 mg/day) +SBT	Placebo+SBT	12 weeks	I, 70.8% vs. C, 76.9%
Ito, 2011 [17]	Open label RCT	NA	51	I, 6.7% vs. C, 6.7%	HD patients	Vildagliptin (50–100 mg/day) +SBT	SBT	24 weeks	I, 100% vs. C, 100%
Nowicki, 2011a [18]	Double blinded RCT	Nowicki 2011b [19]	170	I, 8.5% vs. C, 8.1%	eGFR<50 ml/min, including HD patients	Saxagliptin (2.5 mg/day)+SBT	Placebo+SBT	52 weeks (12+40)	I, 49% vs. C, 58%
Lukashevich, 2011 [20]	Double blinded RCT	Kothny 2012 [21]	369	I, 7.8% vs. C, 7.8%	eGFR<50 ml/min/1.73 m^2, including HD patients	Vildagliptin (50 mg/day)+SBT	Placebo+SBT	52 weeks (24+28)	I, 67.8% vs. C, 60.8%
McGill, 2013 [22]	Double blinded RCT	NA	133	I, 8.2% vs. C, 8.2%	eGFR<30 ml/min/1.73 m^2, not requiring dialysis	Linagliptin (5 mg/day)+SBT	Placebo+SBT	52 weeks	I, 72.1% vs. C, 73.8%
Laakso, 2013 [23]*	Double blinded RCT	NA	235	I, 8.1% vs. C, 8.0%	eGFR<60 ml/min/1.73 m^2, not requiring dialysis	Linagliptin (5 mg/day)+SBT	Placebo+SBT	12 weeks	NR
DPP-4 inhibitor vs. glipizide									
Ferreira, 2013a [24]	Double blinded RCT	NA	422	I, 7.8% vs. C, 7.8%	eGFR<50 ml/min/1.73 m^2, not requiring dialysis	Sitagliptin (25–50 mg/day)+ glipizide matching placebo	Glipizide (2.5–20 mg/day)+ sitagliptin matching placebo	54 weeks	I, 77.7% vs. C, 80.2%
Ferreria, 2013b [25]	Double blinded RCT	NA	129	I, 7.9% vs. C, 7.8%	HD and PD patients	Sitagliptin (25 mg/day)+ glipizide matching placebo	Glipizide (2.5–20 mg/day)+ sitagliptin matching placebo	54 weeks	I, 73% vs. C, 69%
DPP-4 inhibitor vs. GLP-1 receptor agonist albiglutide									
Leiter, 2013 [26]#	Double blinded RCT	NA	231	I, 8.2% vs. C, 8.2%	eGFR 15–60 ml/min/1.73 m^2	Sitagliptin (25–100 mg/day)+ albiglutide matching placebo+SBT	Albiglutide (30 mg/week)+ sitagliptin matching placebo +SBT	26 weeks	NR
Vildagliptin vs. sitagliptin									
Novartis, 2011a [27]	Double blinded RCT	Novartis, 2011b [28]	84	NR	eGFR<30 ml/min/1.73 m^2	Vildagliptin (50 mg/day)+ sitagliptin matching placebo +SBT	Sitagliptin (25 mg/day)+ vildagliptin matching placebo+SBT	52 weeks (24+28)	NR

I, DPP-4 inhibitor group; C, control group; NA, not applicable; NR, not reported; HD, hemodialysis; PD, peritoneal dialysis; eGFR, estimated glomerular filtration rate; SBT, stable background therapy.
*For studies that used placebo as the comparison group for the first period of time (12 weeks) and sulfonylureas for an extended 40–42 weeks, only data from the first period were extracted for the meta-analyses.
#Only data for subjects with moderate to severe renal impairment in this trial were extracted for analysis.

Four studies (or six reports) compared DPP-4 inhibitors with placebo or no treatment in patients who were already treated with a stable antidiabetic therapy [17–22]. Two studies compared DPP-4 inhibitor monotherapy with glipizide monotherapy [24–25]. In addition, two studies used placebo as a control for the first period (12 weeks) followed by an extended 40–42-week sulfonylurea treatment, which was ignored because of the potential influence of the first period [16,23]. The final two studies also compared two different types of DPP-4 inhibitors [27–28] and compared the DPP-4 inhibitor with GLP-1 receptor agonist [26].

Risk of bias in the included studies and quality of the evidence

Random sequence generation was adequate in four of the ten trials (40%). The allocation concealment was stated clearly in one trial (10%). Nine trials (90%) blinded the participants, investigators, and outcome assessors. The outcome data were incomplete in five trials (50%), and selective reporting was not found. The loss to follow-up rate ranged from 0 to 51%. The risk of bias domains of the included studies are shown in Figures 2 and S1. The quality of evidence assessed using the GRADE approach ranged from moderate for any AE to low or very low for all other outcomes (Files S2 and S3).

Glycemic efficacy

HbA1c. The efficacy of the DPP-4 inhibitors was analyzed thoroughly and compared with the placebo or no treatment group. A statistically significant improvement was observed in HbA1c in individuals treated with DPP-4 inhibitors (random MD −0.52, 95%CI −0.64 to −0.39; $p<0.00001$) without heterogeneity ($I^2=0\%$; $p=0.70$) (Figure 3A). The HbA1c change was not significantly different in groups with varied dialysis statuses (test for subgroup differences $p=0.94$). The mean change was −0.50 in the non-dialysis group, compared with −0.49 in the dialysis group (Figure S2). Sensitivity analyses were performed to assess the change in HbA1c by excluding reports at a high risk of bias, eliminating unpublished reports, removing open-label studies, and using fixed-effects models. The results revealed that all the effect sizes were similar in magnitude and direction to the overall estimates (Table S2). The funnel plot (Figure 4) for this outcome was asymmetrical, which was confirmed using Egger's and Begg's tests ($p=0.013$ and $p=0.039$, respectively). The trim and fill method was also used to evaluate the influence of the possible missing studies. However, no trimming was performed and the data were unchanged.

According to the two trials (398 participants) that compared monotherapy using DPP-4 inhibitor or glipizide, there was no significant difference in HbA1c reduction between groups (random MD −0.08, 95%CI −0.40 to 0.25; $p=0.65$). The heterogeneity was moderate ($I^2=52\%$; $p=0.15$) (Figure 3B). A subgroup analysis in another study that compared the efficacy of sitagliptin and albiglutide revealed a significant difference in HbA1c reduction in moderate renal insufficiency patients (−0.53, 95%CI −0.80 to −0.26), whereas no difference was found in the severe renal insufficiency group (−0.47, 95%CI −1.12 to 0.18).

Responder rates: achieving an HbA1c of <7%. Four studies (838 participants) used achieving an HbA1c target of <7% as an outcome. Compared with the placebo or no treatment groups, the DPP-4 inhibitor groups had a higher proportion of patients who achieved the HbA1c goal (461 participants, random RR 1.94, 95%CI 1.40 to 2.70; $p<0.0001$). Heterogeneity was absent ($I^2=0\%$; $p=0.94$) (Figure 5A).

There was no difference in the proportion of patients receiving glipizide monotherapy and DPP-4 inhibitor monotherapy that

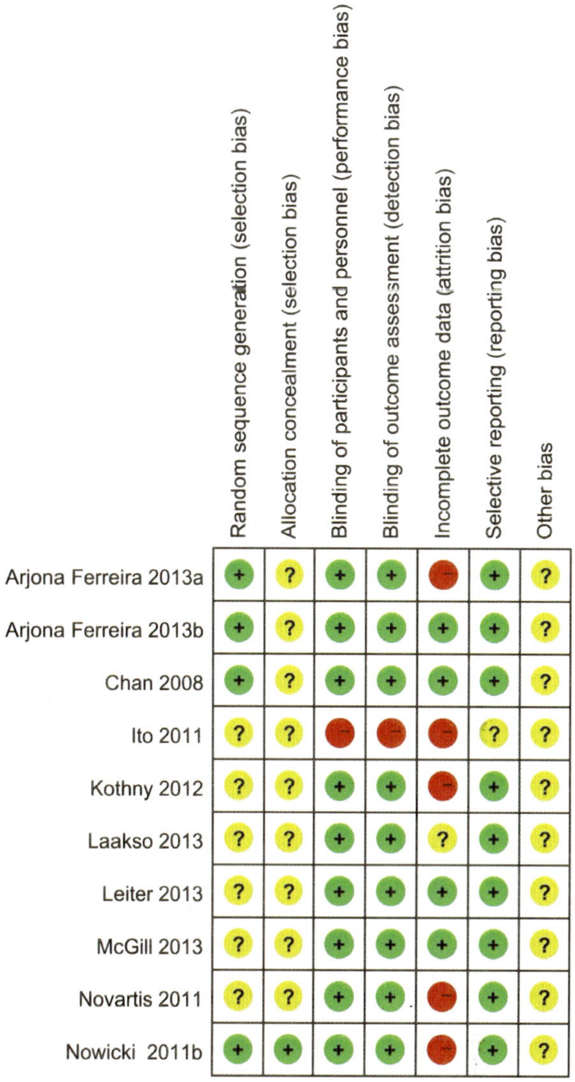

Figure 2. Risk of bias summary of the included studies.

achieved an HbA1c <7% (random RR 0.96, 95%CI 0.66 to 1.40; $p=0.84$); the heterogeneity was moderate ($I^2=64\%$; $p=0.09$) (Figure 5B).

Fasting blood glucose (FBG). Changes in FBG from baseline were described in six studies. As shown in Figure 6A, there was no significant decrease in FBG between the DPP-4 inhibitor and placebo groups, and the heterogeneity was moderate (522 participants, random MD −0.66, 95%CI −1.35 to 0.02, $p=0.06$; $I^2=48\%$). The result remained consistent after excluding reports at a high risk of bias (random MD −0.61, 95%CI −1.95 to 0.73, $p=0.37$; $I^2=76\%$), and dialysis patients (random MD −0.64, 95%CI −1.30 to 0.01, $p=0.05$; $I^2=32\%$). There was also no significant difference between DPP-4 inhibitor monotherapy and glipizide monotherapy (random MD 0.38, 95%CI −0.11 to 0.86; $p=0.13$); there was no heterogeneity ($I^2=0\%$; $p=0.60$) (Figure 6B).

Glycated albumin and 2-h postprandial glucose. Only one study (51 dialysis participants) that compared a DPP-4 inhibitor with a no treatment group reported glycated albumin and 2-h postprandial glucose. After 24 weeks of intervention with vildagliptin, the mean glycated albumin levels were decreased

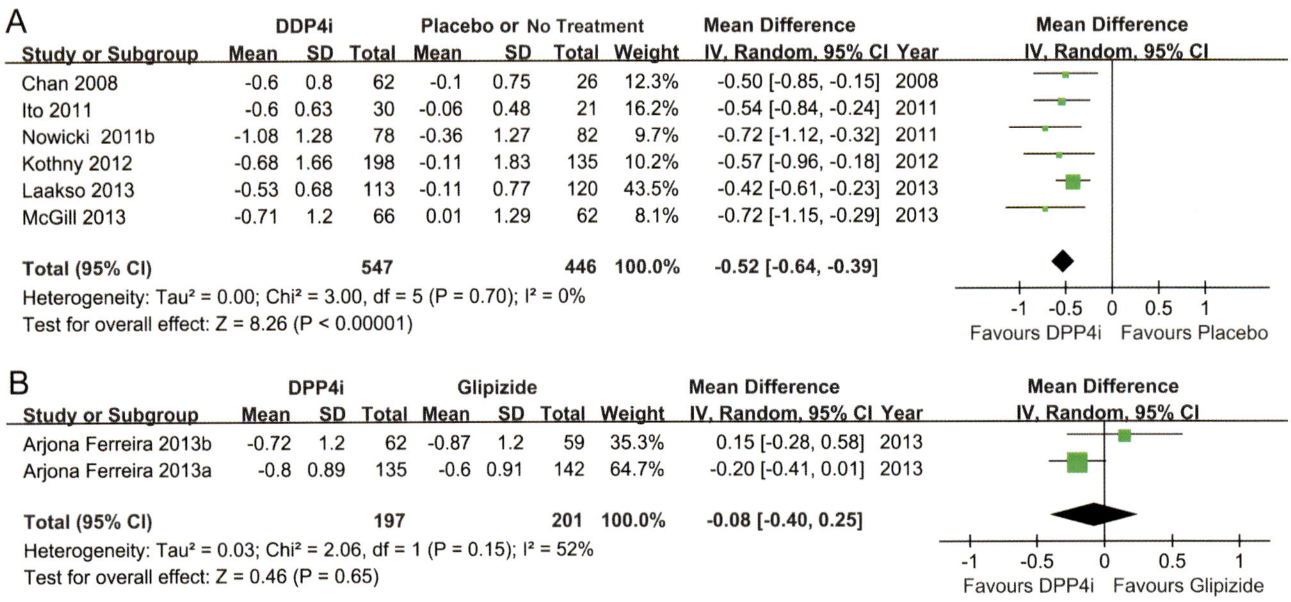

Figure 3. Meta-analysis for changes in HbA1c levels. A, DPP-4 inhibitor vs. placebo or no treatment. B, DPP-4 inhibitor vs. glipizide.

significantly from 24.5% at baseline to 20.5%, and the mean postprandial glucose levels decreased from 186 mg/dl at baseline to 140 mg/dl (all $p<0.0001$) [17].

Safety

Body weight. Seven trials reported changes in body weight, but only five trials (809 participants) were included in the pooled analysis. Compared with the placebo group, the DPP-4 inhibitor group had a neutral weight profile (432 participants, random MD −0.20, 95%CI −1.22 to 0.83; $p=0.71$). The heterogeneity was moderate ($I^2=64\%$; $p=0.06$) (Figure 7A). There were no significant differences in the non-dialysis group (341 participants; random MD −0.61, 95%CI −1.26 to 0.03; $p=0.06$). There was no heterogeneity ($I^2=0\%$; $p=0.46$). The dialysis group was excluded from the analysis because of its effect on dry weight.

DPP-4 inhibitor, but not glipizide monotherapy, treatment resulted in decreased body weight (377 participants, random MD −1.43, 95%CI −2.66 to −0.20; $p=0.02$). There was no heterogeneity ($I^2=0\%$; $p=0.52$) (Figure 7B).

Hypoglycemia. All studies reported the incidence of hypoglycemia, and seven of 10 studies also mentioned severe hypoglycemia; eight cases occurred in the DPP-4 inhibitor groups (464 participants), and ten occurred in the placebo groups (350 participants). Compared with placebo or no treatment, DPP-4

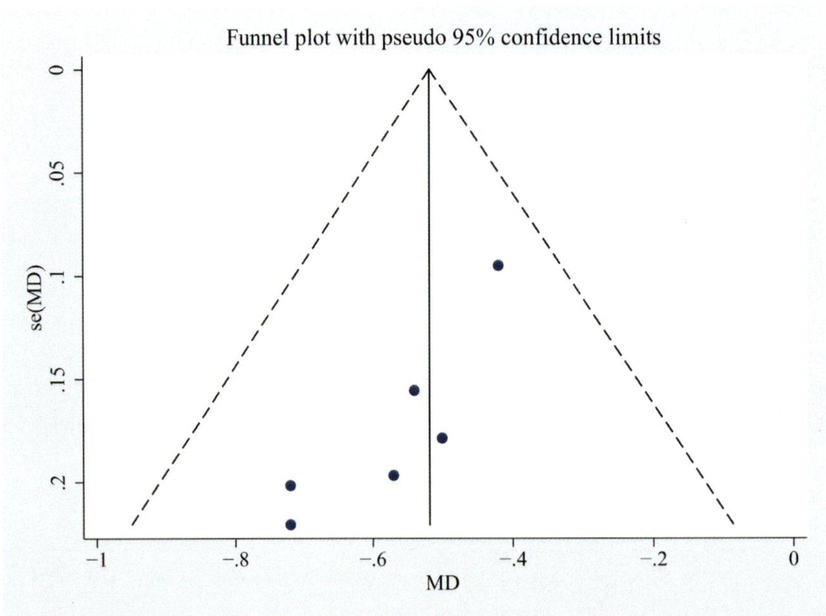

Figure 4. Funnel plot for mean difference (MD) in the change in HbA1c (DPP-4 inhibitor vs. placebo or no treatment).

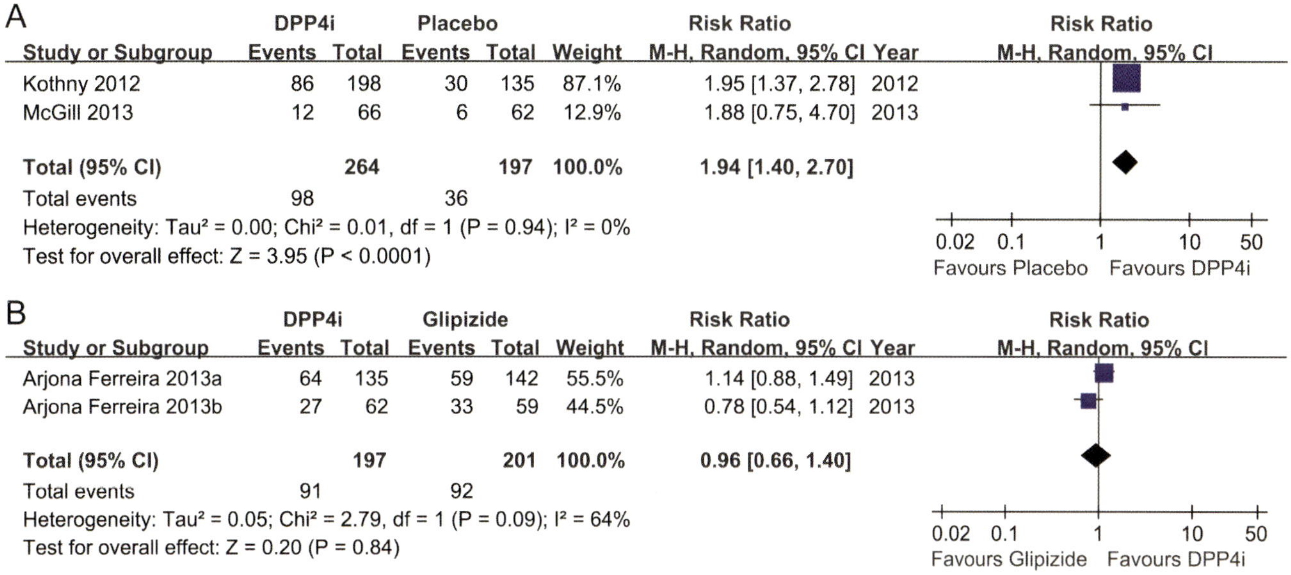

Figure 5. Risk ratio for achieving an HbA1c<7%. A, DPP-4 inhibitor vs. placebo. B, DPP-4 inhibitor vs. glipizide.

inhibitor therapy did not increase the incidence of hypoglycemia (1,049 participants, random RR 1.10, 95%CI 0.92 to 1.32; $p = 0.30$) (Figure 8A), and there was no heterogeneity ($I^2 = 0\%$; $p = 0.43$). Subgroup analyses according to dialysis status were not performed due to insufficient data.

Only two articles compared the effects of DPP-4 inhibitor and glipizide on hypoglycemia. Data revealed that the DPP-4 inhibitor group had a lower incidence of hypoglycemia than did the glipizide group (551 participants, random RR 0.40, 95%CI 0.23 to 0.69; $p = 0.0009$; there was no heterogeneity ($I^2 = 0\%$; $p = 0.42$) (Figure 8B). Compared with glipizide, the DPP-4 inhibitor reduced the incidence of severe hypoglycemia in dialysis patients significantly (five of 64 participants vs. 0 of 64, respectively) but not in non-dialysis patients (six cases of 212 participants vs. three cases of 210 participants). In contrast, there was no significant difference between vildagliptin and sitagliptin regarding their risk of causing hypoglycemia (0 cases of 46 participants vs. two of 38 participants, respectively).

Renal function and cardiovascular disease events. Seven studies assessed the relationship between DPP-4 inhibitors and renal function in non-dialysis patients using several parameters such as changes in eGFR (four studies), serum creatinine (one

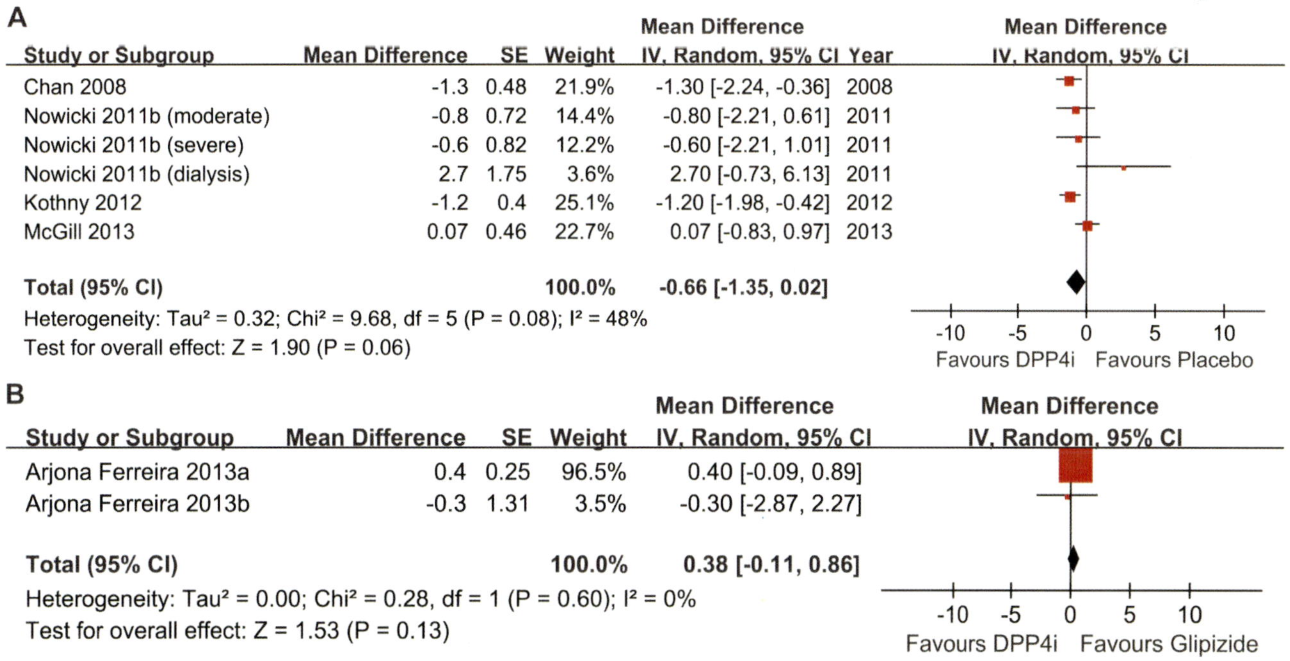

Figure 6. Meta-analysis for the change in fasting blood glucose. A, DPP-4 inhibitor vs. placebo. B, DPP-4 inhibitor vs. glipizide.

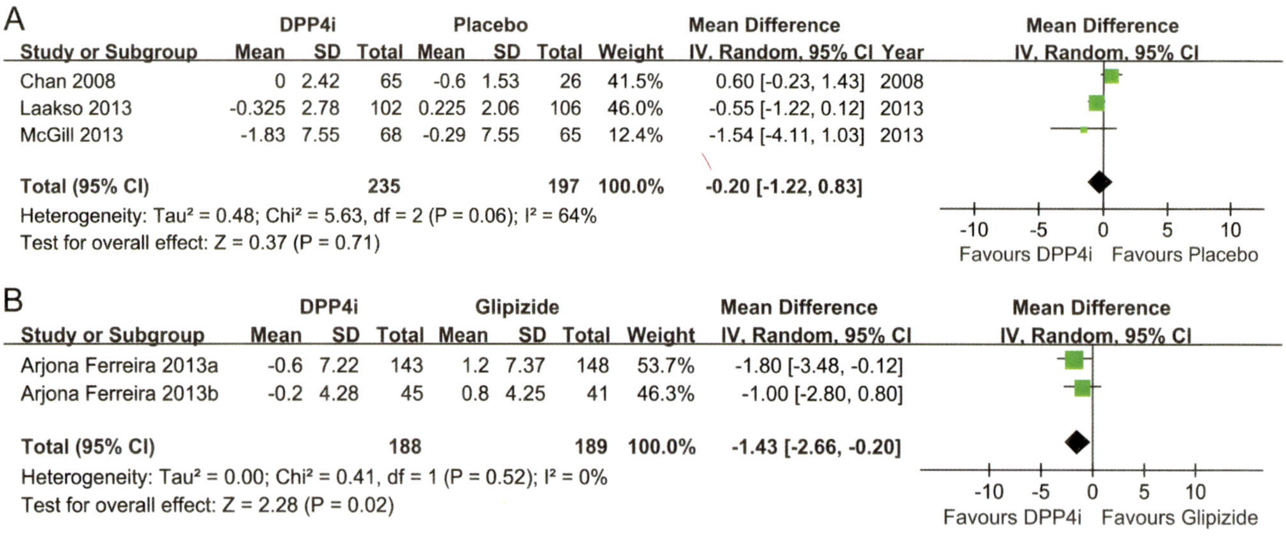

A

Study or Subgroup	DPP4i Mean	DPP4i SD	DPP4i Total	Placebo Mean	Placebo SD	Placebo Total	Weight	Mean Difference IV, Random, 95% CI	Year
Chan 2008	0	2.42	65	-0.6	1.53	26	41.5%	0.60 [-0.23, 1.43]	2008
Laakso 2013	-0.325	2.78	102	0.225	2.06	106	46.0%	-0.55 [-1.22, 0.12]	2013
McGill 2013	-1.83	7.55	68	-0.29	7.55	65	12.4%	-1.54 [-4.11, 1.03]	2013
Total (95% CI)			**235**			**197**	**100.0%**	**-0.20 [-1.22, 0.83]**	

Heterogeneity: Tau² = 0.48; Chi² = 5.63, df = 2 (P = 0.06); I² = 64%
Test for overall effect: Z = 0.37 (P = 0.71)

B

Study or Subgroup	DPP4i Mean	DPP4i SD	DPP4i Total	Glipizide Mean	Glipizide SD	Glipizide Total	Weight	Mean Difference IV, Random, 95% CI
Arjona Ferreira 2013a	-0.6	7.22	143	1.2	7.37	148	53.7%	-1.80 [-3.48, -0.12]
Arjona Ferreira 2013b	-0.2	4.28	45	0.8	4.25	41	46.3%	-1.00 [-2.80, 0.80]
Total (95% CI)			**188**			**189**	**100.0%**	**-1.43 [-2.66, -0.20]**

Heterogeneity: Tau² = 0.00; Chi² = 0.41, df = 1 (P = 0.52); I² = 0%
Test for overall effect: Z = 2.28 (P = 0.02)

Figure 7. Meta-analysis for changes in bodyweight. A, DPP-4 inhibitor vs. placebo. B, DPP-4 inhibitor vs. glipizide.

study), and the progression of renal status (two studies). Although four of the studies focused on a change in eGFR, a reliable pooled estimate could not be performed due to the varied objects used for comparison and a lack of accurate standard deviation values. Nevertheless, the individual studies showed no obvious effect of DPP-4 inhibitors on renal function.

Five studies (1,137 participants) reported cardiovascular disease (CVD) events. However, because different definitions of CVD events were used, a pooled estimate was not available. Table S3 shows the number of participants who experienced CVD events in each trial. There was no difference in CVD incidence between the DPP-4 inhibitor and control groups.

Total mortality and adverse events. Most studies reported total mortality and the incidence of adverse events, as summarized in Table 2. There was no obvious difference in mortality, the incidence of adverse events (any AE, SAE, drug-related AE, and drug-related SAE), and discontinuation rate.

Discussion

The current study used a complete search, integration, and analysis of data to perform a systematic assessment regarding the efficacy and safety of DPP-4 inhibitors in T2DM patients with moderate to severe renal impairment. In contrast to the placebo

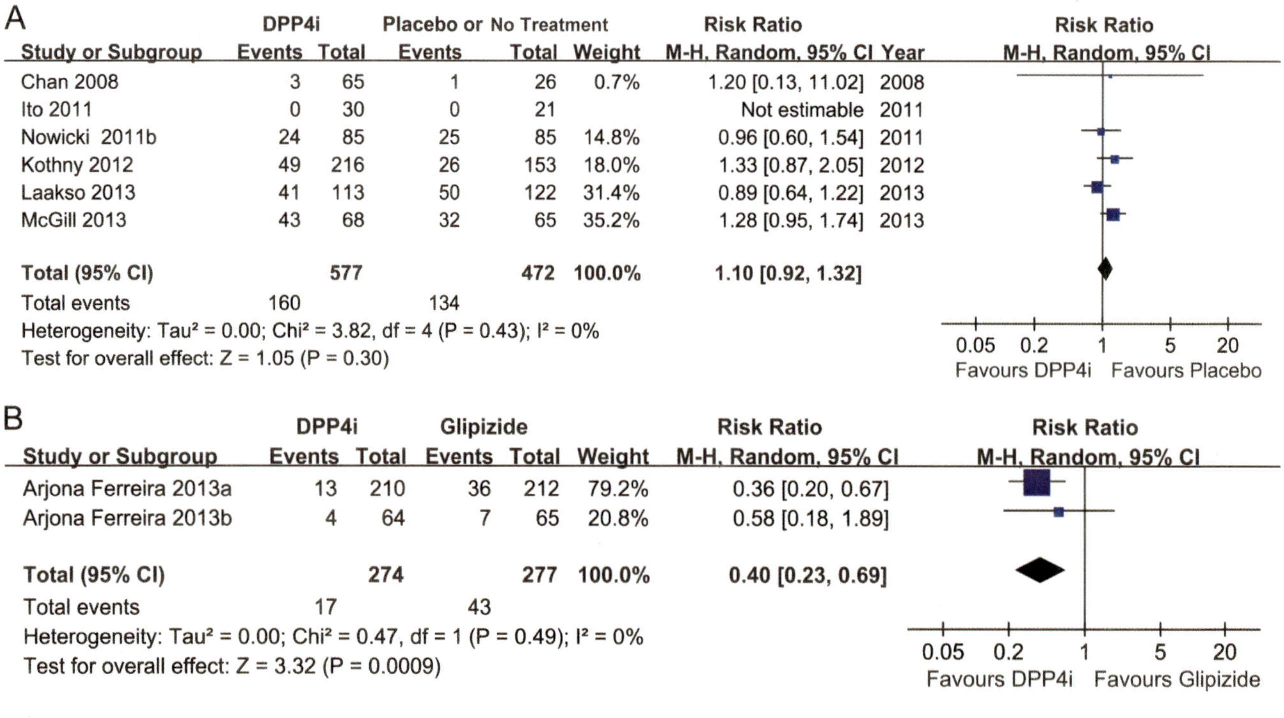

A

Study or Subgroup	DPP4i Events	DPP4i Total	Placebo or No Treatment Events	Placebo or No Treatment Total	Weight	Risk Ratio M-H, Random, 95% CI	Year
Chan 2008	3	65	1	26	0.7%	1.20 [0.13, 11.02]	2008
Ito 2011	0	30	0	21		Not estimable	2011
Nowicki 2011b	24	85	25	85	14.8%	0.96 [0.60, 1.54]	2011
Kothny 2012	49	216	26	153	18.0%	1.33 [0.87, 2.05]	2012
Laakso 2013	41	113	50	122	31.4%	0.89 [0.64, 1.22]	2013
McGill 2013	43	68	32	65	35.2%	1.28 [0.95, 1.74]	2013
Total (95% CI)		**577**		**472**	**100.0%**	**1.10 [0.92, 1.32]**	
Total events	160		134				

Heterogeneity: Tau² = 0.00; Chi² = 3.82, df = 4 (P = 0.43); I² = 0%
Test for overall effect: Z = 1.05 (P = 0.30)

B

Study or Subgroup	DPP4i Events	DPP4i Total	Glipizide Events	Glipizide Total	Weight	Risk Ratio M-H, Random, 95% CI
Arjona Ferreira 2013a	13	210	36	212	79.2%	0.36 [0.20, 0.67]
Arjona Ferreira 2013b	4	64	7	65	20.8%	0.58 [0.18, 1.89]
Total (95% CI)		**274**		**277**	**100.0%**	**0.40 [0.23, 0.69]**
Total events	17		43			

Heterogeneity: Tau² = 0.00; Chi² = 0.47, df = 1 (P = 0.49); I² = 0%
Test for overall effect: Z = 3.32 (P = 0.0009)

Figure 8. Meta-analysis for the risk of hypoglycemia. A, DPP-4 inhibitor vs. placebo. B, DPP-4 inhibitor vs. glipizide.

Table 2. Summary of safety outcomes for DPP-4 Inhibitors compared to comparators.

Outcome	Number of studies	Total number	Events	RR (95%CI)
Death				
PP-4 inhibitor vs. placebo	5	512/446	10/8	1.12 (0.44–2.85)
PP-4 inhibitor vs. glipizide	2	274/277	7/13	0.54 (0.22–1.33)
ildagliptin vs. sitagliptin	1	46/38	0/0	NA
Discontinuation				
PP-4 inhibitor vs. placebo	4	512/446	38/33	1.02 (0.65–1.60)
PP-4 inhibitor vs. glipizide	2	274/277	23/25	0.93 (0.54–1.60)
ildagliptin vs. sitagliptin	1	46/38	6/4	1.24 (0.38–4.07)
Any AE				
PP-4 inhibitor vs. placebo	4	482/425	397/342	1.01 (0.95–1.08)
PP-4 inhibitor vs. glipizide	2	274/277	196/205	0.97 (0.87–1.07)
SAE				
PP-4 inhibitor vs. placebo	4	482/425	105/94	0.97 (0.76–1.23)
PP-4 inhibitor vs. glipizide	2	274/277	57/58	0.99 (0.72–1.37)
ildagliptin vs. sitagliptin	1	46/38	15/10	1.24 (0.63–2.43)
Drug-related AE				
PP-4 inhibitor vs. placebo	3	397/350	113/105	0.96 (0.77–1.20)
PP-4 inhibitor vs. glipizide	2	274/277	37/52	0.72 (0.49–1.06)
Drug-related SAE				
PP-4 inhibitor vs. placebo	2	198/207	8/7	1.16 (0.43–3.10)
PP-4 inhibitor vs. glipizide	2	274/277	2/1	2.02(0.18–22.10)

AE, adverse event; SAE, serious adverse event; NA, not applicable.

and no treatment groups, the DPP-4 inhibitor groups typically had lower HbA1c levels, and a higher proportion of subjects that achieved the HbA1c goal of <7%; dialysis status did not affect these results. Sensitivity analysis indicated that the results were robust. There was no significant difference between the capacity of DPP-4 inhibitors and other active drugs such as sulfonylureas to reduce HbA1c levels. In contrast, DPP-4 inhibitors did not exhibit an FBG lowering effect, probably due to heterogeneity among the studies and an insufficient number of the samples. These results are consistent with those obtained in T2DM patients in similar studies [30–31]. It was reported previously that GLP-1 reduced HbA1c levels to a greater extent than did DPP-4 inhibitors [32–33], yet data in this article showed no difference between DPP-4 inhibitors and GLP-1 in severe renal dysfunction while a relatively poorer reducing effect of DPP-4 inhibitors was indeed observed in moderate renal dysfunction. The results might become more consistent with the previous reports if there was a larger sample size.

Regarding safety, data revealed that there was no change in the incidence of hypoglycemia with DPP-4 inhibitor treatment. The results remained consistent with dialysis patients with severe hypoglycemia. Moreover, there was no increase in weight gain, incidence of severe adverse effects, and total mortality. Although the definition of CVD was different among the trials included in this systematic review, no studies reported an increase in the incidence of CVD events as a result of DPP-4 inhibitor therapy. This is consistent with recent evidence showing that DPP-4 inhibitors did not increase CVD events in T2DM patients [34–35].

Although individual studies indicated that there was no deterioration in renal status during DPP-4 inhibitor administration, this conclusion could be strengthened by a pooled estimation on renal function. However, this could not be accomplished in the current study due to variations in the comparison objects and a lack of accurate standard deviation values. In addition, the effect of DDP-4 inhibitors on renal function in CKD patients remains unclear. Previous reports found either the progression of renal status or no affect on renal deterioration in patients treated with these agents [36–37]. Recently, studies assessing the attenuation of renal dysfunction in an ischemia-reperfusion injury model and remnant kidneys revealed that there might be a potential nephroprotective effect of DPP-4 inhibitors [38–39]. The mechanism for this might be associated with a reduction in apoptosis and inflammation and an increase in antioxidant production. Although a large number of ongoing trials have assessed the proteinuria-lowering effect of DPP-4 inhibitors [40–41], few primary articles have investigated the effect of these agents on renal status, particularly in individuals at an early stage of renal impairment. Therefore, there is little evidence that DPP-4 inhibitors could help delay the progression of renal status.

This is the first meta-analysis to assess the safety and efficacy of DPP-4 inhibitors in T2DM patients with moderate to severe renal impairment. The strength of this article is that it reports a comprehensive search that enrolled almost all the published and unpublished articles, including conferences abstracts, clinical trials registries, company websites, and FDA and EMA websites. In addition, a transparent GRADE approach provided an accurate assessment of the quality of evidence for each outcome.

However, the study also has some limitations. Notably, no studies at a low risk of bias were found, which could be attributed to several factors. For example, some studies might have inadequate random sequence generation and allocation sequence concealment. Moreover, the included open label study might have affected the results due to the lack of blinding. Articles with incomplete outcome data might have overestimated the efficacy of DPP-4 inhibitors on lowering HbA1c. In addition, all the above studies were sponsored by pharmaceutical companies, which might increase the risk of bias. A summary of the findings and the quality of evidence for this review are shown in Files S2 and S3. Although GRADE analysis indicated that the quality of evidence for each outcome was mostly low, 'any adverse events' were graded moderate. Due to insufficient data, our subgroup analyses were based on dialysis status rather than CKD stages. In addition, the dialysis group focused mainly on hemodialysis patients, with few data on peritoneal dialysis. However,it is quite necessary and difficult to establish good glycemic control for peritoneal dialysis patients due to the clinical use of glucose-containing dialysis solution [42]. Therefore, it is important to conduct further testing on the efficacy and safety of DPP-4 inhibitors in patients at various CKD stages and peritoneal dialysis. In addition, more attention should be paid to glycated albumin, which is a new and potentially better indicator of glycemic control, particularly in ESRD patients [43–44].

There are several different types of DPP-4 inhibitors, and each lacks sufficient testing. Therefore, we were unable to perform a detailed meta-analysis. The same problem exists for assessing the difference between DPP-4 inhibitors and other active agents, and for subgroup analyses based on different antidiabetic backgrounds.

Funnel plot asymmetry was observed and confirmed using Egger's and Begg's tests. This is recognized as a sign of potential publication bias. However, several alternative factors might also lead to asymmetry [45], including selection bias, poor methodological design, inadequate analysis in smaller studies, and true heterogeneity induced by factors such as different durations of intervention [46]. As shown in Figure 4, three studies in the lower left quadrant contributed to the asymmetry because of a long follow-up period and a high risk of bias (due to the inclusion of incomplete outcome data in two studies). Therefore, the asymmetry in our analysis might be attributed to true heterogeneity caused by clinical and methodological heterogeneity, even though no statistical heterogeneity was detected. Finally, it is inevitable that some unpublished articles might have been missed from the search.

This comprehensive analysis revealed that DPP-4 inhibitors lowered HbA1c, and did not increase the incidence of adverse events. Therefore, they represent a feasible treatment option for T2DM patients with moderate to severe renal impairment. However, considering the overall low quality of the data in this study, as judged by GRADE, DPP-4 inhibitors should be tested further in better-designed randomized trials. Additional attention should be paid to a comparison between DPP-4 inhibitors and other active drugs in patients at different stages of CKD, particularly including dialysis patients.

Conclusions

DPP-4 inhibitors are effective at lowering HbA1c in T2DM patients with moderate to severe renal impairment, and might lower the risk of adverse events. Further well-designed randomized trials focusing on the safety and efficacy of DPP-4 inhibitors in patients at different CKD stages are needed urgently because of the low quality of evidence in the current meta-analysis.

Supporting Information

Figure S1 Risk of bias graph of all included studies.

Figure S2 Subgroup analysis for change in HbA1c (DPP-4 inhibitor vs placebo or no treatment).

Table S1 PRISMA Checklist.

Table S2 Sensitivity analyses comparing DPP-4 inhibitors with placebo on HbA1c.

Table S3 Findings of comparing DPP-4 inhibitors with comparators on CVD.

File S1 Search strategies.

File S2 Summary of findings: Efficacy of DPP-4 inhibitors in type 2 diabetes mellitus patients with moderate to severe renal impairment.

File S3 Summary of findings: Safety of DPP-4 inhibitors in type 2 diabetes mellitus patients with moderate to severe renal impairment.

Acknowledgments

We thank all the members of our study team for their cooperation and the authors of the included trials for their wonderful work. We thank LetPub (www.letpub.com) for its linguistic assistance during the preparation of this manuscript.

Author Contributions

Conceived and designed the experiments: DC YF YL JL YC XW NW. Performed the experiments: DC YL JL YC XW NW. Analyzed the data: DC YF YL. Contributed reagents/materials/analysis tools: DC YL. Wrote the paper: DC YF NW.

References

1. National Kidney Foundation (2012) KDOQI Clinical Practice Guideline for Diabetes and CKD: 2012 update. Am J Kidney Dis 60:850–886.
2. Perkovic V, Heerspink HL, Chalmers J, Woodward M, Jun M, et al. (2013) Intensive glucose control improves kidney outcomes in patients with type 2 diabetes. Kidney Int 83:517–523.
3. Kidney Disease: Improving Global Outcomes (KDIGO) CKD Work Group (2013) KDIGO Clinical Practice Guideline for the Evaluation and Management of Chronic Kidney Disease. Kidney Int Suppl 3: 1–150.
4. Inzucchi SE (2002) Oral antihyperglycemic therapy for type 2 diabetes: scientific review. JAMA 287:360–372.
5. Nesto RW, Bell D, Bonow RO, Fonseca V, Grundy SM, et al. (2004) Thiazolidinedione use, fluid retention, and congestive heart failure: a consensus statement from the American Heart Association and American Diabetes Association. Diabetes Care 27:256–263.
6. Iglesias P, Diez JJ (2008) Insulin therapy in renal disease. Diabetes Obes Metab 10:811–823.
7. Drucker DJ, Nauck MA (2006) The incretin system: glucagon-like peptide-1 receptor agonists and dipeptidyl peptidase-4 inhibitors in type 2 diabetes. Lancet 368:1696–1705.
8. Park H, Park C, Kim Y, Rascati KL (2012) Efficacy and safety of dipeptidyl peptidase-4 inhibitors ,in type 2 diabetes: meta-analysis. Ann Pharmacother 46:1453–1469.
9. Giorda CB, Nada E, Tartaglino B (2014) Pharmacokinetics, safety, and efficacy of DPP-4 inhibitors and GLP-1 receptor agonists in patients with type 2 diabetes mellitus and renal or hepatic impairment. A systematic review of the literature. Endocrine DOI 10.1007/s12020-014-0179-0.

10. Ramirez G, Morrison AD, Bittle PA (2013) Clinical practice considerations and review of the literature for the Use of DPP-4 inhibitors in patients with type 2 diabetes and chronic kidney disease. Endocr Pract 19:1025–1034.
11. Liberati A, Altman DG, Tetzlaff J, Mulrow C, Gøtzsche PC, et al. (2009) The PRISMA statement for reporting systematic reviews and meta-analyses of studies that evaluate health care interventions: explanation and elaboration. Ann Intern Med 151:W65–W94.
12. Higgins JP, Altman DG, Gotzsche PC, Juni P, Moher D, et al. (2011) The Cochrane Collaboration's tool for assessing risk of bias in randomised trials. BMJ 343:d5928.
13. Guyatt G, Oxman AD, Akl EA, Kunz R, Vist G, et al. (2011) GRADE guidelines: 1. Introduction-GRADE evidence profiles and summary of findings tables. J Clin Epidemiol 64:383–394.
14. Deeks JJ, Higgins JPT, Altman DG (2011) Analysing data and undertaking meta-analyses. In: Higgins JPT, Green S, eds. Cochrane handbook for systematic reviews of interventions. Version 5.1.0. Oxford, UK:Cochrane Collaboration.
15. Higgins JP, Thompson SG, Deeks JJ, Altman DG (2003) Measuring inconsistency in meta-analyses. BMJ 327:557–560.
16. Chan JC, Scott R, Arjona Ferreira JC, Sheng D, Gonzalez E, et al. (2008) Safety and efficacy of sitagliptin in patients with type 2 diabetes and chronic renal insufficiency. Diabetes Obes Metab 10:545–555.
17. Ito M, Abe M, Okada K, Sasaki H, Maruyama N, et al. (2011) The dipeptidyl peptidase-4 (DPP-4) inhibitor vildagliptin improves glycemic control in type 2 diabetic patients undergoing hemodialysis. Endocr J 58:979–987.
18. Nowicki M, Rychlik I, Haller H, Warren ML, Suchower L, et al. (2011) Saxagliptin improves glycaemic control and is well tolerated in patients with type 2 diabetes mellitus and renal impairment. Diabetes Obes Metab 13:523–532.
19. Nowicki M, Rychlik I, Haller H, Warren M, Suchower L, et al. (2011) Long-term treatment with the dipeptidyl peptidase-4 inhibitor saxagliptin in patients with type 2 diabetes mellitus and renal impairment: a randomised controlled 52-week efficacy and safety study. Int J Clin Pract 65:1230–1239.
20. Lukashevich V, Schweizer A, Shao Q, Groop PH, Kothny W (2011) Safety and efficacy of vildagliptin versus placebo in patients with type 2 diabetes and moderate or severe renal impairment: a prospective 24-week randomized placebo-controlled trial. Diabetes Obes Metab 13:947–954.
21. Kothny W, Shao Q, Groop PH, Lukashevich V (2012) One-year safety, tolerability and efficacy of vildagliptin in patients with type 2 diabetes and moderate or severe renal impairment. Diabetes Obes Metab 14:1032–1039.
22. McGill JB, Sloan L, Newman J, Patel S, Sauce C, et al. (2013) Long-term efficacy and safety of linagliptin in patients with type 2 diabetes and severe renal impairment: a 1-year, randomized, double-blind, placebo-controlled study. Diabetes Care 36:237–244.
23. Laakso M, Rosenstock J, Groop PH, Hehnke U, Tamminen I, et al.(2013) Linagliptin vs placebo followed by glimepiride in Type 2 Diabetes patients with moderate to severe renal impairment. American Diabetes Association (ADA) 73rd Scientific Sessions, Chicago, USA.
24. Arjona Ferreira JC, Marre M, Barzilai N, Guo H, Golm GT, et al. (2013) Efficacy and safety of sitagliptin versus glipizide in patients with type 2 diabetes and moderate-to-severe chronic renal insufficiency. Diabetes Care 36:1067–1073.
25. Arjona Ferreira JC, Corry D, Mogensen CE, Sloan L, Xu L, et al. (2013) Efficacy and safety of sitagliptin in patients with type 2 diabetes and ESRD receiving dialysis: a 54-week randomized trial. Am J Kidney Dis 61:579–587.
26. Leiter L, Carr MC, Stewart M, Jones-Leone A, Yang F, et al. (2013) HARMONY 8: once-weekly glucagon-like peptide 1 receptor agonist albiglutide vs sitagliptin for patients with type 2 diabetes with renal impairment: week 26 results. European Association for the Study of Diabetes (EASD) 49th Annual Meeting, Barcelona, Spain.
27. Novartis Clinical Trial Results Database website. Available: http://www.novctrd.com/ctrdWebApp/clinicaltrialrepository/displayFile.do?trialResult=5924. Accessed: 2014 Jun 20.
28. Novartis Clinical Trial Results Database website. Available: http://www.novctrd.com/ctrdWebApp/clinicaltrialrepository/displayFile.do?trialResult=5923. Accessed: 2014 Jun 20.
29. Clinicaltrials.gov website. Available: http://www.clinicaltrials.gov./ct2/show/NCT01968044. Accessed: 2014 Jun 20.
30. Karagiannis T, Paschos P, Paletas K, Matthews DR, Tsapas A (2012) Dipeptidyl peptidase-4 inhibitors for treatment of type 2 diabetes mellitus in the clinical setting: systematic review and meta-analysis. BMJ 344:e1369.
31. Monami M, Iacomelli I, Marchionni N, Mannucci E (2009) Dipeptydil peptidase-4 inhibitors in type 2 diabetes: a meta-analysis of randomized clinical trials. Nutr Metab Cardiovasc Dis 20:224–235.
32. Pratley RE, Nauck M, Bailey T, Montanya E, Cuddihy R, et al. (2010) Liraglutide versus sitagliptin for patients with type 2 diabetes who did not have adequate glycaemic control with metformin: a 26-week, randomised, parallel-group, open-label trial. Lancet 375:1447–1456.
33. Wang T, Gou Z, Wang F, Ma M, Zhai SD (2014) Comparison of GLP-1 Analogues versus Sitagliptin in the Management of Type 2 Diabetes: Systematic Review and Meta-Analysis of Head-to-Head Studies. PLoS One 9:e103798.
34. White WB, Cannon CP, Heller SR, Nissen SE, Bergenstal RM, et al. (2013) EXAMINE Investigators. Alogliptin after acute coronary syndrome in patients with type 2 diabetes. N Engl J Med 369:1327–1335.
35. Scirica BM, Bhatt DL, Braunwald E, Steg PG, Davidson J, et al. (2013) SAVOR-TIMI 53 Steering Committee and Investigators.Saxagliptin and cardiovascular outcomes in patients with type 2 diabetes mellitus. N Engl J Med 369:1317–1326.
36. Kao DP, Kohrt HE, Kugler J (2008) Renal failure and rhabdomyolysis associated with sitagliptin and simvastatin use. Diabet Med 25:1229–1230.
37. Pendergrass M, Fenton C, Haffner SM, Chen W (2012) Exenatide and sitagliptin are not associated with increased risk of acute renal failure: a retrospective claims analysis. Diabetes Obes Metab 14:596–600.
38. Glorie LL, Verhulst A, Matheeussen V, Baerts L, Magielse J, et al. (2012) DPP4 inhibition improves functional outcome after renal ischemia-reperfusion injury, associated with antiapoptotic, immunological, and antioxidative changes. Am J Physiol Renal Physiol 303:F681–F688.
39. Joo KW, Kim S, Ahn SY, Chin HJ, Chae DW, et al. (2013) Dipeptidyl peptidase IV inhibitor attenuates kidney injury in rat remnant kidney. BMC Nephrol 14:98
40. Clinicaltrials.gov website. Available: http://www.clinicaltrials.gov./ct2/show/NCT01792518. Accessed: 2014 Jun 20.
41. Clinicaltrials.gov website. Available: http://www.clinicaltrials.gov./ct2/show/NCT02048904. Accessed: 2014 Jun 20.
42. Mehrotra R, de Boer IH, Himmelfarb J (2013) Adverse effects of systemic glucose absorption with peritoneal dialysis: how good is the evidence? Curr Opin Nephrol Hypertens 22:663–668.
43. Inaba M, Okuno S, Kumeda Y, Yamada S, Imanishi Y, et al. (2007) Glycated albumin is a better glycemic indicator than glycated hemoglobin values in hemodialysis patients with diabetes: effect of anemia and erythropoietin injection. J Am Soc Nephrol 18:896–903.
44. Freedman BI, Andries L, Shihabi ZK, Rocco MV, Byers JR, et al. (2011) Glycated albumin and risk of death and hospitalizations in diabetic dialysis patients. J Am Soc Nephrol 6:1635–1643.
45. Deeks JJ, Higgins JPT, Altman DG (2011) Addressing reporting biases. In: Higgins JPT, Green S, eds. Cochrane handbook for systematic reviews of interventions.Version 5.1.0. Oxford, UK: Cochrane Collaboration.
46. Egger M, Davey Smith G, Schneider M, Minder C (1997) Bias in meta-analysis detected by a simple, graphical test. BMJ 315: 629–634.

Associations between the Duration of Dialysis, Endotoxemia, Monocyte Chemoattractant Protein-1, and the Effects of a Short-Dwell Exchange in Patients Requiring Continuous Ambulatory Peritoneal Dialysis

Chia-Lin Wu[1,2,3]⁹, Hung-Ming Wu[4]⁹, Ping-Fang Chiu[1,2], Hung-Hsiang Liou[5], Chirn-Bin Chang[1,2], Der-Cherng Tarng[3,6,7]*, Chia-Chu Chang[1,2]*

1 Division of Nephrology, Department of Internal Medicine, Changhua Christian Hospital, Changhua, Taiwan, **2** School of Medicine, Chung-Shan Medical University, Taichung, Taiwan, **3** Institute of Clinical Medicine, National Yang-Ming University, Taipei, Taiwan, **4** Inflammation Research and Drug Development Center, Changhua Christian Hospital, Changhua, Taiwan, **5** Division of Nephrology, Department of Internal Medicine, Hsin Jen Hospital, Taipei, Taiwan, **6** Division of Nephrology, Department of Medicine, Taipei Veterans General Hospital, Taipei, Taiwan, **7** Department and Institute of Physiology, National Yang-Ming University, Taipei, Taiwan

Abstract

Background: Endotoxemia is exaggerated and contributes to systemic inflammation and atherosclerosis in patients requiring continuous ambulatory peritoneal dialysis (CAPD). The risk of mortality is substantially increased in patients requiring CAPD for >2 years. However, little is known about the effects of long-term CAPD on circulating endotoxin and cytokine levels. Therefore, the present study evaluated the associations between plasma endotoxin levels, cytokine levels, and clinical parameters with the effects of a short-dwell exchange on endotoxemia and cytokine levels in patients on long-term CAPD.

Methods: A total of 26 patients were enrolled and divided into two groups (short-term or long-term CAPD) according to the 2-year duration of CAPD. Plasma endotoxin and cytokine levels were measured before and after a short-dwell exchange (4-h dwell) during a peritoneal equilibration test (a standardized method to evaluate the solute transport function of peritoneal membrane). These data were analyzed to determine the relationship of circulating endotoxemia, cytokines and clinical characteristics between the two groups.

Results: Plasma endotoxin and monocyte chemotactic protein-1 (MCP-1) levels were significantly elevated in the long-term group. PD duration was significantly correlated with plasma endotoxin ($r = 0.479$, $P = 0.016$) and MCP-1 ($r = 0.486$, $P = 0.012$). PD duration was also independently associated with plasma MCP-1 levels in multivariate regression. Plasma MCP-1 levels tended to decrease (13.3% reduction, $P = 0.077$) though endotoxin levels did not decrease in the long-term PD group after the 4-h short-dwell exchange.

Conclusion: Long-term PD may result in exaggerated endotoxemia and elevated plasma MCP-1 levels. The duration of PD was significantly correlated with circulating endotoxin and MCP-1 levels, and was an independent predictor of plasma MCP-1 levels. Short-dwell exchange seemed to have favorable effects on circulating MCP-1 levels in patients on long-term PD.

Editor: Cordula M. Stover, University of Leicester, United Kingdom

Funding: This study was funded by grants 100-CCH-IRP-17 and 102-CCH-IRP-010 from the Changhua Christian Hospital Research Foundation. The funder had no role in study design, data collection and analysis, the decision to publish the results, or the preparation of the manuscript.

Competing Interests: The authors have declared that no competing interests exist.

* Email: dctarng@vghtpe.gov.tw (DCT); Chiachu@cch.org.tw (CCC)

⁹ These authors contributed equally to this work.

Introduction

Peritoneal dialysis (PD) is a well-established treatment modality for patients with end-stage renal disease. In Taiwan, about 6000 (10% of all patients undergoing dialysis) patients received PD in 2009 (Taiwan Renal Registry Data System, 2009) [1,2]. Patients treated with PD may have better independence, mobility, and quality of life than patients treated with hemodialysis (HD) [3]. Prior studies also revealed that PD confers a survival advantage compared with HD during the first 2 years of dialysis [4,5]. However, beyond 2 years, PD was associated with greater risk of mortality compared with HD [4]. Indeed, the long-term survival rate of patients undergoing PD is still poor (about 42% at 5 years) despite continued developments in modern medicine [6].

Cardiovascular disease, infection, and peritoneal fibrosis are common and clinically important complications of PD. Cardiovascular diseases are the most common causes of death in dialysis patients. Cardiovascular risk factors in PD patients include traditional (age, male gender, smoking, hypertension, diabetes and dyslipidemia), non-traditional (anemia, calcium-phosphate complex, inflammation, oxidative stress, etc.), and dialysis-related (bacteremia, hyperglycemia, and fluid overload) risk factors [7,8].

Endotoxin, also known as a bacterial lipopolysaccharide (LPS), is expressed on the outer membrane of the cell wall of Gram-negative bacterial pathogens, especially *Escherichia coli* [9,10]. Circulating endotoxin levels are higher in patients with advanced chronic kidney disease (CKD) and in dialysis patients than in other groups of patients [10]. Endotoxemia is also indicative of systemic inflammation, accelerated atherosclerosis, and malnutrition, and contributes to high rates of cardiovascular disease and mortality in dialysis patients [10–12]. Endotoxin was considered to be a modifiable factor for inflammation and nutrition in HD patients [13,14], although no interventional studies for reducing endotoxin levels in PD patients have been performed.

Proinflammatory cytokines, such as interleukin-6 (IL-6) and tumor necrosis factor (TNF), are elevated and are associated with hypoalbuminemia, left ventricular diastolic dysfunction, and mortality in PD patients [15–18]. Some studies have also demonstrated that the levels of anti-inflammatory cytokines, such as IL-10 and IL-1 receptor antagonist (IL-1RA), are elevated in PD patients [19,20].

The dwell time (the period of the dialysis solution in abdomen) has an important impact on dialysis adequacy (i.e., Kt/V_{urea}) and ultrafiltration. Long-dwell exchanges may enhance the clearance of uremic toxins such as creatinine and phosphate. However, a prolonged dwell time with a glucose-based solution actually decreases ultrafiltration because of the progressive reduction of the osmotic gradient. In a recent study, a longer daily dwell time was associated with peritoneal epithelial-to-mesenchymal transition [21]. Short-dwell exchanges (dwell time below 4 hours) may provide greater ultrafiltration, and improvements in blood pressure and fluid control, especially in patients with ultrafiltration failure [22]. However, it is unclear whether short- or long-dwell time has better effects on reducing peritoneal fibrosis, inflammation, and atherosclerosis.

To our knowledge, there is little information regarding the relationship between long-term PD, circulating endotoxin levels, and pro- and anti-inflammatory cytokine levels. Furthermore, no studies have demonstrated whether short-dwell dialysis reduces endotoxemia or inflammatory mediators. We hypothesized that endotoxin and proinflammatory cytokines may accumulate in patients requiring long-term CAPD and that their levels would be attenuated by a shorter dwell time compared with a longer dwell time.

Materials and Methods

Patients

Between October 1, 2011 and July 31, 2012, we performed an interventional, non-randomised, single-arm, pilot clinical study of 26 stable patients on CAPD at Changhua Christian Hospital PD center. The study was approved by the Institutional Review Board of Changhua Christian Hospital (approval number: 110317). All of the patients were treated with usual dwell time (4–6 hours during the day and 8–10 hours at night), clinically stable and without evidence of an active infection, and all received conventional glucose-based dialysates (Dianeal; Baxter Healthcare SA, Singapore Branch, Singapore). None of the patients were being treated with non-glucose-based PD solutions (e.g., icodextrin), immunosuppressants, non-steroidal anti-inflammatory drugs, iron supplements, or antioxidants such as vitamins C or E. All of the participants provided written informed consent before two blood tests to measure endotoxin and cytokine levels on the day of a peritoneal equilibration test (PET). All patients visited the clinic after an overnight fast and underwent conventional blood tests as well as additional tests to measure circulating endotoxin and cytokine levels.

Blood and urine sampling

Complete blood cell count, blood urea nitrogen, urinary urea nitrogen, serum creatinine, dialysate creatinine, urinary creatinine, serum high-sensitivity C-reactive protein (hs-CRP), total cholesterol, triglyceride, low-density lipoprotein cholesterol, high-density lipoprotein cholesterol, serum glucose, dialysate glucose, glycated hemoglobin, serum albumin, ferritin, iron, transferrin, and intact parathormone levels were measured using standardized procedures at the Department of Laboratory Medicine at Changhua Christian Hospital.

PET

Peritoneal equilibration test (PET) is a well-established method to determine the small solute transport function of peritoneal membrane [23]. Higher peritoneal solute transport rate has been linked to worse survival in PD patients [15]. We used a standardized procedure for PET, as proposed by Twardowski et al. [23]. In brief, the collection of peritoneal dialysate samples at several time intervals (0 hour, 2 hours and 4 hours) and a mid-point (2 hours) blood sample for measurement of urea, glucose and creatinine were obtained during the 4-hour exchange with 2 liter of 2.5% glucose dialysate. Dialysate to plasma ratios (D/P) at 4 hours for creatinine were used to quantify and classify individual peritoneal membrane characteristics.

Circulating endotoxin and cytokine levels

Blood samples for plasma endotoxin and various cytokines were obtained twice on the day of the PET. The first sample was collected after a long overnight dwell and the second sample was obtained after a subsequent short, 4-h dwell. Serum endotoxin levels were measured by a chromogenic Limulus Amebocyte Lysate assay (QCL-1000; Lonza, Walkersville, MD) as previously described [24]. The lower limit of detection was 0.1 endotoxin units (EU)/mL. Plasma levels of the proinflammatory cytokines IL-1β, IL-6, IL-8, IL-12p70, granulocyte-macrophage colony-stimulating factor (GM-CSF), interferon-γ (IFN-γ), and TNF were measured using a highly sensitive magnetic bead-based assay kit (MILLIPLEX MAP Kit, High Sensitivity Human Cytokine Magnetic Bead Kit – Premixed; EMD Millipore, Billerica, MA, USA) [25]. The levels of the proinflammatory cytokine monocyte chemoattractant protein-1 (MCP-1) and the anti-inflammatory mediators IL-10 and IL-1 receptor antagonist (IL-1RA) were assessed using another magnetic bead-based kit (MILLIPLEX MAP Kit, Human Cytokine/Chemokine Magnetic Bead Panel; EMD Millipore) [26]. All assays were performed in accordance with the manufacturers' instructions.

Statistical analysis

Results are expressed as the percentage, median (interquartile range) or mean ± standard error of the mean. Each variable was tested for normal distribution using the Shapiro-Wilk test.

Table 1. Demographics and clinical characteristics of the study patients.

Variable	Value
n	26
Sex (men/women)	17/9
Age (years)	46.4±1.9
Time on PD (months)	23.6 (7.1–67.7)
Primary renal diagnosis, n (%)	
Glomerulonephritis	13 (50)
Diabetic nephropathy	3 (11.5)
Hypertension	2 (7.7)
Tubulointerstitial disease	2 (7.7)
Polycystic kidney disease	2 (7.7)
Unknown	4 (15.4)
Comorbidities, n (%)	
Diabetes	8 (30.8)
Cardiovascular disease	8 (30.8)
CCI	2.5 (2–4)
BSA (/m^2)	1.76 (1.51–1.85)
BMI (kg/m^2)	23.6±0.7
WBC (/μL)	6550 (4850–8950)
Hemoglobin (g/dL)	9.9±0.3
Albumin (g/dL)	3.1±0.1
HbA1c (%)	5.6±0.2
Cholesterol (mg/dL)	182.7±8.0
Triglyceride (mg/dL)	92 (67–128.3)
LDL-C (mg/dL)	150.8±12.5
HDL-C (mg/dL)	48.8±4.4
Uric acid (mg/dL)	6.0±0.3
BUN (mg/dL)	61.2±3.3
Serum creatinine (mg/dL)	12.0±0.7
Serum Ca (mg/dL)	9.4±0.2
Serum P (mg/dL)	5.7±0.3
iPTH (pg/mL)	367.7 (182.8–666.1)
4-h D/P creatinine	0.67±0.028

Values are median (interquartile range), means±standard error of the mean or n (%).
4-h D/P creatinine, dialysate/plasma creatinine ratio at 4 hours; BSA, body surface area; BMI, body mass index; BUN, blood urea nitrogen; CCI, Charlson's comorbidity index; Ca, calcium; HbA1c, glycated hemoglobin; HDL-C, high-density lipoprotein cholesterol; iPTH, intact parathyroid hormone; LDL-C, low-density lipoprotein cholesterol; P, phosphorus; PD, peritoneal dialysis; WBC, white blood cell count.

Variables were analyzed using nonparametric statistical tests. Comparisons between two groups were made using the Mann–Whitney U test for continuous variables or the χ^2 test for categorical variables. The Wilcoxon signed-rank test was used to compare paired data. Correlations between pairs of continuous variables were determined by the Spearman rank correlation test. The multivariate regression analysis was performed to predict the independent influence of clinical/biological parameters on duration of PD. The significant variables in correlation analysis (age, Charlson's comorbidity index) and gender, diabetes, serum albumin, hs-CRP, plasma IL-1b, IL-6 and duration of PD were forced into the model to predict circulating endotoxin and MCP-1. All statistical analyses (including principal component analysis) were performed using SPSS Statistics for Windows, version 15 (SPSS Inc., Chicago, IL, USA). In all analyses, P-values of <0.05 were considered statistically significant.

Results

Patient characteristics

Twenty-six patients (17 men, 9 women) at our PD center were enrolled in this study and their data were suitable for statistical analysis. The mean age was 46.4 years (range, 21.1–62.7 years) and the median time on PD was 23.6 months (range, 1.1–134.4 months). Table 1 shows the baseline demographic and clinical characteristics of these patients. A principal-component analysis (PCA) was performed to reveal the major sources of variation of demographic, clinical and laboratory profiles in the dataset (Figure S1).

Table 2. Comparison of demographic and laboratory data between the short- and long-term PD groups.

	Short-term PD (n = 14)		Long-term PD (n = 12)		*P*-value
	Average±SD	**Range**	**Average±SD**	**Range**	
Demographic data					
Age (years)	49.4±10.8	21.1–62.7	43.0±7.2	28–57	0.02
Male gender (%)	78.6		50.0		0.22
BMI (kg/m^2)	24.3±3.7	16.1–30.3	22.8±3.8	17.4–29.4	0.20
SBP (mmHg)	133.1±21.1	80–150	139.7±12.7	120–150	0.54
DBP (mmHg)	81.3±12.1	60–100	80.1±9.9	65–96	0.69
CCI	3.43±1.40	2–6	2.42±0.67	2–4	0.049
Diabetes, n (%)	6 (42.9)		2 (16.7)		0.22
History of CAD, n (%)	5 (35.7)		3 (25.0)		0.68
PD duration (months)	10.9±8.6	1.1–23.7	72.8±34.0	32.6–134.4	<0.01
Laboratory data					
WBC (/μL)	8278.6±5139.3	3200–23900	6433.3±3575.3	600–15100	0.34
Hemoglobin (g/dL)	9.7±1.9	6.4–12.2	10.0±1.3	7.1–11.6	0.86
Albumin (g/dL)	3.1±0.4	2.3–3.7	3.3±0.3	2.9–3.7	0.25
hs-CRP (mg/dL)	1.05±1.71	0.01–5.90	0.77±1.73	0.01–6.18	0.51
HbA1c (%)	5.8±1.0	3.7–7.9	5.3±0.4	4.9–6.0	0.09
Creatinine (mg/dL)	11.9±4.0	7.0–19.3	12.0±2.9	6.6–15.7	0.82
Ferritin (ng/mL)	284.3±311.4	16.6–1188.6	308.8±376.0	13.7–1331.0	0.88
TSAT (%)	25.5±10.3	11.0–49.7	30.0±14.0	3.4–52.9	0.24
Dialysis-related variables					
4-h D/P creatinine	0.72±0.14	0.53–0.93	0.61±0.13	0.40–0.82	0.05
Weekly CrCL (L/week)	66.6±15.4	50.7–94.1	61.9±12.9	44.0–94.7	0.64
iPTH (pg/mL)	320.9±275.7	26.0–907.3	580.7±272.3	277.0–1324.4	0.02
nPNA (g/kg/day)	0.96±0.28	0.66–1.64	1.00±0.18	0.79–1.49	0.44
Endotoxin (EU/mL)	9.5±15.4	0–58.8	22.6±24.6	2.5–82.2	0.02
Cytokines					
MCP-1 (pg/mL)	301.0±111.5	159–563	489.4±263.7	270–1004	0.04
IL-1β (pg/mL)	4.3±4.0	0–11.9	4.6±5.2	0–16.4	0.92
IL-1RA (pg/mL)	129.3±53.6	42.3–236.0	157.4±102.4	4.8–390.0	0.46
IL-1β/IL-1RA ratio	0.030±0.026	0–0.066	0.027±0.027	0–0.068	0.88
IL-6 (pg/mL)	18.4±13.2	1.9–51.2	15.2±13.9	1.6–53.7	0.22
IL-8 (pg/mL)	21.6±6.7	7.5–31.5	23.5±8.4	12.6–46.0	0.96
IL-10 (pg/mL)	52.0±38.1	9.0–151.0	59.7±70.1	3.0–256.0	0.84
IL-12p70 (pg/mL)	16.39±13.13	0.01–42.38	15.29±14.57	0.01–40.37	0.80
TNF (pg/mL)	28.8±10.2	14.2–49.4	30.6±10.6	16.5–53.5	0.72
GM-CSF (pg/mL)	14.70±12.20	0.01–39.28	14.72±15.30	0.01–43.34	0.88
IFN-γ (pg/mL)	35.8±29.2	5.2–103.0	35.0±33.0	1.4–93.5	0.84

Values are means±standard deviation (SD), range or n (%).
CAD, coronary artery disease; CrCL, creatinine clearance; DBP, diastolic blood pressure; GM-CSF, granulocyte-macrophage colony-stimulating factor; hs-CRP, high-sensitivity C-reactive protein; IFN-γ, interferon-γ; IL, interleukin; IL-1RA, interleukin-1 receptor antagonist; MCP-1, monocyte chemoattractant protein-1; nPNA, normalized protein nitrogen appearance; SBP, systolic blood pressure; TNF, tumor necrosis factor; TSAT, transferrin saturation.

Comparisons between the short-term and long-term PD groups

Patients whose duration of PD was greater than 2 years (long-term PD group) were younger, had a lower Charlson's comorbidity index (CCI), and higher circulating intact parathyroid hormone (iPTH), endotoxin and MCP-1 levels than patients with short-term PD. Table 2 compares the demographic, laboratory, and dialysis-related data, as well as circulating endotoxin and cytokine levels between the short-term and long-term PD groups.

Correlations between patient characteristics and blood parameters

Age (49.4±2.9 years in short-term PD and 43.0±2.1 years in long-term PD, $P = 0.02$), CCI (3 (2–5) in short-term PD and 2 (2–3) in long-term PD, $P = 0.049$), and circulating iPTH (246.1

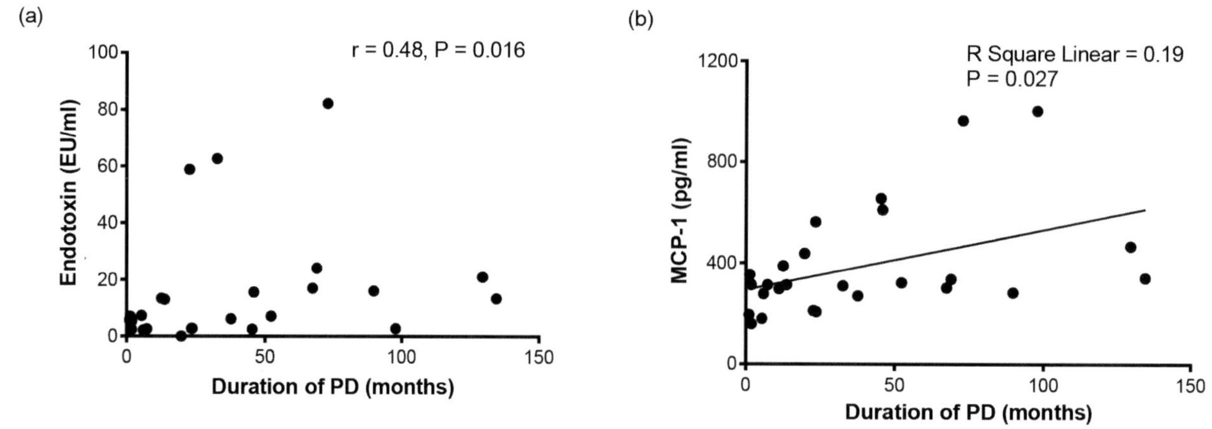

Figure 1. Correlations between the duration of peritoneal dialysis and serum endotoxin (a) and serum MCP-1 (b). A positive association between the duration of PD and serum endotoxin (a) and linear association between the duration of PD and serum monocyte chemoattractant protein-1 (b) levels in patients on CAPD.

(132.9–447.3) pg/ml in short-term PD and 537 (397.7–684.8) pg/ml in long-term PD, $P = 0.02$), endotoxin (5.4 (2.5–10.2) EU/ml in short-term PD and 15.9 (6.4–23.3) EU/ml in long-term PD, $P = 0.02$) and MCP-1 (306 (204–362.5) pg/ml in short-term PD and 339.5 (304.8–644.8) pg/ml in long-term PD, $P = 0.04$) levels were significantly different between the short-term and long-term PD groups (Table 2). PD duration was positively correlated with plasma endotoxin ($r = 0.479$, $P = 0.016$) and MPC-1 ($r = 0.486$, $P = 0.012$) levels and was negatively correlated with age ($r = -0.500$, $P = 0.009$) and CCI ($r = -0.389$, $P = 0.049$) (Figure 1 and Table 3). PD duration was not correlated with serum iPTH, albumin, cholesterol, triglyceride, low-density lipoprotein cholesterol, high-density lipoprotein cholesterol, uric acid, normalized protein nitrogen appearance, total weekly creatinine clearance, or plasma IL-1β, IL-1RA, IL-6, IL-8, IL-10, IL-12p70, TNF, GM-CSF, or IFN-γ levels (Table 3, Figure S2 and S3).

Multivariate analyses of plasma endotoxin and MCP-1 levels

The multivariate linear regression models for endotoxin and MCP-1 levels are shown in Table 4. PD duration was independently associated with elevated plasma MCP-1 (beta coefficient $= 0.545$, $P = 0.039$; Table 4).

Effects of short-dwell exchange on plasma endotoxin and MCP-1 levels

After a 4-h dwell, circulating endotoxin and cytokine levels were not significantly different between the short-term and long-term PD groups (Table 5). In the short-term PD group, plasma endotoxin and MCP-1 levels were not significantly different between before and after the 4-h exchange (Figure 2). In the long-term PD group, plasma endotoxin levels were not significantly different between before and after the exchange (Figure 2a). Plasma MCP-1 levels tended to decrease in the long-term PD group from 339.5 (304.8–644.8) pg/mL before the exchange to 294.5 (234.5–395.8) pg/mL after the exchange (13.3% reduction; $P = 0.077$; Figure 2b).

Discussion

The current study revealed that patients receiving CAPD for > 24 months had higher plasma endotoxin and MCP-1 levels than patients with a shorter PD duration. Circulating endotoxin and MCP-1 levels were also significantly correlated with the duration of PD. In addition, a short-dwell exchange was associated with a trend towards a decrease in plasma MCP-1 levels in patients on long-term PD.

Table 3. Correlations between PD duration, clinical parameters, and cytokine levels.

	Age	CCI	iPTH	Endotoxin	MCP-1
PD duration	$r = -0.500$ $P = 0.009$	$r = -0.389$ $P = 0.049$	$r = 0.373$ $P = 0.061$	$r = 0.479$ $P = 0.016$	$r = 0.486$ $P = 0.012$
Age	1	$r = 0.339$ $P = 0.09$	$r = -0.266$ $P = 0.188$	$r = -0.313$ $P = 0.128$	$r = -0.100$ $P = 0.628$
CCI		1	$r = -0.357$ $P = 0.073$	$r = -0.235$ $P = 0.259$	$r = -0.091$ $P = 0.657$
iPTH			1	$r = 0.022$	$r = 0.069$
				$P = 0.919$	$P = 0.736$
Endotoxin				1	$r = 0.030$
					$P = 0.887$

CCI, Charlson's comorbidity index; iPTH, intact parathyroid hormone; MCP-1 monocyte chemoattractant protein-1; PD, peritoneal dialysis; *r*, Spearman's rank correlation coefficient.

Table 4. Multivariate linear regression analyses of factors associated with circulating endotoxin and MCP-1 levels.

	β coefficient	95% CI	P value
Dependent variable: MCP-1			
PD duration	0.545	0.17, 5.85	0.039
Dependent variable: Endotoxin			
PD duration	0.208	−0.18, 0.40	0.430

CI, confidence interval; MCP-1 monocyte chemoattractant protein-1; PD, peritoneal dialysis.
Age, gender, diabetes, Charlson's comorbidity index, serum albumin, high-sensitivity C-reactive protein; interleukin-1β, and interleukin-6 were included as variables in this model.

Endotoxemia seems to be exaggerated by long-term PD and is associated with the peritoneal transport status. Elevated circulating endotoxin levels were also reported in patients with periodontal disease [27], diabetes mellitus [28], severe hepatic disease [29], or decompensated heart failure [30]. High endotoxin levels were also found in patients with advanced CKD and in patients on dialysis [10,12]. Circulating endotoxin levels were almost 6 times higher in patients on dialysis compared with those who were not [10]. A population-based chronic disease risk survey demonstrated that high endotoxin level increased the risk for incident cardiovascular disease at 10 years (hazard ratio 1.82) [27]. Additionally, circulating endotoxemia was associated with systemic inflammation, malnutrition, atherosclerosis, and increased mortality in patients with advanced CKD and in patients on dialysis [10,12]. Endotoxemia is thought to involve the translocation of endotoxin by a number of mechanisms. The authors [10] postulated that HD-induced splanchnic hypoperfusion may contribute to endotoxemia in HD patients while enteric venous congestion or edema may contribute to endotoxemia in PD patients. In addition, it is currently unknown which cytokine is involved or plays a dominant role in the etiology of systemic inflammation in patients on long-term PD. Our study revealed that circulating endotoxin and proinflammatory MCP-1 levels were elevated in patients on long-term PD. Conventional peritoneal dialysate fluids abolished in vivo leukocyte recruitment in response to lipopolysaccharide and may adversely affect the peritoneal host defense [31]. Additionally, patients who require PD for a long time may have severe periodontal disease [32], venous congestion or gastrointestinal edema because of reduced ultrafiltration, and the presence of more co-morbidities could exacerbate endotoxemia. LPS monomers are released from LPS aggregates by LPS-binding protein. These monomers are transferred to CD14 expressed on the membrane of circulating monocytes, resulting in monocyte activation and the production of proinflammatory mediators [33,34]. The binding of LPS monomers to soluble CD14 expressed by endothelial cells induces cytokine production and atherosclerosis through the Toll-like receptor 4 signaling pathway [33,35]. This signaling pathway induces MCP-1 production in murine peritoneal mesothelial cells and recruits leukocytes into the peritoneal cavity [36]. Higher endotoxin levels are associated with increased mortality risk in patients with CKD and dialysis patients [10]. Therefore, it seems feasible that patients on long-term PD may have more advanced atherosclerosis and cardiovascular disease, conferring increased risk of mortality.

Peritoneal fibrosis is a major cause of encapsulating peritoneal sclerosis, the most serious complications in patients on long-term PD, and is linked to ultrafiltration failure and higher mortality [37]. MCP-1 is closely related to inflammation and fibrosis induced by LPS, and is believed to be a good target for treating endotoxemia, sepsis, and peritoneal fibrosis [36,38,39]. Circulating MCP-1 level predicts LPS-induced murine systemic inflammation [40]. MCP-1 induces proliferation in human smooth muscle cells and is crucial to the initiation of atherosclerosis [41,42]. Elevated circulating MCP-1 levels were associated with

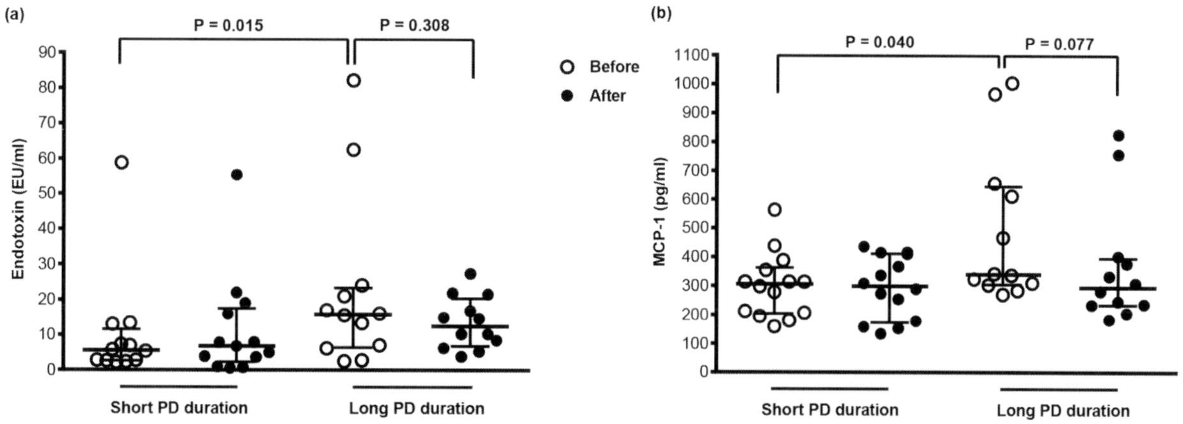

Figure 2. Comparison of circulating endotoxin (a) and MCP-1 (b) levels before and after a 4-h exchange between the short- and long-term PD groups. Circulating endotoxin and MCP-1 levels before a 4-hour exchange were significantly elevated in the long PD duration group. In the short PD duration group, plasma endotoxin and MCP-1 levels were not significantly different between before and after a 4-hour exchange. In the long PD duration group, plasma endotoxin levels were not significantly different after a 4-hour exchange (a). Plasma MCP-1 levels tended to decrease after a 4-hour exchange (b).

Table 5. Comparison of circulating endotoxin and cytokine levels after a 4-h exchange between the short- and long-term PD groups.

	PD duration				*P*-value
	Short (n = 14)	Baseline (% change)	Long (n = 12)	Baseline (% change)	
Endotoxin (EU/mL)	6.8 (2.4–17.6)	5.4 (2.5–10.2) (25.9%)	12.5 (6.9–20.4)	15.9 (6.4–23.3) (21.4%)	0.14
MCP-1 (pg/mL)	298.5 (173–411.3)	306 (204–362.5) (2.5%)	294.5 (234.5–395.8)	339.5 (304.8–644.8) (13.3%)	0.78
IL-1β (pg/mL)	5.7 (0–8.2)	4.8 (0–7.2) (18.8%)	3.1 (0.3–8.6)	2.7 (0.2–8.3) (14.8%)	0.86
IL-1RA (pg/mL)	149.6±18.5	129.3±14.3 (15.7%)	148±21.6	157.4±29.6 (6%)	0.64
IL-1β/IL-1RA ratio	0.027 (0–0.058)	0.027 (0–0.054) (0%)	0.028 (0.002–0.046)	0.012 (0.002–0.054) (133.3%)	0.94
IL-6 (pg/mL)	16.1 (10.1–21.6)	17.1 (9–21.5) (5.8%)	10.9 (5.4–16.4)	12.5 (6.9–16.5) (12.8%)	0.30
IL-8 (pg/mL)	22.1±2.3	21.6±1.8 (2.3%)	23.6±2.6	23.5±2.4 (0.4%)	1.00
IL-10 (pg/mL)	53.1 (22.6–93.9)	48.8 (21–69.9) (8.8%)	32.7 (13.6–85.7)	31.6 (18.1–73.3) (3.5%)	0.72
IL-12p70 (pg/mL)	18.8 (2–28.4)	16.8 (4.1–25.3) (11.9%)	10.2 (3.7–26.6)	10.6 (2.8–26.9) (3.8%)	0.86
TNF (pg/mL)	31.9±3.2	28.8±2.7 (10.8%)	32.7±3.3	30.6±3.0 (6.9%)	0.94
GM-CSF (pg/mL)	17.2 (0–29)	13.9 (3–24.6) (23.7%)	12.5 (1.2–29.8)	8.9 (0.8–26.4) (40.4%)	0.92
IFN-γ (pg/mL)	39.6 (4.7–68.6)	31.0 (10.4–54.2) (27.7%)	24.2 (9.9–63.2)	22.8 (9.9–62.9) (6.1%)	0.84

Values are median (interquartile range) or means±standard error of the mean.
% change, percentage change; GM-CSF, granulocyte-macrophage colony-stimulating factor; IFN-γ, interferon-γ; IL, interleukin; IL-1RA, interleukin-1 receptor antagonist; MCP-1, monocyte chemoattractant protein-1; TNF, tumor necrosis factor.

traditional risk factors for atherosclerosis and an increased risk of myocardial infarction or death in patients with acute coronary syndromes [43]. MCP-1 was also associated with an increased risk of recurrent cardiovascular events in diabetic patients with acute ischemic stroke [44]. In a previous study [45], plasma MCP-1 levels were 1.8-fold elevated in patients on dialysis compared with controls and the duration of dialysis was associated with elevated plasma MCP-1 levels and oxidative stress. Another study showed that MCP-1 concentrations in the PD effluent were positively related to serum MCP-1 and duration of PD [46]. Administration of LPS increases plasma MCP-1 levels *in vivo* [47,48]. Endotoxin was also capable of inducing MCP-1 production in peritoneal mesothelial cells and may play an important role in peritoneal fibrosis according to prior *in vitro* studies [36,49]. In the current study, we found that the PD duration was independently associated with plasma MCP-1 levels. Taken together, the higher circulating endotoxin and MCP-1 levels may reflect the inflammatory and fibrotic environment in the peritoneum, and might contribute to the poor outcomes in these patients.

Despite the increased levels of circulating endotoxin and MCP-1, we did not observe elevated levels of the anti-inflammatory mediators IL-10 and IL-1RA in patients on long-term PD. This imbalance between proinflammatory and anti-inflammatory cytokines had been reported in patients with chronic renal failure and dialysis patients [50,51].

Previous studies have showed that epidermal growth factor, L-glutamine, oats supplementation, or zinc may reduce circulating endotoxin by preserving intestinal integrity in alcoholic liver disease [52]. Administration of rosiglitazone was also associated with a reduction in circulating endotoxin levels in patients with type 2 diabetes [28]. Additionally, sevelamer, a non-calcium-based phosphate binder, was reported to reduce plasma endotoxin levels in HD patients [13]. CAPD was thought to be associated with a slow but relatively constant clearance rate of large molecules [53]. MCP-1 has a much smaller molecular weight (13 kDa) than the LPS–LPS binding protein complex (70–80 kDa) or LPS aggregates (>1000 kDa) and is thought to be readily removed from the peritoneum by PD [54–56]. In the current study, we observed a trend towards a decrease in plasma MCP-1 levels ($P = 0.077$) but not in plasma endotoxin levels after a short-dwell exchange. Because of progressive ultrafiltration loss, gastrointestinal venous congestion or edema may be exaggerated during an overnight dwell with conventional glucose solutions in long-term PD patients. It is likely that endotoxin and MCP-1 are released during overnight dwells and MCP-1 may be removed by short-dwell exchanges in these patients. Automated peritoneal dialysis (APD) with short-dwell exchanges enhances ultrafiltration in many patients, especially in patients with high peritoneal solute transport [57]. Further studies are needed to clarify whether short-dwell exchange with APD reduces endotoxemia or MCP-1 and reduces the risk of atherosclerosis, peritoneal membrane failure, and mortality.

There are several limitations of our study. First, we only enrolled 26 patients and used a cross-sectional design rather than a longitudinal design. We did not perform a prospective follow-up and the small sample size reduced the statistical power of this study. Second, although the duration of PD was associated with circulating endotoxin and MCP-1 levels, we did not measure their levels in the PD effluent. Third, there may be some selection bias because patients on long-term PD were younger and their CCI was lower than patients on short-term PD. This selection bias may result in an underestimate of the true associations in both groups of PD patients. Fourth, single-point measurements of endotoxin and cytokine levels may result in the lack of a true 'baseline' or the possible inter-individual variability. Finally, we did not perform a pathological study of the peritoneum or determine the extent of peritoneal inflammation or fibrosis. Further studies such as multiple measurements of endotoxin and cytokine levels or obtaining serial blood/effluent samples during the short-dwell exchange would be needed to clarify these issues.

Conclusions

This was the first study to show the effect of short-dwell exchange in terms of lowering circulating MCP-1 levels in patients on long-term PD. We found that the duration of PD was positively and significantly correlated with plasma endotoxin and proinflammatory MCP-1 levels, and that the duration of PD was independently associated with the MCP-1 level. Anti-inflammatory cytokine levels might not be significantly different between the short-term and long-term PD patients. Short-dwell exchange seemed to have favorable effects on circulating MCP-1 levels in patients on long-term PD. Further studies are warranted to elucidate whether short-dwell exchange reduces endotoxemia and MCP-1 and is a preferable regimen in patients on long-term PD.

Supporting Information

Figure S1 Principal-component analysis (PCA) loading plot (a) and scores plot (b). (a) The first principal component (PC-1) accounts for 23.3% of the variance and is primarily defined by dialysate/plasma creatinine ratio at 4 hours (4-h D/P creatinine), body mass index (BMI), body surface area (BSA), Charlson's comorbidity index (CCI), glycated hemoglobin (HbA1c) and hemoglobin (Hb). The second principal component (PC-2) accounts for 16.9% of the variance and is defined by serum creatinine, phosphorus (P), age, weekly creatinine clearance (CrCL), uric acid, intact parathyroid hormone (iPTH), PD duration, ferritin, and albumin. The third principal component (PC-3) accounts for 11.2% of the variance and is defined by normalized protein nitrogen appearance (nPNA), serum calcium (Ca), cholesterol and white blood cell count (WBC). (b) Scores plot of 26 patients in a three-dimensional space derived from PCA. The scores plot shows grouping of the demographic and laboratory profiles between short (blue open circle) and long (green open triangle) PD duration groups.

Figure S2 Correlations between the duration of PD and biological (a–f) and dialysis-related (g–i) parameters in patients on CAPD. Duration of PD was not correlated with serum albumin (a), cholesterol (b), triglyceride (c), low-density lipoprotein cholesterol (d), high-density lipoprotein cholesterol (e), uric acid (f), normalized protein nitrogen appearance (g), or total weekly creatinine clearance (h).

Figure S3 Correlations between the duration of PD and various serum cytokine levels except MCP-1 in patients on CAPD. Duration of PD was not correlated with plasma interleukin-1β (a), interleukin-1 receptor antagonist (b), interleukin-6 (c), interleukin-8 (d), interleukin-10 (e), interleukin-12p70 (f), tumor necrosis factor (g), granulocyte-macrophage colony-stimulating factor (h), or interferon-γ (i) levels.

Author Contributions

Conceived and designed the experiments: HMW CCC. Performed the experiments: HMW CBC. Analyzed the data: CLW HMW PFC CCC. Contributed reagents/materials/analysis tools: CLW HMW PFC HHL DCT CCC. Wrote the paper: CLW HMW.

References

1. Wu M-S, Wu I-W, Shih C-P, Hsu K-H (2011) Establishing a Platform for Battling End-Stage Renal Disease and Continuing Quality Improvement in Dialysis Therapy in Taiwan-Taiwan Renal Registry Data System (TWRDS). Acta Nephrologica 25: 148–153.
2. Wu M-S, Wu I-W, Hsu K-H (2012) Survival Analysis of Taiwan Renal Registry Data System (TWRDS) 2000–2009. Acta Nephrologica 26: 104–108.
3. Chaudhary K, Sangha H, Khanna R (2011) Peritoneal dialysis first: rationale. Clinical journal of the American Society of Nephrology: CJASN 6: 447–456.
4. Termorshuizen F, Korevaar JC, Dekker FW, Van Manen JG, Boeschoten EW, et al. (2003) Hemodialysis and peritoneal dialysis: comparison of adjusted mortality rates according to the duration of dialysis: analysis of The Netherlands Cooperative Study on the Adequacy of Dialysis 2. Journal of the American Society of Nephrology: JASN 14: 2851–2860.
5. Jaar BG, Coresh J, Plantinga LC, Fink NE, Klag MJ, et al. (2005) Comparing the risk for death with peritoneal dialysis and hemodialysis in a national cohort of patients with chronic kidney disease. Annals of internal medicine 143: 174–183.
6. U.S. Renal Data System, USRDS 2013 Annual Data Report: Atlas of Chronic Kidney Disease and End-Stage Renal Disease in the United States, National Institutes of Health, National Institute of Diabetes and Digestive and Kidney Diseases, Bethesda, MD.
7. Rucker D, Tonelli M (2009) Cardiovascular risk and management in chronic kidney disease. Nature reviews Nephrology 5: 287–296.
8. Chiu YW, Mehrotra R (2010) Can we reduce the cardiovascular risk in peritoneal dialysis patients? Indian journal of nephrology 20: 59–67.
9. Raetz CR, Whitfield C (2002) Lipopolysaccharide endotoxins. Annual review of biochemistry 71: 635–700.
10. McIntyre CW, Harrison LE, Eldehni MT, Jefferies HJ, Szeto CC, et al. (2011) Circulating endotoxemia: a novel factor in systemic inflammation and cardiovascular disease in chronic kidney disease. Clinical journal of the American Society of Nephrology: CJASN 6: 133–141.
11. Lassenius MI, Pietilainen KH, Kaartinen K, Pussinen PJ, Syrjanen J, et al. (2011) Bacterial endotoxin activity in human serum is associated with dyslipidemia, insulin resistance, obesity, and chronic inflammation. Diabetes care 34: 1809–1815.
12. Szeto CC, Kwan BC, Chow KM, Lai KB, Chung KY, et al. (2008) Endotoxemia is related to systemic inflammation and atherosclerosis in peritoneal dialysis patients. Clinical journal of the American Society of Nephrology: CJASN 3: 431–436.
13. Navarro-Gonzalez JF, Mora-Fernandez C, Muros de Fuentes M, Donate-Correa J, Cazana-Perez V, et al. (2011) Effect of phosphate binders on serum inflammatory profile, soluble CD14, and endotoxin levels in hemodialysis patients. Clinical journal of the American Society of Nephrology: CJASN 6: 2272–2279.
14. Kubotera N, Prokopienko AJ, Garba AO, Pai AB (2013) Endotoxin binding by sevelamer: potential impact on nutritional status. International journal of nephrology 2013: 954956.
15. Lambie M, Chess J, Donovan KL, Kim YL, Do JY, et al. (2013) Independent effects of systemic and peritoneal inflammation on peritoneal dialysis survival. Journal of the American Society of Nephrology: JASN 24: 2071–2080.
16. Okyay GU, Er RE, Tekbudak MY, Pasaoglu O, Inal S, et al. (2013) Novel inflammatory marker in dialysis patients: YKL-40. Therapeutic apheresis and dialysis: official peer-reviewed journal of the International Society for Apheresis, the Japanese Society for Apheresis, the Japanese Society for Dialysis Therapy 17: 193–201.
17. Lee JK, Lin HH, Tsai CT, Chen JJ, Kuo CC, et al. (2012) Differential association of proinflammatory cytokines with left ventricular diastolic dysfunction in subjects with and without continuous ambulatory peritoneal dialysis. Nutrition, metabolism, and cardiovascular diseases: NMCD 22: 974–980.
18. Shioya M, Yoshida T, Kasai K, Furuya R, Kato A, et al. (2013) Inflammatory factors for hypoalbuminemia in Japanese peritoneal dialysis patients. Nephrology 18: 539–544.
19. Borazan A, Ustun H, Ustundag Y, Aydemir S, Bayraktaroglu T, et al. (2004) The effects of peritoneal dialysis and hemodialysis on serum tumor necrosis factor-alpha, interleukin-6, interleukin-10 and C-reactive-protein levels. Mediators of inflammation 13: 201–204.
20. Pereira BJ, Shapiro L, King AJ, Falagas ME, Strom JA, et al. (1994) Plasma levels of IL-1 beta, TNF alpha and their specific inhibitors in undialyzed chronic renal failure, CAPD and hemodialysis patients. Kidney international 45: 890–896.
21. Lee YC, Tsai YS, Hung SY, Lin TM, Lin SH, et al. (2014) Shorter daily dwelling time in peritoneal dialysis attenuates the epithelial-to-mesenchymal transition of mesothelial cells. BMC nephrology 15: 35.
22. Strauss FG, Holmes DL, Dennis RL, Nortman DF (1993) Short-dwell peritoneal dialysis: increased use and impact on clinical outcome. Advances in peritoneal dialysis Conference on Peritoneal Dialysis 9: 49–51.
23. Twardowski ZJ, Nolph KD, Khanna R, Prowant BF, Ryan LP, et al. (1987) PERITONEAL EQUILIBRATION TEST. Peritoneal Dialysis Bulletin 7: 138–147.
24. Jialal I, Huet BA, Kaur H, Chien A, Devaraj S (2012) Increased toll-like receptor activity in patients with metabolic syndrome. Diabetes care 35: 900–904.
25. Lucas R, Parikh SJ, Sridhar S, Guo DH, Bhagatwala J, et al. (2013) Cytokine profiling of young overweight and obese female African American adults with prediabetes. Cytokine 64: 310–315.
26. Tang X, Peng R, Phillips JE, Deguzman J, Ren Y, et al. (2013) Assessment of Brd4 inhibition in idiopathic pulmonary fibrosis lung fibroblasts and in vivo models of lung fibrosis. The American journal of pathology 183: 470–479.

27. Pussinen PJ, Tuomisto K, Jousilahti P, Havulinna AS, Sundvall J, et al. (2007) Endotoxemia, immune response to periodontal pathogens, and systemic inflammation associate with incident cardiovascular disease events. Arteriosclerosis, thrombosis, and vascular biology 27: 1433–1439.
28. Al-Attas OS, Al-Daghri NM, Al-Rubeaan K, da Silva NF, Sabico SL, et al. (2009) Changes in endotoxin levels in T2DM subjects on anti-diabetic therapies. Cardiovascular diabetology 8: 20.
29. Lumsden AB, Henderson JM, Kutner MH (1988) Endotoxin levels measured by a chromogenic assay in portal, hepatic and peripheral venous blood in patients with cirrhosis. Hepatology 8: 232–236.
30. Anker SD, Egerer KR, Volk HD, Kox WJ, Poole-Wilson PA, et al. (1997) Elevated soluble CD14 receptors and altered cytokines in chronic heart failure. The American journal of cardiology 79: 1426–1430.
31. Mortier S, De Vriese AS, McLoughlin RM, Topley N, Schaub TP, et al. (2003) Effects of conventional and new peritoneal dialysis fluids on leukocyte recruitment in the rat peritoneal membrane. Journal of the American Society of Nephrology: JASN 14: 1296–1306.
32. Cengiz MI, Bal S, Gokcay S, Cengiz K (2007) Does periodontal disease reflect atherosclerosis in continuous ambulatory peritoneal dialysis patients? Journal of periodontology 78: 1926–1934.
33. Heumann D, Roger T (2002) Initial responses to endotoxins and Gram-negative bacteria. Clinica chimica acta; international journal of clinical chemistry 323: 59–72.
34. Estruch M, Bancells C, Beloki L, Sanchez-Quesada JL, Ordonez-Llanos J, et al. (2013) CD14 and TLR4 mediate cytokine release promoted by electronegative LDL in monocytes. Atherosclerosis 229: 356–362.
35. Dunzendorfer S, Lee HK, Soldau K, Tobias PS (2004) Toll-like receptor 4 functions intracellularly in human coronary artery endothelial cells: roles of LBP and sCD14 in mediating LPS responses. FASEB journal: official publication of the Federation of American Societies for Experimental Biology 18: 1117–1119.
36. Kato S, Yuzawa Y, Tsuboi N, Maruyama S, Morita Y, et al. (2004) Endotoxin-induced chemokine expression in murine peritoneal mesothelial cells: the role of toll-like receptor 4. Journal of the American Society of Nephrology: JASN 15: 1289–1299.
37. Braun N, Alscher MD, Kimmel M, Amann K, Buttner M (2011) Encapsulating peritoneal sclerosis - an overview. Nephrologie & therapeutique 7: 162–171.
38. Aoyama T, Paik YH, Seki E (2010) Toll-like receptor signaling and liver fibrosis. Gastroenterology research and practice 2010.
39. Ramnath RD, Ng SW, Guglielmotti A, Bhatia M (2008) Role of MCP-1 in endotoxemia and sepsis. International immunopharmacology 8: 810–818.
40. Juskewitch JE, Knudsen BE, Platt JL, Nath KA, Knutson KL, et al. (2012) LPS-induced murine systemic inflammation is driven by parenchymal cell activation and exclusively predicted by early MCP-1 plasma levels. The American journal of pathology 180: 32–40.
41. Viedt C, Vogel J, Athanasiou T, Shen W, Orth SR, et al. (2002) Monocyte chemoattractant protein-1 induces proliferation and interleukin-6 production in human smooth muscle cells by differential activation of nuclear factor-kappa B and activator protein-1. Arteriosclerosis, thrombosis, and vascular biology 22: 914–920.
42. Gosling J, Slaymaker S, Gu L, Tseng S, Zlot CH, et al. (1999) MCP-1 deficiency reduces susceptibility to atherosclerosis in mice that overexpress human apolipoprotein B. The Journal of clinical investigation 103: 773–778.
43. de Lemos JA, Morrow DA, Sabatine MS, Murphy SA, Gibson CM, et al. (2003) Association between plasma levels of monocyte chemoattractant protein-1 and long-term clinical outcomes in patients with acute coronary syndromes. Circulation 107: 690–695.
44. Davi G, Tuttolomondo A, Santilli F, Basili S, Ferrante E, et al. (2009) CD40 ligand and MCP-1 as predictors of cardiovascular events in diabetic patients with stroke. Journal of atherosclerosis and thrombosis 16: 707–713
45. Pawlak K, Pawlak D, Mysliwiec M (2007) Impaired renal function and duration of dialysis therapy are associated with oxidative stress and proatherogenic cytokine levels in patients with end-stage renal disease. Clinical biochemistry 40: 81–85.
46. Malik AR, Little MA, Henriksson M, Tam FW, Brown EA (2007) Peritonitis, peritoneal inflammation and membrane permeability: a longitudinal study of dialysate and serum MCP-1 in stable patients on peritoneal dialysis. Journal of nephrology 20: 340–349.
47. Heesen M, Renckens R, de Vos AF, Kunz D, van der Poll T (2006) Human endotoxemia induces down-regulation of monocyte CC chemokine receptor 2. Clinical and vaccine immunology: CVI 13: 156–159.
48. Mehta NN, McGillicuddy FC, Anderson PD, Hinkle CC, Shah R, et al. (2010) Experimental endotoxemia induces adipose inflammation and insulin resistance in humans. Diabetes 59: 172–181.
49. Lee SH, Kang HY, Kim KS, Nam BY, Paeng J, et al. (2012) The monocyte chemoattractant protein-1 (MCP-1)/CCR2 system is involved in peritoneal dialysis-related epithelial-mesenchymal transition of peritoneal mesothelial cells. Laboratory investigation; a journal of technical methods and pathology 92: 1698–1711.
50. Goldstein SL, Leung JC, Silverstein DM (2006) Pro- and anti-inflammatory cytokines in chronic pediatric dialysis patients: effect of aspirin. Clinical journal of the American Society of Nephrology: CJASN 1: 979–986.
51. Descamps-Latscha B, Herbelin A, Nguyen AT, Roux-Lombard P, Zingraff J, et al. (1995) Balance between IL-1 beta, TNF-alpha, and their specific inhibitors in chronic renal failure and maintenance dialysis. Relationships with activation markers of T cells, B cells, and monocytes. Journal of immunology 154: 882–892.
52. Purohit V, Bode JC, Bode C, Brenner DA, Choudhry MA, et al. (2008) Alcohol, intestinal bacterial growth, intestinal permeability to endotoxin, and medical consequences: summary of a symposium. Alcohol 42: 349–361.
53. Leypoldt JK (2002) Solute transport across the peritoneal membrane. Journal of the American Society of Nephrology: JASN 13 Suppl 1: S84–91.
54. Deshmane SL, Kremlev S, Amini S, Sawaya BE (2009) Monocyte chemoattractant protein-1 (MCP-1): an overview. Journal of interferon & cytokine research: the official journal of the International Society for Interferon and Cytokine Research 29: 313–326.
55. Gegner JA, Ulevitch RJ, Tobias PS (1995) Lipopolysaccharide (LPS) signal transduction and clearance. Dual roles for LPS binding protein and membrane CD14. The Journal of biological chemistry 270: 5320–5325.
56. Tobias PS, Soldau K, Iovine NM, Elsbach P, Weiss J (1997) Lipopolysaccharide (LPS)-binding proteins BPI and LBP form different types of complexes with LPS. The Journal of biological chemistry 272: 18682–18685.
57. Mujais S (1999) Ultrafiltration management in automated peritoneal dialysis. Contributions to nephrology 129: 255–266.

High Peritoneal Transport Status Was Not Associated with Mortality in Peritoneal Dialysis Patients with Diabetes

Naya Huang[1], Jiehui Chen[1,2]**, Li Fan[1], Qian Zhou[3], Qingdong Xu[1], Ricong Xu[1], Liping Xiong[1], Xueqing Yu[1], Haiping Mao[1*]**

1 Department of Nephrology, The First Affiliated Hospital, Sun Yat-sen University, Key Laboratory of Nephrology, Ministry of Health of China, Guangdong Provincial Key Laboratory of Nephrology, Guangzhou, Guangdong, China, **2** Department of Nephrology, The Sixth People's Hospital of Shenzhen, Shenzhen, Guangdong, China, **3** Epidemiology Research Unit, Translational Medicine Research Center, The First Affiliated Hospital, Sun Yat-sen University, Guangzhou, Guangdong, China

Abstract

Background: Continuous ambulatory peritoneal dialysis (CAPD) patients with diabetes are at increased risk of mortality and high peritoneal transporters appear to contribute to poor survival. However, little is known about the combined impacts of high peritoneal transporters and diabetes on mortality.

Methods: This was a prospective observational cohort study. 776 incident CAPD patients were enrolled. Unadjusted and adjusted Cox proportional regression models were used to evaluate the association and interaction of peritoneal transport and diabetic status with mortality

Results: In the entire cohort, high peritoneal transport status was associated with an increased risk of all-cause mortality in unadjusted model [hazard ratio (HR) 2.35, 95% confidence interval (CI) 1.30 to 4.25, $P = 0.01$], but this association was not significant in multivariable model. There was an interaction between peritoneal membrane transport status and diabetes ($P = 0.028$). Subgroup analyses showed that compared to low and low average transporters, high transporters was associated with a higher risk of all-cause mortality (adjusted HR 1.78, 95% CI 1.07 to 4.70, $P = 0.04$) in CAPD patients without diabetes, but not in those with diabetes (adjusted HR 0.79, 95%CI 0.33 to 1.89, $P = 0.59$). Results were similar when transport status was assessed as a continuous variable.

Conclusions: The association between high peritoneal transport and all-cause mortality was likely to vary with diabetes status. High peritoneal transport was associated with an elevated risk of death among CAPD patients without diabetes, but not in those with diabetes.

Editor: Zhanjun Jia, University of Utah School of Medicine, United States of America

Funding: This work was supported by the National Key Technology Research and Development Program of the Ministry of Science and Technology of China (2011BAI10B05), the National Basic Research Program of China (2012CB517700-2012CB517706), the Guangzhou Committee of Science and Technology, China (2010U1-E00831), and 5010 Clinical Program of Sun Yat-sen University (2007007). The funders had no role in study design, data collection and analysis, decision to publish, or preparation of the manuscript.

Competing Interests: The authors have declared that no competing interests exist.

* Email: haipingmao@126.com

These authors contributed equally to this work.

Introduction

Peritoneal transport characteristics, as assessed by the dialysate to plasma ratio of creatinine (D/P Cr) from a peritoneal equilibration test (PET), is traditionally used to evaluate peritoneal permeability in peritoneal dialysis (PD) setting [1]. However, peritoneal transport status has been demonstrated to have a paradoxical association with mortality in PD patients. Many previous studies [2–6], such as the CANUSA study and the study from Australian and New Zealand, indicated that high peritoneal transporters had adverse impacts on both mortality and technique failure in PD patients. However, these findings have not been confirmed by other studies [7–10]. In the ADEMEX trial, a prospective study, showed that high transport had no impact on patient survival in PD patients. Meanwhile, a Korean study has shown that peritoneal protein clearance, which is positively correlated with D/P Cr, is not associated with increased all-cause mortality in multivariate Cox analysis in PD patients [11]. The discrepancy between the conflicting results is not clearly demonstrated, but may due to difference in the primary cause of end stage of renal disease (ESRD), a mixture of incident and prevalent patients, racial origin, the methodology of transport test, and comorbid illness burden.

Table 1. Baseline demographic and clinical characteristics of the study population.

Variables	Total (n = 776)	NDM (n = 600)	DM (n = 176)	*P*
PET classes				**0.002**
L&LA	237 (30.5%)	193 (32.2%)	44 (25.0%)	
HA	373 (48.1%)	296 (49.3%)	77 (43.8%)	
H	166 (21.4%)	111 (18.5%)	55 (31.2%)	
D/P Cr 4h	0.71±0.12	0.70±0.11	0.75±0.12	**<0.001**
Age (year)	46.85±15.12	43.54±14.70	58.17±10.25	**<0.001**
Male gender	451 (58.1%)	350 (58.3%)	101 (57.1%)	0.77
Dialysis vintage	26.3(16.5, 40.2)	26.0(16.4, 39.3)	27.0(17.3, 42.4)	0.21
History of cardiovascular disease	361 (46.5%)	253 (41.9%)	108 (61.4%)	**<0.001**
BMI (kg/m^2)	21.05±3.93	20.65±3.79	22.42±4.08	**<0.001**
SBP (mmHg)	137.38±17.07	136.71±17.20	139.56±16.47	0.06
DBP (mmHg)	82.84±12.28	84.51±12.40	77.14±9.96	**<0.001**
Hemoglobin (g/L)	109.9±21.5	111.0±21.7	106.3±20.0	**0.01**
Serum albumin (g/L)	37.6±5.9	38.3±5.6	35.3±6.1	**<0.001**
Serum prealbumin(mg/L)	347.48±102.92	365.32±99.34	289.10±92.58	**<0.001**
nPCR (g/kg/d)	0.94±0.23	0.96±0.23	0.86±0.22	**<0.001**
Uric acid (μmol/L)	406.2±91.0	412.2± 86.8	381.3±98.7	**<0.001**
Calcium (mmol/L)	2.30±0.36	2.30±0.29	2.29 ±0.56	0.93
Phosphate(mmol/L)	1.46± 0.48	1.48±0.51	1.37 ±0.34	**0.002**
iPTH (pg/mL)	241 (103, 416)	247 (108, 433)	210 (82, 371.5)	**0.02**
Glucose (mmol/L)	6.34±1.13	5.85±1.07	8.02±1.32	0.26
Haemoglobin A1c(%)	6.29 ±1.26	6.58±1.23	6.08±1.27	**0.008**
Cholesterol (mmol/L)	5.29±2.97	5.12±2.05	5.89±4.87	**0.05**
Triglyceride(mmol/L)	1.71±1.17	1.58±0.90	2.12±1.73	**<0.001**
hs-CRP (mg/L)	1.74 (0.66, 6.47)	1.64 (0.66, 5.74)	2.23 (0.65, 8.58)	0.30
UF on PET (ml)	280 (160, 380)	300 (160, 380)	240 (120, 380)	0.20
WCCr(L/w/1.73 m^2)	88.83±35.37	88.42±5.54	90.20±28.61	0.82
Weekly total Kt/V urea	2.40±0.64	2.38±0.67	2.46±0.57	0.16
RRF (ml/min/1.73 m^2)	3.13 (1.86, 5.02)	3.02 (1.74, 4.56)	4.06 (2.39, 5.90)	**0.001**

Results are expressed as mean ± SD, median (interquartile range) or number (%).
Abbreviations: BMI, body mass index; SBP, systolic blood pressure; DBP, diastolic blood pressure; nPCR, normalized protein catabolic rate; iPTH, intact parathyroid hormone; hs-CRP, high-sensitivity C-reactive protein; PET, peritoneal equilibration test; UF, ultrafitration; WCCr, total weekly creatinine clearance; RRF, residual renal function; NDM, non-diabetes mellitus, DM, diabetes mellitus; H, high transport; HA, high average transport; LA, low average transport; L, low transport.

Diabetes mellitus (DM) is increasing to be the second cause of ESRD in China. Compared with PD patients without diabetes, those with diabetes generally have poorer patient survival. A number of studies have suggested that diabetes *per se* is associated with a high risk of mortality [12–14]. Meanwhile, high peritoneal transporters have been shown to be more prevalent in PD patients with diabetes [2], [15]. However, it is unknown whether high peritoneal transporters contribute additional mortality risk in PD patients with diabetes.

In this study, we evaluated the association of baseline peritoneal transporters and diabetic status on all-cause mortality in CAPD patients and explored whether this association varied by diabetes mellitus.

Materials and Methods

Study Design and Population

This study protocol was approved by the Ethics Committee of The First Affiliated Hospital of Sun Yat-sen University. Written informed consent form was obtained from all participants.

It was a prospective observational cohort study. A total of 776 incident patients who commenced CAPD in our hospital between January 2007 and December 2011 were studied. Patients older than 18 years old undergoing CAPD treatment for more than 3 months were included. Patient who had a history of kidney transplantation, hemodialysis for more than 3 months, and malignant disease was excluded.

A standard PET and total weekly creatinine clearance (peritoneal and residual renal clearance) and urea Kt/V were

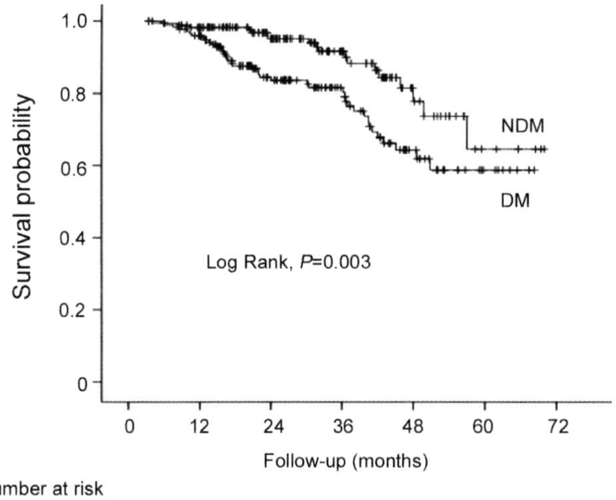

Figure 1. Kaplan-Meier survival curves for age and sex matched CAPD patients with and without diabetes.

performed as previous described [14]. Briefly, a standard 4-hour dwell period was used, with a 2.27% glucose concentration 2 L volume exchange. The results were calculated by using PD Adequest software (Baxter Healthcare Corporation, Chicago, IL, USA). The first PET tests were performed between the first and third month post-PD initiation in patients without significant fluid overload or acute peritonitis and used for analyses. Peritoneal transport status was categorized as low (L), low average (LA), high average (HA), and high (H), according to D/P Cr 4h values defined by Twardowski (L<0.50, LA 0.5–0.64, HA 0.65–0.80, H≥0.81)[16]. We used peritoneal transport status as a categorical variable (PET classes) in our primary analyses, and a continuous variable (D/P Cr 4h) in sensitivity analyses. L transporters (n = 25, 3.2%) were combined into LA transporters (L&LA) for analyses due to relatively few patients.

To investigate whether the relationship between peritoneal transport status and mortality varied in patients with diabetes, subjects were divided into groups with diabetes mellitus (DM) and without diabetes mellitus (NDM) according to the presence or absence of diabetes. Diabetic status was defined if diabetes mellitus was registered as the primary cause of ESRD (included type 1 or 2) or patients with diabetes as comorbidity.

Demographic and Clinical Data

Baseline demographic data included the age, gender, primary cause of ESRD, the presence of cardiovascular disease (CVD) and diabetic status. Cardiovascular disease was defined as myocardial infarction, angina, arrhythmias, valvular heart disease, congestive heart failure, ischemic stroke, transient ischemic attack, peripheral arterial disease [17], [18] . Residual renal function (RRF) was defined as the average of 24-h urinary urea and creatinine clearance, and the ultrafiltration volume (UF) was calculated as the difference of infused and drained dialysate volume during PET. The clinic and biochemical data were collected at the first 3 months after PD initiation.

Outcomes

The primary outcome of this study was all-cause mortality. Survival time was defined as the time from enrollment to death or administrative censoring (transfer to hemodialysis, kidney transplantation, transfer to other dialysis centers, loss of follow-up, or end of the study period) at December 31, 2012.

Statistical analysis

Results of continuous variables were expressed as mean ± standard deviation (SD) for normal distribution, median (interquartile range, IQR) for skewed distribution. For categorical variables, the results were expressed as frequencies and percentages. Comparison of continuous variables and categorical data between two groups in the study were tested by t-test and Chi-Square test.

Survival curves were generated by Kaplan-Meier method. Because patients with diabetes were much older than the non-diabetic ones, we plotted the survival curves both in the entire cohort and in the cohort with age and gender matched patients to demonstrate the patient survival in diabetic and non-diabtetic CAPD patient. Unadjusted and adjusted Cox proportional regression models were used to evaluate the association of peritoneal transport status and all-cause mortality. Variables with *P*-value <0.1 in univariate models and RRF (Table S1) were selected for multivariate Cox regression models.

Table 2. Interaction and association of transport status, diabetes and all-cause mortality in entire cohort.

Variable	Unadjusted model, HR (95% CI)	Adjusted model*, HR (95% CI)	Adjusted interaction *P*-value between transport status and diabetes*
Transport status as a categorical variable			**0.028**
PET Classes			
L&LA	Ref	Ref	
HA	1.07 (0.60, 1.92)	0.74 (0.40, 1.36)	
H	2.35 (1.30, 4.25)	1.31 (0.68, 2.54)	
P- trend	**0.003**	0.13	
Transport status as a continuous variable			**0.048**
D/P Cr 4h (per 0.1 higher)	1.42 (1.17, 1.72)	1.18 (0.95, 1.48)	

*Adjusted for the variables with *P*<0.1 in the univariate model and RRF, including age at initiation of peritoneal dialysis, gender, cardiovascular disease, hemoglobin, serum albumin, DBP, iPTH, total cholesterol, and triglyceride and RRF (Table S1). Transport status was included in the adjusted model as either categorical or continuous variable separately.

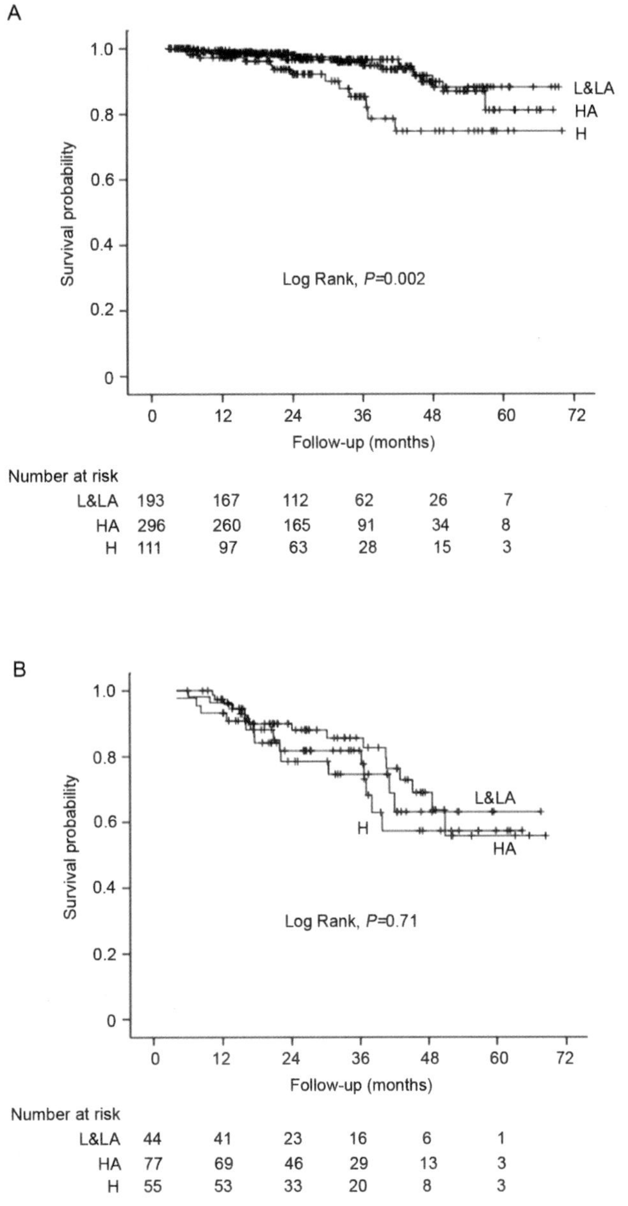

Figure 2. Kaplan-Meier survival curves for CAPD patients without (a) and with diabetes (b) according to PET category.

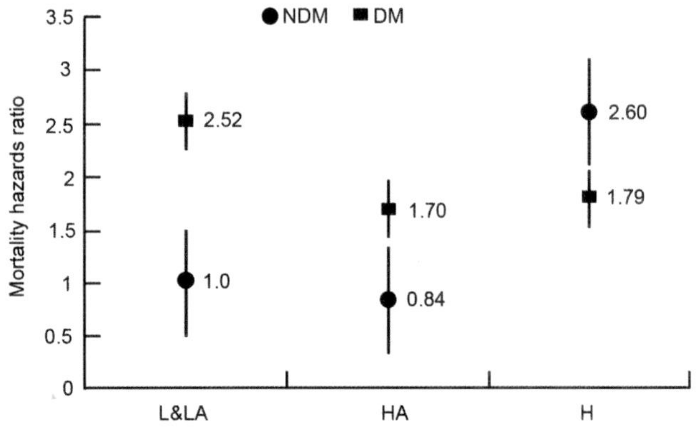

Figure 3. Adjusted hazard ratios of all-cause mortality for CAPD patients with and without diabetes according to PET category. Adjusted for the variables with $P<0.1$ in the univariate model, including age at initiation of peritoneal dialysis, gender, cardiovascular disease, hemoglobin, serum albumin, DBP, iPTH, total cholesterol, and triglyceride.

Given that CAPD patients with diabetes had more proportion of H transporters and poorer survival than those without diabetes, we evaluated *a prior* interaction between peritoneal transport status and diabetes using multivariable Cox regression analyses. Then, we perform subgroup analyses to evaluate the relationship of peritoneal transport status and all-cause mortality in individuals with or without diabetes. All statistical analyses were performed using the SPSS software, version 16.0 (SPSS Inc., Chicago, IL, USA). A P-value<0.05 was considered statistically significant.

Results

Baseline characteristics of the participants

Table 1 showed the baseline demographic and clinical characteristics of the entire cohort and stratified by diabetic status. Overall, the mean age was 46.85±15.12 years, 58.1% were male, and 22.6% had diabetes. The mean D/P Cr 4h was 0.71±0.12 and there were 237 (30.5%) patients with L&LA transport, 373 (48.1%) with HA, and 166 (21.4%) with H transport. The baseline mean D/P Cr 4h was significant higher in patients with diabetes than those without diabetes (0.75±0.12 *vs.* 0.70±0.11; $P<0.001$); and CAPD patients with diabetes had higher proportion of H transporters. In addition, participants with diabetes were more likely to be older, had a greater percentage of CVD, and higher levels of body mass index (BMI), hemoglobin A1c, triglyceride and RRF, and lower diastolic pressure, hemoglobin, serum albumin, serum prealbumin, normalized protein catabolic rate (nPCR), serum uric acid, phosphate and intact parathyroid hormone (iPTH). However, there were no significant differences between DM and NDM group with respect to the total weekly creatinine clearance, total weekly Kt/V urea, and ultrafiltration volume.

Patient survival

During a median follow-up of 26.3 months (IQR: 16.5, 40.2), 76 patients (9.8%) died, in which 35 (5.8%) were in NDM and 41 (23.3%) in DM group. In the cohort with age- and gender-matched patients, Kaplan-Meier curve showed that diabetic CAPD patients had significant poorer patient survival compared to those without diabetes (Figure 1, $P=0.003$). Similar results were shown in the entire cohort (data not shown). The cumulative survival rates at 1-, 3- and 5- year were 96%, 81%, and 56% in diabetic patients, and 99%, 94%, and 83% in non-diabetic patients, respectively.

Interaction of peritoneal transport status and diabetes and their association with mortality

Table 2 demonstrated the association of transport status, diabetes and all-cause mortality in entire cohort. Compared to L&LA transporters, H transporters was associated with an increased risk of all-cause mortality in the unadjusted model [hazard ratio (HR) 2.35, 95% confidence interval (95% CI) 1.30 to 4.25; P-trend = 0.003]. However, this relationship was attenuated and not significant after adjustment for potential confounders (adjusted HR 1.31, 95% CI 0.68 to 2.54; P-trend = 0.13). Results were similar when transport status was evaluated as a continuous variable. Further, we assessed the interaction between peritoneal transporters and diabetes on patient survival. The data demonstrated that a significant interaction between transport status and

Table 3. Association of transport status and all-cause mortality by diabetic status.

Variable	Non-diabetic patients (n = 600)				Diabetic patients (n = 176)			
	Unadjusted model		Adjusted model*		Unadjusted model		Adjusted model*	
	HR (95% CI)	*P*	HR (95% CI)	*P*	HR (95% CI)	*P*	HR (95% CI)	*P*
Transport status as a categorical variable								
PET Class								
L&LA	Ref	–	Ref	–	Ref	–	Ref	–
HA	1.35 (0.54, 3.34)	0.51	0.75 (0.29, 1.93)	0.55	0.78 (0.36, 1.69)	0.53	0.63 (0.27, 1.42)	0.26
H	3.80 (1.53, 9.43)	**0.004**	1.78 (1.07, 4.70)	**0.04**	1.04 (0.47, 2.30)	0.92	0.79 (0.33, 1.89)	0.59
P- trend		**0.004**		**0.01**		0.71		0.56
Transport status as a continuous variable								
D/P Cr 4h (per 0.1 higher)	1.58 (1.18, 2.12)	**0.002**	1.49 (1.05, 2.10)	**0.03**	1.11 (0.87, 1.42)	0.40	1.11 (0.86, 1.42)	0.42

* Adjusted for the variables with $P<0.1$ in the univariate model, including age at initiation of peritoneal dialysis, gender, cardiovascular disease, hemoglobin, serum albumin, DBP, iPTH, total cholesterol, and triglyceride.

diabetes when PET was evaluated as a categorical variable (*P*-interaction = 0.028), and a continuous variable (*P*-interaction = 0.048).

Association of peritoneal transport status and all-cause mortality by diabetic status

As shown in Figure 2, the cumulative patient survival rates among L&LA, HA and H transporters were significant different in CAPD patients without diabetes ($P = 0.002$), but not in those with diabetes ($P = 0.71$). Table 3 showed the hazard ratios of peritoneal transporters and all-cause mortality by diabetic status. In patients without diabetes, H transporters was associated with an increased risk of all-cause mortality both in unadjusted (HR 3.80, 95% CI 1.53 to 9.43; $P = 0.004$) and adjusted (HR 1.78, 95% CI 1.07 to 4.70; $P = 0.04$) analyses compared to L&LA transporters. The HR for all-cause mortality also demonstrated an enhancing trend from the L&LA to the HA to the H transporters (*P*-trend = 0.01). In contrast, mortality in DM group was not associated with transport status, no matter assessed as either categorical (adjusted HR 0.79, 95% CI 0.33 to 1.89; $P = 0.59$) or a continuous variable (D/P Cr, adjusted HR 1.11, 95% CI 0.86 to 1.42; $P = 0.42$, per 0.1 increase). Figure 3 further depicted the adjusted HRs for all-cause mortality by PET category in CAPD patients with and without diabetes. An increase trend was found between peritoneal transport status and mortality risk among patietns without diabetes, whereas no increase trend was observed in those with diabetes.

Discussion

In the present study, we demonstrated that there was an inverse association between high peritoneal transport and all-cause mortality in CAPD population without diabetes, whereas no clear survival disadvantage was observed in those who had diabetes and in the entire cohort. These results suggested that diabetic status may modify the association of peritoneal transport with mortality. In addition, diabetes was independently associated with a higher risk of mortality in CAPD population.

Previous studies have focused on the association between peritoneal transport status and death in overall PD population, which have embraced controversially results. A study by Fried *et al* showed that the 3-yr survival probabilities gradually increased in HA, LA, and L transporters, as compared with H transporters [18]. Thereafter, CANUSA study, a prospective observation of 606 CAPD patients with 82% Caucasian in North America, demonstrated that each 0.1 increment in D/P Cr enhanced the relative risk of death by 19% [2]. Meanwhile, Davies *et al* prospectively identified that high D/P Cr was an independent predictor of mortality [5]. A meta-analysis of 20 studies also indicated there was 15% increase in the overall pooled relative risk of mortality for each 0.1 increment in D/P Cr [4]. It was difficult to apply the findings of this meta-analysis to our study, since two of the pooled studies included only continuous cycler peritoneal dialysis (CCPD) patients, seven studies targeted both CAPD and CCPD patients, and only half studies were focused on CAPD population. On the contrary, more and more investigations have failed to reach consistent results. The best known ADEMEX trial, by far the largest prospective study of 965 CAPD patients with a follow-up of 30 months, found that there was no significant effect of baseline peritoneal transport characteristics on mortality in PD patients [7]. A prospective study by Szeto *et al.* demonstrated that the low transporters had slightly better 2-year patient survival than high/high average transporters (90.2% versus 83.3%) among Chinese CAPD patients, but it was not statistically significant [19].

Similarly, the multicenter European Automated PD Outcome Study prospectively revealed that baseline D/P Cr was not associated with all-cause mortality in PD patients receiving automatic peritoneal dialysis (APD) treatment [20]. Patients using icodextrin solution also favored a significant survival advantage in high transporters [21]. Our results added the previous literature to show that there was no association between baseline peritoneal transport status and all-cause mortality in overall CAPD patients.

To our knowledge, this study is by far the first observation to date to investigate the different association of transport status and mortality between patients with and without diabetes. We found that high transporter was a risk factor for death in CAPD patients without diabetes, but not associated with an increased mortality in those with diabetes. Consistent with previous researches, high transporters showed to have a higher prevalence of hypoalbuminemia [15], [22], [24] and worse in other nutritional surrogates such as nPCR and serum prealbumin (data not shown). These suggested a greater incidence of underlying chronic inflammation and malnutrition among CAPD patients with high transporters. Nevertheless, diabetes *per se* was a significant independent risk factor for patient survival, which was in accordance with previous study [12–15]. Additionally, individuals with diabetes were significantly older, with greater proportion of CVD, and lower levels of serum albumin than those without diabetes, which have been reported as independently factors responsible for the poor outcomes. Thus, the aforementioned risk predictors might surpass the effects of high transporters on mortality in diabetic CAPD population.

Many studies have investigated the interaction between diabetes and inflammation, serum albumin and phosphorus, age and BMI, age and smoking status, as well as diabetes and BMI [23–27]. However, the interaction between transport status and diabetes on mortality risk has not been investigated in PD patients. Our data revealed a significant interaction between high transporter and diabetes, and their interactive effects attenuated the adverse impact of high transporters on patient survival among diabetic CAPD patients, suggesting that diabetes status modified the association of peritoneal transport with mortality. Plausible mechanism of the interaction was not certain. Diabetes is a disease that is strongly associated with microvascular complications, including retinopathy, nephropathy, and neuropathy [28]. The pathogenesis of microvascular disease in diabetes is multifactorial, including the production of advanced glycation end products, abnormal activation of signaling cascades, and elevated production of reactive oxygen species that may increase capillary basement membrane thickening, permeability of endothelial cells, and formation of microaneurysms. A large study by Honda et al. demonstrated that patients with diabetes showed significant increase in average postcapillary venule thickness and decrease in lumen/vessel diameter ratio compared with patients without diabetes in pre-peritoneal dialysis peritoneum [29], suggesting that diabetes-associated vascular alterations may contribute to higher proportion of high transporters in PD patients.

There are some limitations in this study. First, it was a single-center observational study, and a center-specific effect cannot be excluded. In addition, because we only enrolled CAPD patients and icodextrin was not available in the Mainland of China, thus, our results may not necessarily extend to APD patients or patients using icodextrin solution. Second, we excluded a part of patients due to unavailability of baseline PET measurements, which may carry a risk for bias. Third, relatively few patients presented low transporter status and small sample size of diabetes. Finally, our analyses did not study the relationship between the change of peritoneal transport status and mortality.

In conclusion, high peritoneal transport status confers increased all-cause mortality risk in CAPD patients without diabetes. The interaction of transport status and diabetes might modify the risk of death, and high transport did not add adverse effect on patient survival in those with diabetes. Our results should be confirmed by a large cohort of CAPD patients with diabetes and the mechanisms underlying the associations investigated.

Author Contributions

Conceived and designed the experiments: HPM NYH JHC XQY. Performed the experiments: NYH JHC LF QDX RCX LPX. Analyzed the data: NYH JHC LF QZ. Contributed reagents/materials/analysis tools: XQY HPM. Wrote the paper: NYH LF HPM.

References

1. Johnson DW, Hawley CM, McDonald SP, Brown FG, Rosman JB, et al. (2010) Superior survival of high transporters treated with automated versus continuous ambulatory peritoneal dialysis. Nephrol Dial Transplant 25: 1973–1979.
2. Churchill DN, Thorpe KE, Nolph KD, Keshaviah PR, Oreopoulos DG, et al. (1998) Increased peritoneal membrane transport is associated with decreased patient and technique survival for continuous peritoneal dialysis patients. The Canada-USA (CANUSA) Peritoneal Dialysis Study Group. J Am Soc Nephrol 9: 1285–1292.
3. Rumpsfeld M, McDonald SP, Johnson DW (2006) Higher peritoneal transport status is associated with higher mortality and technique failure in the Australian and New Zealand peritoneal dialysis patient populations. J Am Soc Nephrol 17: 271–278.
4. Brimble KS, Walker M, Margetts PJ, Kundhal KK, Rabbat CG (2006) Meta-analysis: peritoneal membrane transport, mortality, and technique failure in peritoneal dialysis. J Am Soc Nephrol 17: 2591–2598.
5. Davies SJ, Phillips L, Russell GI (1998) Peritoneal solute transport predicts survival on CAPD independently of residual renal function. Nephrol Dial Transplant 13: 962–968.
6. Wang T, Heimburger O, Waniewski J, Bergstrom J, Lindholm B (1998) Increased peritoneal permeability is associated with decreased fluid and small-solute removal and higher mortality in CAPD patients. Nephrol Dial Transplant 13: 1242–1249.
7. Paniagua R, Amato D, Vonesh E, Correa-Rotter R, Ramos A, et al. (2002) Effects of increased peritoneal clearances on mortality rates in peritoneal dialysis: ADEMEX, a prospective, randomized, controlled trial. J Am Soc Nephrol 13: 1307–1320.
8. Chang TI, Park JT, Lee DH, Lee JH, Yoo TH, et al. (2010) High peritoneal transport status is not an independent risk factor for high mortality in patients treated with automated peritoneal dialysis. J Korean Med Sci 25: 1313–1317.

9. Park HC, Kang SW, Choi KH, Ha SK, Han DS, et al. (2001) Clinical outcome in continuous ambulatory peritoneal dialysis patients is not influenced by high peritoneal transport status. Perit Dial Int 21 Suppl 3: S80–85.
10. Perl J, Huckvale K, Chellar M, John B, Davies SJ (2009) Peritoneal protein clearance and not peritoneal membrane transport status predicts survival in a contemporary cohort of peritoneal dialysis patients. Clin J Am Soc Nephrol; 4: 1201–1206.
11. Chang TI, Kang EW, Lee YK, Shin SK (2013) Higher peritoneal protein clearance as a risk factor for cardiovascular disease inperitoneal dialysis patient. 208: in press.
12. Yang X, Yi C, Liu X, Guo Q, Yang R, et al. (2013) Clinical outcome and risk factors for mortality in Chinese patients with diabetes on peritoneal dialysis: a 5-year clinical cohort study. Diabetes Res Clin Pract 100: 354–361.
13. Magliano DJ, Soderberg S, Zimmet PZ, Cartensen B, Balkau B, et al. (2010) Mortality, all-cause and cardiovascular disease, over 15 years in multiethnic mauritius: impact of diabetes and intermediate forms of glucose tolerance. Diabetes Care 33: 1983–1989.
14. Morgan CL, Currie CJ, Peters JR (2000) Relationship between diabetes and mortality: a population study using record linkage. Diabetes Care 23: 1103–1107.
15. Cueto-Manzano AM, Correa-Rotter R (2000) Is high peritoneal transport rate an independent risk factor for CAPD mortality? Kidney Int 57: 314–320.
16. Twardowski ZJ, Nolph KD, Khanna R (1987) Peritoneal equilibration test. Perit Dial Bull 7: 134–147.
17. Go AS, Chertow GM, Fan D, McCulloch CE, Hsu CY (2004) Chronic kidney disease and the risks of death, cardiovascular events, and hospitalization. N Engl J Med 351: 1296–1305.
18. Parfrey PS, Foley RN (1999) The clinical epidemiology of cardiac disease in chronic renal failure. J Am Soc Nephrol 10: 1606–1615.
19. Szeto CC, Law MC, Wong TY, Leung CB, Li PK (2001) Peritoneal transport status correlates with morbidity but not longitudinal change of nutritional status of continuous ambulatory peritoneal dialysis patients: a 2-year prospective study. Am J Kidney Dis 37: 329–336.
20. Brown EA, Davies SJ, Rutherford P, Meeus F, Borras M, et al. (2003) Survival of functionally anuric patients on automated peritoneal dialysis: the European APD Outcome Study. J Am Soc Nephrol 14: 2948–2957.
21. Yang X, Fang W, Bargman JM, Oreopoulos DG (2008) High peritoneal permeability is not associated with higher mortality or technique failure in patients on automated peritoneal dialysis. Perit Dial Int 28: 82–92.
22. Margetts PJ, McMullin JP, Rabbat CG, Churchill DN (2000) Peritoneal membrane transport and hypoalbuminemia: cause or effect? Perit Dial Int 20: 14–18.
23. Xu R, Han Q, Zhu T, Ren Y, Chen J, et al. (2013) Diabetic patients could do as well as non-diabetic patients without inflammation onperitoneal dialysis. PLoS One 8: In press.
24. Chung SH, Heimburger O, Stenvinkel P, Wang T, Lindholm B (2003) Influence of peritoneal transport rate, inflammation, and fluid removal on nutritional status and clinical outcome in prevalent peritoneal dialysis patients. Perit Dial Int 23: 174–183.
25. Ma SH, Park BY, Yang JJ, Jung EJ, Yeo Y, et al. (2012) Interaction of body mass index and diabetes as modifiers of cardiovascular mortality in a cohort study. J Prev Med Public Health 45: 394–401.
26. Tobias D, Pan A, Hu FB (2014) BMI and mortality among adults with incident type 2 diabetes. N Engl J Med 370: 1363–1364.
27. Zitt E, Lamina C, Sturm G, Knoll F, Lins F, et al. (2011) Interaction of time-varying albumin and phosphorus on mortality in incident dialysis patients. Clin J Am Soc Nephrol 6: 2650–2656.
28. UK Prospective Diabetes Study (UKPDS) (1991) VIII. Study design, progress and performance. Diabetologia; 34: 877–890.
29. Honda K, Hamada C, Nakayama M, Miyazaki M, Sherif AM, et al. (2008) Impact of uremia, diabetes, and peritoneal dialysis itself on the pathogenesis of peritoneal sclerosis: a quantitative study of peritoneal membrane morphology. Clin J Am Soc Nephrol 3: 720–728.

Association of Versican Turnover with All-Cause Mortality in Patients on Haemodialysis

Federica Genovese[1]*, Morten A. Karsdal[1], Diana J. Leeming[1], Alexandra Scholze[2], Martin Tepel[2]

1 Nordic Bioscience, Fibrosis Biology and Biomarkers, Herlev, Denmark, 2 Odense University Hospital, Department of Nephrology, Institute for Molecular Medicine, Cardiovascular and Renal Research, Institute of Clinical Research, University of Southern Denmark, Odense, Denmark

Abstract

Objective: Cardiovascular diseases are among the most common causes of mortality in renal failure patients undergoing haemodialysis. A high turnover rate of the proteoglycan versican, represented by the increased presence of its fragmentation products in plasma, has previously been associated with cardiovascular diseases. The objective of the study was to investigate the association of versican turnover assessed in plasma with survival in haemodialysis patients.

Methods: A specific matrix metalloproteinase-generated neo-epitope fragment of versican (VCANM) was measured in plasma of 364 haemodialysis patients with a 5-years follow-up, using a robust competitive enzyme-linked immunosorbent assays. Association between VCANM plasma concentration and survival was assessed by Kaplan-Meier analysis and adjusted Cox model.

Results: Haemodialysis patients with plasma VCANM concentrations in the lowest quartile had increased risk of death (odds ratio, as compared to the highest quartile: 7.1, $p<0.001$), with a reduced survival of 152 days compared to 1295 days for patients with plasma VCANM in the highest quartile. Multivariate analysis showed that low VCANM ($p<0.001$) and older age ($p<0.001$) predicted death in haemodialysis patients.

Conclusions: Low concentrations of the versican fragment VCANM in plasma were associated with higher risk of death among haemodialysis patients. A possible protective role for the examined versican fragment is suggested.

Editor: Konradin Metze, University of Campinas, Brazil

Funding: The authors acknowledge the Danish Research Fund (Den Danske Forskningfond) for providing the funding for this research. FG, DJL, and MAK are full-time employees at Nordic Bioscience. Nordic Bioscience provided support in the form of salaries for authors FG, DJL, and MAK, but did not have any additional role in the study design, data collection and analysis, decision to publish, or preparation of the manuscript. The specific roles of these authors are articulated in the 'author contributions' section.

Competing Interests: Federica Genovese has read the journal's policy and the authors of this manuscript have the following competing interests: FG, DJL, and MAK are full-time employees at Nordic Bioscience. All other authors have no competing financial interests.

* Email: fge@nordicbioscience.com

Introduction

Patients with renal failure who undergo haemodialysis have an increased mortality compared to the general population [1,2]. Cardiovascular diseases are frequently a co-morbidity affecting end stage kidney disease (ESKD) patients [3,4], and they are the major cause of death in patients on dialysis [5]. A dysregulated equilibrium between extracellular matrix (ECM) formation and degradation characterizes fibrotic disorders, neoplasia and cardiovascular diseases [6]. Renal fibrosis is the pathological process underlying kidney failure, and most of the co-morbidities affecting ESKD patients can be related to the altered matrix turnover [7]. Thus, novel non-invasive biomarkers able to describe the rate of ECM turnover have the potential to be useful instruments to identify patients with a worse prognosis [8].

Versican is a large extracellular matrix proteoglycan whose role in chronic kidney disease (CKD) has only been described to a certain extent [9]. Versican belongs to the family of the large aggregating proteoglycans, and it has been localized in the ECM of many organs, including kidneys [9,10]. It has a modular structure constituted by a G1 domain at the N-terminal, a glycosaminoglycan (GAG) domain for the attachment of the chondroitin sulphate chains that constitute its carbohydrate fraction, and a G3 domain at the C-terminal end. The G3 domain is further organized in a modular structure containing two EGF-like repeats, a lectin-like subdomain and a complement binding protein (CBP)-like subdomain, which are dedicated to the binding with different ECM components and cytokines [11]. The main protein associated with versican is hyaluronan [12], which interacts with the G1 domain of versican. Moreover versican binds and interacts with elastic fibers, collagen type I, fibronectin and integrins [11]. Versican turnover can be estimated by the amount of fragmentation products released into circulation. A novel neo-epitope specific enzyme-linked immunosorbent assays (ELISA) has been developed to detect a unique fragmentation product generated by the cleavage of matrix metalloproteinases. This fragment of versican variant V0 measurable in plasma (VCANM), has previously been associated with different cardiovascular manifestations [13].

In the present study we tested the hypothesis that versican turnover may be associated with mortality in haemodialysis patients, by measuring plasma levels of VCANM.

Subjects and Methods

Participants

We performed an observational cohort study of 364 haemodialysis patients. The study was approved by the local ethics committee (Ethikkommission Free University Berlin, Reference numbers: ek.211-19, ek.Te2.02) and adhered to the declaration of Helsinki. Inclusion criteria were haemodialysis treatment due to end-stage renal disease and written informed consent.

All patients were routinely dialyzed for four to five hours three times weekly using biocompatible membranes with no dialyser reuse. Blood flow rates were 250 to 300 mL/min, dialysate flow rates were 500 mL/min, dialysate conductivity was 135 mS. Blood pressure was measured pre-dialysis in patients in a recumbent position. Pre-dialysis blood samples were taken at study entry. Blood was collected immediately before the start of the haemodialysis session. Clinical and laboratory data included age, gender, medication (use of angiotensin-converting-enzyme inhibitors, ß-blockers, calcium channel blockers, and erythropoietin), body mass index (calculated as weight in kilograms divided by height in meters squared), systolic and diastolic blood pressure, serum urea, serum calcium, serum potassium, and serum phosphorus. 179 patients (49%) died during the 5-years follow up. The causes of death were classified as cardiovascular, infection, cancer, or unknown. Controls consisted of nineteen age- and sex-matched CKD patients not undergoing dialysis. Among these, two patients had stage two CKD (glomerular filtration rate, GFR, according to MDRD: 90–60 mL/min), and seventeen patients had stage three CKD (GFR according to MDRD: 60–30 mL/min).

Procedures

The neo-epitope peptide generated by matrix metalloproteinase (MMP) degradation of versican (VCANM) was measured in plasma of haemodialysis patients and controls by means of a robust competitive enzyme-linked immunosorbent assays (ELISA) using a specific monoclonal antibody (mAb). The protocols and

Table 1. Baseline clinical and biochemical characteristics of haemodialysis patients stratified by plasma VCANM quartiles (Q1, Q2, Q3, Q4).

Characteristic	Q1	Q2	Q3	Q 4	P-value[a]
Number of patients	92	90	92	90	–
VCANM (range; ng/ml)	0.50 (0.20–0.59)	0.70 (0.60–0.79)	0.80 (0.80–0.99)	1.10 (1.00–1.50)	<0.001
Age (years)	68.0 (60.5–76)	64.2 (56–75)	64.3 (52–76)	64.5 (57–72)	0.12
Gender (% Male)	68%	72%	66%	56%	0.06
Dialysis vintage (months)	25.4 (1.0–35.3)	27.8 (1.0–51.7)	26.5 (1.6–43.0)	23.4 (1.0–30.4)	0.88
Diabetes mellitus (%)	50%	31%	62%	60%	0.30
Weight (kg)	71 (60–80)	74 (63–81)	73 (62–79)	75 (64–83)	0.33
Body mass index[b] (kg/m^2)	24.4 (21–27.7)	25.3 (22–27.8)	24.6 (21.6–26)	25.6 (22.4–29)	0.13
Systolic blood pressure (mmHg)	131 (114–149)	135 (117–153)	134 (114–150)	134 (117–150)	0.73
Diastolic blood pressure (mmHg)	68 (57–80)	71 (59–80)	70 (58–80)	71 (60–82)	0.35
Hemoglobin (mg/dL)	9.9 (8.7–10.8)	10.0 (9.1–11.4)	10.6 (9.3–11.8)	10.6 (9.3–11.9)	0.02
Leukocytes (10^9/L)	10.0 (6.6–12.6)	10.0 (6.5–12.8)	8.4 (6.2–9.7)	7.9 (5.7–9.5)	0.002
Platelets (10^9/L)	243 (173–305)	232 (176–256)	227 (165–271)	248 (187–300)	0.43
Albumin (g/dL)	3.2 (2.6–3.4)	3.2 (2.8–3.6)	3.4 (3.1–3.7)	3.5 (3.1–3.8)	<0.001
High sensitive CRP (mg/dL)	6.7 (2.3–8.0)	4.2 (1.2–4.5)	3.0 (0.75–4.1)	3.8 (0.9–4.7)	<0.001
Urea (mg/dL)	34 (20–36)	33 (20–41)	26 (16–31)	27 (17–35)	0.02
Serum potassium (mmol/L)	4.7 (4.1–5.2)	4.8 (4–5.5)	4.8 (4.3–5.2)	4.8 (4.2–5.4)	0.80
Serum calcium (mmol/L)	2.2 (2–2.4)	2.3 (2.1–2.4)	2.2 (2.1–2.4)	2.2 (2.1–2.4)	0.34
Serum phosphorus (mg/dL)	1.6 (1.2–1.9)	1.7 (1.2–2.1)	1.7 (1.2–2)	1.6 (1.1–2.1)	0.69
Parathyroid hormone (ng/mL)	164 (39–197)	213 (45–272)	199 (43–213)	212 (42–278)	0.96
Serum cholesterol (mg/dL)	142 (108–178)	162 (124–201)	156 (135–181)	166 (137–189)	0.06
LDL-cholesterol (mg/dl)	92 (66–114)	101 (70–129)	98 (79–116)	100 (79–123)	0.55
Dialysis dose (kt/V)	1.2 (1.0–1.3)	1.2 (1.1–1.3)	1.2 (1.0–1.3)	1.2 (1.0–1.3)	0.67
ACE inhibitors (%)	24%	20%	33%	28%	0.23
ß-Blockers (%)	59%	62%	55%	62%	0.87
Calcium channel blockers (%)	23%	29%	38%	29%	0.20
Erythropoietin therapy (%)	48%	42%	62%	45%	0.57

Continuous variables are given as medians (IQR).
[a]Comparisons between groups were made using Kruskal-Wallis test for continuous variables and Chi-square test for categorical variables.
[b]Body mass index was calculated as weight in kilograms divided by height in meters squared.

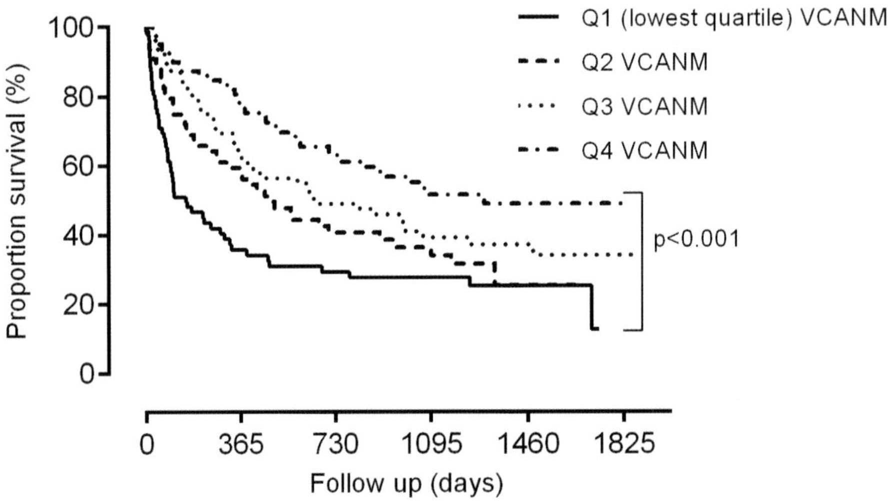

Number at risk

Q1	92	22	18	11	8	0
Q2	90	36	22	16	7	0
Q3	92	43	33	22	15	1
Q4	90	58	44	26	13	1

Figure 1. Kaplan-Meier survival curves for haemodialysis patients stratified in quartiles according to plasma VCANM levels.

technical specifications of the assay have already been described [13]. The VCANM mAb was raised against the sequence KTFGKMKPRY, a neo-epitope generated by *in vitro* proteolytic cleavage at the position 3306 by MMP-12. The antibody was selected to recognize specifically the neo-epitope generated after MMP cleavage, and not the total protein.

Statistical analysis

Continuous variables were expressed as median with interquartile range and compared with Kruskal-Wallis test and Dunn's multiple comparison post-hoc test. Time-to-event analyses were performed using the Kaplan-Meier method. Comparison of survival curves was performed using the log-rank (Mantel-Cox) test. 46 patients (12%) underwent kidney transplantation during the follow up. These patients were censored on the day of

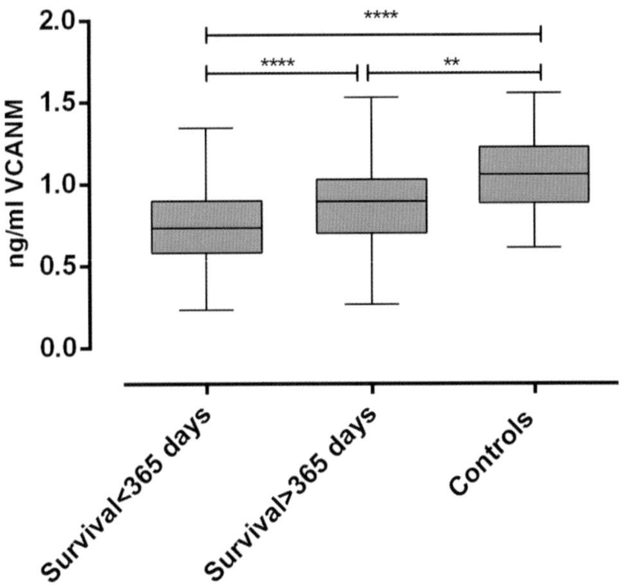

Figure 2. Plasma VCANM levels in haemodialysis patients with survival <365 days and survival >365 days and in the control group. Horizontal line: median; hashed box = IQR; error bars: range of non-outlying values. Significance levels (calculated with one-way ANOVA test, multiple comparison): ** = $p<0.01$; **** = $p<0.001$.

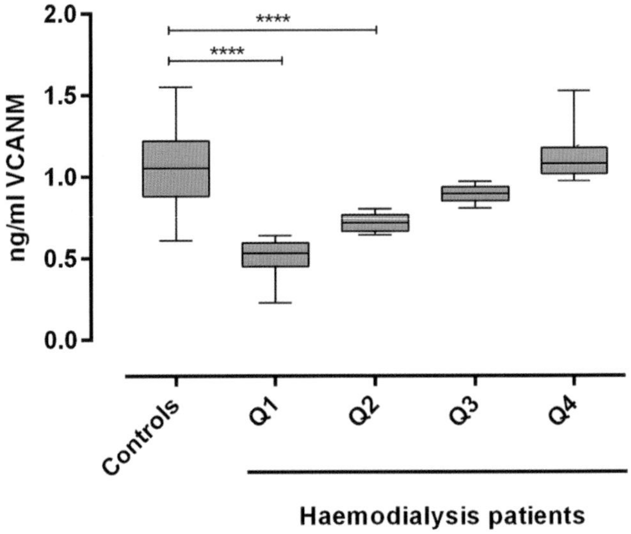

Figure 3. Plasma VCANM levels divided into quartiles in haemodialysis patients and in CKD stage two and three patients (controls). Horizontal line: median; hashed box = IQR; error bars: range of non-outlying values. Significance levels (calculated with Kruskal Wallis test and one-way ANOVA test, multiple comparison): **** = $p<0.001$.

Table 2. Univariate and multivariate Cox regression showing the odds for death in haemodialysis patients.

	Univariate Odds Ratio (95% CI)	P-value	Multivariate Odds Ratio (95% CI)	P-value
VCANM	0.23 (0.12–0.42)	<0.001	0.23 (0.13–0.42)	<0.001
Age	1.06 (1.05–1.08)	<0.001	1.06 (1.05–1.07)	<0.001
Gender (Ref = male)	0.89 (0.66–1.43)	0.31		
High sensitive CRP	1.69 (1.25–2.28)	<0.001		
Albumin	0.67 (0.52–0.86)	0.002		

transplantation. Univariate and multivariate survival analyses were performed using the proportional hazards regression model. The multivariate model was constructed with backward variable selection, using $P<0.05$ for variable retention. Statistical analyses were conducted using GraphPad Prism 5.0 (GraphPad Software, San Diego, CA), SPSS for windows (version 15; SPSS, Chicago, IL) and MedCalc (version 12.3.0.0, MedCalc software bvba for Windows).

Results

Characteristics of cohort at baseline

A total of 364 haemodialysis patients (240 men and 124 women) with a median age of 67 years (IQR, 56 to 75 years), a median time since initiation of dialysis of 247 days (IQR, 31 to 1142 days), and a median dialysis dose (kt/V) of 1.2 (IQR, 1.0 to 1.3) entered into the study. The primary diseases leading to end stage kidney disease were hypertensive nephrosclerosis in 122 cases (34%), diabetic nephropathy in 118 cases (32%), chronic glomerular nephritis in 30 cases (8%), polycystic kidney disease in 10 cases (3%) and other/unknown in 84 cases (23%). Median plasma VCANM concentration was 0.81 ng/mL (IQR, 0.64 to 0.97 ng/mL). Quartiles of plasma VCANM were used for the survival analysis. Table 1 describes the quartiles and summarizes clinical and laboratory variables stratified according to plasma VCANM quartiles.

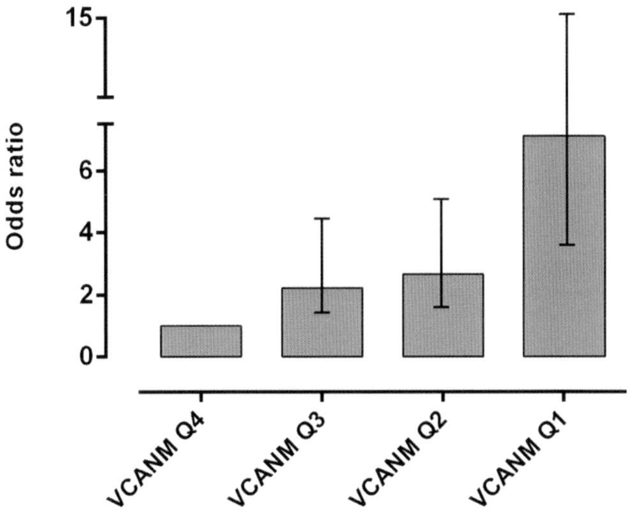

Figure 4. Odds ratio calculated for a cut-off of 365 days in the different VCANM quartiles. Bars: 95% CI.

Plasma VCANM levels are related to mortality

179 patients (49%) died during the 5 year follow up. Death occurred at a median of 201 days (IQR, 63 to 477 days) after study entry. The causes of death were cardiovascular diseases (including sudden death, fatal myocardial infarction, or fatal stroke) in 111 patients (62%), infectious disease (including septicemia) in 35 patients (20%), cancer (any type) in 22 patients (12%), and others/unknown in 11 patients (6%).

When patients were stratified according to quartiles of plasma VCANM, the survival rate differed significantly between the different groups ($p<0.001$). Patients belonging to the lowest VCANM quartile had a survival of 152 days compared to 1295 days for patients with plasma VCNAM in the highest quartile (Figure 1). VCANM was associated to all-cause mortality, and could not distinguish between cardiovascular disease-driven mortality and other mortality causes (data not shown).

The differences in survival rate among the different groups appeared to be evident already at early time points, such as 365 days. Therefore a survival time of 365 days was chosen as cut-off and the haemodialysis patients were divided into two groups: one including patients with survival time below 365 days and the other including patients that survived longer than 365 days. The levels of the analyzed marker in these two groups were compared to those of our control group constituted of patients with chronic kidney disease stage two and three (Figure 2). Plasma VCANM levels were highest in the control group, and lowest in the group of patients with short survival. Figure 3 illustrates the concentration levels in the different quartiles in the haemodialysis patient population and in the controls. VCANM levels were the same in controls and in Q4 and decreased significantly in Q3, Q2 and in the lowest quartile Q1.

The univariate Cox regression analysis showed a significant association of VCANM, age, high sensitive CRP and albumin with survival (Table 2). VCANM and age were retained in the model obtained with a multivariate analysis, showing independency from one another. CRP levels were significantly different in the VCANM quartile groups, decreasing with increasing VCANM concentrations (Table 1).

From the Cox regression analysis it was possible to calculate the odds ratio for an increase of ten years in age (odds = 1.87) and a decrease of 0.5 ng/ml of plasma VCANM (odds = 2.1).

The odds ratio for the different VCANM quartiles was calculated for death at 365 days as outcome (figure 4). VCANM Q1 showed an odds ratio of 7.1 (using as reference the fourth quartile).

Discussion

In the present study we have identified a novel marker of mortality in haemodialysis patients.

This marker represents a fragmentation product of versican, an ECM proteoglycans implicated in vascular remodeling [14], and it was previously associated with cardiovascular diseases caused by dysregulated ECM turnover [13]. The VCANM assay measures a pool of fragments of versican long up to 90 aminoacids, which have a common N-terminal end generated by proteolytic cleavage mediated by matrix metalloproteinases. This fragment is localized in the proximity of the protein C-terminal, in the G3 domain, and belongs to the complement binding protein (CBP)-like motif.

Haemodialysis patients with higher VCANM levels showed better outcome. This finding was strengthened by the observation of higher plasma VCANM levels in CKD patients stage two and three (controls) than in haemodialysis patients with shorter survival. Plasma VCANM concentration and age were retained in a multivariate regression model and were independent from each other. Furthermore, a decrease in plasma VCANM levels of 0.5 ng/ml, which corresponded to the median difference between the lowest and the highest plasma VCANM quartile, described a higher risk of death when compared to an increase of ten years of age. The separation between the different survival curves was maximal at early time points. For this reason we chose a cut-off time point of 365 days to calculate the odds ratio. The odds ratio for mortality for patients in the lowest plasma VCANM quartile was seven times higher compared to that for patients in the highest quartile. Interestingly, levels of VCANM were not exclusively associated to cardiovascular mortality, despite the previous findings that versican fragmentation was increased in cardiovascular diseases such as acute myocardial infarction and coronary calcification [13]. This suggests that in ESKD patients VCANM is not a marker for cardiovascular morbidity. The association of lower plasma levels of this specific fragment with a worse outcome might have different possible explanations: an increased fragmentation of versican in patients with a better prognosis may facilitate its clearance. An upregulated versican mRNA expression in the kidney was associated with the degree of histological damage [15], and histological accumulation of versican was observed in the tubulointerstitium of patients with proteinuric nephropathy [9], and in cellular crescents and periglomerular areas of patients with human crescentic glomerulonephritis [16]; therefore the ability to degrade the accumulated proteoglycan might be a factor that ameliorates the disease burden. Versican has been shown to be produced by stromal cells and leukocytes [17]: the correlation between number of leukocytes and VCANM quartiles (as shown in table 1) suggests that versican formation is more elevated than versican degradation during sustained inflammation. It has been demonstrated that complexes of versican and hyaluronan (HA) promote leukocytes adhesion and that a failed incorporation of versican into the ECM blocks monocyte adhesion and reduces the inflammatory response [17]. Therefore when versican is degraded (hence VCANM presence in plasma increases), the formation of the complex versican-hyaluronan is impaired and inflammation is reduced. This hypothesis is further confirmed by the inverse correlation between serum CRP levels and VCANM levels (table 1). Furthermore, as lower levels of VCANM are associated with higher mortality risk, it can be hypothesized that this fragment may have a protective role in end stage kidney disease patients. Such protective functions have been previously observed for other ECM protein fragments, such as endostatin and tumstatin [18,19]. The paracrine and endocrine functions of the ECM proteins are more and more object of investigation, and the proteins belonging to the matrix are not considered anymore as structural components only. Beside ECM proteins in their native conformation having signaling roles, there are evidences suggesting that ECM proteins that normally don't exert matricellular functions, gain powerful signaling potential after protease cleavage [6,20]. As of today, versican has only been seen as a therapeutic target [21], but the finding that high levels of its degradation product VCANM are associated with longer survival introduces the novel concept of its potential as therapeutic *per se*, which, however, needs to be carefully examined. Further investigations are needed to confirm whether VCANM is not only a fragment generated by proteolytic cleavage of versican, but has also paracrine or endocrine functions.

Acknowledgments

We acknowledge the Danish Research Fund (Den Danske Forskningfond) for providing the funding for this research.

Author Contributions

Conceived and designed the experiments: FG MAK DJL AS MT. Performed the experiments: FG AS MT. Analyzed the data: FG DJL MT. Contributed reagents/materials/analysis tools: MT AS MAK. Contributed to the writing of the manuscript: FG MT DJL MAK.

References

1. Hallan SI, Matsushita K, Sang Y, Mahmoodi BK, Black C, et al. (2012) Age and association of kidney measures with mortality and end-stage renal disease. JAMA 308: 2349–2360.
2. de Jager DJ, Grootendorst DC, Jager KJ, van Dijk PC, Tomas LM, et al. (2009) Cardiovascular and noncardiovascular mortality among patients starting dialysis. JAMA 302: 1782–1789.
3. Raggi P, Boulay A, Chasan-Taber S, Amin N, Dillon M, et al. (2002) Cardiac calcification in adult hemodialysis patients. A link between end-stage renal disease and cardiovascular disease? J Am Coll Cardiol 39: 695–701.
4. Goodman WG, Goldin J, Kuizon BD, Yoon C, Gales B, et al. (2000) Coronary-artery calcification in young adults with end-stage renal disease who are undergoing dialysis. N Engl J Med 342: 1478–1483.
5. Al-Dadah A, Omran J, Nusair MB, Dellsperger KC (2012) Cardiovascular mortality in dialysis patients. Adv Perit Dial 28: 56–59.
6. Karsdal MA, Nielsen MJ, Sand JM, Henriksen K, Genovese F, et al. (2013) Extracellular matrix remodeling: the common denominator in connective tissue diseases. Possibilities for evaluation and current understanding of the matrix as more than a passive architecture, but a key player in tissue failure. Assay Drug Dev Technol 11: 70–92.
7. Gross ML, Ritz E (2008) Hypertrophy and fibrosis in the cardiomyopathy of uremia–beyond coronary heart disease. Semin Dial 21: 308–318.
8. Genovese F, Manresa AA, Leeming DJ, Karsdal MA, Boor P (2014) The extracellular matrix in the kidney: a source of novel non-invasive biomarkers of kidney fibrosis? Fibrogenesis Tissue Repair 7: 4.
9. Rudnicki M, Perco P, Neuwirt H, Noppert SJ, Leierer J, et al. (2012) Increased renal versican expression is associated with progression of chronic kidney disease. PLoS One 7: e44891.
10. Bode-Lesniewska B, Dours-Zimmermann MT, Odermatt BF, Briner J, Heitz PU, et al. (1996) Distribution of the large aggregating proteoglycan versican in adult human tissues. J Histochem Cytochem 44: 303–312.
11. Wu YJ, La Pierre DP, Wu J, Yee AJ, Yang BB (2005) The interaction of versican with its binding partners. Cell Res 15: 483–494.
12. Selbi W, de la Motte CA, Hascall VC, Day AJ, Bowen T, et al. (2006) Characterization of hyaluronan cable structure and function in renal proximal tubular epithelial cells. Kidney Int 70: 1287–1295.
13. Barascuk N, Genovese F, Larsen L, Byrjalsen I, Zheng Q, et al. (2013) A MMP derived versican neo-epitope is elevated in plasma from patients with atherosclerotic heart disease. Int J Clin Exp Med 6: 174–184.
14. Wight TN, Merrilees MJ (2004) Proteoglycans in atherosclerosis and restenosis: key roles for versican. Circ Res 94: 1158–1167.
15. Melk A, Mansfield ES, Hsieh SC, Hernandez-Boussard T, Grimm P, et al. (2005) Transcriptional analysis of the molecular basis of human kidney aging using cDNA microarray profiling. Kidney Int 68: 2667–2679.

16. Stokes MB, Hudkins KL, Zaharia V, Taneda S, Alpers CE (2001) Up-regulation of extracellular matrix proteoglycans and collagen type I in human crescentic glomerulonephritis. Kidney Int 59: 532–542.
17. Wight TN, Kang I, Merrilees MJ (2014) Versican and the control of inflammation. Matrix Biol 35: 152–161.
18. Yamaguchi Y, Takihara T, Chambers RA, Veraldi KL, Larregina AT, et al. (2012) A peptide derived from endostatin ameliorates organ fibrosis. Sci Transl Med 4: 136ra71.
19. Yamamoto Y, Maeshima Y, Kitayama H, Kitamura S, Takazawa Y, et al. (2004) Tumstatin peptide, an inhibitor of angiogenesis, prevents glomerular hypertrophy in the early stage of diabetic nephropathy. Diabetes 53: 1831–1840.
20. Karsdal MA, Henriksen K, Leeming DJ, Woodworth T, Vassiliadis E, et al. (2010) Novel combinations of Post-Translational Modification (PTM) neo-epitopes provide tissue-specific biochemical markers–are they the cause or the consequence of the disease? Clin Biochem 43: 793–804.
21. Merrilees MJ, Wight TN (2012) Targeting the matrix: potential benefits for versican therapeutics. Elsevier Current Opinion doi:10.1016/j.ceb.2013.01.001.

Serum Response Factor Accelerates the High Glucose-Induced Epithelial-to-Mesenchymal Transition (EMT) via Snail Signaling in Human Peritoneal Mesothelial Cells

Lijie He[1,2], Weijuan Lou[1,2], Lihua Ji[1,2,3], Wei Liang[1,2,4], Meilan Zhou[1], Guoshang Xu[1], Lijuan Zhao[1], Chen Huang[1], Rong Li[1], Hanmin Wang[1,2], Xiangmei Chen[1,5]*, Shiren Sun[1,2]*

1 Department of Nephrology, Xijing Hospital, the Fourth Military Medical University, Xi'an, Shaan xi, China, **2** State Key Laboratory of Cancer Biology, Xijing Hospital, the Fourth Military Medical University, Xi'an, Shaan xi, China, **3** Department of Nephrology, Xingyuan Hospital, the Fourth Hospital of Yulin, Yulin, Shaan xi, China, **4** Department of Nephrology, the Ninth Hospital of Xi'an, Xi'an, Shaan xi, China, **5** Department of Nephrology, State Key Laboratory of Kidney Diseases, Chinese PLA General Hospital and Medical College, Beijing, China

Abstract

Background: Epithelial-to-Mesenchymal Transition (EMT) induced by glucose in human peritoneal mesothelial cells (HPMCs) is a major cause of peritoneal membrane (PM) fibrosis and dysfunction.

Methods: To investigate serum response factor (SRF) impacts on EMT-derived fibrosis in PM, we isolated HPMCs from the effluents of patients with end-stage renal disease (ESRD) to analyze alterations during peritoneal dialysis (PD) and observe the response of PM to SRF in a rat model.

Results: Our results demonstrated the activation and translocation of SRF into the nuclei of HPMCs under extensive periods of PD. Accordingly, HPMCs lost their epithelial morphology with a decrease in E-cadherin expression and an increase in α-smooth muscle actin (α-SMA) expression, implying a transition in phenotype. PD with 4.25% glucose solution significantly induced SRF up-regulation and increased peritoneal thickness. In immortal HPMCs, high glucose (HG, 60 mmol/L) stimulated SRF overexpression in transformed fibroblastic HPMCs. SRF-siRNA preserved HPMC morphology, while transfection of SRF plasmid into HPMCs caused the opposite effects. Evidence from electrophoretic mobility shift, chromatin immunoprecipitation and reporter assays further supported that SRF transcriptionally regulated Snail, a potent inducer of EMT, by directly binding to its promoter.

Conclusions: Our data suggested that activation of SRF/Snail pathway might contribute to the progressive PM fibrosis during PD.

Editor: Garyfalia Drossopoulou, National Centre for Scientific Research "Demokritos", Greece

Funding: This study was supported by grants from the National Scientific Foundation of China (81270849, 81270768, 2012K16-08-05, 81170670, 2011BAI10B08). All of the funders had no role in the study design, data collection and analysis, decision to publish, or preparation of the manuscript.

Competing Interests: The authors have declared that no competing interests exist.

* Email: sunshiren@gmail.com (SRS); xmchen301@126.com (XMC)

These authors contributed equally to this work.

Introduction

Peritoneal dialysis (PD) is currently used as a chronic, life-sustaining treatment by approximately 197,000 end-stage renal disease (ESRD) patients, or 11% of the global dialysis population [1]. Long term PD is limited because of the structural and functional changes in the peritoneal membrane (PM) induced by PD fluids (PDFs), which contain high concentrations of glucose that finally lead to a loss of ultrafiltration [2]. The epithelial-to-mesenchymal transition (EMT) is a complex, step-wise phenomenon beneficial for normal wound healing [3] but detrimental in fibrogenic diseases [4], such as peritoneal fibrosis. Biomarkers for EMT have been identified and categorized, including the loss of the epithelial adhesion protein E-cadherin and upregulation of the mesenchymal marker α-smooth muscle actin (α-SMA) [5]. Preventing EMT could ameliorate peritoneal fibrosis, preserving the PM during PD [6].

Serum response factor (SRF), a member of a conserved DNA-binding protein family, is a master switch for the expression of contractile and cytoskeletal genes in virtually all cells across diverse species [7]. SRF plays important roles in diverse pathological processes, including EMT-derived tumor metastasis and fibrosis. For example, SRF expression in hepatocellular carcinoma (HCC) cells that can undergo EMT may play an enhanced role in tumor progression [8]. Overexpression of SRF in colorectal carcinoma cells is associated with the modulation of E-cadherin/β-catenin expression and may enhance metastasis [9]. In addition, SRF translocation into nuclei may contribute to myofibroblast differentiation in human lung fibroblasts and cardiac fibrosis [10–12]. SRF targets, which contain a serum response element (SRE), are activated when SRF is in the nucleus [13,14]. CCG-1423 is a specific inhibitor of Rho pathway-mediated signaling and activation of SRF transcription. CCG-1423 selectively inhibits DNA synthesis, proliferation and invasion of Rho-overexpressing cell lines. Recently, the SRF inhibitor (CCG-1423) was suggested to be a promising compound as a novel pharmacological tool in preventing prostate cancer progression [15].

The high glucose (HG)-induced EMT of HPMCs acts as a key process in peritoneal membrane fibrosis and dysfunction. Mediated by factors including E-cadherin, α-SMA and Snail, epithelial cells may lose their epithelial characteristics and gain mesenchymal cell properties in response to certain stimuli [16,17]. However, to date, whether SRF is involved in EMT-mediated PM deterioration remains incompletely understood. Here, we will firstly demonstrate the role and mechanism of SRF in the EMT-derived peritoneal fibrosis.

Methods

Ethics Statement

The study protocol conformed to the ethical guidelines of the 1975 Declaration of Helsinki and was approved by the ethics committee of Xijing Hospital. Written informed consent was obtained from each patient. The Ethics Committee for Animal Experiments of the Fourth Military Medical University approved all animal work (Permit number: 20120023) and the experimental protocols strictly complied with the institutional guidelines and the criteria outlined in the "Guide for Care and Use of Laboratory Animals". And all efforts were made to minimize the number of animals used and their suffering, in accordance with the ethical guidelines for animal research. All surgery was performed under sodium pentobarbital anesthesia.

HPMC isolation and culture

Human mesothelial cells obtained from the effluents of patients undergoing CAPD in our PD center in the Department of Nephrology, Xijing Hospital were collected and cultured using a previously described method [18–20]. The use of human peritoneal fluid in this study was approved by the institutional review board of the Fourth Military Medical University and was done in accordance with international guidelines for the use of human tissues. The inclusion criteria were age less than 65 years, duration of CAPD longer than 3 months, no peritonitis in the last 6 months, the use of 1.5% glucose dialysis solution, and no history of abdominal surgery or long-term use of an immunosuppressant (Table S1). The CAPD patients were sorted into three groups according to the duration of dialysis (Group 1 was 3-6 months, Group 2 was 7–24 months, and Group 3 was longer than 25 months).

The immortal human HPMC line (ATCC, Rockville, MD), which is an untransformed HPMC line that yields data similar to the results obtained using primary cells, was cultured in Earle's M199 medium. EMT was induced in immortal HPMCs with HG (0.5 ng/mL) (R&D Systems, Minneapolis, MN), as described previously [21–23].

Peritoneal exposure model in rats and immunofluorescence analyses of the peritoneum

A chronic infusion model of non-uremic animal PD was used, as described previously [23]. Briefly, 24 male Sprague-Dawley rats (250 to 300 g) were divided into three groups with eight rats each. The control group was injected with normal saline (100 ml/kg/d) each day for 6 weeks; the HG-PDF group was injected with 4.25% glucose dialysis solution (100 ml/kg/d); and the SRF inhibitor group was injected with 4.25% glucose dialysis solution and CCG-1423 (0.03 mg/kg/d). Lipopolysaccharide (LPS, Sigma, final concentration of 5 μg/L) was used at 8, 9, and 10 days in the HG-PDF and SRF inhibitor groups [6,23]. The SRF inhibitor was purchased from Calbiochem (EMD, Darmstad, Germany). The parietal peritoneum of the abdominal wall was fixed and embedded in paraffin as described in the Concise Methods section. For immunofluorescence microscopy, 3 μm tissue sections were incubated with primary antibodies against E-cadherin, α-SMA or SRF. Rats were manipulated and cared for according to NIH Animal Care and Use Committee guidelines in the Experiment Animal Center of the Fourth Military Medical University (Xi'an, Shanxi, Province, P.R. China).

Western blotting

Total protein extracts from cultured cells were loaded on SDS-PAGE gels, and Western blotting was performed according to a standard protocol. The antibodies used were as follows: anti-p-SRF (Cell Signaling Technology, Inc) diluted 1:500; anti-SRF diluted 1:80; anti-E-cadherin, anti-α-SMA, and anti-Snail diluted 1:50 (Santa Cruz Biotechnology); and anti-β-actin (Sigma) diluted 1:4000. The antibody staining was performed as described previously [23,24].

Confocal microscopy and immunofluorescence

Cultured cells were grown on 0.8 cm×0.8 cm slides, rinsed with ice-cold phosphate-buffered saline and fixed with 4% paraformaldehyde. Immunofluorescence staining was performed on paraffin-embedded sections or cultured cells, as described previously [24]. Samples were immunostained with anti-SRF, anti-α-SMA, anti-E-cadherin or anti-Snail antibodies (Santa Cruz Biotechnology, CA) and then counterstained with FITC-labeled IgG secondary antibodies (Invitrogen). The nuclei were visualized using DAPI. Images were obtained using an Olympus microscope and IM50 imaging software (Leica) or using an FCS confocal laser scanning microscope (LSM510; Carl Zeiss MicroImaging). All sections or slide were examined and scored independently by two investigators without knowledge of the outcome.

Plasmid construction and cell transfection

The siRNA plasmids that recognize human SRF (sc-36563) were purchased from Santa Cruz Biotechnology for the transient transfections. The full-length human SRF plasmids were a gift from Dr. Eric Olson (Department of Molecular Biology, UT Southwestern Medical Center at Dallas, USA). The transfections were performed using Lipofectamine 2000 (Invitrogen, Carlsbad, CA), according to the manufacturer's instructions. Real-time PCR or Western blot analysis was used to assess the transfection efficiency.

Chromatin immunoprecipitation and quantitative PCR

ChIP was performed as previously described [25,26]. Chromatin fragments were co-immunoprecipitated from HG-treated HPMCs and control lysates with the appropriate amount of SRF antibody or an equivalent amount of rabbit IgG (8 μg) as a control. The purified DNA fragments were used as templates for PCR amplification. Real-time PCR was performed using an ABI 7900 Sequence Detection System (Applied Biosystems) and the SYBR Green PCR core reagent kit (Applied Biosystems). The specific primers were as follows: Snail (SRE1) ChIPF1, 5′-CGTCTGTCTCCCTCACTGGACC-3′, Snail (SRE1) ChIPR1, 5′-CTCTCGGCGGCTTGAAATGC-3′, Snail (SRE2) ChIP F2, 5′-GCCCGGGCTCTCACCGCCAC-3′, and Snail (SRE2) ChIP

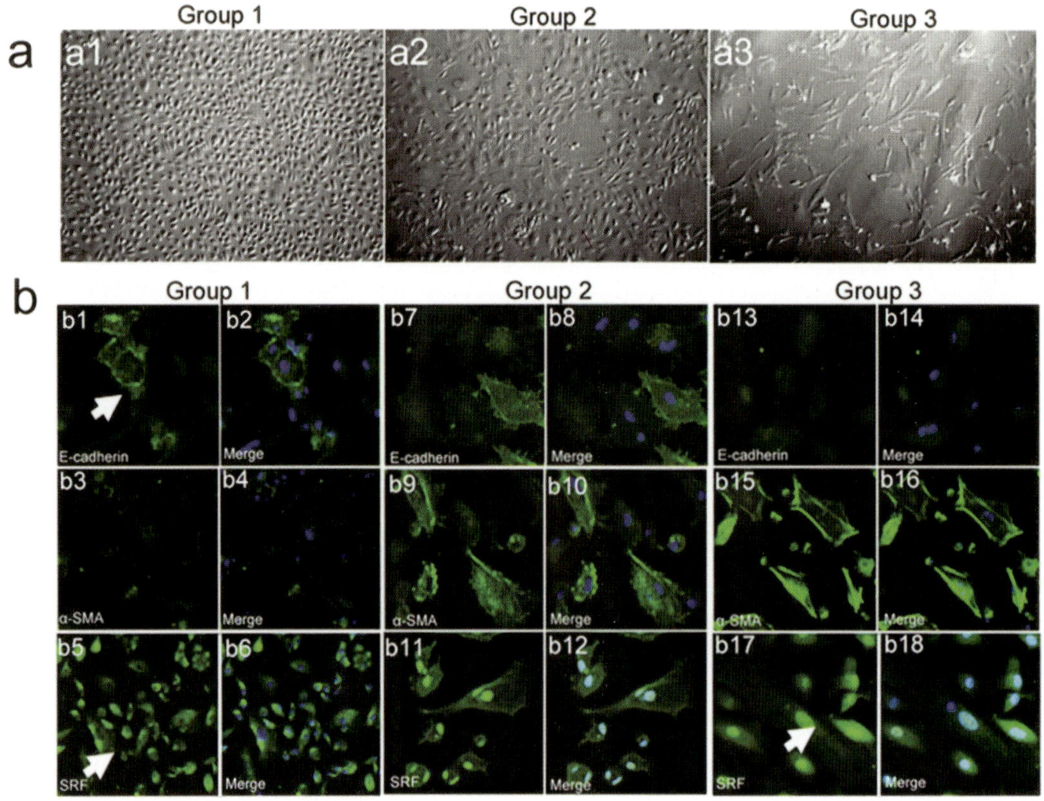

Figure 1. SRF expression in PD effluent-derived HPMCs. (a) Phase contrast microscopy shows different morphological characteristics of HPMCs. (a1) Effluent-derived HPMCs from Group 1 patients with a cobblestone-like morphology. (a2) Effluent-derived HPMCs from Group 2 patients with mixed transitional morphology. (a3) Effluent-derived HPMCs from Group 3 patients with a fibroblast-like morphology. Magnification is 200×. (b) Differences in the EMT markers E-cadherin, α-SMA and SRF expression in HPMCs with different phenotypes from the three groups. Magnification is 200×.

R2, 5′-GCAGCAGCGCCGCCAACTCC-3′. The values were normalized to the input and expressed as a fold increase relative to the IgG control.

DNA sequencing and plasmid construction for the promoter analysis

The snail promoter region from −1 to −1000 was cloned into the pGL3 luciferase vector (Promega) (Promega, Madison, WI, USA). The primers used to create the mutant reporters (MTSNAIL-1, MTSNAIL-2, MTSNAIL-3) are as follows: mutSnailF1: 5′-CGTGCTGGGCGCTCCGTAAACAATCGATCGATCGAGGAACGGGTGCTCTTGGCTAGC-3′, mutSnailR1: 5′-GCTAGCCAAGAGCACCCGTTCCTCGATCGATCGATTGTTTACGGAGCGCCCAGCACG-3′, mutSnailF2: 5′-GCGCGGAGGTGACAAAGGGGCGATCGATCGATCGCCCCGCCCCTCCCACCCCCCACCA-3′, and mutSnailR2: 5′-TGGTGGGGGGTGGGAGGGGCGGGGCGATCGATCGATCGCCCCTTTGTCACCTCCGCGC-3′.

Table 1. Expression and location of SRF in primary HPMCs.

Characteristic	Group 1 (n = 17)	Group 2 (n = 10)	Group 3 (n = 15)	P
CAPD times	3–6 m	6–24 m	>24 m	
Morphology of primary HPMCs				0.000
Cobblestone morphology	13	1		
Mixed morphology	4	7	2	
Fibroblast-like morphology		2	13	
Location of SRF in primary HPMCs				0.000
Located in cytoplasm	12	2	0	
Located both in cytoplasm and nuclei	4	6	4	
Located in nuclei	1	2	11	

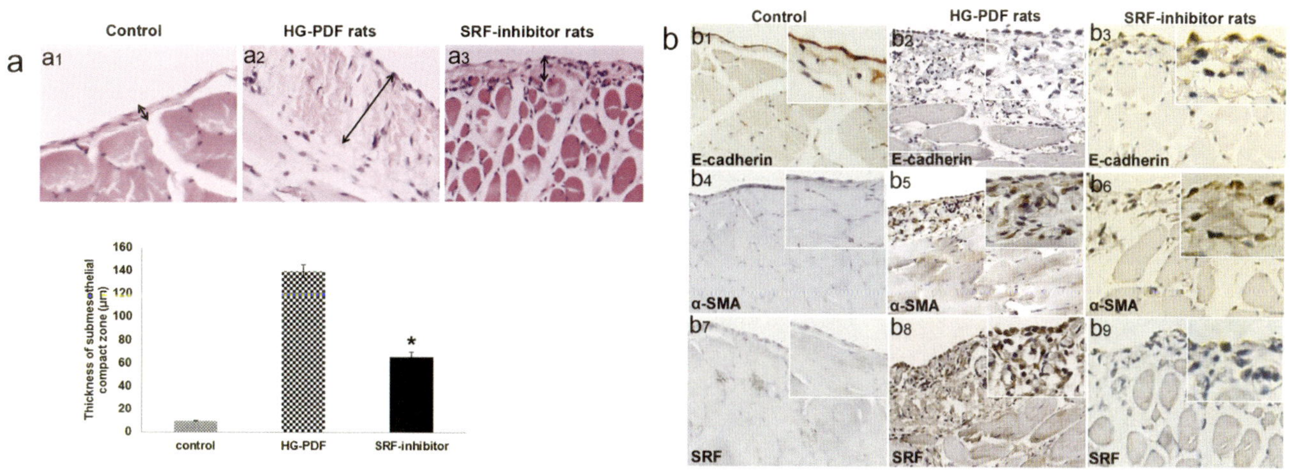

Figure 2. Inhibition of SRF by CCG-1423 ameliorates PD-induced PM fibrosis *in vivo*. (a) Rats received a daily instillation of PD fluid or saline for 6 weeks. After that period, samples were prepared and analyzed as described in the Concise Methods section. (a1) As measured by HE staining, saline exposure resulted in little change in PM. (a2) Exposure to 4.25% PD fluid resulted in an increase in the thickness of the PM. (a3). CCG-1423 treatment significantly reduced HG-PD effects. The histogram showed the thickness for HE staining in the submesothelial compact zone (mean±SE, n = 8). Magnification is 200×. (b) Staining of the EMT markers E-cadherin, α-SMA and SRF in peritoneal samples by immunohistochemistry reveals that PD fluid exposure induces the EMT process, while CCG-1423 treatment significantly ameliorated EMT-derived fibrosis. Magnification is 200×.

Transient transfection luciferase assay

For the transient transfection assays, HG-treated HPMCs or control cells were seeded 48 h before transfection. Then, pGL3-basic was transfected with the PRLsv40 plasmid into cells in the presence of Lipofectamine. The luciferase activity in cell lysates collected 48 h after transfection was measured as relative light units with the Fluoroscan Ascent FL (Labsystems, Franklin, MA, USA) using the Dual-Luciferase Assay System (Promega). The relative luciferase activity was defined as the ratio of the firefly luciferase activity/mean Renilla luciferase activity for each construct relative to the pGL3 control vector (Promega) [24].

Electrophoretic mobility shift assay

Nuclear proteins were isolated using the Nuclear Protein Isolation kit (Panomics). The binding reaction for the electrophoretic mobility shift assay (EMSA) contained 10 mmol/L HEPES (pH 7.5), 80 mmol/L KCl, 1 mmol/L EDTA, 1 mmol/L EGTA, 6% glycerol, 0.5 μg of polydeoxyinosinic-deoxycytidylic acid, 0.5 μg of sonicated salmon sperm DNA, 2 pmol of a double-stranded oligonucleotide of AR/GR HRE conjugated to IR fluorophore IRDye 700 (LI-COR), and 10 μg of the nuclear extract. To verify the specificity of the AR (GR) protein-DNA complexes, a binding reaction was performed using increasing concentrations of non-conjugated HRE (cold probe) and alternating with a mutated HRE conjugated to IRDye 700. A DNA-binding reaction was performed at 16°C for 30 min in a final volume of 20 μL. The DNA-protein complexes were analyzed by Tris-borate EDTA electrophoresis on 6% polyacrylamide gels containing 0.5% glycerol. The DNA-protein complexes were visualized using an Odyssey IR scanner (LI-COR) with a 680-nm scanner channel, and linear graphs were constructed with the LI-COR Odyssey software for quantitative image analysis (LI-COR) [24].

Reverse-transcription PCR

Total RNA was extracted using the RNeasy kit (Qiagen GmbH, Hilden, Germany), and cDNA was obtained from 500 ng of total RNA using an Omniscript RT kit (Qiagen). Quantitative PCR was performed using a LightCycler (Roche Diagnostics GmbH, Mannheim, Germany), SYBR Green kit (Roche Diagnostics GmbH) and the following specific primer sets: GAPDH, F: 5′-CCTCAAGATCATCAGCAAT-3′ and R: 5′-CCATCCACAGTCTTCTGGGT-3′ (used for normalization); SRF, F: 5′-AAACTGCAGCCCATGATCACC-3′ and R: 5′-CTTCAAAGCCAGTGGCACTCA-3′; CDH1, F: 5′-TTCCCTCGACACCCGATTC-3′ and R: 5′-TAGGTGGAGTCCCAGGCGTA-3′; α-SMA, F: 5′-AAGATGACCCAGATCATGTT-3′ and R: 5′-TCAT- AGATGGGGACATTGT-3′; and Snail, F: 5′-ACCCCAATCGGAAGCCTAACT-3′ and R: 5′-GGTCGTAGGGCTGCTGGAA-3′. Experiments were performed in duplicate. After amplification, the PCR products were confirmed by melting curve analysis and gel electrophoresis.

Statistical analysis

The bands from Western blotting or real-time PCR were quantified using Quantity One software (Bio-Rad, Hercules, CA, USA). The numerical data are presented as the mean ± SE using SPSS 12.0 software (Chicago, IL, USA). Differences between the means were assessed using Student's t-test, an ANOVA or the χ^2 test. Significant differences were determined using an analysis of variance followed by a post-hoc comparisons with Fisher's protected least-significant-difference test. The data were significant different if $P<0.05$.

Results

1. Nuclear translocation of SRF occurs in human peritoneal mesothelial cells and morphological and biomarker alterations are consistent with EMT in continuous ambulatory peritoneal dialysis (CAPD) patients

Morphological features of human peritoneal mesothelial cells were markedly variable, ranging from a cobblestone-like appearance to mixed cell populations and fibroblast-like cells (Table 1,

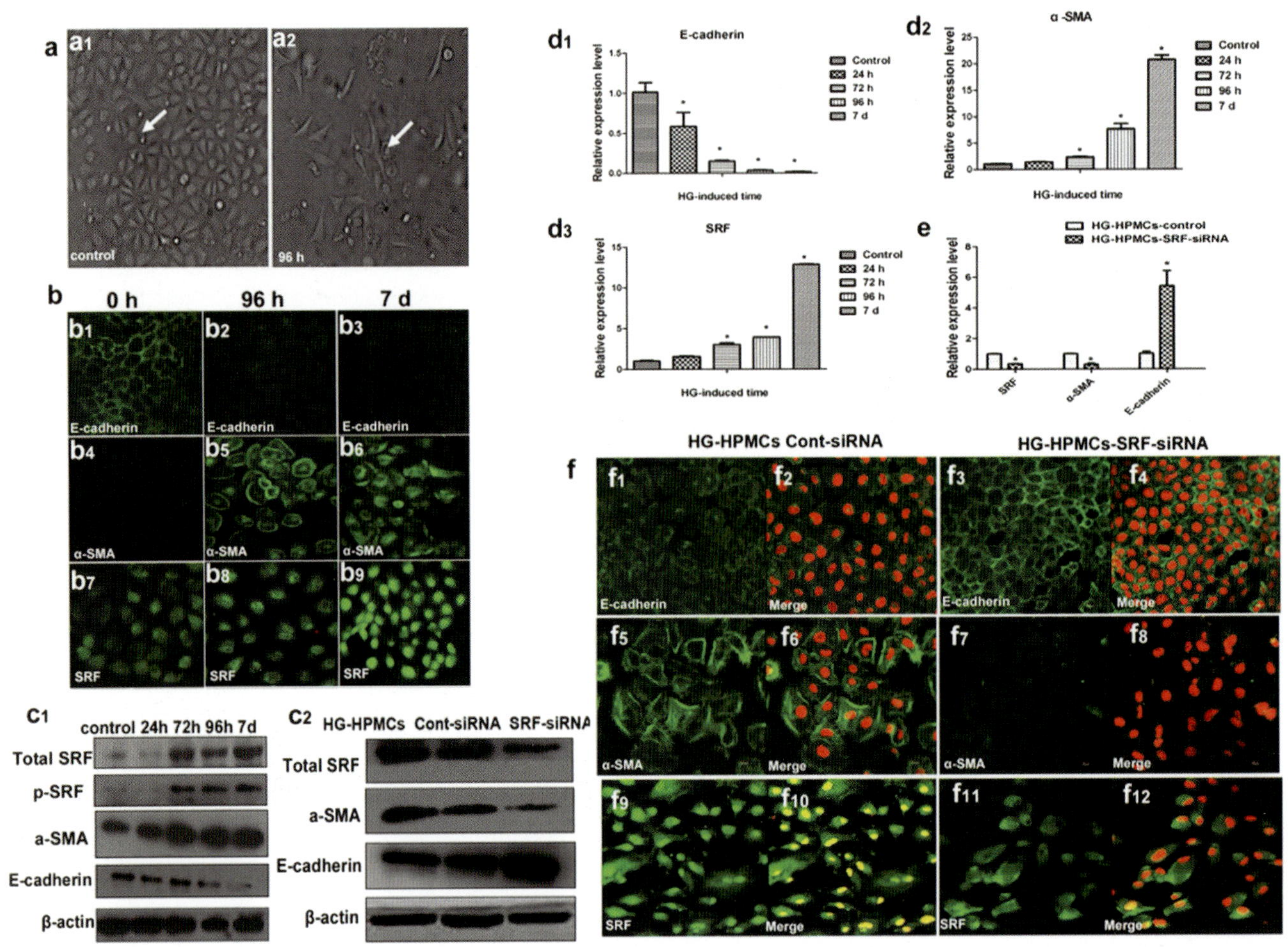

Figure 3. HPMC EMT induced by HG *in vitro* results in increased SRF expression, while knockdown of SRF by SRF-siRNA reverses HPMC EMT *in vitro*. (a) Morphological changes in HPMCs induced by HG stimulation for 96 h compared to the control. Magnification is 200×. (b) Fluorescence microscopy showed the altered location and expression of SRF and EMT markers E-cadherin and α-SMA in HPMCs induced by 0 h, 96 h and 7 d of treatment. Magnification is 200×. (c1) Western blot analysis showing the induction of SRF, p-SRF and EMT marker proteins E-cadherin and α-SMA expression by HG at 0 h, 24 h, 48 h, 72 h, 96 h, and 7 d in immortal HPMCs. (c2) Western blot analysis of SRF in HPMCs which were exposed with HG for 96 h and then transfected with SRF-siRNA or control vector. (d1-3) Induction of E-cadherin, α-SMA and SRF mRNA expression at 0 h, 24 h, 48 h, 72 h, 96 h, and 7 d in immortal HPMCs. Bars in A represent the fold induction over untreated cells and are depicted as the mean +/− S.E. of three independent experiments conducted in duplicate(*$P<0.05$ vs. control HPMCs). (e) Real-time PCR showing mRNA of SRF, E-cadherin and α-SMA in HPMCs transfected with SRF-siRNA or control vector (*$P<0.05$ vs. HG-HPMCs-control). (f) Fluorescence microscopy showed the location and expression of the EMT markers E-cadherin, α-SMA and SRF in HG-induced SRF-siRNA-treated HPMCs and control cells. Magnification, 200×.

Figure 1a). Of the 42 effluent cultures evaluated, 76.47% (13/17) of Group 1 had a cobblestone shape, 70.00% (7/10) of Group 2 showed a mixed morphology (cobblestone and fibroblast-like morphology), and 86.67% (13/15) of Group 3 were fibroblast-like cells. To verify the phenotype of the HPMCs from the PD effluents, we examined expression of E-cadherin, a typical epithelial marker, and α-SMA, a typical mesothelial marker, by immunofluorescence. Effluent cells from Group 1 with a cobblestone-like appearance had higher E-cadherin expression and lower α-SMA expression. In contrast, fibroblast-like cells from Group 3 showed the highest α-SMA expression without E-cadherin expression. The effluent cells from Group 2 patients were in between with a mixed appearance. SRF was primarily localized within the cytoplasm of the HPMCs from Group 1 (70.59%, 12/17). However, SRF translocated to the nuclei of cells from Groups 2 and 3 (Table 1, Figure 1b). These morphological changes, along with the E-cadherin downregulation and α-SMA upregulation in the mesothelial cells derived from the effluent, implied potential EMT after extensive PD.

2. Benefits of SRF inhibition in sustaining PM function in rats undergoing PD

To examine the effect of SRF inhibition in PD, we performed PD in rats with HG-PDF (4.25% glucose dialysis solution) with or without CCG-1423 for 6 weeks. By histopathological examination, the thickness of the submesothelial compact zone in the HG-PDF group (139.9±5.5 μm) was significantly greater than that in the control group (9.7±0.5 μm), significantly less in the SRF-inhibitor group (65.9.7±4.4 μm, $P<0.01$ versus the HG group). So a loss of the mesothelial cell monolayer with a thicker PM was found in the parietal peritoneum from the untreated PD group compared to the saline control (Figure 2a1, a2), while CCG-1423 significantly preserved peritoneal thickness and mesothelium morphology in the treated group (Figure 2a3, Figure S2).

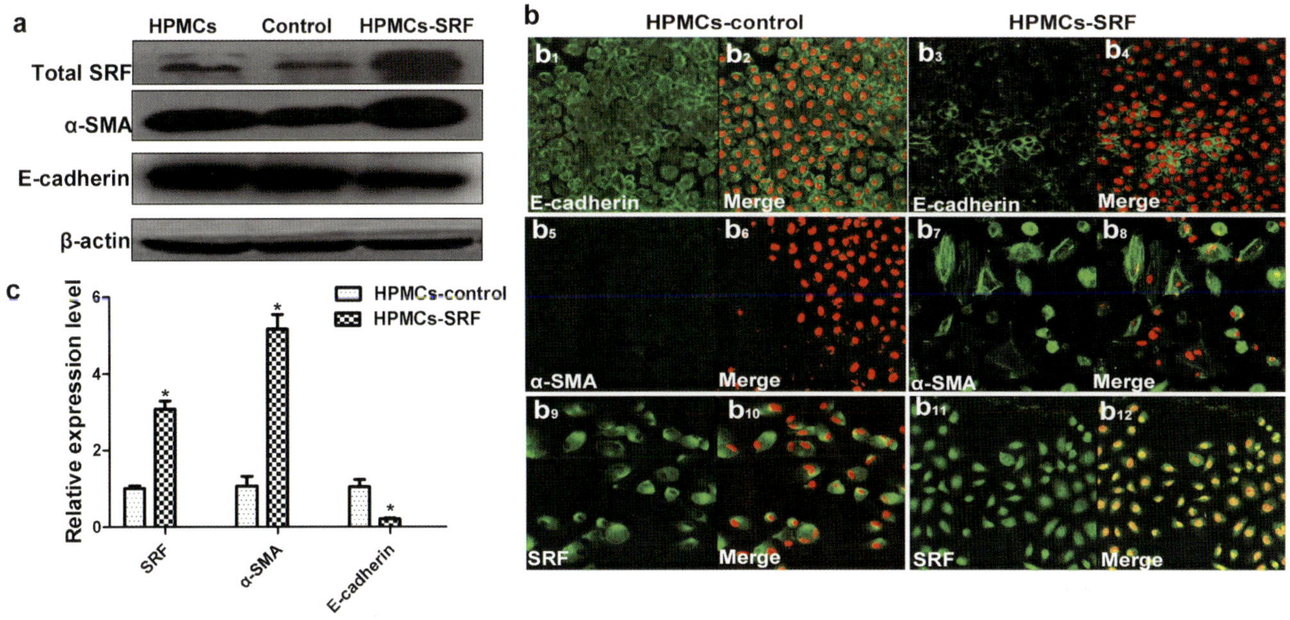

Figure 4. Overexpression of SRF by a SRF plasmid enhances HPMC EMT *in vitro*. (a) Western blot analysis of SRF in HPMCs transfected with a SRF plasmid or control plasmid. (b) Fluorescence microscopy showed the location and expression of the EMT markers E-cadherin, α-SMA and SRF in HPMCs transfected with a SRF plasmid or control plasmid. Magnification is 100×. (c) Real-time PCR showing mRNA of SRF, E-cadherin and α-SMA in HPMCs transfected with a SRF plasmid or control plasmid (*$P<0.05$ vs. control).

EMT markers and fibronectin (FN) analysis by immunohistochemistry indicated that HG-PDF downregulated E-cadherin and upregulated α-SMA levels, which were inhibited by the administration of CCG-1423, suggesting EMT was tempered (Figure 2b1-b6, Figure S3). A correlation between PM thickness and SRF expression is shown in Figure 3b7-b9 and 3c. In addition, CCG-1423 significantly attenuated the HG-PDF-induced SRF expression (Figure 2b7–b9).

3. Small interfering SRF RNA demoted EMT, while transfection of SRF promoted EMT in cultured HPMCs

To pursue direct evidence of SRF on HG-induced EMT, we manipulated SRF gene expression in cultured immortal HPMCs. When the control HPMCs were incubated with HG medium (60 mmol/L) for 72 h, the cells lost intercellular junctions, scattered, and transformed into a spindled fibroblastic shape (Figure 3a, Figure S1). Concordant with our ex vivo and in vivo results, HPMCs lost E-cadherin, gained α-SMA, translocated SRF to nuclei (Figure 3b), and increased SRF at both protein (Figure 3c1) and mRNA levels (Figure 3d1, d2, d3) in response to HG stimulation.

Small interfering SRF RNA (SRF-siRNA) in HPMCs prevented all of the above HG-induced alterations (Figure 3c2, e, f). In contrast, over-expression of SRF by transfecting the full-length human SRF plasmid [26] into immortal HPMCs led to significant downregulation of E-cadherin and upregulation of α-SMA protein levels (Figure 4a, 4b), as well as mRNA levels (Figure 4c), which is consistent with the results from HG-induced primary cultured HPMCs. Therefore, the mediation of SRF on EMT in peritoneal mesothelial cells was further supported.

4. Snail is a downstream target of SRF in EMT-mediated PM fibrosis

To explore the downstream events of SRF-mediated EMT, we assessed target gene sequences for SRF. We found that all possible SRF target genes have one or more highly conserved CArG elements, leading to select Snail as a candidate of the EMT marker in the promoter. Indeed, Snail expression was augmented in HG-induced HPMCs or HPMCs with SRF overexpression both at the protein and mRNA levels, while levels were diminished by siRNA (Figure 5a, b). These data showed that Snail expression might be correlated with SRF expression at the mRNA and protein levels in HPMCs. This upregulation was also found in the Group 3 PD patients compared with Group 1.

In addition, immunohistochemical studies also revealed pronounced Snail staining in the submesothelial layer of the abdominal walls of the PDF rats, which could be attenuated by treatment with the SRF inhibitor CCG-1423 (Figure 5c). Snail translocated from the cytoplasm into the nuclei in ex vivo HPMCs with prolonged PD (Figure 5d). Translocation of Snail expression was recognized in HG-induced HPMCs, SRF-infected HPMCs, and SRF-siRNA-treated HPMC-HG cells in vitro (Figure 5e, f). These findings suggested that Snail could be the downstream target and mediator of SRF in rat peritoneum when exposed to effluent HG-PD.

5. SRF transcriptionally regulated Snail expression by directly binding the SNAIL promoter

In hunting for the molecular basis of the regulation of Snail by SRF, we performed chromatin immunoprecipitation (ChIP) to examine the binding of SRF to CArG elements in Snail in HPMCs. Two serum response elements, SRE1 and SRE2, in the promoter regions of the Snail gene were predicted as candidate binding sites of SRF. Fifty-fold enrichment was set as a threshold

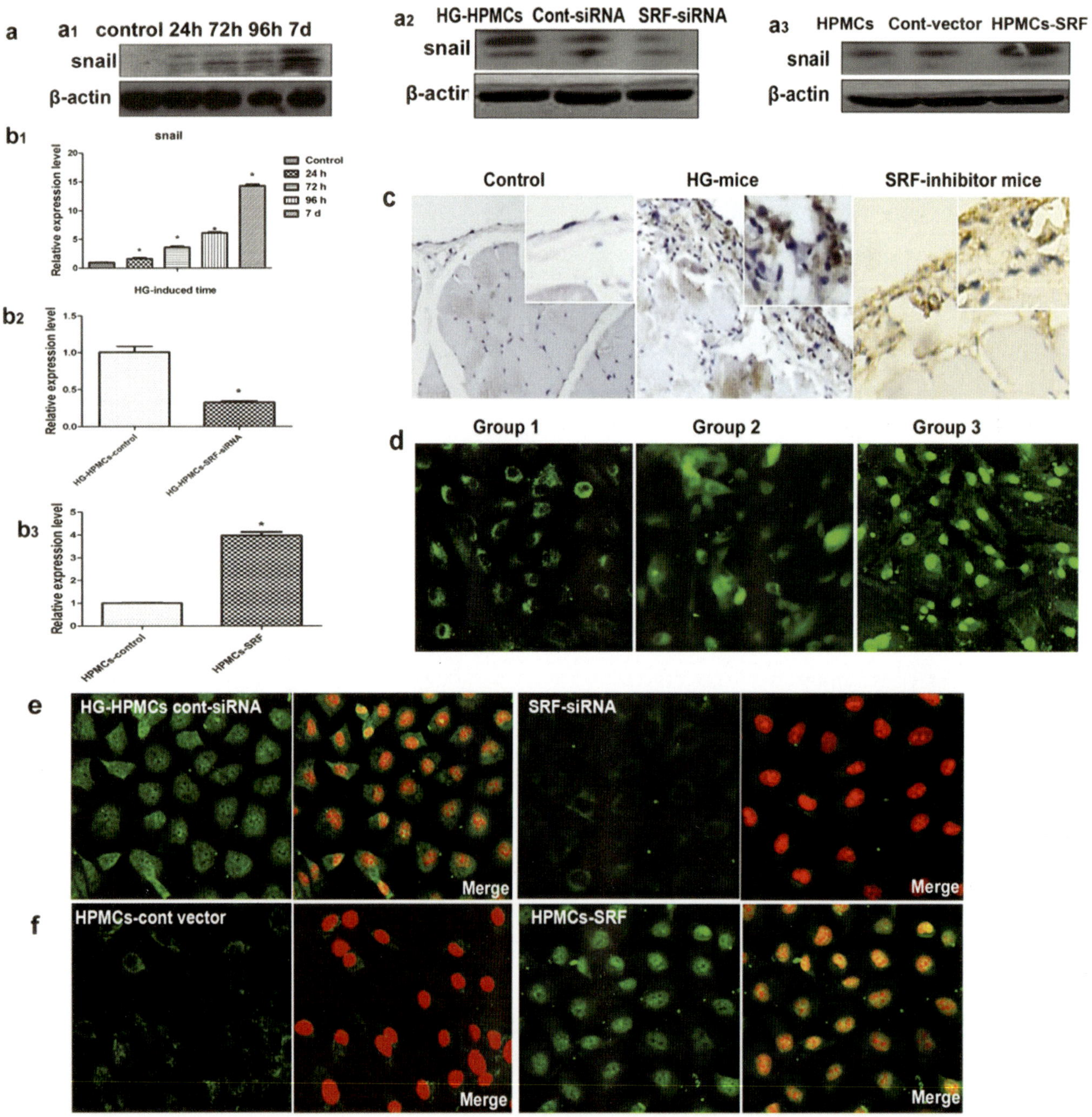

Figure 5. SRF regulates the expression of Snail in HG-induced HPMCs. (a1) Western blot analysis of expression of Snail in HG-induced HPMCs in vitro compared to control HPMCs at 0 h, 24 h, 48 h, 72 h, 96 h, and 7 d. (a2) Western blot analysis of Snail in HPMCs transfected with SRF-siRNA or control vector. (a3) Western blot analysis of Snail in HPMCs transfected with a SRF plasmid or control plasmid. (b1) Real-time PCR showing the expression of Snail in HG-induced HPMCs at 0 h, 24 h, 48 h, 72 h, 96 h, and 7 d. (b2) Real-time PCR showing the expression level of Snail in HG-induced SRF-siRNA-treated HPMCs compared to HG-induced HPMCs. (b3) Real-time PCR showing the expression level of Snail in HPMCs infected with SRF plasmid compared with control HPMCs (*$P<0.05$ vs. control). (c) The results from immunohistochemistry showed Snail staining in the peritoneal samples of normal rats treated with HG or HG+SRF inhibitor (CCG-1423). Magnification is 200×. (d) Location and expression of Snail in ex vivo HPMCs from patients with different phenotypes from Groups 1, 2 or 3. (e) Fluorescence microscopy showed the location and expression of Snail in HG-induced in vitro HPMCs transfected with SRF-siRNA vector compared with the control vector. Magnification is 200×. (f) Fluorescence microscopy showed the location and expression of Snail in HPMCs transfected with a SRF plasmid or the control plasmid in vitro. Magnification is 200×.

for positive SRF binding. Our results showed positive SRF binding at SRE2 in HPMCs. Moreover, the binding signal greatly increased in the HG-induced HPMCs, in agreement with their higher SRF expression (Figure 6a). Electrophoretic mobility shift assays (EMSA) further confirmed that SRF was active and bound to an intronic CArG element after HG incubation for 72 or 96 h (Figure 6b), compared with fewer SRF-containing complexes from the HPMCs in normal medium.

Up-regulated Snail by SRF was further confirmed by luciferase activity assays. In the control HPMCs, transfected full-length SRE

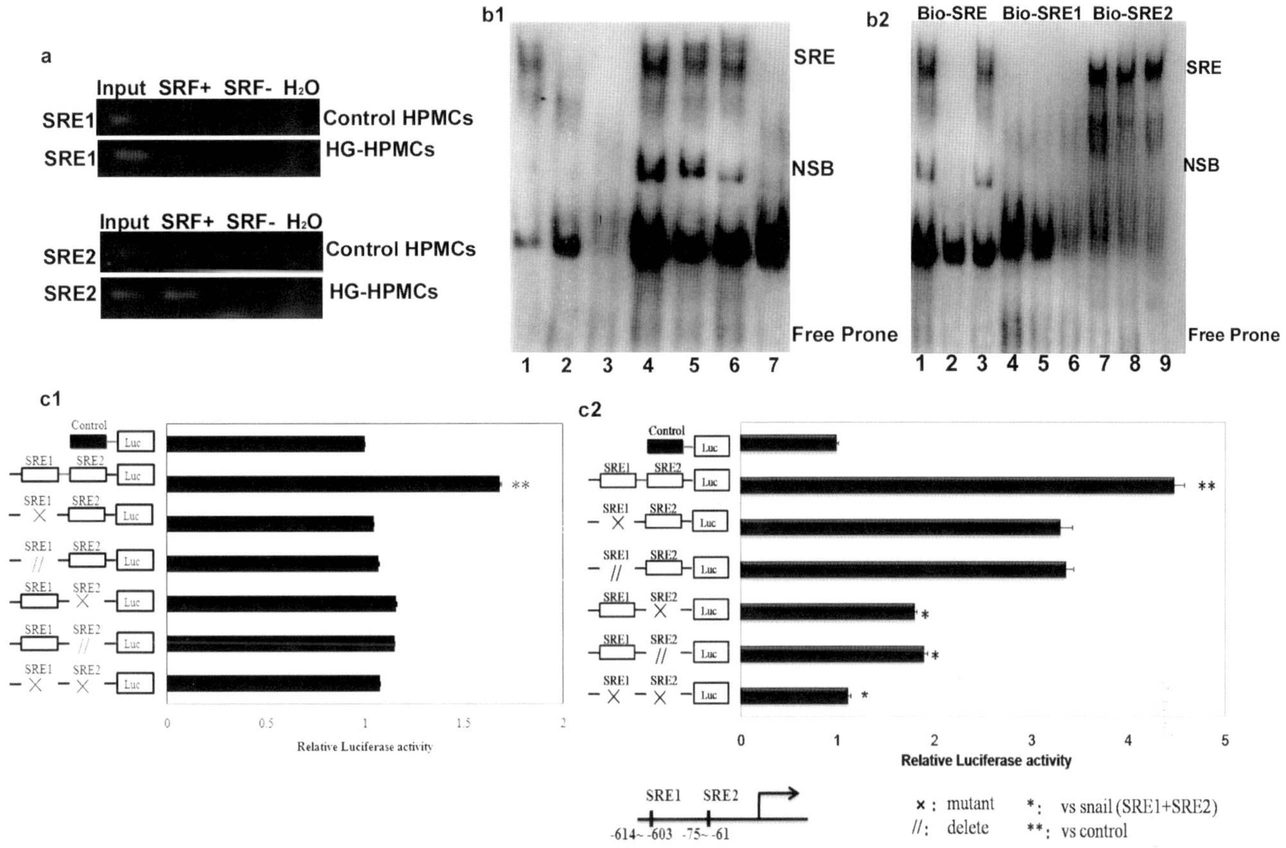

Figure 6. SRF directly induced Snail expression and transcriptional activation in HPMCs. (a) Identification of SRE1 and SRE2 in the SNAIL promoter. Chromatin immunoprecipitation was used to examine SRF binding to the SNAIL promoter in HG-induced HPMCs and the control. Reaction controls included immunoprecipitations performed using a nonspecific IgG monoclonal antibody; PCR was performed using whole cell genomic DNA (Input). A representative example of three independent experiments is shown. (b) EMSA was used to analyze the SRF-binding site induced by HG. (b1) Samples 1 to 7 were induced by HG for 0 h, 5 h, 18 h, 72 h, and 96 h and compared with a positive control and negative control. SRE was bound after inducing for 72 h. (b2) Analysis of the SRF-binding site in the SNAIL promoter by EMSA. Biotin-labeled SRE1 and SRE2 oligonucleotides were used as a probe. Of the two examined putative SRE-binding sites within the SNAIL gene promoter, only SRE2 displayed specific SRF binding in HPMCs induced by HG. Samples 1 to 7 were 72 h+SRE, 72h+SRE + cold-SRE, 72h+SRE + cold SER Mut, 72h+SRE1, 72 h+SRE1+ cold-SRE1, 72h+SRE1+ cold-SRE1 Mut, 72h+SER2, 72h+SER2 +cold-SRE2, and 72h+SER2 +cold-SRE2 Mut. Cold probe, unlabeled SRE; SRE mut, mutated SRE. (c) For the competition assays with SRE1 and SRE2, 200-fold molar excess of the Snail plasmid and mutant SRE1, deleted SRE1, mutant SRE2, deleted SRE2 and mutant SRE1 and SRE2 were used in HPMCs (c1) and HG-induced HPMCs (c2). All results shown are representative of at least three independent experiments. * $P<0.05$ vs. Snail (SRE1+SRE2) plasmid; ** $P<0.05$ vs. control plasmid.

(SRE1+SRE2) plasmids could stimulate their luciferase activity from the basal level either in normal medium ($P=0.030$) or high glucose medium ($P=0.007$) compared to control vectors. Mutation of SRE1 moderately affected their response but without statistical significance ($P=0.061$). However, mutation of SRE2 alone or a double mutation of both SRE1+SRE2 eliminated the luciferase activity response to HG ($P=0.013$ and $P=0.001$ vs. SRE1+SRE2, respectively) (Figure 6c1, c2). These results suggested that the activation of the SRF-Snail signaling occurs via the binding of SRF to Snail predominately at the SRE2 site in its promoter region.

Discussion

Our results demonstrate that HPMCs from ex vivo effluents or from PD rats in vivo undergo EMT during PD. We determined that SRF promotes EMT-mediated fibrosis and acts as a critical transcription factor for HPMCs. Moreover, infection with SRF-siRNA vectors demonstrated the HG-induced upregulation of E-cadherin and downregulation of α-SMA during EMT in HPMCs in vitro. Furthermore, we predicted and demonstrated that Snail is regulated by SRF, which can directly promote Snail transcription via SRE2. Thus, a novel SRF/Snail pathway promotes EMT-mediated peritoneal fibrosis and acts as a critical transcription factor during HPMC EMT.

Increasing evidence shows that EMT, which was originally thought to be limited to tumor development and metastasis, occurs in other diseases, including kidney, liver and lung fibrosis [27–29]. Recently, HPMCs EMT in the peritoneum and effluents of patients undergoing PD was associated with the recurrent use of HG and has been linked to a decline in peritoneal function due to peritoneal fibrosis [4,30]. Using HG, we sought to reproduce the damage caused by the PD effluent and the profibrotic stimuli induced during peritoneal EMT in vivo and in vitro. HG in the PD effluent may induce EMT in HPMCs and has additional effects on cell morphology [30]. Our results revealed that HG could change HPMC morphology and EMT markers, which as an available model for peritoneal EMT in vitro. We could see that HPMCs lost their epithelial morphology with a decrease in E-cadherin expression and an increase in α-SMA expression, implying a transition in phenotype. Several transcription factors, such as twist, were proved to induce EMT in our previous work [23]. In our study, we found that HG treatment induced SRF expression and increased α-SMA but decreased E-cadherin expression. The activation and translocation of SRF into the nuclei of HPMCs was found under extensive periods of PD. In immortal HPMCs, high glucose stimulated SRF overexpression in transformed fibroblastic HPMCs. SRF-siRNA preserved HPMC morphology, while transfection of SRF plasmid into HPMCs caused the opposite effects. PD with 4.25% glucose solution significantly induced SRF up-regulation and increased peritoneal thickness in rats. According to this, SRF translocation may be linked to HPMC EMT during the development of peritoneal fibrosis, suggesting that active SRF is necessary for EMT.

We also found that the inhibition of SRF signaling could prevent HPMCs from acquiring a spindle-like phenotype, reverse EMT, downregulate α-SMA and upregulate E-cadherin. To our knowledge, this report is the first to demonstrate a link between the translocation and activation of SRF in HPMCs and HG-induced EMT. In addition, SRF phosphorylation, which promotes SRF transcriptional activity, may have a role in EMT.

Snail is a zinc finger transcription factor expressed in cells and is the core EMT regulator that plays essential roles in fibrosis [31,32]. The main mechanism by which Snail induces EMT is by downregulating E-cadherin [33–35]. In our study, we found cytoplasmic SRF translocated to the nucleus to induce Snail expression. We conclude that the subcellular localization of SRF and Snail may affect the changes in cellular morphology and behavior, which may be associated with altered signaling pathways, and the subsequent EMT-mediated fibrosis in the development of PD. We demonstrated high Snail expression in the peritoneal fibroblasts, confirming that such expression may play a substantial role in fibrosis progression. Evidence from electrophoretic mobility shift, chromatin immunoprecipitation and reporter assays further supported that SRF transcriptionally regulated Snail, a potent inducer of EMT, by directly binding to its promoter. Both SRE1 and SRE2, which can bind SRF, were predicted to be in the Snail promoter. However, SRE2 is the main binding site for SRF, and SRE1 plays a supporting role.

Moreover, there is still some limitation needed to show in our study. CCG-1423, a specific inhibitor of Rho pathway-mediated signaling and activation of SRF transcription, selectively inhibits DNA synthesis, proliferation and invasion of Rho-overexpressing cell lines. However, HG solutions could directly induce Rho kinases. Although a nuclear translocation of SRF in PD patients and a preservation of the peritoneal membrane in animals undergoing PD with HG solutions and receiving the inhibitor were shown in our study, any blockade of Rho kinases would reduce EMT and fibrosis, possibly irrespective of its specific SRF-dependent effects. So we added supplement data to demonstrate that Rho kinase inhibitor CCG-1423 has similar effects with SRF siRNA in vitro (Figure S2). It showed that inhibition of Rho kinase downstream SRF, has a similar effect with inhibition of Rho kinase per se on EMT and fibrosis, which are implied most of these are SRF-specific effect. In addition, so far we did not found any inhibitors to Rho kinase downstream, independent of SRF, so knockdown of SRF with SRF siRNA lentivirus in vivo is needed in future work.

In all, this study is the first extensive characterization of a signaling pathway that controls EMT in a non-tumor primary cell culture model and provides basic knowledge and clinical relevance. Our results from rats experiment reveal that, CCG-1423 could weaken the EMT happening of peritoneal mesothelial cells when stimulated by glucose contained in PD fluid, and protect peritoneal member function. These results could form the rationale for developing drugs that can counteract the progressive deterioration of the PM that occurs in CAPD patients. However, lots of work is needed to explore deeply molecular mechanism and to identify the safety and detail usage of drugs.

Supporting Information

Figure S1 The expression of SRF, E-cadherin and α-SMA were tested by Western blot after transfection by siRNA or SRF up-regulated plasmid in HPMCs which were stimulated by HG for 96 h.

Figure S2 CCG-1423 is stable in high glucose *in vitro* and *in vivo*. (a) For in vivo study, we injected high glucose PDF after 2 hours of DMSO with CCG-1423 injection. The other progress is the same as before. The results by immunohistochemistry with PBS show that CCG-1423 still has a strong inhibition for peritoneal membrane proliferation even in high glucose solution. Magnification is 200×. (b) We demonstrated that Rho kinase inhibitor CCG-1423 has similar effects with SRF siRNA in vitro. Treated HPMCs with CCG-1423 after high glucose treatment (G1), before high glucose treatment (G2), as well as simultaneously treatment with high glucose (G3), CCG-1423 has a similar effect on SRF inhibition, and this result could be repeated with SRF siRNA (G4). Total incubation time of CCG-1423 or SRF-siRNA for each group was 72 hours.

Figure S3 Inhibition of SRF by CCG-1423 ameliorates PD-induced PM fibrosis *in vivo*. (a) Masson staining and expression of FN showed PD-induced PM fibrosis in Rats in vivo by immunohistochemistry. Magnification is 200×. (b) Westren blot staining of FN in HPMCs stimulated by HG reveals that PD fluid exposure induces the EMT and fibrosis process.

Table S1 Characteristics of CAPD patients with ESRD in our study.

Acknowledgments

We thank Yongqiang Ding (LAND) for suggestions and technical support with ChIP and the reporter assay.

Author Contributions

Conceived and designed the experiments: LJH. Performed the experiments: WJL LHJ WL. Analyzed the data: LJH HMW XMC SRS. Contributed reagents/materials/analysis tools: MLZ GSX LJZ CH RL. Wrote the paper: LJH.

References

1. Jain AK, Blake P, Cordy P, Garg AX. (2012) Global trends in rates of peritoneal dialysis. J Am Soc Nephrol 23: 533–544.

2. Williams JD, Craig KJ, Topley N, Von Ruhland C, Fallon M, et al. (2002) Morphologic changes in the peritoneal membrane of patients with renal disease. J Am Soc Nephrol 13: 470–479.

3. Weber CE, Li NY, Wai PY, Kuo PC. (2012) Epithelial-mesenchymal transition, tgf-beta, and osteopontin in wound healing and tissue remodeling after injury. J Burn Care Res 33: 311–318.
4. Aroeira LS, Aguilera A, Sanchez-Tomero JA, Bajo MA, Del PG et al. (2007) Epithelial to mesenchymal transition and peritoneal membrane failure in peritoneal dialysis patients: pathologic significance and potential therapeutic interventions. J Am Soc Nephrol 18: 2004–2013.
5. Zeisberg M, Neilson EG. (2009) Biomarkers for epithelial-mesenchymal transitions. J Clin Invest 119: 1429–1437.
6. Yu MA, Shin KS, Kim JH, Kim YI, Chung SS, et al. (2009) Hgf and bmp-7 ameliorate high glucose-induced epithelial-to-mesenchymal transition of peritoneal mesothelium. J Am Soc Nephrol. 20: 567–581.
7. Miano JM, Long X, Fujiwara K. (2007) Serum response factor: master regulator of the actin cytoskeleton and contractile apparatus. Am J Physiol Cell Physiol. 292:C70–C81.
8. Park MY, Kim KR, Park HS, Park BH, Choi HN, et al. (2007) Expression of the serum response factor in hepatocellular carcinoma: implications for epithelial-mesenchymal transition. Int J Oncol. 31: 1309–1315.
9. Choi HN, Kim KR, Lee JH, Park HS, Jang KY, et al. (2009) Serum response factor enhances liver metastasis of colorectal carcinoma via alteration of the e-cadherin/beta-catenin complex. Oncol Rep 21: 57–63.
10. Sandbo N, Kregel S, Taurin S, Bhorade S, Dulin NO. (2009) Critical role of serum response factor in pulmonary myofibroblast differentiation induced by tgf-beta. Am J Respir Cell Mol Biol 41: 332–338.
11. Saka M, Obata K, Ichihara S, Cheng XW, Kimata H, et al. (2006) Attenuation of ventricular hypertrophy and fibrosis in rats by pitavastatin: potential role of the rhoa-extracellular signal-regulated kinase-serum response factor signalling pathway. Clin Exp Pharmacol Physiol 33: 1164–1171.
12. Yang Y, Zhe X, Phan SH, Ullenbruch M, Schuger L. (2003) Involvement of serum response factor isoforms in myofibroblast differentiation during bleomycin-induced lung injury. Am J Respir Cell Mol Biol 29: 583–590.
13. Zhang SX, Garcia-Gras E, Wycuff DR, Marriot SJ, Kadeer N, et al. (2005) Identification of direct serum-response factor gene targets during me2so-induced p19 cardiac cell differentiation. J Biol Chem 280: 19115–19126.
14. Niu Z, Iyer D, Conway SJ, Martin JF, Ivey K, et al. (2008) Serum response factor orchestrates nascent sarcomerogenesis and silences the biomineralization gene program in the heart. Proc Natl Acad Sci U S A 105: 17824–17829.
15. Evelyn CR, Wade SM, Wang Q, Wu M, Iniguez-Lluhi JA, et al. (2007) Ccg-1423: a small-molecule inhibitor of rhoa transcriptional signaling. Mol Cancer Ther 2007;6: 2249–2260.
16. Peinado H, Olmeda D, Cano A: Snail, zeb and bhlh factors in tumour progression: an alliance against the epithelial phenotype? Nat Rev Cancer 7: 415–428.
17. Vega S, Morales AV, Ocana OH, Valdes F, Fabregat I, et al. (2004) Snail blocks the cell cycle and confers resistance to cell death. Genes Dev 18: 1131–1143.
18. Stylianou E, Jenner LA, Davies M, Coles GA, Williams JD. (1990) Isolation, culture and characterization of human peritoneal mesothelial cells. Kidney Int 37: 1563–1570.
19. Lopez-Cabrera M, Aguilera A, Aroeira LS, Ramirez-Huesca M, Perez-Lozano ML, et al. (2006) Ex vivo analysis of dialysis effluent-derived mesothelial cells as an approach to unveiling the mechanism of peritoneal membrane failure. Perit Dial Int 26: 26–34.
20. Yanez-Mo M, Lara-Pezzi E, Selgas R, Ramirez-Huesca M, Dominguez-Jimenez C, et al. (2003) Peritoneal dialysis and epithelial-to-mesenchymal transition of mesothelial cells. N Engl J Med 348: 403–413.
21. Aroeira LS, Aguilera A, Selgas R, Ramirez-Huesca M, Perez-Lozano ML, et al. (2005) Mesenchymal conversion of mesothelial cells as a mechanism responsible for high solute transport rate in peritoneal dialysis: role of vascular endothelial growth factor. Am J Kidney Dis 46: 938–948.
22. Bidmon B, Endemann M, Arbeiter K, Ruffingshofer D, Regele H, et al. (2004) Overexpression of hsp-72 confers cytoprotection in experimental peritoneal dialysis. Kidney Int 66: 2300–2307.
23. Li C, Ren Y, Jia X, Liang P, Lou W, et al. (2012) Twist overexpression promoted epithelial-to-mesenchymal transition of human peritoneal mesothelial cells under high glucose. Nephrol Dial Transplant. Nov;27(11):4119–4124.
24. Sun S, Ning X, Zhang Y, Lu Y, Nie Y, et al. (2009) Hypoxia-inducible factor-1alpha induces twist expression in tubular epithelial cells subjected to hypoxia, leading to epithelial-to-mesenchymal transition. Kidney Int 75: 1278–1287.
25. Arva NC, Gopen TR, Talbott KE, Campbell LE, Chicas A, et al. (2005) A chromatin-associated and transcriptionally inactive p53-mdm2 complex occurs in mdm2 snp309 homozygous cells. J Biol Chem 280: 26776–26787.
26. Kuwahara K, Barrientos T, Pipes GC, Li S, Olson EN. (2005) Muscle-specific signaling mechanism that links actin dynamics to serum response factor. Mol Cell Biol 25: 3173–3181.
27. Thiery JP, Sleeman JP. (2006) Complex networks orchestrate epithelial-mesenchymal transitions. Nat Rev Mol Cell Biol 7: 131–142.
28. Kalluri R, Neilson EG. (2003) Epithelial-mesenchymal transition and its implications for fibrosis. J Clin Invest 112: 1776–1784.
29. Iwano M, Plieth D, Danoff TM, Xue C, Okada H, et al. (2002) Evidence that fibroblasts derive from epithelium during tissue fibrosis. J Clin Invest 110: 341–350.
30. Del PG, Jimenez-Heffernan JA, Bajo MA, Aroeira LS, Aguilera A, et al. (2008) Epithelial-to-mesenchymal transition of mesothelial cells is an early event during peritoneal dialysis and is associated with high peritoneal transport. Kidney Int Suppl S26–S33.
31. Harney AS, Meade TJ, LaBonne C. (2012) Targeted inactivation of snail family emt regulatory factors by a co(iii)-ebox conjugate. PLoS One 7:e32318.
32. Foubert E, De Craene B, Berx G. (2010) Key signalling nodes in mammary gland development and cancer. The snail1-twist1 conspiracy in malignant breast cancer progression. Breast Cancer Res 12: 206.
33. Bezdekova M, Brychtova S, Sedlakova E, Langova K, Brychta T, et al. (2012) Analysis of snail-1, e-cadherin and claudin-1 expression in colorectal adenomas and carcinomas. Int J Mol Sci 13: 1632–1643.
34. Dong C, Wu Y, Wang Y, Wang C, Kang T, et al. (2012) Interaction with suv39h1 is critical for snail-mediated e-cadherin repression in breast cancer. Oncogene
35. Dennis M, Wang G, Luo J, Lin Y, Dohadwala M, et al. (2012) Snail controls the mesenchymal phenotype and drives erlotinib resistance in oral epithelial and head and neck squamous cell carcinoma cells. Otolaryngol Head Neck Surg 147: 726–732.

Patients with Encapsulating Peritoneal Sclerosis Have Increased Peritoneal Expression of Connective Tissue Growth Factor (CCN2), Transforming Growth Factor-β1, and Vascular Endothelial Growth Factor

Alferso C. Abrahams[1]*, Sayed M. Habib[2], Amélie Dendooven[3], Bruce L. Riser[4], Jan Willem van der Veer[1], Raechel J. Toorop[5], Michiel G. H. Betjes[2], Marianne C. Verhaar[1], Christopher J. E. Watson[6], Tri Q. Nguyen[3], Walther H. Boer[1]

1 Department of Nephrology and Hypertension, University Medical Center Utrecht, Utrecht, The Netherlands, **2** Department of Internal Medicine, Division of Nephrology and Transplantation, Erasmus Medical Center, Rotterdam, The Netherlands, **3** Department of Pathology, University Medical Center Utrecht, Utrecht, The Netherlands, **4** Department of Physiology and Biophysics, Rosalind Franklin University of Medicine and Science, IL, United States of America, **5** Department of Vascular Surgery, University Medical Center Utrecht, Utrecht, The Netherlands, **6** Department of Surgery, Box 202, Addenbrooke's Hospital, and Cambridge NIHR Biomedical Research Centre, Cambridge, United Kingdom

Abstract

Introduction: Encapsulating peritoneal sclerosis (EPS) is a devastating complication of peritoneal dialysis (PD). The pathogenesis is not exactly known and no preventive strategy or targeted medical therapy is available. CCN2 has both pro-fibrotic and pro-angiogenic actions and appears an attractive target. Therefore, we studied peritoneal expression of CCN2, as well as TGFβ1 and VEGF, in different stages of peritoneal fibrosis.

Materials and methods: Sixteen PD patients were investigated and compared to 12 hemodialysis patients and four pre-emptively transplanted patients. Furthermore, expression was investigated in 12 EPS patients in comparison with 13 PD and 12 non-PD patients without EPS. Peritoneal tissue was taken during kidney transplantation procedure or during EPS surgery. In a subset of patients, CCN2 protein levels in peritoneal effluent and plasma were determined. Samples were examined by qPCR, histology, immunohistochemistry, and ELISA.

Results: Peritoneal CCN2 expression was 5-fold higher in PD patients compared to pre-emptively transplanted patients ($P < 0.05$), but did not differ from hemodialysis patients. Peritoneal expression of TGFβ1 and VEGF were not different between the three groups; neither was peritoneal thickness. Peritoneum of EPS patients exhibited increased expression of CCN2 (35-fold, $P<0.001$), TGFβ1 (24-fold, $P<0.05$), and VEGF (77-fold, $P<0.001$) compared to PD patients without EPS. In EPS patients, CCN2 protein was mainly localized in peritoneal endothelial cells and fibroblasts. CCN2 protein levels were significantly higher in peritoneal effluent of EPS patients compared to levels in dialysate of PD patients (12.0 ± 4.5 vs. 0.91 ± 0.92 ng/ml, $P<0.01$), while plasma CCN2 levels were not increased.

Conclusions: Peritoneal expression of CCN2, TGFβ1, and VEGF are significantly increased in EPS patients. In early stages of peritoneal fibrosis, only CCN2 expression is slightly increased. Peritoneal CCN2 overexpression in EPS patients is a locally driven response. The potential of CCN2 as biomarker and target for CCN2-inhibiting agents to prevent or treat EPS warrants further study.

Editor: Philip C. Trackman, Boston University Goldman School of Dental Medicine, United States of America

Funding: This study was supported by a grant from the Dutch Kidney Foundation (C10.2344) and a Clinical Evidence Council grant from Baxter Healthcare (10CECEU1007). The funders had no role in study design, data collection and analysis, decision to publish, or preparation of the manuscript.

Competing Interests: BLR is founder and president of BLR Bio LLC, which focuses on fibrosis directed therapies. ACA has received a grant from Baxter Healthcare. All other authors have declared that no competing interests exist.

* Email: A.C.Abrahams@umcutrecht.nl

Introduction

Chronic treatment with peritoneal dialysis (PD) results in morphological changes in the peritoneal membrane. These alterations include progressive fibrosis and neo-angiogenesis and are associated with increased solute transport and loss of ultrafiltration [1–10]. Encapsulating peritoneal sclerosis (EPS) could be considered as a severe, advanced form of peritoneal fibrosis for which a second hit is mandatory [11–13]. This condition, for which no preventive strategy or targeted medical therapy is available, is a significant threat to patients on PD with a reported mortality of 25 to 55% [14,15].

The human pathogenesis of EPS is not fully understood, but animal studies strongly suggest that both transforming growth factor-β1 (TGFβ1) and vascular endothelial growth factor (VEGF) are key players in the early peritoneal membrane changes and are potential targets for intervention [16–23]. This was recently illustrated by Loureiro *et al.* [24], who demonstrated that intraperitoneal administration of TGF-β1-blocking peptides to mice exposed to PD fluid significantly decreased peritoneal fibrosis and angiogenesis and improved peritoneal ultrafiltration.

Although this study suggests that TGFβ1 inhibition could be a tool to prevent or treat EPS, direct and chronic inhibition of systemic TGFβ1 activity is probably not desirable in humans given the important role of TGFβ1 in immune regulation and tumor suppression [25–31]. In this respect, the main downstream pro-fibrotic mediator of TGFβ1 activity, connective tissue growth factor (CCN2), might be a more attractive target. This protein, which is also involved in neo-angiogenesis [32], is overexpressed in a variety of fibrotic disorders [33–35] and some studies also suggest a pathogenic role for CCN2 in the peritoneal membrane alterations caused by long term PD [36–38].

Peritoneal biopsy studies in humans, which investigate the expression of pro-fibrotic and pro-angiogenic factors including CCN2, are scarce. In the current study, we investigated the peritoneal gene expression of CCN2, TGFβ1, and VEGF in different stages of peritoneal fibrosis. We hypothesized that CCN2, TGFβ1, and VEGF are already upregulated in early stages of peritoneal fibrosis and further overexpressed in EPS. For this purpose, we compared peritoneal expression of these factors in PD patients to PD naive patients with end stage kidney disease (ESKD) and in EPS patients in comparison to PD patients without EPS.

Materials and Methods

Study design

We performed two cross-sectional studies between October 2008 and September 2012. In study 1, we investigated peritoneal CCN2, TGFβ1, and VEGF gene expression and peritoneal thickness in three groups of patients with ESKD. In study 2, we determined peritoneal mRNA levels for CCN2, TGFβ1, and VEGF in EPS patients in comparison to two groups of patients without EPS (PD patients and non-PD patients).

Study populations

Study 1. We obtained biopsies of the parietal peritoneum during kidney transplant procedures performed in the University Medical Center Utrecht in 16 PD patients, in 12 hemodialysis (HD) patients, and in four patients who received a pre-emptive kidney transplant. In PD patients, peritonitis was excluded at the time of biopsy by effluent cell count of $<0.1\times10^9$/L and negative culture.

Study 2. We performed a study in collaboration with Addenbrooke's Hospital in Cambridge, UK, which is one of the two referral centers in the UK for EPS surgery. Peritoneal tissue was obtained in 12 consecutive EPS patients who underwent surgery to resolve severe bowel obstruction. These EPS patients were compared with 25 ESKD patients without EPS who underwent kidney transplantation in the University Medical Center Utrecht; 13 patients who were on PD (PD group) and 12 ESKD patients who were never treated with PD (non-PD patients). None of these patients had symptoms of intestinal obstruction or had macroscopic signs of EPS (evaluated during kidney transplantation).

All EPS patients fulfilled the criteria for EPS developed by the Ad Hoc Committee of the International Society for Peritoneal Dialysis [39] and had severe clinical symptoms related to intestinal obstruction in combination with radiological evidence. In all EPS patients, the diagnosis was confirmed macroscopically. None of the PD patients had peritonitis at the time of biopsy.

Demographic and clinical data were collected from all patients. Both studies were conducted in accordance with the Declaration of Helsinki and the Good Clinical Practice guidelines set by the International Conference on Harmonization. Study protocols were approved by the Ethics Committees of the University Medical Center Utrecht and of the Addenbrooke's Hospital. All study participants provided written informed consent.

Sample collection and processing

Collection of peritoneal tissue during kidney transplantation was done using a standardized procedure. In brief, a suture loop was inserted through the outer layer of the parietal peritoneum. By using the suture to lift the peritoneum, an ellipse of 2 cm in length was excised and pinned onto a paraffin wax plate with the mesothelial surface uppermost. Afterwards, the peritoneal cavity was closed with a suture.

In EPS patients, peritoneal tissue was taken during a decortication procedure which was performed to release obstructed small bowel segments. This sample included the falciform ligament and adjacent parietal peritoneum since this is typically excised and discarded.

Immediately after sampling, half of the biopsy was snap frozen in liquid nitrogen for isolation of RNA. The other half was fixed with 4% formaldehyde. After fixation for 24 hours at room temperature, samples were routinely processed for light microscopy and embedded in paraffin.

For study 2, we collected plasma samples before the surgical procedure whenever possible. If ascites fluid was present in EPS patients during surgery, this was also collected for analysis. In PD patients, a standard four-hour peritoneal equilibration test was performed [40] with a 3.86% glucose solution just before transplantation when time allowed this. Plasma and peritoneal fluid samples were stored at −80°C.

Samples were examined by quantitative PCR, histology, immunohistochemistry, and sandwich enzyme-linked immunosorbent assay (ELISA).

Quantitative PCR

Total RNA was extracted from frozen peritoneal tissue using RNeasy columns (Qiagen, Venlo, The Netherlands). After cDNA synthesis, determination of CCN2 (Hs00170014_m1), TGFβ1 (Hs00998133_m1), and VEGF (Hs00900055_m1) mRNA levels were assessed by quantitative real-time PCR using TaqMan Gene Expression Assays with commercially pre-designed probe and primers (Applied Biosystems, Foster City, CA, USA). TATA box binding protein (TBP) (Hs00427620_m1) and glyceraldehyde 3-phosphate dehydrogenase (GAPDH) (Hs02758991_g1) were used as internal reference in study 1 and 2, respectively.

Histological analysis

Peritoneal thickness was determined by measuring the thickness of the submesothelial compact (SMC) zone on hematoxylin and eosin stained formalin-fixed four-μm-thick tissue sections. The SMC zone is the submesothelial interstitial layer between the basal border of surface mesothelial cells and upper border of peritoneal adipose tissue. All biopsies were digitalized using a microscope camera (Nikon Eclipse E800 microscope with DXM1200 digital camera, Tokyo, Japan) and analyzed by image analysis software (ImageJ 1.45, NIH, Bethesda, MY, USA). Peritoneal thickness was measured perpendicular to the serosal surface at ten randomly selected points by two independent, blinded examiners, and then the average peritoneal thickness (APT) was calculated as described by Honda *et al.* [9]. The mean of the two APT values obtained in this fashion was used for further analysis.

CCN2 immunohistochemistry

To validate CCN2 expression at the protein level and to determine its exact localization, CCN2 immunohistochemistry was performed in EPS patients on four-µm-thick paraffin embedded sections and compared to non-EPS PD patients. These samples were treated with endogenous peroxidase block. Antigen retrieval was achieved by predigestion with Protease XXIV (Sigma, St. Louis, MO, USA). Sections were incubated with a goat-anti-CCN2 antibody (sc-14939, Santa Cruz Biotechnology, Heidelberg, Germany), followed by rabbit-anti-goat IgG (Dako, Glostrup, Denmark) and goat-anti-rabbit BrightVision-PO (Klinipath, Duiven, Netherlands). Bound antibody was visualized with NovaRed (Vector Laboratories, Burlingame, CA, USA).

CCN2 ELISA

Plasma and peritoneal fluid samples were thawed on the day of use and any solids pelleted by centrifugation. Afterwards, the supernatant was diluted 1:10 in assay buffer. CCN2 present in the plasma or peritoneal fluid was then quantified using an ELISA as previously reported [41]. Briefly, the ELISA plate was first coated with CCN2 L-20 antibody, as a specific trapping antibody (sc-14939, Santa Cruz Biotechnology Inc., Dallas, TX, USA). The plates were incubated with sample or CCN2 standard and afterwards washed before the addition of 20a anti-CCN2 antibody. After further washing, horseradish peroxidase-conjugated secondary antibody (goat anti-rabbit; Jackson ImmunoResearch, West Grove, PA, USA) was added, followed by horseradish peroxidase substrate (Enhanced K-Blue TMB substrate, 308175; Neogen Corp., Lexington, KY, USA). The color intensity was allowed to develop, and read at 650 nm using a microplate reader. All CCN2 levels are expressed as ng/ml.

Statistical analysis

Data are presented as mean ± SD or median (interquartile range). Difference between groups were analysed by one way ANOVA or Kruskal-Wallis test where appropriate, with Bonferroni correction or Dunn's test for multiple post-hoc comparisons.

Spearman's rank correlation test was used to assess correlation coefficients.

For all comparisons, a P-value <0.05 was considered to be significant (two-tailed). Statistical analysis was performed using GraphPad Prism software version 5.02 for Windows.

Results

Patient characteristics

The clinical characteristics of the study population are summarized in table 1 and 2.

In study 1, none of the PD patients had a history of ultrafiltration failure (UFF) and HD patients were predominantly male. In study 2, EPS patients were younger (P<0.05) and had a longer cumulative duration of PD (P<0.001) compared to PD patients without EPS. At the time of diagnosis, none of the EPS patients were treated with PD, nine were on HD and three had a functioning kidney graft. Four EPS patients and none of the PD patients without EPS had a known history of UFF.

Peritoneal CCN2, TGFβ1, and VEGF gene expression and peritoneal thickness in PD patients, HD patients, and pre-emptively transplanted patients (study 1)

Peritoneal gene expression of CCN2 was 5-fold higher in PD patients compared to pre-emptively transplanted patients (P< 0.05), but did not significantly differ from HD patients (figure 1A). Peritoneal gene expression of TGFβ1 and VEGF were not significantly different between the three groups (figure 1B and 1C). Peritoneal thickness also did not differ significantly between groups (figure 2A). In PD patients, no correlation was found between CCN2 gene expression and peritoneal thickness (figure 2B) or between CCN2 gene expression and PD duration (figure 2C). Also TGFβ1 and VEGF gene expression did not correlate with peritoneal thickness.

Peritoneal CCN2, TGFβ1, and VEGF gene expression in EPS patients and PD and non-PD patients without EPS (study 2)

Peritoneal gene expression of CCN2 was 35-fold higher in EPS patients compared to PD patients without EPS (P<0.001, figure 3A). CCN2 gene expression did not differ between the two groups of patients without EPS (figure 3A).

Peritoneal gene expression of TGFβ1 and VEGF were also higher in EPS patients compared to non-EPS PD patients (24-fold, P<0.05 and 77-fold, P<0.001, respectively), while this did not differ between the two groups of patients without EPS (figure 3B and 3C).

Peritoneal CCN2 protein expression and CCN2 protein concentrations in ascites and plasma of EPS patients

CCN2 immunohistochemistry could be performed on peritoneal samples of six EPS patients. In agreement with the increased CCN2 gene expression, we found a clear, prominent elevation in CCN2 staining in EPS patients compared to PD patients without EPS (n = 13) with localization mainly in endothelial cells and interstitial fibroblasts (figure 4).

Mean CCN2 protein concentration in ascites of EPS patients obtained in seven patients during surgery was 12.0±4.5 ng/ml. These levels were approximately 12-fold higher than levels measured in dialysate of four PD patients without EPS obtained from a standard four-hour peritoneal equilibration test (mean 0.91±0.92 ng/ml, P<0.01, figure 5A). In contrast, CCN2 protein levels determined in plasma did not differ between patient groups (40.4±19.5 ng/ml in EPS versus 34.1±16.5 ng/ml in PD without EPS versus 23.7±13.8 ng/ml in non-PD without EPS, P=0.11, figure 5B). It should be noted that plasma samples were obtained in only six EPS patients.

Discussion

Our study shows markedly increased gene expression of CCN2 (35-fold), TGFβ1 (24-fold), and VEGF (77-fold) in the peritoneal membrane of EPS patients compared to PD patients without EPS. In the latter group, we could at best demonstrate a very mildly (5-fold) increased peritoneal gene expression of CCN2 in patients with a median dialysis duration of 34 months compared to pre-emptively transplanted patients with ESKD, while TGFβ1 and VEGF gene expression were not increased. Peritoneal CCN2 protein expression, which was also markedly increased in EPS

Table 1. Baseline characteristics of patients in study 1.

	Peritoneal dialysis patients (n = 16)	Hemodialysis patients (n = 12)	Pre-emptively transplanted patients (n = 4)	P-value
Age (years)	56 (42–62)	57 (47–63)	43 (35–48)	0.10
Gender (F/M)	9/7	2/10	2/2	0.10
Cause of kidney disease				
Glomerulonephritis	6 (37%)	5 (41%)	0 (0%)	
Renal vascular disease	1 (6%)	0 (0%)	0 (0%)	
Cystic kidney disease	4 (25%)	2 (17%)	3 (75%)	
Diabetic nephropathy	0 (0%)	0 (0%)	0 (0%)	
Congenital and hereditary kidney disease	1 (6%)	0 (0%)	0 (0%)	
Other	2 (13%)	2 (17%)	0 (0%)	
Unknown	2 (13%)	3 (25%)	1 (25%)	
Dialysis duration (months)	34 (12–55)	45 (6–60)	N/A	0.82
Residual renal function (yes)	6 (38%)	5 (42%)	4 (100%)	0.07
History of peritonitis (yes)	8 (50%)	N/A	N/A	
Ultrafiltration failure (yes)	0 (0%)	N/A	N/A	

Data are median (IQR) or number of patients (%)
Abbreviations: F, female; M, male; N/A, not applicable.

patients, was most prominent in endothelial cells and interstitial fibroblasts.

EPS is the most severe complication of treatment with PD and its pathogenesis is not exactly known. A two-hit theory has been proposed, with long term PD itself and the chronic use of bioincompatible PD solutions as first hits, leading to peritoneal fibrosis and possibly UFF. Severe peritonitis, discontinuation of PD or kidney transplantation have been proposed as second hits provoking fulminant EPS [13,42].

Table 2. Baseline characteristics of patients in study 2.

	EPS patients (n = 12)	Peritoneal dialysis patients (n = 13)	Non peritoneal dialysis patients (n = 12)	P-value
Age (years)	47 (40–54)	56 (52–62)	52 (45–62)	<0.05*
Gender (F/M)	4/8	7/6	3/9	0.31
Cause of kidney disease				
Glomerulonephritis	3 (25%)	3 (23%)	4 (33%)	
Renal vascular disease	1 (8%)	0 (0%)	0 (0%)	
Cystic kidney disease	1 (8%)	5 (38%)	4 (33%)	
Diabetic nephropathy	3 (25%)	0 (0%)	0 (0%)	
Congenital and hereditary kidney disease	2 (17%)	1 (8%)	0 (0%)	
Other	0 (0%)	1 (8%)	2 (17%)	
Unknown	2 (17%)	3 (23%)	2 (17%)	
PD duration (months)	67 (53–98)	26 (12–45)	N/A	<0.001
History of peritonitis (yes)	7 (58%)	6 (46%)	N/A	0.54
Ultrafiltration failure (yes)	4 (31%)	0 (0%)	N/A	<0.05
Renal replacement therapy when EPS				
Peritoneal dialysis	0 (0%)	N/A	N/A	
Hemodialysis	9 (75%)	N/A	N/A	
Kidney transplantation	3 (25%)	N/A	N/A	

Data are median (IQR) or number of patients (%).
* EPS vs. PD.
Abbreviations: F, female; M, male; PD, peritoneal dialysis; EPS, encapsulating peritoneal sclerosis; N/A, not applicable.

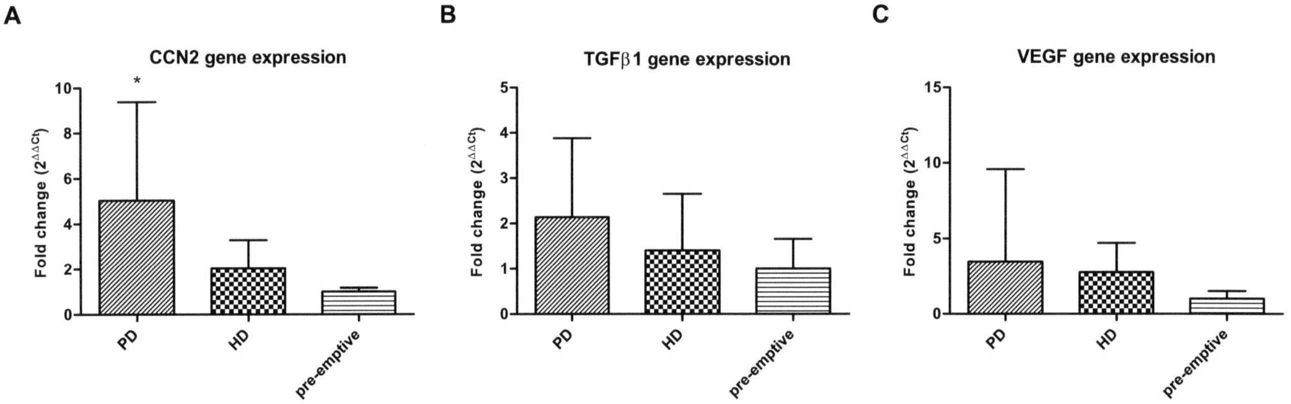

Figure 1. Peritoneal CCN2, TGFβ1, and VEGF gene expression in end stage kidney disease. Gene expression of CCN2 (**1A**), TGFβ1 (**1B**), and VEGF (**1C**) in peritoneum of peritoneal dialysis (PD), hemodialysis (HD), and pre-emptively transplanted patients. Mean±SD. * $P<0.05$ versus pre-emptive.

Several *in vitro* and animal studies have focused on the pathogenesis of peritoneal fibrosis and sclerosis. These preclinical studies indicate that TGFβ1 and VEGF are key players in the development of both peritoneal fibrosis and EPS [16,19,21–24,43] and that CCN2 expression in cultured human peritoneal mesothelial cells (HPMCs) and peritoneal fibroblasts could be induced by exposing these cells to PD solutions, glucose, glucose degradation products, and advanced glycation end products [36,37]. However, biopsy studies in humans investigating the role of TGFβ1, VEGF, and CCN2 in peritoneal fibrosis and EPS in humans are scarce.

Using immunohistochemistry, Braun *et al.* studied the protein expression of TGFβ1, CCN2, and VEGF in the peritoneum of nine EPS patients who underwent surgery for bowel obstruction after a PD duration of 103±32 months [44]. For comparison, they studied patients on PD (n = 10, mean PD duration 19±28 months) and 10 non-renal surgical controls with normal peritoneum. Peritoneal tissue was obtained in the PD patients during elective surgery for hernias, leakage or catheter reinsertion. Compared to the surgical controls, peritoneal TGFβ1 was upregulated in patients on PD and in EPS patients, but the expression between the latter groups was not different. The peritoneal CCN2 expression was increased in PD patients compared to the surgical controls but did not differ from that in EPS patients. Interestingly, the peritoneal thickness in the PD patients without EPS was considerable (~2000 μm) and comparable to that in EPS patients (~2500 μm), indicating that the PD patients had a rather "sick" peritoneal membrane despite the relatively short PD duration. This may explain the lack of difference in TGFβ1 and CCN2 expression between PD patients and those suffering from EPS. Despite this similarity in peritoneal damage in the EPS and non-EPS groups in the study of Braun, the increase in VEGF expression was much more pronounced in the EPS group, pointing to an important role for this cytokine in the development of EPS. In agreement with this observation, the increase in VEGF mRNA expression was also more pronounced than that of TGFβ1 or CCN2 in the EPS patients in our study.

In PD patients with UFF, but without EPS, Mizutani *et al.* specifically investigated the peritoneal expression of CCN2 [38]. They studied the CCN2 mRNA levels in ESKD patients at the time of PD catheter implantation (uremic controls, n = 26), in incidental PD patients at the time of catheter removal for reasons other than UFF (n = 23) and in patients with UFF (n = 7). The peritoneal CCN2 mRNA expression in patients with UFF, who

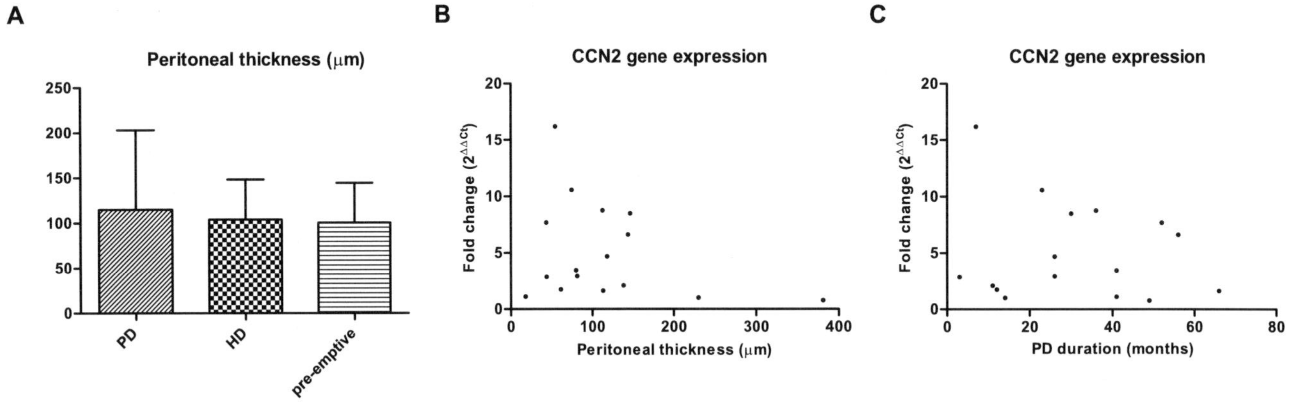

Figure 2. Peritoneal thickness, PD duration, and CCN2 expression in end stage kidney disease. Peritoneal thickness did not differ between peritoneal dialysis (PD), hemodialysis (HD), and pre-emptively transplanted patients (**2A**). Mean ±SD. In PD patients no correlation was found between CCN2 gene expression and peritoneal thickness ($R = -0.24$, $P = 0.36$) (**2B**) and between CCN2 gene expression and PD duration ($R = -0.11$, $P = 0.67$) (**2C**).

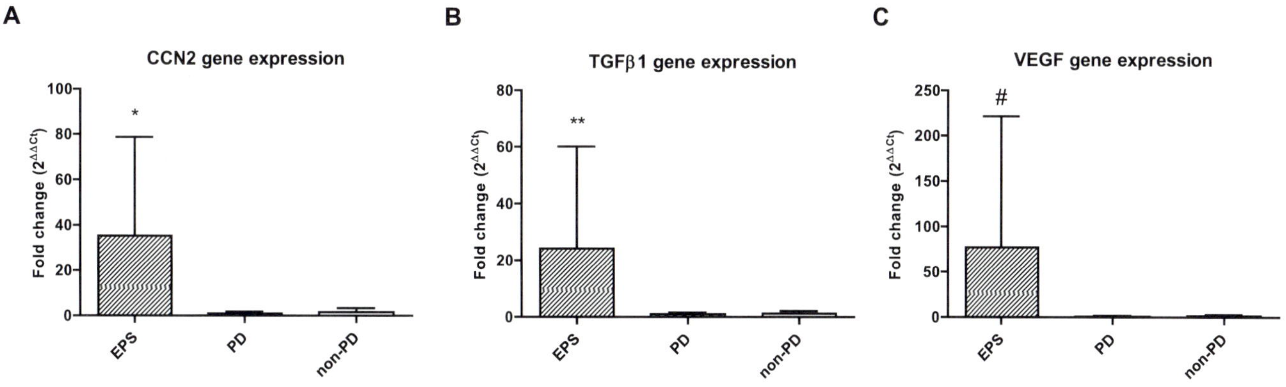

Figure 3. Peritoneal CCN2, TGFβ1, and VEGF gene expression in encapsulating peritoneal sclerosis. Gene expression of CCN2 (**3A**), TGFβ1 (**3B**), and VEGF (**3C**) in peritoneum of patients with encapsulating peritoneal sclerosis (EPS) compared to peritoneal dialysis (PD) and non-PD patients without EPS. Mean ±SD. * $P<0.001$ versus PD patients without EPS. ** $P<0.05$ versus PD patients without EPS. # $P<0.001$ versus PD patients without EPS.

had been on PD for 9.4 years, was found to be increased 11.4-fold compared to the uremic controls, who also had a less thickened peritoneum than the UFF group (157 µm versus 308 µm). Interestingly, the CCN2 gene expression as well as the peritoneal thickness (155 µm) in the group of PD patients with normal ultrafiltration, who had been on PD for a mean of 3.7 years, were similar to that in the uremic control group, indicating that these patients had sustained little peritoneal damage despite PD treatment. This agrees with the very mild increase in CCN2 gene expression observed in our non-EPS PD patients.

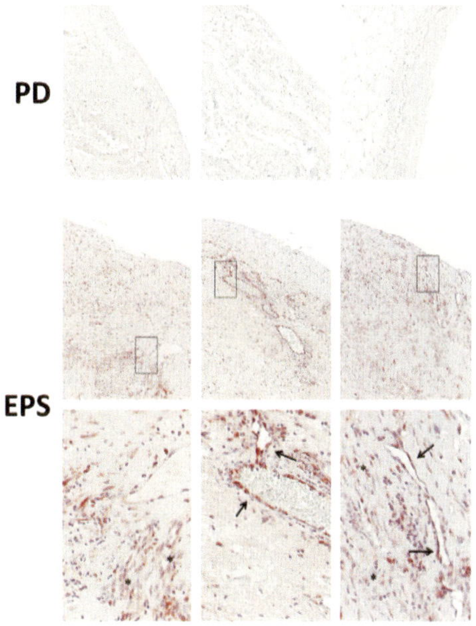

Figure 4. Peritoneal CCN2 protein expression in encapsulating peritoneal sclerosis. Immunohistochemistry for CCN2 in representative peritoneal biopsies of three peritoneal dialysis (PD) patients shows no significant staining (**upper panel**). In representative peritoneal biopsies of three patients with encapsulating peritoneal sclerosis (EPS), strong CCN2 staining is observed (**middle panel**). At higher magnification (**lower panel**), it is seen that CCN2 protein is mainly localized in endothelial cells (arrows) and interstitial fibroblasts (asterisks).

The results of the above mentioned studies and our findings indicate that the fibrotic pathway involving TGFβ1 and CCN2 is markedly activated in the peritoneal tissues of patients with advanced peritoneal damage, resulting in either UFF (CCN2 in Mizutani's study) or EPS (both factors in the Braun *et al*. study and in ours). In addition, a very pronounced peritoneal upregulation of VEGF seems to be specific for EPS patients (Braun *et al.* and present study). In contrast, these growth factors are apparently not or only mildly (CCN2 in present study) upregulated in patients with a PD duration of 3 to 4 years who have a peritoneal thickness comparable to that of uremic and HD patients. It is of note that neither our study nor that of Mizutani *et al.* included a substantial number of patients with a PD duration intermediate between the 3 to 4 years of the control patients and the longer interval after which UFF or EPS develops. Therefore, it remains uncertain if activation of the fibrotic pathway involving overexpression of TGFβ1 and CCN2 occurs gradually or is a relatively abrupt and late phenomenon provoked by a second hit.

Our observation that both TGFβ1 and CCN2 are highly expressed in the peritoneum of EPS patients is in accordance with the current view that CCN2 is induced by TGFβ1 and acts as a cofactor to enhance the fibrotic actions of TGFβ1 [45–47]. The close interaction between CCN2 and TGFβ in the development of EPS was clearly demonstrated in an experiment by Wang *et al.* [46], in which only simultaneous intraperitoneal administration of TGFβ and CCN2 produced an EPS like phenotype in neonatal mice, whereas administration of either cytokine alone failed to produce any fibrosis. Although blocking of TGFβ1 seems a rational and effective approach to ameliorate peritoneal fibrosis [24], this may be unwarranted in view of the important favourable role that TGFβ1 plays in cell immunity, proliferation and differentiation [25–31]. Therefore, CCN2 may be a more appropriate target to prevent or reduce peritoneal fibrosis. Using small interfering RNA (siRNA) of CCN2, Liu *et al.* showed that the expression of CCN2 and VEGF induced by TGFβ1 can be inhibited in cultured HPMCs [48]. The same group showed that CCN2 knockdown using interference RNA also attenuated TGFβ1-induced extracellular matrix production and VEGF expression in HPMCs [49]. Phase 2 studies have indicated that EXC 001, an antisense oligonucleotide targeting CCN2, may be efficacious in reducing hypertrophic scar formation following surgery. Also, a humanized monoclonal antibody (FG-3019) directed at CCN2 has undergone safety trials in patients with diabetes mellitus and microalbuminuria [50], and is currently

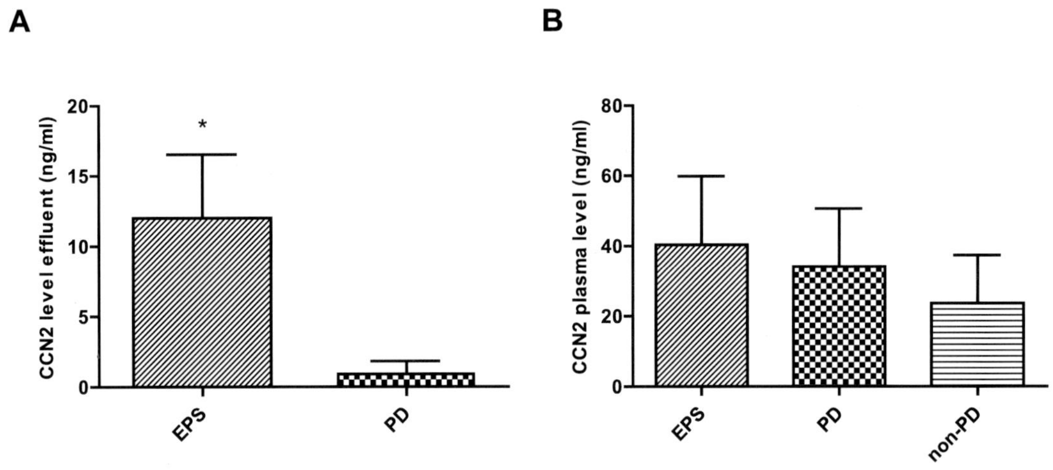

Figure 5. CCN2 protein levels in encapsulating peritoneal sclerosis. CCN2 protein levels in ascites of patients with encapsulating peritoneal sclerosis (EPS, n = 7) were higher compared to levels in dialysate of peritoneal dialysis (PD) patients without EPS obtained from a peritoneal equilibration test (n = 4) (**5A**). CCN2 protein levels in plasma of EPS patients (n = 6), in peritoneal dialysis (PD) patients (n = 13), and in PD naïve patients (non-PD, n = 12) did not differ between the groups (**5B**). Mean±SD. * P<0.01 versus PD.

being tested in patients with idiopathic pulmonary fibrosis and liver fibrosis. Finally, it has recently been shown that CCN3, another CCN family member, works in a yin/yang manner to regulate CCN2 production and activity. In cell-based models of renal and skin disease, TGFβ1 and platelet-derived growth factor stimulated CCN2 activity and collagen deposition leading to progression of fibrosis. Exogenous CCN3 was able to block these effects [51,52]. These findings with CCN3 have provided the basis for a third CCN2-targeted biological currently being developed as an anti-fibrosis therapy. Collectively, these data suggest that the application one or more of these biologicals, perhaps by the intraperitoneal route, may also be feasible in the PD patient to prevent or block progression of EPS.

Early detection of the development of EPS would be very important, especially in view of the potential preventive or therapeutic interventions. CCN2 is locally produced and present in dialysate [38,53] and appears to correlate with the dialysate-to-plasma ratio of creatinine [38]. In addition, a positive relation was reported between the CCN2 concentration in PD fluid after an overnight dwell and PD duration in a cross-sectional study, albeit with a very low R^2 value of 0.07. However, whether longitudinal follow-up of peritoneal CCN2 concentration or appearance rate has any value in predicting the development of peritoneal fibrosis or sclerosis remains to be studied. In view of the prominent overexpression of VEGF in EPS biopsies in our study and that of Braun *et al.* [44], it is disappointing that the longitudinally obtained dialysate VEGF concentration could not predict the development EPS in patients on PD [54], which makes it difficult to apply any preventive anti-VEGF therapy. Finally, TGFβ1 is also not a useful diagnostic marker for EPS as only an inactive soluble form is present in peritoneal effluent [55,56]. To date, no study has measured CCN2 levels in ascites or in peritoneal effluent of EPS patients. We obtained ascites in 7 of the 12 EPS patients and found considerably higher CCN2 concentrations in ascites of EPS patients than in the effluent of non-EPS PD patients. In contrast, plasma concentrations of CCN2 did not differ. These high CCN2 levels in ascites in combination with peritoneal CCN2 overexpression agree with a locally driven response in EPS. However, we cannot rule out the effect of a difference in dwelling time on the local CCN2 levels in these groups. While the dwelling time in non-EPS patients was four hours, the "dwelling time" of ascites in our EPS patients was, for obvious reasons, unknown but undoubtedly longer than that.

In conclusion, peritoneal CCN2, TGFβ1, and VEGF expression are markedly increased in the peritoneal membrane of PD patients with EPS. Whether this increased expression is a late, sudden phenomenon induced by a second hit or a more gradual process correlated with PD duration remains to be determined. As CCN2 appears an attractive target for antifibrotic therapy, prospective, longitudinal studies are needed to determine whether the dialysate CCN2 concentration or appearance rate combined with peritoneal transport studies can predict the development of peritoneal fibrosis and sclerosis.

Acknowledgments

We thank Dionne van der Giezen, Roel Broekhuizen, and Kendra Garchow for technical assistance.

Author Contributions

Conceived and designed the experiments: ACA MCV CJEW TQN WHB. Performed the experiments: ACA SMH AD BLR JWV TQN. Analyzed the data: ACA SMH AD BLR JWV MCV TQN WHB. Contributed reagents/materials/analysis tools: BLR RJT MGHB CJEW TQN. Wrote the paper: All authors.

References

1. Di Paolo N, Sacchi G, de Mia M, Gaggiotti E, Capotondo L, et al. (1986) Morphology of the peritoneal membrane during continuous ambulatory peritoneal dialysis. Nephron 44: 204–211.
2. Dobbie JW. (1989) Morphology of the peritoneum in CAPD. Blood Purif 7: 74–85.
3. Pollock CA, Ibels LS, Eckstein RP, Graham JC, Caterson RJ, et al. (1989) Peritoneal morphology on maintenance dialysis. Am J Nephrol 9: 198–204.
4. Honda K, Nitta K, Horita S, Yumura W, Nihei H (1996) Morphological changes in the peritoneal vasculature of patients on CAPD with ultrafiltration failure. Nephron 72: 171–176.
5. Mateijsen MAM, Van Der Wal AC, Hendriks PMEM, Zweers MM, Mulder J, et al. (1999) Vascular and interstitial changes in the peritoneum of CAPD patients with peritoneal sclerosis. Perit Dial Int 19: 517–525

6. Di Paolo N, Sacchi G (2000) Atlas of peritoneal histology. Perit Dial Int 20 Suppl 3: S5–96.
7. Williams JD, Craig KJ, Topley N, Von Ruhland C, Fallon M, et al. (2002) Morphologic changes in the peritoneal membrane of patients with renal disease. J Am Soc Nephrol 13: 470–479.
8. Williams JD, Craig KJ, Von Ruhland C, Topley N, Williams GT (2003) The natural course of peritoneal membrane biology during peritoneal dialysis. Kidney Int Suppl 64: S43–S49.
9. Honda K, Hamada C, Nakayama M, Miyazaki M, Sherif AM, et al. (2008) Impact of uremia, diabetes, and peritoneal dialysis itself on the pathogenesis of peritoneal sclerosis: A quantitative study of peritoneal membrane morphology. Clin J Am Soc Nephrol 3: 720–728.
10. Krediet RT, Struijk DG (2013) Peritoneal changes in patients on long-term peritoneal dialysis. Nat Rev Nephrol 9: 419–429.
11. Honda K, Oda H (2005) Pathology of encapsulating peritoneal sclerosis. Perit Dial Int 25 Suppl 4: S19–29.
12. Braun N, Fritz P, Ulmer C, Latus J, Kimmel M, et al. (2012) Histological criteria for encapsulating peritoneal sclerosis - A standardized approach. PLoS ONE 7.
13. Kawanishi H, Watanabe H, Moriishi M, Tsuchiya S (2005) Successful surgical management of encapsulating peritoneal sclerosis. Perit Dial Int 25: S39–S47.
14. Habib SM, Betjes MGH, Fieren MWJA, Boeschoten EW, Abrahams AC, et al. (2011) Management of encapsulating peritoneal sclerosis: A guideline on optimal and uniform treatment. Neth J Med 69: 500–507.
15. Korte MR, Sampimon DE, Betjes MGH, Krediet RT (2011) Encapsulating peritoneal sclerosis: The state of affairs. Nat Rev Nephrol 7: 528–538.
16. Margetts PJ, Kolb M, Galt T, Hoff CM, Shockley TR, et al. (2001) Gene transfer of transforming growth factor-ß1 to the rat peritoneum: Effects on membrane function. J Am Soc Nephrol 12: 2029–2039.
17. Margetts PJ, Bonniaud P (2003) Basic mechanisms and clinical implications of peritoneal fibrosis. Perit Dial Int 23: 530–541.
18. Margetts PJ, Oh K-, Kolb M (2005) Transforming growth factor-ß: Importance in long-term peritoneal membrane changes. Perit Dial Int 25 Suppl 3: S15–S17.
19. Liu L, Shi CX, Ghayur A, Zhang C, Su JY, et al. (2009) Prolonged peritoneal gene expression using a helper-dependent adenovirus. Perit Dial Int 29: 508–516.
20. Summers AM (2009) Encapsulating peritoneal sclerosis-have we found the perpetrator? Perit Dial Int 29: 499–501.
21. Io H, Hamada C, Ro Y, Ito Y, Hirahara I, et al. (2004) Morphologic changes of peritoneum and expression of VEGF in encapsulated peritoneal sclerosis rat models. Kidney Int 65: 1927–1936.
22. Yoshio Y, Miyazaki M, Abe K, Nishino T, Furusu A, et al. (2004) TNP-470, an angiogenesis inhibitor, suppresses the progression of peritoneal fibrosis in mouse experimental model. Kidney Int 66: 1677–1685.
23. Tanabe K, Maeshima Y, Ichinose K, Kitayama H, Takazawa Y, et al. (2007) Endostatin peptide, an inhibitor of angiogenesis, prevents the progression of peritoneal sclerosis in a mouse experimental model. Kidney Int 71: 227–238.
24. Loureiro J, Aguilera A, Selgas R, Sandoval P, Albar-Vizcaíno P, et al. (2011) Blocking TGF-ß1 protects the peritoneal membrane from dialysate-induced damage. J Am Soc Nephrol 22: 1682–1695.
25. Yoshimura A, Muto G (2010) TGF-ß function in immune suppression. Curr Top in Microbiol Immunol 350: 127–147.
26. Yoshimura A, Wakabayashi Y, Mori T (2010) Cellular and molecular basis for the regulation of inflammation by TGF-ß. J Biochem 147: 781–792.
27. Wang X, Nie J, Jia Z, Feng M, Zheng Z, et al. (2010) Impaired TGF-ß signalling enhances peritoneal inflammation induced by E. coli in rats. Nephrol Dial Transplant 25: 399–412.
28. Derynck R, Akhurst RJ, Balmain A (2001) TGF-ß signaling in tumor suppression and cancer progression. Nat Genet 29: 117–129.
29. Pardali E, Ten Dijke P (2009) Transforming growth factor-beta signaling and tumor angiogenesis. Front Biosci 14: 4848–4861.
30. Pardali K, Moustakas A (2007) Actions of TGF-ß as tumor suppressor and pro-metastatic factor in human cancer. Biochim Biophys Acta 1775: 21–62.
31. Katz LH, Li Y, Chen JS, Muñoz NM, Majumdar A, et al. (2013) Targeting TGF-ß signaling in cancer. Expert Opin Ther Targets 17: 743–760.
32. Hall-Glenn F, de Young RA, Huang BL, van Handel B, Hofmann JJ, et al. (2012) CCN2/Connective tissue growth factor is essential for pericyte adhesion and endothelial basement membrane formation during angiogenesis. PLoS ONE 7.
33. Leask A, Parapuram SK, Shi-Wen X, Abraham DJ (2009) Connective tissue growth factor (CTGF, CCN2) gene regulation: A potent clinical bio-marker of fibroproliferative disease? J Cell Commun Signal 3: 89–94.
34. Dendooven A, Gerritsen KG, Nguyen TQ, Kok RJ, Goldschmeding R (2011) Connective tissue growth factor (CTGF/CCN2) ELISA: A novel tool for monitoring fibrosis. Biomarkers 16: 289–301.
35. Hall-Glenn F, Lyons KM (2011) Roles for CCN2 in normal physiological processes. Cell Mol Life Sci 68: 3209–3217.
36. Sakamoto N, Sugimura K, Kawashima H, Tsuchida K, Takemoto Y, et al. (2005) Influence of glucose and inflammatory cytokines on TGF-beta1 and CTGF mRNA expressions in human peritoneal mesothelial cells. Int J Mol Med 15: 907–911.
37. Leung JCK, Chan LYY, Tam KY, Tang SCW, Lam MF, et al. (2009) Regulation of CCN2/CTGF and related cytokines in cultured peritoneal cells under conditions simulating peritoneal dialysis. Nephrol Dial Transplant 24: 458–469.
38. Mizutani M, Ito Y, Mizuno M, Nishimura H, Suzuki Y, et al. (2010) Connective tissue growth factor (CTGF/CCN2) is increased in peritoneal dialysis patients with high peritoneal solute transport rate. Am J Physiol Renal Physiol 298: F721–F733.
39. Kawaguchi Y, Kawanishi H, Mujais S, Topley N, Oreopoulos DG (2000) Encapsulating peritoneal sclerosis: Definition, etiology, diagnosis, and treatment. international society for peritoneal dialysis ad hoc committee on ultrafiltration management in peritoneal dialysis. Perit Dial Int 20 Suppl 4: S43–55.
40. La Milia V (2010) Peritoneal transport testing. J Nephrol 23: 633–647.
41. Tsoutsman T, Wang X, Garchow K, Riser B, Twigg S, et al. (2013) CCN2 plays a key role in extracellular matrix gene expression in severe hypertrophic cardiomyopathy and heart failure. J Mol Cell Cardiol 62: 164–178.
42. Habib SM, Dor FJMF, Korte MR, Hagen SM, Betjes MGH (2013) Post-transplantation encapsulating peritoneal sclerosis without inflammation or radiological abnormalities. BMC Nephrol 14. 1
43. Liu Y, Li JF, Liu H, Liu FY, Peng Y, et al. (2014) Functional and structural alterations of peritoneum and secretion of fibrotic cytokines in rats caused by high glucose peritoneal dialysis solutions. Ren Fail 36: 292–299.
44. Braun N, Reimold F, Biegger D, Fritz P, Kimmel M, et al. (2009) Fibrogenic growth factors in encapsulating peritoneal sclerosis. Nephron Clin Pract 113: c88–c95.
45. Mori T, Kawara S, Shinozaki M, Hayashi N, Kakinuma T, et al. (1999) Role and interaction of connective tissue growth factor with transforming growth factor-ß in persistent fibrosis: A mouse fibrosis model. J Cell Physiol 181: 153–159.
46. Wang Q, Usinger W, Nichols B, Gray J, Xu L, et al. (2011) Cooperative interaction of CTGF and TGF-ß in animal models of fibrotic disease. Fibrogenesis Tissue Repair 4.
47. Riser BL, Denichilo M, Cortes P, Baker C, Grondin JM, et al. (2000) Regulation of connective tissue growth factor activity in cultured rat mesangial cells and its expression in experimental diabetic glomerulosclerosis. J Am Soc Nephrol 11: 25–38.
48. Liu FY, Xiao L, Peng Y, Duan SB, Liu H, et al. (2007) Inhibition effect of small interfering RNA of connective tissue growth factor on the expression of vascular endothelial growth factor and connective tissue growth factor in cultured human peritoneal mesothelial cells. Chin Med J 120: 231–236.
49. Xiao L, Sun L, Liu FY, Peng YM, Duan SB (2010) Connective tissue growth factor knockdown attenuated matrix protein production and vascular endothelial growth factor expression induced by transforming growth factor-ß1 in cultured human peritoneal mesothelial cells. Ther Apher Dial 14: 27–34.
50. Adler SG, Schwartz S, Williams ME, Arauz-Pacheco C, Bolton WK, et al. (2010) Phase 1 study of anti-CTGF monoclonal antibody in patients with diabetes and microalbuminuria. Clin J Am Soc Nephrol 5: 1420–1428.
51. Riser BL, Najmabadi F, Perbal B, Peterson DR, Rambow JA, et al. (2009) CCN3 (NOV) is a negative regulator of CCN2 (CTGF) and a novel endogenous inhibitor of the fibrotic pathway in an in vitro model of renal disease. Am J Pathol 174: 1725–1734.
52. Riser BL, Bhagavathula N, Perone P, Garchow K, Xu Y, et al. (2012) Gadolinium-induced fibrosis is counter-regulated by CCN3 in human dermal fibroblasts: A model for potential treatment of nephrogenic systemic fibrosis. Journal of Cell Communication and Signaling 6: 97–105.
53. Zarrinkalam KH, Stanley JM, Gray J, Oliver N, Faull RJ (2003) Connective tissue growth factor and its regulation in the peritoneal cavity of peritoneal dialysis patients. Kidney Int 64: 331–338.
54. Sampimon DE, Korte MR, Barreto DL, Vlijm A, de Waart R, et al. (2010) Early diagnostic markers for encapsulating peritoneal sclerosis: A case-control study. Perit Dial Int 30: 163–169.
55. Zweers MM, De Waart DR, Smit W, Struijk DG, Krediet RT (1999) Growth factors VEGF and TGF-ß1 in peritoneal dialysis. J Lab Clin Med 134: 124–132.
56. Lopes Barreto D, Krediet RT (2013) Current status and practical use of effluent biomarkers in peritoneal dialysis patients. Am J Kidney Dis 62: 823–833.

Outcomes and Characteristics of Patients Undergoing Percutaneous Angioplasty Followed by Below-Knee or Above-Knee Amputation for Peripheral Artery Disease

Chun-Tai Mao[1,4¶], Ming-Lung Tsai[2,4¶], Chao-Yung Wang[2,4], Ming-Shien Wen[2,4], I-Chang Hsieh[2,4], Ming-Jui Hung[1,4], Chao-Hung Wang[1,4], Chun-Chi Chen[2,4], Tien-Hsing Chen[2,3,4*]

1 Heart Failure Center, Division of Cardiology, Department of Internal Medicine, Chang Gung Memorial Hospital, Keelung, Taiwan, **2** Division of Cardiology, Department of Internal Medicine, Chang Gung Memorial Hospital, Taipei, Taiwan, **3** Department of cardiology, Chang Gung Memorial Hospital, Xiamen, China, **4** College of Medicine, Chang Gung University, Taoyuan, Taiwan

Abstract

Objective: Little is known about long-term outcomes among patients who receive percutaneous angioplasty (PTA) for peripheral artery disease (PAD) then undergo below-knee or above-knee amputations. We sought to determine clinical outcomes associated with below-knee or above-knee amputation, along with possible explanatory factors and treatment strategies.

Methods: Using data from Taiwan's National Health Insurance Research Database from 1997 to 2010, 7,568 adult patients were divided into three groups: lower extremity preserved (LE), below-knee amputation (BK) and above-knee amputation (AK). We assessed outcomes including major adverse cardiovascular events (MACE) and associated risk factors.

Results: Overall MACE was significantly higher in the AK group compared to the LE and BK groups, over a mean follow-up of 2.45 years (hazard ratio [HR]: 1.81; 95% confidence interval [CI]: 1.50–2.18 for AK vs. LE; HR: 1.67; 95% CI: 1.36–2.06 for AK vs. BK). However MACE were similar for the BK and LE groups (HR: 1.08; 95% CI: 0.98–1.20). Overall mortality was highest in the AK group (HR: 1.65, 95% CI: 1.34–2.04 for AK vs. BK). As for patient characteristics, atrial fibrillation was more prevalent in the AK group than in the BK group (17% vs. 7%). Independent risk factors associated with death after above- or below-knee amputation included advanced age, heart failure, dialysis, male gender and high patient volume.

Conclusion: The MACE rate was highest in the AK group, whereas the LE and BK groups were similar in this regard. Furthermore, overall mortality increased with larger area of amputation.

Editor: Ryuichi Morishita, Osaka University Graduate School of Medicine, Japan

Funding: The authors have no support or funding to report.

Competing Interests: The authors have declared that no competing interests exist.

* Email: mr7599@outlook.com

¶ These authors contributed equally to this work.

Introduction

As societies age, the incidence of peripheral artery disease (PAD) has been increasing, along with the increase in patients with risk factors for atherosclerosis, especially diabetes mellitus [1,2]. Patients with PAD have a high probability of suffering from critical limb ischemia (CLI) which may require major lower extremity amputation, including above-knee (AK) or below-knee (BK) amputations [2]. Prior studies have revealed that such patients face high morbidity and health costs [3–7]. Furthermore, major lower extremity amputations may contribute to high mortality [8–10]. Therefore revascularization, including bypass surgery and percutaneous angioplasty (PTA), should be considered before amputation, according to the American College of Cardiology/American Heart Association guideline recommendations [11]. In the real world, however, bypass surgery is rarely applied to patients with CLI, because such patients commonly have higher incidence of comorbidities and advanced age, making PTA the preferred treatment [2,12]. After PTA, patients may be able to keep their lower extremity, or they may receive BK or AK amputation. Little is known about long-term and short-term outcomes for these three groups of patients–those receiving only PTA, and those receiving PTA followed by BK, or receiving PTA followed by AK amputation. We evaluated the outcomes in terms of myocardial infarction (MI), stroke, and all causes of mortality. The clinical prognoses of these patients vary based on a number of factors, some of which are patient specific, but no comprehensive report thus far has evaluated the effect of such factors on cardiovascular outcomes.

To evaluate outcomes among PTA patients who kept their lower extremity or received AK or BK amputation, we analyzed data from Taiwan's National Healthcare Insurance (NHI) Program. Our specific aims were to (1) determine rates of death, MI, and stroke among patients who kept their leg or received AK or BK amputation following PTA; (2) determine factors associated with clinical outcomes in the three groups; and (3) determine the major causes of death.

Methods

1. Data source

We conducted a nationwide population-based cohort study using Taiwan's National Health Insurance Research Database (NHIRD), which consists of standard computerized claims documents submitted by medical institutions seeking reimbursement through the NHI Program. PTA is an option covered by the NHI, and patients with PAD who received PTA are recorded in the NHIRD.

The NHI program covers medical needs for 99.19% of the population in Taiwan, more than 25 million people. The accuracy and validation of NHIRD data is based on regular auditing of claims by the NHI Bureau [13–16]. False reimbursement claims result in substantial penalties. Minor infractions involve fines of 100 times the amount of the false claim, while serious infractions may result in revoking physicians' licenses or criminal charges.

This study was approved by the Ethics Institutional Review Board of Chang Gung Memorial Hospital. The information and records of patients were anonymized and de-identified prior to analysis.

2. Study Cohorts and Follow-up

We identified all patients in the NHIRD who received PTA between January 1, 1997 and December 31, 2010 and considered first time admission for PTA as the index hospitalization. The study excluded patients with arterio-venous shunt dysfunction in end stage renal disease who may have received PTA for this clinical event. After we selected this initial cohort of PAD patients receiving PTA, we divided them into three groups according to the results of their index hospitalization. The lower extremity preserved (LE) group consisted of patients whose lower extremity were preserved after PTA. The BK group included patients who received BK amputation following PTA. The AK group included patients receiving AK amputation after PTA (Fig. 1). Follow-up was from the date of index hospitalization to date of death or December 31th, 2010.

3. Outcomes and covariate measurements

Baseline comorbidities were identified by ICD-9-CM (International Classification of Diseases, 9th Revision, Clinical Modification) diagnosis codes and medication during index hospitalization. Primary outcomes were major adverse cardiovascular events (MACE) including death, MI and stroke.

4. Statistical methods

We used the chi-square test to examine the difference in proportions of categorical variables among the LE, AK and BK groups, and tested continuous variables by one-way ANOVA. Associations between the three groups and complications were identified by multivariate logistic regression analysis. We performed multivariate Cox regressions to reveal the association between the three groups and outcomes (prognoses). In a further subgroup analysis, we created a multivariate Cox model to identify the factors associated with overall mortality for patients receiving major amputations. The results are presented as adjusted odds ratios (OR) for logistic regression, or as adjusted hazard ratios (HR) for Cox regressions, with corresponding 95% confidence

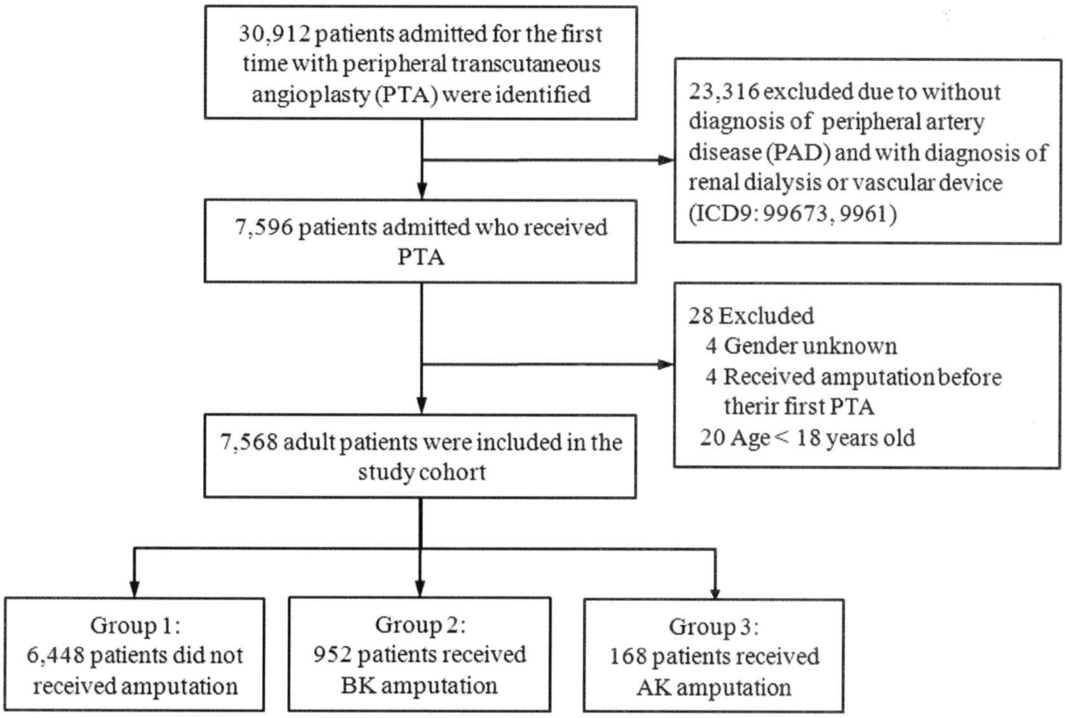

Figure 1. Enrollment flow chart.

Table 1. Clinical characteristics and comorbidities of the study patients.

		Amputation at the admission			
Characteristics	**All patients**	**LE group**	**BK group**	**AK group**	***P***
Number of patients	7568	6448	952	168	–
Age, year	71.3±11.1	71.5±11.1	69.8±10.9	73.6±11.4	<0.001
Male sex	4694 (62)	4052 (63)	539 (57)	103 (61)	0.001
Indication					
Type2 DM foot	857 (11)	432 (7)	392 (41)	33 (20)	<0.001
Type1 DM foot	4 (0)	0 (0)	4 (0)	0 (0)	<0.001
Chronic ulceration	513 (7)	398 (6)	108 (11)	7 (4)	<0.001
Gangrene	1279 (17)	689 (11)	529 (56)	61 (36)	<0.001
Comorbidities					
Hypertension	6976 (92)	5927 (92)	884 (93)	165 (98)	0.008
Diabetes	5003 (66)	4040 (63)	845 (89)	118 (70)	<0.001
Dyslipidemia	2998 (40)	2655 (41)	304 (32)	39 (23)	<0.001
Gout	721 (10)	617 (10)	79 (8)	25 (15)	0.026
Stroke	2161 (29)	1830 (28)	277 (29)	54 (32)	0.524
Atrial fibrillation	855 (11)	756 (12)	71 (7)	28 (17)	<0.001
Malignancy	586 (8)	508 (8)	67 (7)	11 (7)	0.559
COPD	828 (11)	705 (11)	102 (11)	21 (13)	0.791
Uremia	1798 (24)	1440 (22)	314 (33)	44 (26)	<0.001
Congestive heart failure	1792 (24)	1501 (23)	242 (25)	49 (29)	0.083
Old myocardial infarction	1003 (13)	872 (14)	110 (12)	21 (13)	0.237
Coronary artery disease	3608 (48)	3194 (50)	349 (37)	65 (39)	<0.001
CABG	552 (7)	478 (7)	60 (6)	14 (8)	0.409
Carotid stenting	103 (1)	98 (2)	4 (0)	1 (1)	0.016
Dialysis	1348 (18)	1072 (17)	243 (26)	33 (20)	<0.001

Abbreviations: COPD = chronic obstructive pulmonary disease; CABG = coronary artery bypass graft; DM = diabetes; LE = Lower extremity preserved; BK = below knee; AK = above knee.

intervals (CI). All data analyses were conducted using SPSS software version 15 (SPSS Inc., Chicago, Illinois).

Results

1. Patient characteristics

For our study cohort, we identified a total of 7,588 patients diagnosed with PAD who underwent PTA. Twenty patients under age 18 when undergoing PTA were excluded, resulting in a total of 7,568 adult patients. In the whole cohort there were 4,694 (62%) male patients and 2,874 (38%) female ones. The mean age for the overall cohort was 71.3 years ($SD = 11.1$). The mean follow-up period was 2.45 years ($SD = 2.54$). At the index hospitalization where the patient received PTA, 6,448 patients who remained free of amputation were designated as the LE group, 952 patients who received BK amputation were designated as the BK group, and 168 patients who suffered AK amputation were designated as the AK group.

Table 1 shows the clinical characteristics and comorbidities of the patients. AK patients were older than patients in the two other groups. The prevalence of diabetes, dyslipidemia and end stage renal disease was substantially higher in the BK group compared to the AK group (89% *vs.* 70%; 32% *vs.* 23%; 26% *vs.* 20%, respectively). In contrast, the prevalence of atrial fibrillation was higher in the AK group when compared to the BK group (17% *vs.* 7%).

2. Events during index hospitalization

Table 2 shows the case number and proportion of various complications for the three groups. The risk of acute renal failure was higher in the AK group than the LE and BK groups (OR = 5.57, 3.90, $P<0.001$). Both the AK and BK groups had a higher risk of newly initiated dialysis compared to the LE group (OR = 1.79, $P = 0.003$, for BK; OR = 3.10, $P = 0.001$, for AK). A significantly higher risk of in-hospital mortality was observed for the AK group when compared to the LE and BK groups (OR = 4.18, 3.28, $P<0.001$). In contrast, these three groups did not differ in the risk of new occurrence of MI or stroke. Results for risk of MACE were similar to the pattern for in-hospital mortality.

3. Outcomes during Follow-up

Table 3 displays the numbers of cases and proportion of various prognoses one year after PTA and overall for the three groups. No risk of second amputation above the knee or newly initiated dialysis was found for the AK and BK groups. The BK group were at higher risk of suffering a second BK after PTA compared to the LE group (HR = 1.19, $P = 0.028$), whereas the AK group were less likely to suffer BK compared to the LE and BK groups (HR = 0.35, $P = 0.003$; HR = 0.30, $P = 0.001$). One year after

Table 2. The association of amputation status after PTA with complication at same admission.

	Number of event (%)			Adjusted odds ratio and 95% CI					
Variable	**LE (*n*=6448)**	**BK (*n*=952)**	**AK (*n*=168)**	**BK *vs.* LE**		**AK *vs.* LE**		**AK *vs.* BK**	
				OR (95% CI)	***P***	**OR (95% CI)**	***P***	**OR (95% CI)**	***P***
ARF	93 (1.4)	22 (2.3)	14 (8.3)	1.43 (0.88–2.32)	0.150	5.57 (3.04–10.20)	<0.001	3.90 (1.92–7.94)	<0.001
New onset of dialysis	113 (1.8)	38 (4.0)	10 (6.0)	1.79 (1.21–2.65)	0.003	3.10 (1.56–6.19)	0.001	1.73 (0.82–3.63)	0.147
MACE	498 (7.7)	69 (7.2)	25 (14.9)	1.00 (0.76–1.32)	0.991	2.11 (1.34–3.32)	0.001	2.11 (1.26–3.51)	0.004
In-hospital death	177 (2.7)	39 (4.1)	20 (11.9)	1.27 (0.88–1.84)	0.195	4.18 (2.52–6.94)	<0.001	3.28 (1.82–5.90)	<0.001
Myocardial infarction	124 (1.9)	17 (1.8)	4 (2.4)	1.08 (0.64–1.84)	0.767	1.33 (0.48–3.67)	0.584	1.23 (0.40–3.72)	0.718
Stroke	222 (3.4)	19 (2.0)	3 (1.8)	0.79 (0.47–1.32)	0.361	0.53 (0.16–1.77)	0.302	0.68 (0.19–2.44)	0.550

The odds ratio were adjusted for age, gender, diabetes, hypertension, dyslipidemia, previous cerebral vascular accident, heart failure, coronary artery disease, chronic kidney disease, gout, AF, malignancy, chronic obstructive pulmonary disease, center volume and level of hospital.

Abbreviations: ARF = acute renal failure; MACE = major adverse cardiac events; LE = Lower extremity preserved; BK = below knee; AK = above knee; OR = odds ratio; CI = confidence interval.

Table 3. The association of amputation status after PTA with prognoses.

	Number of event (%)			Adjusted hazard ratio and 95% CI					
Variable	**LE (*n*=6448)**	**BK (*n*=952)**	**AK (*n*=168)**	**BK *vs.* LE**		**AK *vs.* LE**		**AK *vs.* BK**	
				HR (95% CI)	***P***	**HR (95% CI)**	***P***	**HR (95% CI)**	***P***
Above knee amputation	236 (3.7)	48 (5.0)	9 (5.4)	1.23 (0.89–1.70)	0.206	1.83 (0.94–3.59)	0.077	1.49 (0.73–3.06)	0.276
Below knee amputation	945 (14.7)	216 (22.7)	8 (4.8)	1.19 (1.02–1.39)	0.028	0.35 (0.18–0.71)	0.003	0.30 (0.15–0.60)	0.001
New onset of dialysis	179 (2.8)	33 (3.5)	3 (1.8)	1.32 (0.89–1.94)	0.162	1.10 (0.35–3.48)	0.867	0.84 (0.26–2.75)	0.771
MACE (1 year)	1427 (22.1)	239 (25.1)	74 (44.0)	1.00 (0.87–1.15)	0.959	1.94 (1.53–2.45)	<0.001	1.93 (1.49–2.51)	<0.001
Death	1134 (17.6)	218 (22.9)	69 (41.1)	1.14 (0.98–1.32)	0.083	2.18 (1.70–2.78)	<0.001	1.91 (1.45–2.51)	<0.001
Myocardial infarction	122 (1.9)	12 (1.3)	3 (1.8)	0.70 (0.38–1.29)	0.253	1.15 (0.37–3.65)	0.807	1.64 (0.46–5.84)	0.444
Stroke	279 (4.3)	26 (2.7)	4 (2.4)	0.63 (0.42–0.95)	0.026	0.61 (0.23–1.63)	0.322	0.97 (0.34–2.78)	0.948
MACE (Overall)	2983 (46.3)	467 (49.1)	116 (69.0)	1.08 (0.98–1.20)	0.128	1.81 (1.50–2.18)	<0.001	1.67 (1.36–2.06)	<0.001
Death	2529 (39.2)	430 (45.2)	112 (66.7)	1.20 (1.08–1.33)	0.001	1.98 (1.63–2.40)	<0.001	1.65 (1.34–2.04)	<0.001
Myocardial infarction	310 (4.8)	38 (4.0)	8 (4.8)	1.00 (0.70–1.41)	0.985	1.49 (0.74–3.03)	0.265	1.50 (0.70–3.23)	0.301
Stroke	675 (10.5)	69 (7.2)	9 (5.4)	0.83 (0.64–1.07)	0.142	0.71 (0.37–1.37)	0.304	0.86 (0.43–1.72)	0.662

The hazard ratio were adjusted for age, gender, diabetes, hypertension, dyslipidemia, previous cerebral vascular accident, heart failure, coronary artery disease, chronic kidney disease, gout, AF, malignancy, chronic obstructive pulmonary disease, center volume and level of hospital.
Abbreviations: MACE = major adverse cardiac events; LE = Lower extremity preserved; BK = below knee; AK = above knee; HR = hazard ratio; CI = confidence interval.

Table 4. Cause of mortality (*n* = 2531).

	Overall	LE	BK	AK
Cause of mortality	*n* (%)	*n* (%)	*n* (%)	*n* (%)
Cannot be specified	258 (10.2)	216 (10.4)	36 (10.3)	6 (6.1)
DM and PAD related	435 (17.2)	331 (15.9)	74 (21.1)	30 (30.6)
Sepsis*	362 (14.3)	279 (13.4)	64 (18.3)	19 (19.4)
Pneumonia	290 (11.5)	240 (11.5)	39 (11.1)	11 (11.2)
COPD	20 (0.8)	18 (0.9)	2 (0.6)	0 (0.0)
Cardiovascular disease	395 (15.6)	340 (16.3)	41 (11.7)	14 (14.3)
Stroke	148 (5.8)	127 (6.1)	17 (4.9)	4 (4.1)
Respiratory failure	253 (10.0)	211 (10.1)	37 (10.6)	5 (5.1)
Renal failure	64 (2.5)	53 (2.5)	10 (2.9)	1 (1.0)
GI bleeding and GI system	75 (3.0)	60 (2.9)	11 (3.1)	4 (4.1)
Fall and related mortality	10 (0.4)	7 (0.3)	2 (0.6)	1 (1.0)
Malignancy	162 (6.4)	150 (7.2)	12 (3.4)	0 (0.0)
Others	59 (2.3)	51 (2.4)	5 (1.4)	3 (3.1)

*included UTI, septic septicemia, gangrene, decubitus ulcer.
Abbreviations: DM = diabetes; PAD = peripheral artery disease; COPD = chronic obstructive pulmonary disease; GI = Gastrointestinal; LE = Lower extremity preserved; BK = below knee; AK = above knee.

index hospitalization with PTA, the risk of death as well as MACE was significantly higher in the AK group than in the LE and BK groups. The BK group had a lower risk of stroke than the LE group (HR = 0.63, $P<0.05$), but there was no statistically significant difference in risk of MI among the three groups.

The AK group had higher risk of overall mortality and MACE than the other two groups. The rate of MACE was similar for the LE and BK groups, but the BK group had a higher risk of death than the LE group (HR = 1.20, $P<0.01$).

4. Death causes analysis

Table 4 tabulates the most common causes of death in PAD patients after PTA. For the whole cohort, the leading cause of death was diabetes mellitus (DM) and PAD-related complications (17.2%), followed by cardiovascular disease (15.6%), sepsis (14.3%), pneumonia (11.5%) and respiratory failure (10%), respectively. DM- and PAD-related death is defined as the death due to complications or sequelae induced or aggravated by DM and PAD, including gangrene-related sepsis and complications during PTA or amputation. Patients in the AK group were more

Table 5. Factors associated with death after major amputation of the lower extremity (*n* = 1120).

Variable	HR (95% CI)	*P*
Age (per 10 years)	1.38 (1.26–1.51)	<0.001
Male gender	1.19 (1.00–1.42)	0.049
Diabetes	1.13 (0.88–1.44)	0.342
Hypertension	1.10 (0.77–1.58)	0.606
Dyslipidemia	1.06 (0.86–1.29)	0.593
Previous stroke	1.08 (0.89–1.31)	0.428
Heart failure	1.62 (1.32–1.98)	<0.001
Coronary artery disease	0.98 (0.81–1.18)	0.837
Dialysis	1.98 (1.62–2.42)	<0.001
Gout	1.10 (0.82–1.46)	0.535
Atrial fibrillation	1.23 (0.92–1.64)	0.169
Malignancy	1.31 (0.98–1.77)	0.072
Chronic obstructive pulmonary disease	1.04 (0.79–1.37)	0.785
High center volume‡	1.23 (1.02–1.49)	0.029
Medical center	0.92 (0.77–1.11)	0.393

‡defined as greater than 27 procedures per year.
Abbreviations: HR = hazard ratio; CI = confidence interval.

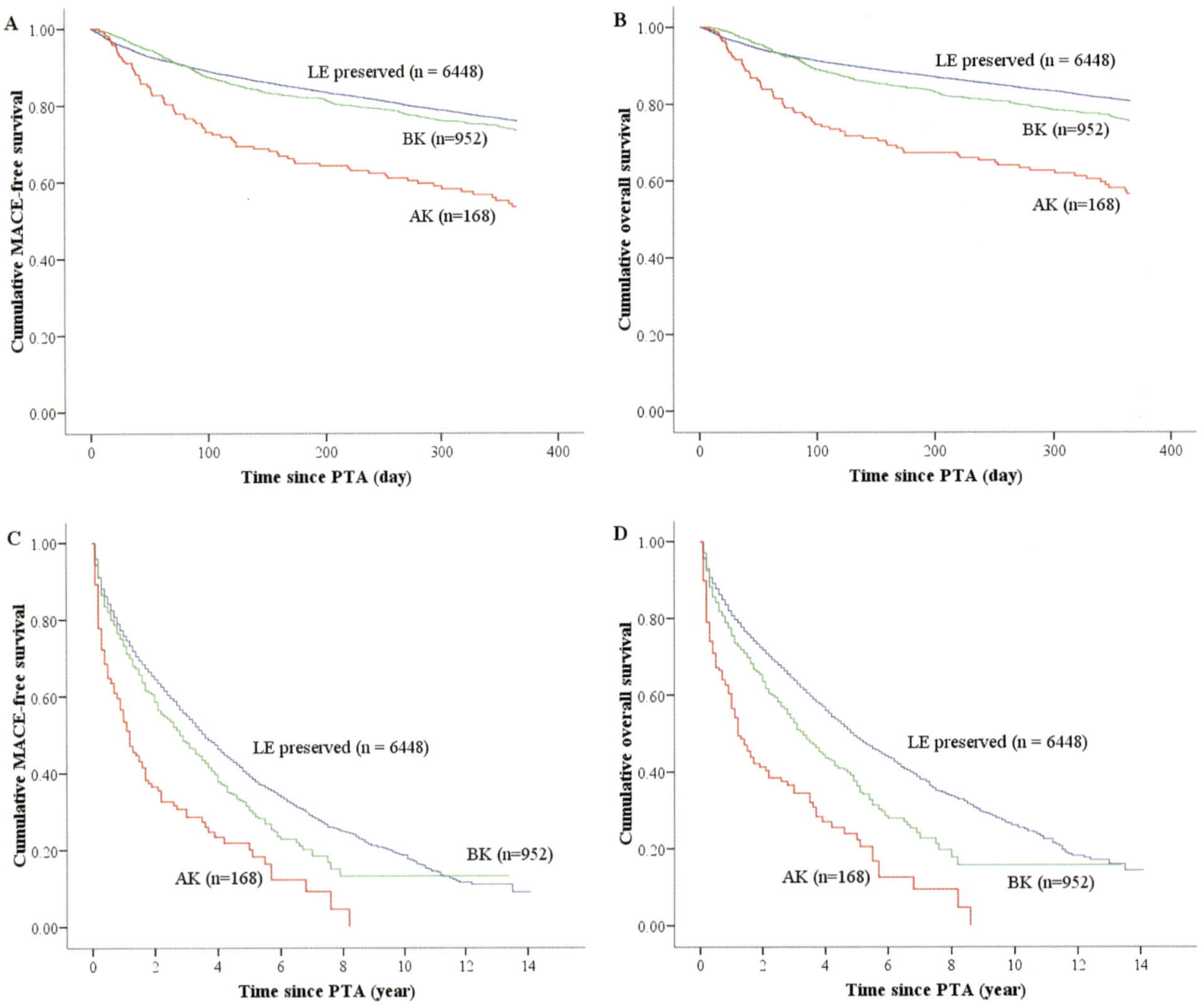

Figure 2. Comparison of prognostics among the study groups. (A) major adverse cardiac events in one year, (B) 1-year mortality, (C) overall major adverse cardiac events, and (D) overall mortality.

likely to expire due to DM and PAD-related complications (30.6%) and less likely to die of respiratory failure (5.1%) and malignancy (0%), when compared to the other groups. DM- and PAD-related complications and sepsis were substantially lower in the LE group (15.9%, 13.4%) compared to the AK and BK groups.

5. Clinical factors associated with death after major amputation of the lower extremity

Table 5 reveals the results of Cox models designed to identify the clinical predictors of overall mortality after BK or AK amputation. Older age (HR = 1.38, $P<0.001$), male gender (HR = 1.19, $P<0.05$), history of heart failure (HR = 1.62, $P<0.001$), history of dialysis (HR = 1.98, $P<0.001$) and receiving PTA in a hospital with high patient volume (HR = 1.23, $P<0.05$) were independently associated with higher risk of death after BK or AK amputation. In the subgroup analysis for patients receiving major amputation at large volume medical centers and low volume centers, the proportion of AK amputations at large volume centers is significantly higher than at low volume centers (19.7% vs. 11.3%, $p<0.001$). The baseline characteristics, including age and gender, were similar at large volume centers and low volume centers. The comorbidities, including hypertension, diabetes, stroke, malignancy, heart failure, coronary artery disease and myocardial infarction history, were not different between these two groups.

Discussion

The previous literature [10] demonstrated that the overall MACE rate was high in the AK and BK groups; however, in our study, the MACE rate was not significantly different for the LE and BK groups. Additionally, the incidence of atrial fibrillation (AF) was higher in the AK group than the two other groups, which may imply different disease mechanisms and treatment strategies for patients undergoing AK amputations.

1. Patient characteristics

In our cohort, patients with PAD undergoing PTA were predominantly male, consistent with findings from the previous study [17]. Because risk factors for PAD, such as smoking and hyperlipidemia, are more common among males, the incidence of PAD is higher for them. In addition, male gender was a predisposing factor for mortality in our cohort study. Meanwhile, comorbidities such as hypertension, stroke, coronary artery disease and myocardial infarction had the same prevalence across the three groups, which implied that atherosclerosis may be the common disease mechanism affecting those patients [8]. In coronary artery disease studies, many medications, including those for lipid profile modification [18], blood sugar control [19] or blood pressure control [20], have been used to promote atherosclerotic plaque regression. According to a previous study [21], regression of atherosclerotic coronary plaque volume may represent a surrogate for myocardial infarction and repeat revascularization. Medication that modifies lipid profiles, and those that act on blood sugar metabolism and blood pressure may also induce regression of atherosclerotic plaque in peripheral artery disease, consequently reducing the rate of re-stenosis in peripheral vessels and repeat revascularization.

2. Events during index hospitalization and outcomes after discharge

During the index hospitalization, the prevalence of acute renal failure was higher in the AK group than the BK and LE groups. Newly initiated dialysis occurred more frequently in the two amputation groups compared to the LE group (Table 2). However, after long-term follow up, the rate of new dialysis occurring was the same for the three groups (Table 3). So the transient renal function impairment showing in the AK group did not indicate increased risk of dialysis in the long term.

During following up, the frequency of a second amputation, BK, was much higher in the AK and BK groups than the LE group (Table 3). This result reveals that patients undergoing AK or BK amputation at index hospitalization are more likely to have the other leg amputated in the future. However MACE in the BK group was the same as in the LE group.

During one-year follow up, the incidence of stroke was a little lower in the BK group than the LE group, and a slightly higher mortality rate was noted in the BK group compared to the LE group, although the difference was not significant. Higher mortality rates may reduce the incidence of stroke due to the competitive outcome effect. The same scenario was also observed for the AK and LE groups, however the result was not statistically significant (HR: 0.61; 95% CI: 0.23–1.63) because of the relatively small sample size of the AK group.

Consistent with the previous literatures [9,10], despite undergoing PTA, high mortality among PAD patients was observed in our study, with or without major amputation. However it was surprising that all-cause mortality showed no statistically significant differences between the LE and BK groups at one-year follow up, but significantly higher mortality was observed in the AK group (Fig. 2B). In long-term follow up, mortality was higher in the BK group than the LE group, but it was highest in AK group (Fig. 2D). However there was no significant difference in MACE between the BK and LE groups in short-term (Fig. 2A) or long-term follow up (Fig. 2C). MACE was unequivocally highest in the AK group.

Although BK amputation, like AK amputation, has been defined as a major amputation [9,10,22], the outcomes were very different for those two groups. According to a previous study [23], survival among patients with BK amputations was not better than those with AK amputations, but our results show better outcomes for the BK amputation group and LE group than for the AK group. Our results are compatible with those from the latest study that has been done [10]. Our study shows that avoiding AK amputation should be a key treatment strategy for PAD patients who receive PTA.

3. Risk factors associated with outcomes and causes of death

Since avoiding AK amputation is the most important strategy following PTA, it is worth noting some different baseline characteristics of patients in the AK and BK groups. As mentioned previously, AF was more prevalent among the patients in the AK group compared to those in the BK group (17% vs. 7%, $p<0.001$), which could suggest that arterial embolisms induced by AF may be the cause of some severely ischemic legs needing AK amputation [8,17,24], On the other hand, the higher prevalence of DM and dyslipidemia among the patients in the BK group compared to the AK group (89% vs. 70%, $p<0.001$; 32% vs. 23%, $p<0.001$) may indicate that atherosclerosis may be a more important cause of PAD in the BK group than in the AK group. So anticoagulation and thrombolysis may be important treatment strategies for avoiding AK amputation in patients who have PAD and AF [22,25,26].

Consistent with findings from the existing literature [10,27], the factors associated with higher mortality included advanced age, heart failure, dialysis, and male gender, all of which could contribute to these extremely high short- and long-term event rates following AK or BK amputation. Unlike other study which revealed better outcomes at medical centers with higher patient volume [28], receiving PTA at high volume medical centers in Taiwan was associated with a higher risk of death after major amputation. According to subgroup analysis for large volume and low volume centers, the proportion of AK amputations in large volume centers is significantly greater than in low volume centers (19.7% vs. 11.3%, $p<0.001$). The baseline characteristics and comorbidities are similar for the two groups. This means that patients with more severe PAD are sent to large volume centers for peripheral angioplasty, so the proportion of AK amputations is higher in large volume centers, with the result that there seem to be more unfavorable outcomes in large volume centers.

Our study also reviewed the causes of mortality. DM or PAD was the most important cause of death in patients with PAD, even when they received aggressive treatment such as PTA. The risk of sepsis was higher in patients with PAD [29], and was an important cause of mortality. Consistent with previous literature [11,22], we found that cardiovascular disease is also a major cause of death in patients with PAD. Pneumonia also poses a threat to their lives. In order to reduce mortality among such patients, effective infection prevention and control are very important, in addition to treating the PAD itself. Some PAD patients may suffer walking impairment or even immobility due to lower limb dysfunction. As with stroke patients, immobility can predispose them to pneumonia [30]. Declining ability to walk is also known to affect mortality [31]. Rehabilitation to increase mobility may thus improve both daily activity levels and medical outcomes [32].

Study Limitations

Our study has a number of limitations. First, the NHI data do not include information about the severity of disease, such as the numbers of diseased vessels and TASC classifications, which may influence both the rate of AK or BK amputation and long-term outcomes following AK or BK amputation. Second, our study cannot distinguish whether new endovascular intervention devices such as stents or drug-eluting balloons, which may affect the prognosis of PAD, were used during PTA. Lastly, our study only suggests trends and possible treatment strategies for improving outcomes among patients with PAD. Randomized controlled trials should be designed to test these different treatment strategies.

Conclusion

Mortality rates among patients with PAD undergoing PTA remain high. MACE were much higher among patients receiving AK amputation than among those receiving BK amputation or those whose lower extremity were preserved, whether in both long-term or short-term follow up. Short-term and overall MACE were the same for the LE and BK groups. Furthermore, overall mortality increased with increasing area of amputation. Sepsis, cardiovascular disease and pneumonia are the major causes of mortality, in addition to DM and PAD-related complications.

Author Contributions

Conceived and designed the experiments: CTM MLT THC. Performed the experiments: CYW MSW. Analyzed the data: ICH MJH. Contributed reagents/materials/analysis tools: CHW CCC. Contributed to the writing of the manuscript: CTM MLT THC.

References

1. Tseng CH, Tai TY, Chen CJ, Lin BJ (1994) Ten-year clinical analysis of diabetic leg amputees. J Formos Med Assoc 93: 388–392.
2. Iida O, Nakamura M, Yamauchi Y, Kawasaki D, Yokoi Y, et al. (2013) Endovascular treatment for infrainguinal vessels in patients with critical limb ischemia: OLIVE registry, a prospective, multicenter study in Japan with 12-month follow-up. Circ Cardiovasc Interv 6: 68–76.
3. McDermott MM, Liu K, Greenland P, Guralnik JM, Criqui MH, et al. (2004) Functional decline in peripheral arterial disease: associations with the ankle brachial index and leg symptoms. JAMA 292: 453–461.
4. Margolis J, Barron JJ, Grochulski WD (2005) Health care resources and costs for treating peripheral artery disease in a managed care population: results from analysis of administrative claims data. J Manag Care Pharm 11: 727–734.
5. Hirsch AT, Criqui MH, Treat-Jacobson D, Regensteiner JG, Creager MA, et al. (2001) Peripheral arterial disease detection, awareness, and treatment in primary care. JAMA 286: 1317–1324.
6. Diehm C, Allenberg JR, Pittrow D, Mahn M, Tepohl G, et al. (2009) Mortality and vascular morbidity in older adults with asymptomatic versus symptomatic peripheral artery disease. Circulation 120: 2053–2061.
7. Peacock JM, Keo HH, Duval S, Baumgartner I, Oldenburg NC, et al. (2011) The incidence and health economic burden of ischemic amputation in Minnesota, 2005–2008. Prev Chronic Dis 8: A141.
8. Hirsch AT, Haskal ZJ, Hertzer NR, Bakal CW, Creager MA, et al. (2006) ACC/AHA 2005 guidelines for the management of patients with peripheral arterial disease (lower extremity, renal, mesenteric, and abdominal aortic): executive summary a collaborative report from the American Association for Vascular Surgery/Society for Vascular Surgery, Society for Cardiovascular Angiography and Interventions, Society for Vascular Medicine and Biology, Society of Interventional Radiology, and the ACC/AHA Task Force on Practice Guidelines (Writing Committee to Develop Guidelines for the Management of Patients With Peripheral Arterial Disease) endorsed by the American Association of Cardiovascular and Pulmonary Rehabilitation; National Heart, Lung, and Blood Institute; Society for Vascular Nursing; TransAtlantic Inter-Society Consensus; and Vascular Disease Foundation. J Am Coll Cardiol 47: 1239–1312.
9. Cruz CP, Eidt JF, Capps C, Kirtley L, Moursi MM (2003) Major lower extremity amputations at a Veterans Affairs hospital. Am J Surg 186: 449–454.
10. Jones WS, Patel MR, Dai D, Vemulapalli S, Subherwal S, et al. (2013) High mortality risks after major lower extremity amputation in Medicare patients with peripheral artery disease. Am Heart J 165: 809–815, 815 e801.
11. Rooke TW, Hirsch AT, Misra S, Sidawy AN, Beckman JA, et al. (2011) 2011 ACCF/AHA Focused Update of the Guideline for the Management of Patients With Peripheral Artery Disease (updating the 2005 guideline): a report of the American College of Cardiology Foundation/American Heart Association Task Force on Practice Guidelines. J Am Coll Cardiol 58: 2020–2045.
12. Goodney PP, Beck AW, Nagle J, Welch HG, Zwolak RM (2009) National trends in lower extremity bypass surgery, endovascular interventions, and major amputations. J Vasc Surg 50: 54–60.
13. Yang YW, Chen YH, Xirasagar S, Lin HC (2011) Increased risk of stroke in patients with bullous pemphigoid: a population-based follow-up study. Stroke 42: 319–323.
14. Wu CY, Wu MS, Kuo KN, Wang CB, Chen YJ, et al. (2010) Effective reduction of gastric cancer risk with regular use of nonsteroidal anti-inflammatory drugs in Helicobacter pylori-infected patients. J Clin Oncol 28: 2952–2957.
15. Wu CY, Chen YJ, Ho HJ, Hsu YC, Kuo KN, et al. (2012) Association between nucleoside analogues and risk of hepatitis B virus-related hepatocellular carcinoma recurrence following liver resection. JAMA 308: 1906–1914.
16. Cheng CL, Kao YH, Lin SJ, Lee CH, Lai ML (2011) Validation of the National Health Insurance Research Database with ischemic stroke cases in Taiwan. Pharmacoepidemiol Drug Saf 20: 236–242.
17. Chen JJ, Lin LY, Lee CH, Liau CS (2012) Age, male gender, and atrial fibrillation predict lower extremity amputation or revascularization in patients with peripheral artery diseases: a population-based investigation. Int J Angiol 21: 35–40.
18. Ballantyne CM, Raichlen JS, Nicholls SJ, Erbel R, Tardif JC, et al. (2008) Effect of rosuvastatin therapy on coronary artery stenoses assessed by quantitative coronary angiography: a study to evaluate the effect of rosuvastatin on intravascular ultrasound-derived coronary atheroma burden. Circulation 117: 2458–2466.
19. Nissen SE, Nicholls SJ, Wolski K, Nesto R, Kupfer S, et al. (2008) Comparison of pioglitazone vs glimepiride on progression of coronary atherosclerosis in patients with type 2 diabetes: the PERISCOPE randomized controlled trial. Jama 299: 1561–1573.
20. Hirohata A, Yamamoto K, Miyoshi T, Hatanaka K, Hirohata S, et al. (2010) Impact of olmesartan on progression of coronary atherosclerosis a serial volumetric intravascular ultrasound analysis from the OLIVUS (impact of OLmesarten on progression of coronary atherosclerosis: evaluation by intravascular ultrasound) trial. J Am Coll Cardiol 55: 976–982.
21. D'Ascenzo F, Agostoni P, Abbate A, Castagno D, Lipinski MJ, et al. (2013) Atherosclerotic coronary plaque regression and the risk of adverse cardiovascular events: a meta-regression of randomized clinical trials. Atherosclerosis 226: 178–185.
22. Kinlay S (2013) Outcomes for clinical studies assessing drug and revascularization therapies for claudication and critical limb ischemia in peripheral artery disease. Circulation 127: 1241–1250.
23. Harris JP, Page S, Englund R, May J (1988) Is the outlook for the vascular amputee improved by striving to preserve the knee? J Cardiovasc Surg (Torino) 29: 741–745.
24. Menke J, Luthje L, Kastrup A, Larsen J (2010) Thromboembolism in atrial fibrillation. Am J Cardiol 105: 502–510.
25. Ouriel K, Veith FJ, Sasahara AA (1998) A comparison of recombinant urokinase with vascular surgery as initial treatment for acute arterial occlusion of the legs. Thrombolysis or Peripheral Arterial Surgery (TOPAS) Investigators. N Engl J Med 338: 1105–1111.
26. Ouriel K, Veith FJ (1998) Acute lower limb ischemia: determinants of outcome. Surgery 124: 336–341; discussion 341–332.
27. Abou-Zamzam AM, Jr., Teruya TH, Killeen JD, Ballard JL (2003) Major lower extremity amputation in an academic vascular center. Ann Vasc Surg 17: 86–90.
28. Kontos MC, Wang Y, Chaudhry SI, Vetrovec GW, Curtis J, et al. (2013) Lower Hospital Volume Is Associated With Higher In-Hospital Mortality in Patients Undergoing Primary Percutaneous Coronary Intervention for ST-Segment-Elevation Myocardial Infarction: A Report From the NCDR. Circ Cardiovasc Qual Outcomes 6: 659–667.
29. Wang HE, Shapiro NI, Griffin R, Safford MM, Judd S, et al. (2012) Chronic medical conditions and risk of sepsis. PLoS One 7: e48307.
30. Westendorp WF, Nederkoorn PJ, Vermeij JD, Dijkgraaf MG, van de Beek D (2011) Post-stroke infection: a systematic review and meta-analysis. BMC Neurol 11: 110.
31. Jain A, Liu K, Ferrucci L, Criqui MH, Tian L, et al. (2013) Declining walking impairment questionnaire scores are associated with subsequent increased mortality in peripheral artery disease. J Am Coll Cardiol 61: 1820–1829.
32. Titsworth WL, Hester J, Correia T, Reed R, Guin P, et al. (2012) The effect of increased mobility on morbidity in the neurointensive care unit. J Neurosurg 116: 1379–1388.

Multidisciplinary Predialysis Education Reduced the Inpatient and Total Medical Costs of the First 6 Months of Dialysis in Incident Hemodialysis Patients

Yu-Jen Yu[1,2], I-Wen Wu[1,2], Chun-Yu Huang[3], Kuang-Hung Hsu[3], Chin-Chan Lee[1,2], Chio-Yin Sun[1,2], Heng-Jung Hsu[1,2], Mai-Szu Wu[1,4,5]*

1 Department of Nephrology, Chang Gung Memorial Hospital, Keelung, Taiwan, **2** College of Medicine, Chang Gung University, Tao-Yuan, Taiwan, **3** Laboratory for Epidemiology, Department of Health Care Management, Chang Gung University, Tao-Yuan, Taiwan, **4** Division of Nephrology, Taipei Medical University Hospital, Taipei, Taiwan, **5** School of Medicine, Taipei Medical University, Taipei, Taiwan

Abstract

Background: The multidisciplinary pre-dialysis education (MPE) retards renal progression, reduce incidence of dialysis and mortality of CKD patients. However, the financial benefit of this intervention on patients starting hemodialysis has not yet been evaluated in prospective and randomized trial.

Methods: We studied the medical expenditure and utilization incurred in the first 6 months of dialysis initiation in 425 incident hemodialysis patients who were randomized into MPE and non-MPE groups before reaching end-stage renal disease. The content of the MPE was standardized in accordance with the National Kidney Foundation Dialysis Outcomes Quality Initiative guidelines.

Results: The mean age of study patients was 63.8±13.2 years, and 221 (49.7%) of them were men. The mean serum creatinine level and estimated glomerular filtration rate was 6.1±4.0 mg/dL and 7.6±2.9 mL·min^{-1}·1.73 m^{-2}, respectively, at dialysis initiation. MPE patients tended to have lower total medical cost in the first 6 months after hemodialysis initiation (9147.6±0.1 USD/patient vs. 11190.6±0.1 USD/patient, p = 0.003), fewer in numbers [0 (1) vs. 1 (2), p<0.001] and length of hospitalization [0 (15) vs. 8 (27) days, p<0.001], and also lower inpatient cost [0 (2617.4) vs. 1559,4 (5019.6) USD/patient, p< 0.001] than non-MPE patients, principally owing to reduced cardiovascular hospitalization and vascular access–related surgeries. The decreased inpatient and total medical cost associated with MPE were independent of patients' demographic characteristics, concomitant disease, baseline biochemistry and use of double-lumen catheter at initiation of hemodialysis.

Conclusions: Participation of multidisciplinary education in pre-dialysis period was independently associated with reduction in the inpatient and total medical expenditures of the first 6 months post-dialysis owing to decreased inpatient service utilization secondary to cardiovascular causes and vascular access–related surgeries.

Editor: Emmanuel A. Burdmann, University of Sao Paulo Medical School, Brazil

Funding: Chang Gung Memorial Hospital at Keelung provided grant support for this research (CMRPG260323/CMRPG2A0422). The funder had no role in study design, data collection and analysis, decision to publish, or preparation of the manuscript.

Competing Interests: The authors have declared that no competing interests exist.

* Email: maiszuwu@gmail.com

These authors contributed equally to this work.

Introduction

The number of patients worldwide with chronic kidney disease (CKD) and end-stage renal disease (ESRD) being treated with renal replacement therapy has been continuously increasing in recent years, with a 7% rate of increase per year [1]. Aging and type 2 diabetes mellitus are the two most important factors [2]. Taiwan is the leading country in terms of ESRD prevalence, with a rate of 2447 per million population [3]. The implementation of National Health Insurance (NHI) has helped drive the growth of the ESRD populations in Taiwan [4]. However, the official prohibition of the use of aristolochic acid–containing herbs and the introduction of the nationwide CKD Preventive Project with a multidisciplinary care program have proved their effectiveness in decreasing the incidence of dialysis, and mortality and medical costs of CKD patients [5]. However, the financial benefit of this intervention has not yet been evaluated in prospective and randomized manner on patients starting hemodialysis.

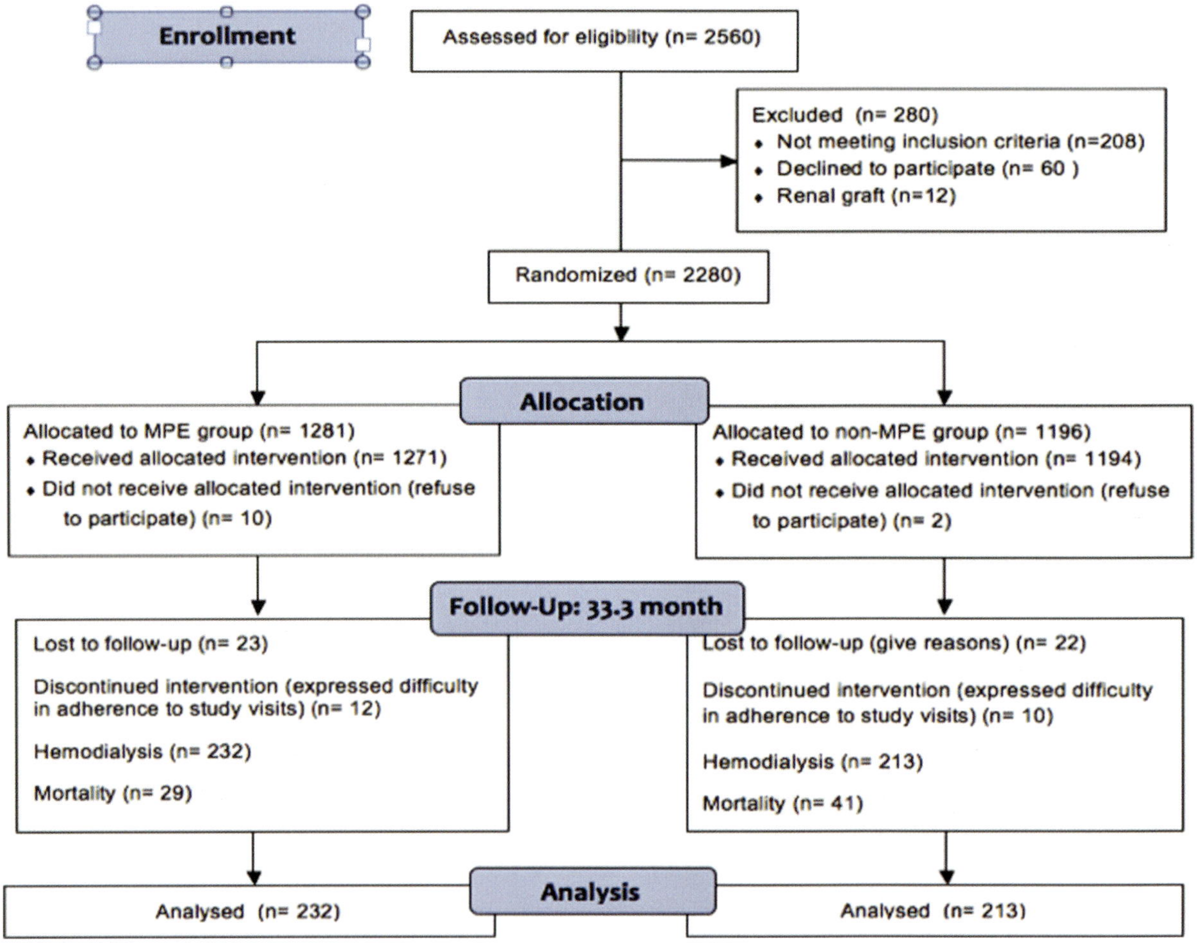

Figure 1. Enrolment scheme and patient status. MPE: multidisciplinary predialysis education.

High ESRD prevalence constitutes a large economic burden for the patient, society, and the country. Renal insufficiency represents a status of increased cardiovascular disease risk, comorbidities, and mortality [6], demanding high medical expenditures and health-care utilization [1]. The cost for ESRD has increased to $34.3 billion, accounting for 6.3% of the total Medicare budget according to the 2013 US Renal Data System Annual Data Report [7]. Similarly, in Taiwan, the annual dialysis costs have accounted for 5.0–7.52% of the total budget of the NHI in recent years [8]. Optimal and efficient treatment strategies to combat the high prevalence of ESRD and its high cost of care are thus urgently needed.

Predialysis education can decrease the ESRD incidence and mortality in the first year of dialysis [9,10]. Nephrology-based care has also significantly improved the clinical outcomes of CKD patients in both the predialysis and postdialysis periods [11,12], especially in type 2 diabetes patients [13,14]. It has been associated with better biochemical variables, shorter hospitalization length, a higher percentage of elective construction of the arteriovenous fistula, and the availability of alternative dialysis modality [15]. Our previous controlled cohort study has confirmed that multidisciplinary predialysis education (MPE) based on the National Kidney Foundation Dialysis Outcomes Quality Initiative (NKF/DOQI) guidelines provides a better outcome with a significantly reduced incidence of ESRD and all-cause mortality [16]. The MPE program has effectively improved the quality of pre-ESRD care, increased patients' self-care ability, and has retarded renal progression and reduced morbidities in late-stage CKD patients [17]. Multidisciplinary predialysis team care was found to decreased service utilization and saved medical costs in the 6 months before dialysis initiation and at dialysis initiation, being secondary to the early preparation of vascular access and the lack of hospitalization at dialysis initiation [18]. Predialysis nephrology–based care has been associated with reduced costs in elderly patients after the initiation of dialysis [19]. Most of these controlled or randomized trials have used the renal or patient outcome as their endpoints. However, randomized studies to evaluate the cost-saving effect of MPE in the post-dialysis period have been seldom reported to date.

Most of the medical costs associated with caring for CKD patients are incurred for the treatment of comorbidities, hospitalization, and transition into ESRD [20]. After dialysis initiation, most of the adverse outcomes occurred within the first year of hemodialysis. The all-cause mortality and mortality due to cardiovascular disease or other causes is found to peaked in the second month after initiation, and then decreased [20]. It is unclear whether the MPE program could extend the financial benefit to after the initiation of dialysis and reduces the medical costs during the first 6 months of hemodialysis initiation. We hypothesize that knowledge acquisition from MPE in the predialysis period may have a "legacy effect" during the postdialysis period. This beneficial effect of MPE may result in differences in disease patterns, reduced medical expenditure and utilization, and reduced medical costs in the immediate post-dialysis period. To further clarify this issue, we studied the medical expenditure and utilization incurred during the first 6 months of dialysis initiation in 425 incident hemodialysis patients who were randomized into MPE and non-MPE groups before reaching ESRD.

Materials and Methods

Patient cohort and settings The protocol for this trial and supporting CONSORT checklist are available as supporting information; see Checklist S1 and Protocol S1. This is an analysis of a subset population from our previously reported randomized cohort (Clinical Trials.gov NCT00644046) [16]. Briefly, the cohort includes predialysis CKD patients with an estimated glomerular filtration rate (eGFR) of <60 mL·min^{-1}·1.73 m^{-2} (determined by using the Modification of Diet in Renal Disease equation) who visited the nephrology outpatient clinics of the Department of Nephrology, Chang Gung Memorial Hospital, Keelung, from July 2007 and followed up to June 30, 2011. Patients aged 18–80 years and without renal graft failure were included in the study after obtaining informed consent from them. A total of 2280 patients were enrolled in the study and were randomly divided into the MPE group and the non-MPE group by using a random table at study entry. Four hundred and five patients reached ESRD needing hemodialysis after a mean follow-up of 33±2.6 months (232 patients in the MPE group and 213 patients in the non-MPE group, as shown in Figure 1). The medical expenditure and utilization in the first 6 months of initiation of hemodialysis in these 425 patients were accurately recorded and compared between MPE and non-MPE patients. Medical service utilization was calculated as the frequency of outpatient visits and the frequency and length of hospitalization. Outpatient visits were categorized as outpatient services, preventive care (e.g., influenza vaccination and dietary counseling), and emergency services. Medical service expenditures included outpatient expenditures (all costs including physicians' and nursing fees, examinations, surgery, and medication) and inpatient expenditures (all costs including laboratory testing, imaging testing, medications, surgery and consulting, ward and administrative, nasogastric tube feeding, and hemodialysis fees). The expenditures for each participant were totaled to compute the sum of ambulatory and inpatient medical service utilization costs and expenditures. The analysis of costs in this study only included those medical costs for which our hospitals made reimbursement claims to the NHI. The salaries, overheads, and administrative costs of the care team were not included. This study was approved by the ethics committee of

Table 1. baseline characteristics of study patients.

Parameter	MPE group (n = 232)	Non-MPE group (n = 213)	p
Age, years	67.5±11.4	61.8±15.0	<0.001
Male, n (%)	116 (50.0%)	105 (49.3%)	0.882
Diabetes, n (%)	153 (65.9%)	127 (59.6%)	0.168
Hypertension, n (%)	202 (87.1%)	171 (80.3%)	0.052
Coronary artery disease, n (%)	30 (12.9%)	41 (19.2%)	0.069
Cerebrovascular disease, n (%)	30 (12.9%)	29 (13.6%)	0.832
Gout, n (%)	61 (26.3%)	44 (20.7%)	0.162
eGFR, ml/min	7.49±3.1	7.87±3.6	0.228
Serum albumin, mg/dL	3.1±0.7	3.2±0.8	0.062
Hemoglobin, g/dL	9.4±1.6	9.0±2.7	0.100
Urea reduction rate, %	0.74±0.7	0.76±0.8	0.464
Kt/V, Daugirdas	1.66±0.36	1.71±0.38	0.509
nPCR, g/Kg/day	1.13±0.37	1.20±0.32	0.371
Systolic blood pressure, mmHg	144.3±22.7	147.2±25.9	0.221
Primary renal disease			0.135
Diabetes, n (%)	139 (59.9%)	118 (55.4%)	
Hypertension, n (%)	6 (2.6%)	5 (2.3%)	
Chronic glomerulonephritis, n %	16 (6.9%)	13 (6.1%)	
Others, n %	71 (30.6%)	77 (36.2%)	
Education levels			0.650
Below elementary	42 (18.1%)	3 (1.4%)	
Elementary	151 (65.1%)	207 (97.2%)	
High school	31 (13.4%)	3 (1.4%)	
University	8 (3.4%)	0 (0%)	
Vascular access at initiation of dialysis			
Patients with vascular access created, n (%)	143 (61.6%)	100 (46.9%)	0.002
Patients without insertion of double-lumen catheter, n (%)	129 (55.6%)	96 (45.1%)	0.029

Abbreviation: eGFR, estimated glomerular filtration rate; nPCR, normalized protein catabolic rate.

the institutional review board of Chang Gung Memorial Hospital (Number: 100-0040A3, 96-0408B) and was conducted according to the principles expressed in the Declaration of Helsinki. All patients provided written informed consent. The registration of our cohort at Clinical Trials.gov was delayed by administrative issues (set up of Core Lab, employment of research assistance). The authors confirm that all ongoing and related trials for this drug/intervention were registered.

MPE

The MPE program was implemented in May 2006 at the Keelung Center. The team comprised a nurse for case management, social workers, dietitians, hemodialysis, peritoneal dialysis patient volunteers and 10 nephrologists. The program consisted of an integrated course involving individual lectures on renal health, delivered by the case-management nurse, according to the guidelines given in a standardized instruction booklet. The lectures focused on nutrition, lifestyle, nephrotoxin avoidance, dietary principles, and pharmacological regimens. Furthermore, the case-management nurse contacted the patients to ensure timely follow-up. Standardized interactive educational sessions were periodically conducted wherein all patients were interviewed depending on their CKD stage, determined earlier by using the NKF/DOQI guideline. Stage III or IV CKD patients were followed up every 3 months, and stage V CKD patients were followed up on a monthly basis. For stage III CKD patients, the program consisted of lectures on healthy renal function, the clinical presentation of uremia, risk factors and complications associated with renal progression, and an introduction to the various renal replacement therapies (i.e., hemodialysis, peritoneal dialysis, and renal transplantation). For stage IV CKD patients, the program included discussions on the management of complications associated with CKD, indications of renal replacement therapy, and the evaluation of vascular or peritoneal access. Patients with stage V CKD were monitored for timely initiation of renal replacement therapies, the care of vascular or peritoneal access, dialysis-associated complications, and registration for inclusion in the renal transplantation waiting list. All patients received dietary counseling biannually from a dietitian. In addition, the case-management nurse often contacted the participants by telephone to encourage them to inform their nephrologists of their symptoms and to reinforce the importance of medical visits. The MPE program was discontinued once renal replacement therapies were initiated for these patients.

Customary care

The same group of nephrologists instructed all participants about renal function, the evaluation of laboratory data, and clinical indicators of chronic renal failure, as well as about the strategies for its management and treatment. Furthermore, the nephrologists explained the general principles of hemodialysis and peritoneal dialysis when the patients exhibited an eGFR of $< 30\ mL{\cdot}min^{-1}{\cdot}1.73\ m^{-2}$ (stage IV CKD). All patients were provided with written instructions. The nephrologists evaluated the comorbidity factors influencing each patient's condition before referral to a nurse specializing in hemodialysis or peritoneal dialysis. The nursing staff provided instructions for daily living and explained the criteria used for hemodialysis and peritoneal dialysis selection, and the difference between the two modalities.

Statistical analysis

Descriptive statistics were expressed as the mean (standard deviation) or median (interquartile range). Discrete variables were presented in terms of frequencies and percentages. The normality of numerical variables was tested using the Kolmogorov-Smirnov method, and an appropriate transformation was considered before statistical testing. The Student t-test or Mann-Whitney U-test was applied to compare mean or median values among the groups. The association between categorical variables was analyzed by using the χ^2 test. Multiple linear regression analysis was applied to calculate the unstandardized coefficients associated with MPE in both inpatient and total medical cost. All statistical tests were two-tailed, and a p value <0.05 was considered to be statistically significant. Data were analyzed by using SPSS 17.0 for Windows XP (SPSS Inc., Chicago, IL, USA).

Results

The mean age of study patients was 63.8±13.2 years, and 221 (49.7%) of them were men. The mean serum creatinine level and eGFR was 6.1±4.0 mg/dL and $7.6{\pm}mL{\cdot}min^{-1}{\cdot}1.73\ m^{-2}$, respectively, at dialysis initiation. Diabetes mellitus was identified as the leading cause of renal disease in both groups, followed by chronic glomerulonephritis. Table 1 shows the demographic and clinical characteristics of the patients in the MPE and non-MPE

Table 2. Medical utilization and expenditure between groups.

Parameter	MPE group (n = 232)	Non-MPE group (n = 213)	p
No. outpatient visits, times/patient	15.1±11.6	17.9±11.1	0.009
No. of hospitalization, times/patient	0.00 (1.00)	1.00 (2.00)	<0.001*
Frequency of hospitalization, n (%)			<0.001
Never	144 (62.1%)	86 (40.4%)	
1 time	47 (20.2%)	73 (34.2%)	
2 times	31 (13.4%)	30 (14.1%)	
≥3 times	10 (4.3%)	24 (11.3%)	
Length of hospitalization, days/patient	0.00 (15.00)	8.00 (27.00)	<0.001*
Cost of outpatient service, mean, USD/patient	6885.7±5201.2	7491.8±4200.2	0.175
Log cost of inpatient service, mean, USD/patient	3.09±4.02	4.95±4.15	<0.001
Log total cost of medical service, mean, USD/patient	6.75±4.21	8.58±2.43	<0.001

*p value using Mann-Whitney U test.

Table 3. Costs of outpatient service between groups.

Variables	MPE group (n = 232)	Non-MPE group (n = 213)	p
Hemodialysis, laboratory and imagen	6258.8±4647.2	6841.5±3883.1	0.154
Physician fee	94.4±80.1	116.9±93.4	0.007
Medication fee	512.6±120.1	510.8±75.4	0.985
Pharmacist, nursing and administrative fee	19.9±16.4	22.5±17.4	0.107

Costs were expressed in mean ± SD, USD/patient.

groups at the initiation of hemodialysis. These patients received 4 hours of hemodialysis 3 times weekly. Hemodialysis for these patients used single-use hollow-fiber dialyzers equipped with modified cellulose-based, polyamide, or polysulfone membranes. The dialysate used in all patients was a standard ionic composition and bicarbonate-based buffer. Many indices of dialysis adequacy (Urea reduction rate, Kt/V and normalized protein catabolic rate) were similar at baseline for the two groups of patients. However, the MPE group patients were more likely to have permanent vascular access created (61.6% vs. 46.9%, p = 0.002) and less insertion of double-lumen catheter at initiation of hemodialysis (55.6% vs. 45.1%, p = 0.029, Table 1).

MPE patients tended to have lower total medical cost in the first 6 months after hemodialysis initiation (9147.6±0.1 USD/patient vs. 11190.6±0.1 USD/patient, p = 0.003, Table 2). Despite the fewer outpatient visits of MPE patients, the cost of outpatient service did not differ between the groups. Most of the costs of outpatient service were spent for treatment (including hemodialysis, laboratory, and image study; Table 3). However, MPE patients were significantly fewer in numbers [mean (SD) 0.61±0.9 vs. 1.0±1.2, p<0.001; median (IQR) 0 (1) vs. 1 (2), p<0.001] and had shorter lengths [mean (SD) 10.6±21.9 days vs. 19.3±29.3 days, p<0.001; median (IQR) 0 (15) vs. 8 (27) days, p<0.001] of hospitalization than non-MPE patients. Therefore, the medical cost of inpatient service was significantly lower in MPE patients [median 0 (2617.4) or (mean 2261.8±5635.8) USD/patient in MPE patients vs. median 1559, 4 (5019.6) or (mean 3698.8±5540.9) USD/patient in non-MPE patients, respectively, p<0.001, Table 2]. The reduced cost of inpatient service observed in MPE patients was attributed to the reduction in the costs of physicians, wards, nasogastric feeding, radiology examination, nursing, blood transfusion, hemodialysis, medication, and pharmacist service fees. Most of the costs of inpatient service were spent on hemodialysis treatment in both groups of patients (Table 4). Eighty-eight (37.9%) patients in the MPE group had at least one hospitalization, compared with 127 patients (59.6%) in the non-MPE group (p<0.001). In all first hospitalizations, 66 (75%) patients in the MPE group were admitted to the nephrology ward. Similarly, 94 (74%) of the non-MPE patients were admitted to the nephrology ward at their first hospitalization. Table 5 lists the main causes of the first hospitalization and surgery in both groups of patients. Cardiovascular disease (including uncontrolled hypertension, coronary artery disease, stroke, heart failure, and peripheral artery occlusive disease) was the main cause of first hospitalization in all patients. Participation in the MPE program reduced cardiovascular hospitalization during the first 6 months postdialysis (18.53% vs. 29.58%, p = 0.007). Among all patients, those in the MPE group were more likely to have fewer vascular access related surgeries during the first admission [35 patients (15.09%) vs. 55 (25.82%), p = 0.005]. Most first surgeries were performed for Hickman catheter–related intervention (implantation, exchange, and removal) and arteriovenous fistula/graft–related intervention (creation, thrombectomy, repair, and excision; Table 5).

Participation in MPE was independently associated with reduced inpatient cost and total medical cost in the first 6 months of dialysis initiation by using various adjustment strategies, including demographic characteristics (age and gender) in model 2, concomitant disease (diabetes mellitus and number of comorbidities) in model 3, baseline biochemistry at entry to hemodialysis

Table 4. Log-transformed costs of inpatient service between groups.

Variables	MPE group (n = 232)	Non-MPE group (n = 213)	p*
Physician fee	2.03±2.67	3.28±2.79	<0.001
Ward fee	2.49±3.26	3.99±3.38	<0.001
Laboratory examination fee	5.22±1.32	5.52±1.15	0.126
Nasogastric tube feeding fee	0.56±1.61	1.40±2.36	<0.001
Radiology examination fee	1.17±2.05	1.84±2.29	<0.001
Nursing fee	1.78±2.69	2.83±2.91	<0.001
Surgery fee	1.89±3.82	3.31±4.58	<0.001
Blood transfusion fee	1.04±1.93	1.89±2.39	<0.001
Hemodialysis fee	2.65±3.46	4.13±3.58	<0.001
Medication fee	2.16±2.94	3.45±3.08	<0.001
Pharmacist service fee	1.48±1.98	2.32±2.04	<0.001

Costs were expressed in mean ± SD, USD/patient.

Table 5. Main cause of first hospitalization and surgery.

	MPE group	Non-MPE group
Cause of first hospitalization, n		
Renal-related disease	12 (5.17%)	26 (12.21%)
Cardiovascular disease	43 (18.53%)	63 (29.58%)
Vascular access infection	9 (3.88%)	11 (5.16%)
Acute pulmonary edema	3 (1.29%)	4 (1.88%)
Other	21 (9.05%)	23 (10.8%)
No hospitalization	144 (62.07%)	86 (40.38%)
Cause of first surgery, n		
Hickman catheter related	25 (10.78%)	36 (16.9%)
Arteriovenous fistula/graft related	24 (10.34%)	39 (18.31%)
Limb amputation	2 (0.86%)	3 (1.41%)
Hemothorax/pneumothorax	1 (0.43%)	6 (2.82%)
Other	15 (6.47%)	4 (1.88%)
No surgery	165 (71.12%)	125 (58.69%)

Cardiovascular disease includes uncontrolled hypertension, coronary artery disease, stroke, heart failure, and peripheral artery occlusive disease.

(eGFR, hemoglobin, and serum albumin levels) in model 4 and status of use of double-lumen catheter at initiation of hemodialysis (model 5, Table 6).

Discussion

In this prospective study, we examined the medical expenditure and utilization incurred in the first 6 months of dialysis initiation in 425 incident hemodialysis patients who were randomized into MPE and non-MPE groups before reaching ESRD. We found that participation in a multidisciplinary education program at the predialysis period was associated with reduced inpatient service utilization, reduced inpatient cost, and reduced total medical cost in the first 6 months of hemodialysis. The reduction of cost in inpatient service was attributed to the reduction in cardiovascular disease and vascular access–related surgery during hospitalization. The decreased inpatient cost and total medical cost of service associated with MPE were independent of patients' demographic characteristics, concomitant disease, baseline biochemistry at entry to hemodialysis and use of double-lumen catheter at initiation of hemodialysis. The findings of the present study provide evidence supporting the implementation of MPE as part of integrative CKD care to combat the high economic burden and financial impact of hemodialysis on patients.

A previous prospective controlled study demonstrated that MPE based on the NKF/DOQI guidelines effectively reduced the incidence of ESRD and all-cause mortality with a significantly reduced overall hospitalization rate among MPE patients [16]. In our study, the delivery of MPE was stopped once the patient started hemodialysis therapy. After the initiation of hemodialysis, all patients received dietary counseling in the hemodialysis room on a monthly basis. On the basis of these assumptions, knowledge acquisition from a multidisciplinary education program in the predialysis period might be one of the factors that influence the disease pattern and health-care utilization in the postdialysis period. The positive effect of MPE in the postdialysis period could be the result of many factors, such as increased knowledge about self-care [17], better diet and fluid control, medication compliance, better preparation of vascular access, the adoption of a healthier lifestyle, and greater awareness about the use of

Table 6. Multiple linear regression analysis of effect of MPE on inpatient and total medical cost.

	Inpatient cost		Total cost	
	Unstandardized Coefficients	p	Unstandardized Coefficients	p
Model 1	−43109.74	0.007	−61289.80	0.003
Model 2	−46226.19	0.005	−60200.11	0.005
Model 3	−44575.46	0.005	−62959.92	0.003
Model 4	−44447.13	0.001	−54490.22	0.013
Model 5	−33826.85	0.029	−52241.43	0.011

Both of the two dependent variables in these models were the log transformation of inpatient costs and total costs.
Model 1: crude.
Model 2: adjusted for age and gender.
Model 3: adjusted for diabetes status and number of comorbidities.
Model 4: adjusted for eGFR, hemoglobin and serum albumin levels at initation of hemodialysis.
Model 5: adjusted for insertion of double-lumen catheter at initiation of hemodialysis.

nephrotoxin. The transition period into ESRD and the first year of dialysis therapy represented the most vulnerable point that demands the highest health-care expenditure and utility in CKD patients [20]. The cost-saving effect of MPE in terms of inpatient and total medical service in this immediate postdialysis period was confirmed by the regression models with the adjustment of different covariates. The total medical cost of the first 6 months of hemodialysis in MPE participants was 18% less than that of nonparticipants (9147.6 USD/patient vs. 11190.6 USD/patient). For a total of 8000 incident hemodialysis patients each year in Taiwan [3], the crude estimation of cost-saving could be up to 16.3 million USD per 6 months if each incident patient was to be provided with the MPE program before reaching ESRD.

MPE is certainly beneficial in lowering the enormous cost for the care of hemodialysis patients. Although the long-term economic impact of MPE has not been studied, the findings of the present study suggest the need for a universal and efficient delivery of multidisciplinary education to all CKD patients as early as possible.

Several studies have reported on the cost-saving effect of MPE in the hospitalization of CKD patients; however, only a few retrospective studies have addressed the financial benefits of MPE in the postdialysis period [18,19]. From this prospective study, we have found that hemodialysis and the diseases associated with this treatment (cardiovascular disease and noninfectious vascular access complication) were responsible for most of the health-care cost incurred in both inpatient and outpatient services (Tables 3 and 4). Taking into account the beneficial effect of MPE in reducing renal progression [17], the incidence of ESRD [16], and cardiovascular hospitalization and vascular access surgery in the postdialysis period in our study, the implementation of MPE could result in an overall reduction in the medical utilization and expenditure of CKD patients. Similarly, Wei et al., in their retrospective observational study, found that participants in the CKD care program had lower medical costs at dialysis initiation and lower medical cost for the total period of observation than nonparticipants because of the early preparation of vascular access and the lack of hospitalization at dialysis initiation [18]. A retrospective observational study described fewer hospital days and lower total health-care costs during the year after dialysis initiation in patients receiving predialysis nephrology care [19]. We have reported a reduction in the 1-year hospitalization rate (2.8% vs. 16.4%) in recipients of MPE in a controlled prospective cohort. However, the reason for hospitalization for these patients did not differ significantly between them [16]. In a 3-year prospective study, participation in multidisciplinary care was associated with a 40% reduction in the risk of infection-related hospitalization in the predialysis period [21]. A propensity score matched cohort study found that MPE participants had less unplanned urgent dialysis, shorter hospital days, and a lower incidence of cardiovascular events than non-MPE patients during the observation period [22]. A novel finding of our study was that patients with MPE had reduced cardiovascular-related hospitalization in their postdialysis period. This finding could possibly be attributed to better control of cardiovascular risk factors, better medical adherence, fluid control, and compliance with dietary restriction in the postdialysis period with a prior acquisition of renal knowledge.

Our study included a comprehensive analysis of medical service utilization and expenditures with detailed information about outpatient and inpatient costs in patients with comparable baseline characteristics derived from a randomized cohort. The delivery of MPE was standardized according to the NKF/DOQI guidelines. A single nurse conducted the MPE program for all patients to limit interpersonal variability. This single-center study has been conducted in a university-afflicted teaching hospital. All enrolled participants were patients who visited the nephrology outpatient clinics of Chang Gung Memorial Hospital at Keelung and underwent dialysis treatment at the hemodialysis unit of the same hospital. This hospital is a group practice institution comprised 10 nephrologists and only one hemodialysis unit. Furthermore, variation within dialysis units did not exist, because the single hemodialysis unit setting. In this group practice setting, all nephrologists followed the same institutional regulation. All nephrologists were subject to the same criteria of reimbursement under a single NHI system of government of Taiwan. These 10 nephrologists took care of all renal patients at outpatient and inpatient departments. The same group of 10 nephrologists instructed the MPE and non-MPE patients at their predialysis education and also continuous their medical care in the post-dialysis period at our hemodialysis unit. For these reasons, confounding effects by practice pattern of individual nephrologists might be neglected. Despite the several advantages of MPE presented in our investigation, several limitations should be addressed. First, the study represented a secondary cost analysis of a subset of patients who started hemodialysis and were randomized into MPE and non-MPE groups before reaching ESRD. Second, patients who had died before reaching ESRD were excluded. It was unclear how MPE could influence the postdialysis health-care expenditure and utility costs of these critically ill patients. Third, the age of patients in the two groups was not comparable at the baseline. However, despite the older age of the MPE patients, the outcome of interest was consistently better than that of the non-MPE patients. In addition, the adjustment for age in the regression model has indicated no significance of this factor in our outcome. Finally, although this study examined the economic impact of MPE for the first 6 months of dialysis, its long-term effect remains unclear. Further investigations with a large-scale population, including other treatment modalities (peritoneal dialysis or renal transplantation) and a longer duration would be needed to demonstrate the cost benefit of MPE for an extended period.

In conclusion, in this prospective study, we demonstrated the lowered inpatient and total medical costs in the first 6 months postdialysis in patients receiving the MPE program. This cost reduction was attributed to decreased inpatient service utilization, and principally concerning services used because of cardiovascular causes and vascular access–related surgeries. This reduction in cost was independent of the patients' demographic characteristics, concomitant disease, baseline biochemistry and status of use of double-lumen catheter at entry to hemodialysis. This valuable information confirmed the legacy effect of the MPE program on the economic outcome in the postdialysis period. Although the optimal dose and duration of MPE remains debated, an efficient and universal delivery of multidisciplinary education should be considered as part of the integrative care of CKD patients. This simple strategy could be an ideal resolution to the problem of the increasing financial burden of renal failure worldwide.

Author Contributions

Conceived and designed the experiments: YJU IWW MSW. Performed the experiments: YJU IWW. Analyzed the data: IWW CYH KHH. Contributed reagents/materials/analysis tools: YJU IWW CCL CYS HJH. Wrote the paper: YJU IWW.

References

1. Lysaght MJ (2002) Maintenance dialysis population dynamics: current trends and long-term implications. J Am Soc Nephrol 13 Suppl 1: S37–40.
2. Meguid El Nahas A, Bello AK (2005) Chronic kidney disease: the global challenge. Lancet 365: 331–340.
3. Wu MS, Wu IW, Shih CP, Hsu KH (2011) Establishing a platform for battling end-stage renal disease and continuing quality improvement in dialysis therapy in Taiwan - Taiwan Renal Registry Data System (TWRDS). Acta Nephrologica 25: 148–153.
4. Yang WC, Hwang SJ, Taiwan Society of Nephrology (2008) Incidence, prevalence and mortality trends of dialysis end-stage renal disease in Taiwan from 1990 to 2001: the impact of national health insurance. Nephrol Dial Transplant 23: 3977–3982.
5. Hwang SJ, Tsai JC, Chen HC (2010) Epidemiology, impact and preventive care of chronic kidney disease in Taiwan. Nephrology (Carlton) 15 Suppl 2: 3–9.
6. Muntner P, He J, Hamm L, Loria C, Whelton PK (2002) Renal insufficiency and subsequent death resulting from cardiovascular disease in the United States. J Am Soc Nephrol 13: 745–753.
7. Collins AJ, Foley RN, Chavers B, Gilbertson D, Herzog C, et al. (2014) US Renal Data System 2013 Annual Data Report. Am J Kidney Dis 63: A7.
8. Department of Health. National Health Insurance Annual Statistical Report 2012. Taiwan: Department of Health, 2014. Available: http://www.nhi.gov.tw. Accessed 2014 September 2.
9. Goldstein M, Yassa T, Dacouris N, McFarlane P (2004) Multidisciplinary predialysis care and morbidity and mortality of patients on dialysis. Am J Kidney Dis 44: 706–714.
10. Devins GM, Mendelssohn DC, Barre PE, Taub K, Binik YM (2005) Predialysis psychoeducational intervention extends survival in CKD: a 20-year follow-up. Am J Kidney Dis 46: 1088–1098.
11. Bradbury BD, Fissell RB, Albert JM, Anthony MS, Critchlow CW, et al. (2007) Predictors of early mortality among incident US hemodialysis patients in the Dialysis Outcomes and Practice Patterns Study (DOPPS). Clin J Am Soc Nephrol 2: 89–99.
12. Jungers P, Massy ZA, Nguyen-Khoa T, Choukroun G, Robino C, et al. (2001) Longer duration of predialysis nephrological care is associated with improved long-term survival of dialysis patients. Nephrol Dial Transplant 16: 2357–2364.
13. Wu MS, Lin CL, Chang CT, Wu CH, Huang JY, et al. (2003) Improvement in clinical outcome by early nephrology referral in type II diabetics on maintenance peritoneal dialysis. Perit Dial Int 23: 39–45.
14. Tseng CL, Kern EF, Miller DR, Tiwari A, Maney M, et al. (2008) Survival benefit of nephrologic care in patients with diabetes mellitus and chronic kidney disease. Arch Intern Med 168: 55–62.
15. Dogan E, Erkoc R, Sayarlioglu H, Durmus A, Topal C (2005) Effects of late referral to a nephrologist in patients with chronic renal failure. Nephrology (Carlton) 10: 516–519.
16. Wu IW, Wang SY, Hsu KH, Lee CC, Sun CY, et al. (2009) Multidisciplinary predialysis education decreases the incidence of dialysis and reduces mortality–a controlled cohort study based on the NKF/DOQI guidelines. Nephrol Dial Transplant 24: 3426–3433.
17. Chen SH, Tsai YF, Sun CY, Wu IW, Lee CC, et al. (2011) The impact of self-management support on the progression of chronic kidney disease–a prospective randomized controlled trial. Nephrol Dial Transplant 26: 3560–3566.
18. Wei SY, Chang YY, Mau LW, Lin MY, Chiu HC, et al. (2010) Chronic kidney disease care program improves quality of pre-end-stage renal disease care and reduces medical costs. Nephrology (Carlton) 15: 108–115.
19. Stroupe KT, Fischer MJ, Kaufman JS, O'Hare AM, Sohn MW, et al. (2011) Predialysis nephrology care and costs in elderly patients initiating dialysis. Med Care 49: 248–256.
20. U.S. Renal Data System, USRDS 2013. Annual Data Report: Atlas of Chronic Kidney Disease and End-Stage Renal Disease in the United States, National Institutes of Health, National Institute of Diabetes and Digestive and Kidney Diseases, Bethesda, MD, 2013.
21. Chen YR, Yang Y, Wang SC, Chiu PF, Chou WY, et al. (2013) Effectiveness of multidisciplinary care for chronic kidney disease in Taiwan: a 3-year prospective cohort study. Nephrol Dial Transplant 28: 671–682.
22. Cho EJ, Park HC, Yoon HB, Ju KD, Kim H, et al. (2012) Effect of multidisciplinary pre-dialysis education in advanced chronic kidney disease: Propensity score matched cohort analysis. Nephrology (Carlton) 17: 472–479.

Effect of Cholecalciferol Supplementation on Inflammation and Cellular Alloimmunity in Hemodialysis Patients

Lily Li[1,2], Marvin Lin[1,2], Maria Krassilnikova[1,2], Katya Ostrow[1,2], Amanda Bader[1,2], Brian Radbill[1,2], Jaime Uribarri[1,2], Joji Tokita[1,2], Staci Leisman[1,2], Vijay Lapsia[1,2], Randy A. Albrecht[5,6], Adolfo García-Sastre[2,5,6], Andrea D. Branch[2,7], Peter S. Heeger[1,2,3,4¶], Anita Mehrotra[1,2*¶]

1 Division of Nephrology, Icahn School of Medicine at Mount Sinai, New York, New York, United States of America, **2** Department of Medicine, Icahn School of Medicine at Mount Sinai, New York, New York, United States of America, **3** Recanati Miller Transplantation Institute, Icahn School of Medicine at Mount Sinai, New York, New York, United States of America, **4** Immunology Institute, Icahn School of Medicine at Mount Sinai, New York, New York, United States of America, **5** Department of Microbiology, Icahn School of Medicine at Mount Sinai, New York, New York, United States of America, **6** Global Health and Emerging Pathogens Institute, Icahn School of Medicine at Mount Sinai, New York, New York, United States of America, **7** Division of Liver Diseases, Icahn School of Medicine at Mount Sinai, New York, New York, United States of America

Abstract

Background: Memory T-cells are mediators of transplant injury, and no therapy is known to prevent the development of cross-reactive memory alloimmunity. Activated vitamin D is immunomodulatory, and vitamin D deficiency, common in hemodialysis patients awaiting transplantation, is associated with a heightened alloimmune response. Thus, we tested the hypothesis that vitamin D_3 supplementation would prevent alloreactive T-cell memory formation in vitamin D-deficient hemodialysis patients.

Methods and Findings: We performed a 12-month single-center pilot randomized, controlled trial of 50,000 IU/week of cholecalciferol (D_3) versus no supplementation in 96 hemodialysis patients with serum 25(OH)D$<$25 ng/mL, measuring effects on serum 25(OH)D and phenotypic and functional properties of T-cells. Participants were randomized 2:1 to active treatment versus control. D_3 supplementation increased serum 25(OH)D at 6 weeks (13.5 [11.2] ng/mL to 42.5 [18.5] ng/mL, $p<0.001$) and for the duration of the study. No episodes of sustained hypercalcemia occurred in either group. Results of IFNγ ELISPOT-based panel of reactive T-cell assays (PRT), quantifying alloreactive memory, demonstrated greater increases in the controls over 1 year compared to the treatment group (delta PRT in treatment 104.8+/−330.8 vs 252.9+/−431.3 in control), but these changes in PRT between groups did not reach statistical significance ($p = 0.25$).

Conclusions: D_3 supplements are safe, effective at treating vitamin D deficiency, and may prevent time-dependent increases in T-cell alloimmunity in hemodialysis patients, but their effects on alloimmunity need to be confirmed in larger studies. These findings support the routine supplementation of vitamin D-deficient transplant candidates on hemodialysis and highlight the need for large-scale prospective studies of vitamin D supplementation in transplant candidates and recipients.

Editor: Kathrin Eller, Medical University of Graz, Austria

Funding: This work was supported by grants from the Doris Duke Charitable Foundation (LL), National Kidney Foundation (PSH), American Heart Association (AM), and National Institute of Health: DK090317, DA0301095 (ADB), U01AI063594 (PSH), U19AI089987 (AG-S, RA), and UL1TR000067 from the National Center for Advancing Translational Sciences. The funders had no role in study design, data collection and analysis, decision to publish, or preparation of the manuscript.

Competing Interests: The authors have declared that no competing interests exist.

* Email: anita.mehrotra@mssm.edu

These authors contributed equally to this work.

¶ These authors are co-senior authors on this work.

Introduction

Alloreactive memory T-cells are pathogenic mediators of transplant injury. They are among the first cells to injure vascularized allografts in animal models [1], prevent tolerance induction in mice [2], and are associated with inferior transplant outcomes both in non-human primates and in human kidney transplant recipients [3–6].

Memory T-cells can be induced by direct exposure to alloantigens through transplantation, pregnancy, or blood transfusion. Evidence also indicates that heterologous (cross-reactive) immune responses initiated by environmental pathogens and homeostatic proliferation can facilitate the induction and expansion of alloreactive memory T-cells [7,8]. Interventions to reduce graft injury caused by T-cell memory are not yet available.

The biologically active form of vitamin D, 1,25-dihydroxyvitamin D [1,25(OH)$_2$D] has immune-modulatory properties. T-cells and dendritic cells (DCs), express the vitamin D receptor (VDR) and the 1α-hydroxylase needed to convert 25-hydroxyvitamin D [25(OH)D] to 1,25(OH)$_2$D [9]. 1,25(OH)$_2$D can directly modulate the function of T-cells and DCs through a variety of mechanisms [10–13], and can enhance tolerance induction in mice [14]. Importantly, many of the immune effects of vitamin D require local, immune cell production of 1,25(OH)$_2$D from its immediate precursor, 25(OH)D, which circulates in blood [9,15,16].

Vitamin D deficiency is widespread among the general population [17], and is prevalent in patients with end-stage renal disease (ESRD) on hemodialysis (HD). The concentration of 25(OH)D is the main clinical indicator of vitamin D status and is used to define vitamin D deficiency. According to the Institute of Medicine (IOM), there is an elevation in the risk of experiencing adverse health consequences of vitamin D deficiency at 25(OH)D levels <20 ng/mL [18]. Over 80% of HD patients have serum 25(OH)D concentrations within the insufficient/deficient range despite ongoing treatment with activated vitamin D [1,25(OH)$_2$D] for prevention of uremic bone disease [19,20]. While there have been uncontrolled studies of nutritional vitamin D (D$_2$ or D$_3$) supplementation in HD patients and one short-term (3 week) randomized, controlled trial of D$_3$ supplementation [20–23], the safety, efficacy, and *immunological* impact of nutritional vitamin D repletion in HD patients, particularly in patients already receiving 1,25(OH)$_2$D, has not been tested in controlled studies.

Observational studies of kidney transplant recipients show an association between 25(OH)D deficiency and inferior graft outcomes [24,25]. Our previously published data show a strong correlation between 25(OH)D deficiency and elevated memory T-cell alloimmunity in dialysis patients, many of whom are on the transplant waiting list, independent of known sensitizing events [19]. We hypothesized that inadequate concentrations of 25(OH)D contribute to the development of alloreactive memory T-cells by reducing the local synthesis of the 1,25(OH)$_2$D that is needed to achieve optimal levels in immune cells. To test this hypothesis and to obtain preliminary data for power calculations for a larger multi-center study, we performed a pilot, single-center, randomized, controlled trial (RCT) of oral cholecalciferol (D$_3$) (versus no supplementation) to assess the impact of increased 25(OH)D on memory T-cell alloimmunity, in patients already receiving 1,25(OH)$_2$D as clinically indicated. Our data indicate that D$_3$ supplementation is safe and effective at correcting vitamin D deficiency in this setting, and may prevent the time-dependent increase of peripheral cellular alloimmunity that occurs in many dialysis patients, establishing a strong rationale for conducting a larger, multi-center RCT to confirm these findings.

Methods

Clinical Trial Design

The protocol for this trial, sample case report form, and supporting CONSORT checklist are available as supporting information; see Protocol S1, Sample Case Report Form S1, and CONSORT Checklist S1. We recruited adults (≥18 years) on hemodialysis for ≥2 months at the Icahn School of Medicine at Mount Sinai (ISMMS) and Terrence Cardinal Cooke outpatient dialysis units in New York City from August 2010 to October 2011, excluding patients with a history of acute renal failure with potential for recovery, a history of HIV/AIDS, or inability to provide informed consent. All participants gave written informed consent, and the study was conducted according to the principles expressed in the Declaration of Helsinki. The study was approved by the Icahn School of Medicine at Mount Sinai (ISMMS) Institutional Review Board (IRB #09-2275) and registered at clinicaltrials.gov (NCT01175798).

Peripheral blood was obtained during the hemodialysis procedure. All study subjects were being dialyzed using biocompatible dialysis membranes. Serum 25(OH)D concentrations were determined commercially in a CLIA-certified laboratory (Nationwide Laboratories, Ft. Lauderdale, FL) by the chemiluminescent Diasorin method (www.diasorin.com, Stillwater, MN). Subjects with serum 25(OH)D<25 ng/mL were eligible for randomization. This cut-off for randomization was pre-determined based on previous data showing the distribution of vitamin D concentrations in the population [19].

The study was an open-label pilot RCT of nutritional Vitamin D- therapy (D$_3$: cholecalciferol, purchased from BioTech Pharmacal, Inc: http://www.biotechpharmacal.com/). Participants were randomized in a 2:1 ratio using Random Allocation Software (Version 1.0.0) [26] into one of two groups: oral cholecalciferol or no treatment (currently the standard of care at the dialysis units, as routine screening for and treatment of 25(OH)D deficiency are not part of practice guidelines for this population). Randomization was stratified by baseline 25(OH)D (10–24 ng/mL and <10 ng/mL). Within each stratum, randomization occurred in permuted 12-subject blocks. Implementation of randomization was performed by a study investigator.

Those participants randomized to D$_3$ had a target 25(OH)D concentration of >35 ng/ml. The initial dose of D$_3$ was 50,000/ week for 6 weeks, at which time 25(OH)D was re-measured. Subjects whose 25(OH)D remained ≤35 ng/ml continued on 50,000 IU weekly for another 6 weeks, at which point 25(OH)D concentrations were repeated. Those subjects who achieved 25(OH)D concentrations >35 ng/ml were transitioned to 10,000 IU/week. D$_3$ therapy was directly observed by a study coordinator or investigator. 25(OH)D was measured at baseline, 6 weeks, 3 months, and 6 months following randomization in both treatment and control groups, and other clinical information (routine labs, medication dosage) was collected at the same time-points.

The primary outcome was change in 25(OH)D at 6 weeks, 3 months, and 6 months. Secondary outcomes included change in clinical laboratory values (intact parathyroid hormone [PTH], serum calcium, and phosphorus), activated vitamin D requirements (mcg/treatment), and laboratory-based phenotypic and functional T-cell assays.

All study subjects continued to receive routine care at their hemodialysis unit including monthly laboratory testing of calcium, phosphorus, and intact parathyroid hormone. Dosing of hemodialysis-related intravenous medications (activated vitamin D analog) continued as per pre-specified, standardized protocols in the hemodialysis units. Nursing staff adjusting hemodialysis-related intravenous medications were blinded to treatment assignment. Study subjects undergoing kidney transplantation during the study period were not included in the final analysis (Figure 1).

Laboratory Procedures

Peripheral blood was collected during the hemodialysis procedure into BD Vacutainer tubes (BD, Franklin Lakes, NJ)

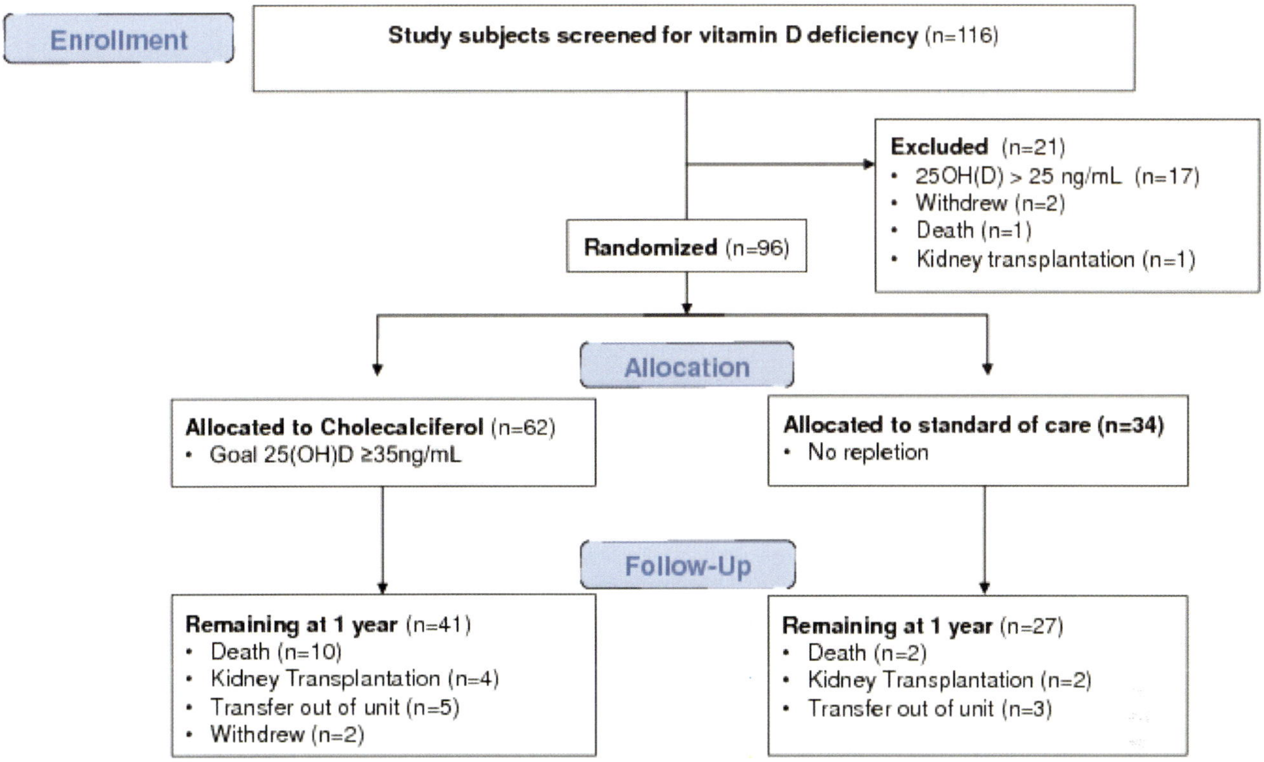

Figure 1. Study flow diagram. A total of 116 hemodialysis patients were screened, and 96 were randomized in a 2:1 ratio to receive oral cholecalciferol (n = 62) or no repletion (n = 34). There were no differences in dropout rates from transplantation (6.6% vs 5.9% at 1 year, p = .90) or death (16.4% vs 5.9% at 1 year, p = .14) between groups. A total of 68 subjects completed follow-up to 1 year. Of those 68 subjects, 51 (34 in the treatment group and 17 in the control group) had sufficient PBMC samples meeting predetermined quality-assurance criteria for immunologic assessment.

containing sodium heparin for plasma or no additive for serum. PBMCs were isolated by Ficoll gradient centrifugation, cryopreserved at a concentration of 10^7 cells/mL, and placed in a −80°C freezer for ≥24 hours prior to transfer to liquid nitrogen for long-term storage for ELISPOT assays. Serum separator tubes were left for one hour at room temperature before centrifugation at 1500 rpm for 15 minutes at 20°C, and serum was immediately divided into 0.5 mL aliquots and stored at −80°C until analysis.

10^6 PBMCs were treated overnight with Streck Cell Preservative (Streck, Omaha, Nebraska) and stained with fluorochrome-labeled antibodies the following day as per the manufacturers' recommendations for each antibody. Antibodies used for differentiation of T-cell subsets included: anti-CD4-FITC, anti-CD25-APC, anti-CD8-PE, anti-CD45RA-APC, anti-CD45RO-FITC (BD, Franklin Lakes, NJ), anti-CD4-PE-Cy7 and anti-Foxp3-PE (eBioscience, San Diego, CA). Stained cells were analyzed on a

Table 1. Baseline patient characteristics.

Characteristic	Treatment (n = 62)	Control (n = 34)	p-value
Baseline 25(OH)D, ng/mL (median, [IQR])	13.4 [9.3, 19.7]	13.1 [9.9, 18.6]	0.97
Age, years	60.2 [14.3]	58.9 [14.9]	0.66
Gender: Female	26 (41.9)	14 (41.2)	0.94
Race: Black	42 (67.7)	17 (50)	0.09
Dialysis Vintage, years (median, [IQR])	4.0 [1.3,8.0]	3.5 [1.2,7.9]	0.86
Diabetes	26 (41.9)	15 (44.1)	0.84
Current or Former Smoker	25 (40.3)	15 (44.1)	0.71
Dialysis Access: Catheter	12 (19.4)	8 (23.5)	0.45
Prior transplant	13 (21.0)	7 (20.6)	0.97
Prior blood transfusion	30 (48.4)	21 (61.8)	0.14
Prior pregnancy	20 (32.3)	13 (38.2)	0.31

Mean [SD] or count (%) unless otherwise specified.

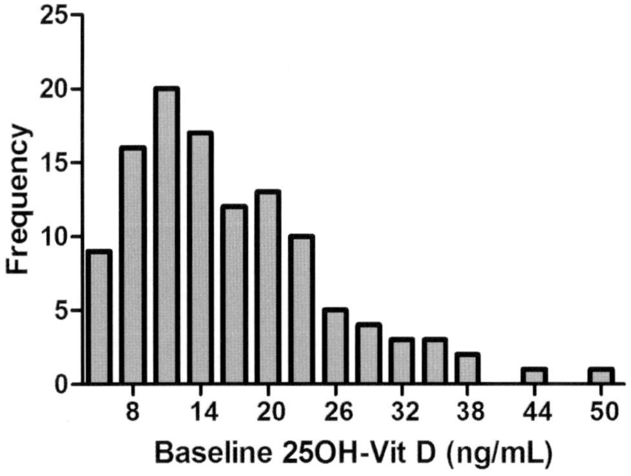

Figure 2. Baseline serum 25(OH)D concentrations in the study cohort. Distribution of serum 25(OH)D in the entire study cohort (n = 116) is shown. Median (IQR) 25(OH)D was 14.7 (10.5–21.6) ng/mL. 17 subjects with a baseline vitamin D level >25 ng/mL were excluded from randomization.

FACS Canto II flow cytometry (BD Bioscience, San Jose, CA, see Foxp3stainingeBioscience S1) and comparative results processed using FlowJo software (Tree Star, Inc, Ashland, OR).

IFNγ ELISPOT PRT assays were performed as previously described [5,19,27]. A total of 3×10^5 live responder cells were incubated with 1×10^5 of each allogeneic B cell line in duplicate or triplicate for 24 hours. Phytohemagglutinin (0.02 mg/mL) was used as a positive control. ELISPOT assays were developed according to standard operating protocol and spots quantified using an automated Immunospot Reader and CTL Immunospot Software (Cellular Technology Limited, Shaker Heights, OH). Mean numbers of IFNγ ELISPOTS from control wells (responder cells plus media only, typically <10 spots per well) were subtracted from the total number of spots in stimulated wells. Results are reported as the sum of the mean responses to each set of six stimulators [19].

Plasma anti-HLA antibody was assessed using HLA class I and class II antigen-coated microbeads (LABScreen Mixed, One Lambda Inc., Canoga Park, CA) and a flow analyzer (BioPlex 200 System with HTF, Bio-Rad, Hercules, CA) as previously described [28]. Determination of cut-off for reactivity was based on calculations as per the manufacturer's software. A new reactivity was defined by an MFI <1000 at baseline that increased to ≥5000 at one year. Results were analyzed using HLA fusion software (One Lambda Inc., Canoga Park, CA).

Statistical Analysis

Although the primary outcome was change in 25(OH)D concentrations, we attempted to power the study to detect differences in PRT results within groups over time, based on a standard deviation of 375 spots from our previous work [19], so as to provide estimates for power calculations for a larger, multi-center study. 30 subjects per group would provide 80% power to detect a difference of 200 spots in the PRT assay over time (alpha = 0.05). 30 study subjects per group would also provide 80% power to detect a difference in 25(OH)D levels *between* groups of 11 ng/mL at the 1 year time-point, based on a conservative estimate of the standard deviation of 15 ng/mL. Because we were unsure of how patients would respond to D_3 supplementation, randomization was performed in a 2:1 ratio to ensure an adequate number of patients had an increase in 25(OH)D levels over time, leading us to target an enrollment of 60 patients in the intervention group and 30 patients in the control group.

Statistical analysis was performed using SPSS version 20.0 (Chicago, IL) and GraphPad Prism 5 (GraphPad Software, Inc., La Jolla, CA). All analysis was performed on a per-protocol basis. There was no group cross-over, but, only patients reaching the 1-year time point were included in the 1-year data analysis in order to minimize the effect of missing data from patients lost to follow-up in the interim. Data are reported as medians and interquartile ranges or means and standard deviations for continuous variables, as appropriate, and as percentages of total for categorical variables. Baseline characteristics of the groups were compared using parametric (student's t-test) or non-parametric (Mann-Whitney) tests for continuous variables, as appropriate, and Chi-square or Fisher's exact tests for categorical variables, as appropriate. Changes over time were compared between groups using parametric (t-test) or non-parametric (Wilcoxon signed-rank test) tests, as appropriate. A two-tailed p-value<0.05 was considered statistically significant.

Results

Oral D_3 supplementation is safe and effective

Of 116 chronic hemodialysis patients screened, 99 (85.3%) had 25(OH)D concentrations <25 ng/mL and qualified for randomization (**Figure 1**). The median (IQR) 25(OH)D concentration of the 116 patients (**Figure 2**) was 14.7 (10.5–21.6) ng/mL. 25(OH)D concentration was independent of month (time of year)

Table 2. Laboratory parameters of bone and mineral metabolism and activated Vitamin D requirements.

	Treatment		Control		P-value*
	Baseline	12 Months	Baseline	12 Months	
25OH-D,** ng/mL (median, [IQR])	13.5 [9.8, 20.9]	40.9 [32.2, 45.5]	13.0 [10.9, 20.4]	15.8 [9.5, 19.5]	<0.001
PTH, pg/mL	465.0 (360.5)	555.9 (436.6)	434.3 (380.7)	637.4 (645.5)	0.35
Calcium, mg/dL	9.2 (0.6)	9.0 (0.7)	8.8 (1.0)	9.0 (1.0)	0.09
Phosphorus, mg/dL	5.8 (1.2)	5.3 (1.4)	5.4 (1.8)	5.1 (1.4)	0.95
Activated Vitamin D dose, mcg/treatment (median, [IQR])	4.0 [0, 9.1]	4.0 [2.5, 5.0]	3.5 [0, 5.6]	5.0 [2.3, 7.5]	0.22

Mean (SD) unless otherwise specified.
*p-values for comparison of change from baseline to 12 months between groups (treatment vs control).
**n = 41 in treatment group and 27 in control group.

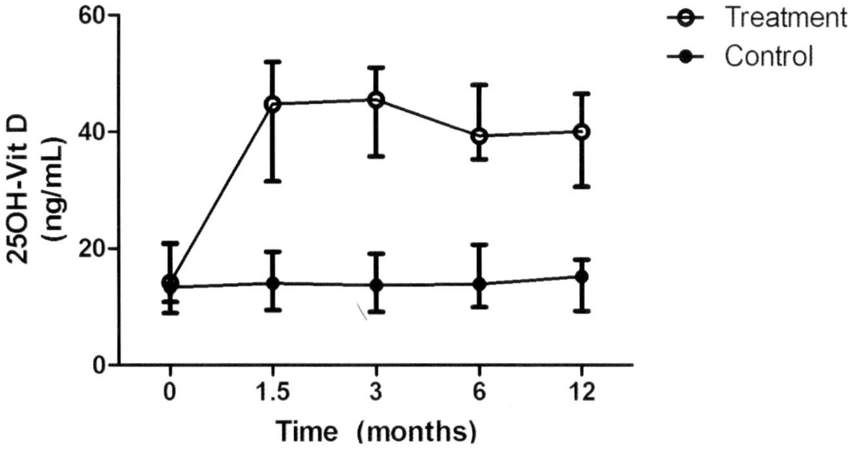

Figure 3. Effects of Vitamin D supplementation on serum 25(OH)D concentrations. Values increased by six weeks in the treatment group (13.5 [11.2] ng/mL to 42.5 [18.5] ng/mL, $p<0.001$), but remained low in the control group throughout the study duration. Median (IQR) are displayed on the graph.

of testing (data not shown). Reflecting the 2:1 enrollment design, 62/99 (62.6%) were randomized to treatment with cholecalciferol (D_3), and 34/99 (34.3%) were randomized to standard of care (control, no treatment); two patients withdrew, and one patient died prior to randomization (**Figure 1**). As randomization was stratified by baseline 25(OH)D concentration (10–24 ng/mL and<10 ng/mL), there were similar numbers of study subjects with baseline 25(OH)D<10 ng/mL in both groups (27.4% in the D_3 group and 23.5% in the control group, $p = 0.68$). Demographics of the randomized patients (**Table 1**) showed no differences between treatment and control groups in baseline 25(OH)D, age, gender, race, dialysis vintage, history of diabetes, smoking status, and dialysis access (catheter vs. arteriovenous fistula/arteriovenous graft). The majority (61.5%) of randomized patients were of self-reported African ancestry.

Therapy with oral D_3 resulted in a significant rise in serum 25(OH)D by 6 weeks (**Figure 3**), which was sustained throughout the 12 months of study. Serum 25(OH)D in the control group did not change (**Figure 3**). We did not observe any adverse events attributable to D_3 supplementation (see AdverseEventsTable S1). There were no differences in dropout rates from transplantation (6.6% vs 5.9% at 1 year, $p = .90$) or death (16.4% vs 5.9% at 1 year, $p = .14$) between groups (**Figure 1**), and importantly, the overall mortality of 11.6% at 1 year was not higher than expected for the general dialysis population based on previous reports (approximately 20%) [29]. Serum calcium, phosphorus, intact PTH, and activated vitamin D requirements (paricalcitol) were similar in the control and intervention arms through the trial (**Table 2**), and no episodes of sustained hypercalcemia occurred in either group during the study (**Table 2**, see RawData S1).

Effect of D_3 supplementation on T-cell phenotype

We used flow cytometry to analyze and quantify PBMCs collected at baseline and 1 year. Gating strategies are shown in **Figure 4** and the data are summarized in **Table 3 and Table 4**. Of 96 subjects randomized, 51 patients (34 in the treatment group and 17 in the control group) were available for 12 month follow-up, had sufficient PBMC, and were included in this analysis. None of the study subjects included in this analysis received packed red blood cell (PRBC) transfusions during the study period. At baseline, the median 25(OH)D concentration for these 51 patients was 14.1 ng/mL (IQR: 10.9–21.0 ng/mL), a value that did not differ from the parent cohort (14.7 ng/mL, IQR: 10.5–21.6 ng/mL). The baseline demographics of these subjects did not differ from those of the parent cohort ($p>0.05$ for each), supporting random and equal loss from the treatment and control groups, without evidence of bias.

Table 3. Effects of Vitamin D supplementation on T cell phenotypes†.

	Oral D_3 (n = 34)		Control (n = 17)	
	Baseline	**1 Year**	**Baseline**	**1 Year**
CD4%	37.0 [29.0,45.4]	40.6 [29.9,47.1]	34.5 [22.3,39.5]	35.7 [27.8,40.6]
Naïve CD45RA+	33.6 [20.4,44.5]	32.9 [16.8,44.8]	31.3 [19.4,49.7]	34.7 [17.3,50.1]
Memory CD45RO+	52.7 [41.0,64.9]	50.6 [39.0,66.3]	61.9 [39.9,70.4]	49.2 [41.4,72.5]
Foxp3+CD25+	7.9 [5.9,9.3]	5.9 [2.8,9.0]	7.8 [4.6,10.9]	3.9 [1.4,7.6]
CD8%	17.1 [12.8,25.8]	14.0 [9.8,22.9]	17.7 [11.6,22.8]	15.8 [13.0,18.6]
Naïve CD45RA+	64.5 [55.8,80.0]	67.7 [52.3,77.0]	68.8 [51.5,79.5]	65.8 [47.6,79.9]
Memory CD45RO+	14.6 [7.1,19.3]	14.2 [8.0,21.7]	14.6 [8.8,26.7]	20.0 [9.0,27.9]

Values are expressed as median [IQR].
†no statistically significant differences in baseline, 1 year, or change from baseline to 1 year between groups.

Table 4. Effects of Vitamin D supplementation on monocyte subsets†.

	Oral D_3 (n = 34)		Control (n = 17)	
	Baseline	**1 Year**	**Baseline**	**1 Year**
Total % Monocytes (CD19−/HLA-DR+)	6.4 [3.7,11.8]	6.2 [3.6,8.6]	5.5 [3.1,9.7]	5.9 [5.5,8.7]
Classical CD14++/CD16− % of monocytes	67.2 [53.4,78.5]	66.8 [57.2,78.2]	72.0 [64.2,79.5]	67.8 [52.5,73.4]
Nonclassical CD14lo/CD16+ % of monocytes	9.0 [4.8,16.4]	10.6 [6.6,16.7]	9.5 [6.4,13.8]	10.3 [5.3,16.4]
CCR2−/M-DC8−	2.5 [0.6,4.3]	2.1 [1.0,3.6]	1.5 [0.6,2.9]	2.0 [1.7,5.1]
CCR2−/MDC-8+	1.8 [0.6,4.5]	0.9 [0.5,1.8]	1.2 [0.5,3.3]	1.3 [0.6,2.9]

†no statistically significant differences in baseline, 1 year, or change from baseline to 1 year between groups.
doi:10.1371/journal.pone.0109998.t004

We examined the percentages of CD4 and CD8 T-cells including their naïve (CD45RA+/CD45RO^{neg}) and memory (CD45RA^{neg}/CD45RO+) subsets and quantified CD4+Foxp3+ T-cells. These analyses showed no differences in memory or naïve CD4 or CD8 cell subsets between the groups at baseline and at 1 year (**Table 3**). The percentages of CD4+Foxp3+ T-cells were lower in both groups at 1 year versus baseline, but the values did not differ between groups at either time point (**Table 3**).

D_3 supplementation may prevent time-dependent increases in cellular alloimmunity

We used an IFNγ ELISPOT-based panel of reactive T-cell (PRT) assay to quantify the frequencies of alloreactive memory T-

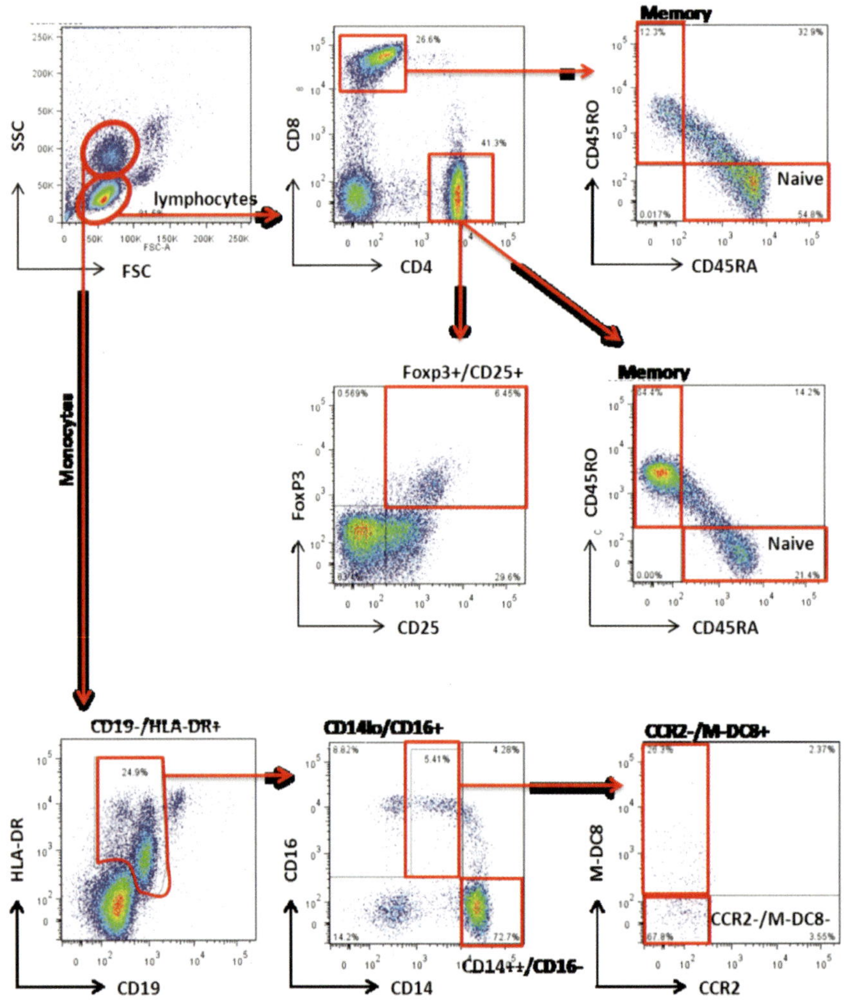

Figure 4. Gating strategy for enumeration of T cell and monocyte subsets. CD4 and CD8 memory (CD45RO+/CD45RA^{neg}) and naïve (CD45RO^{neg}/CD45RA+) T cells, and the Foxp3+/CD25+/CD4+ population containing regulatory cells were evaluated. Monocytes were identified by a CD19^{neg}/HLA-DR+ phenotype, and further characterized into the CD14++/CD16^{neg} classical subset, and the CD14^{lo}/CD16+ non-classical M-DC8+ and M-DC8^{neg} subsets.

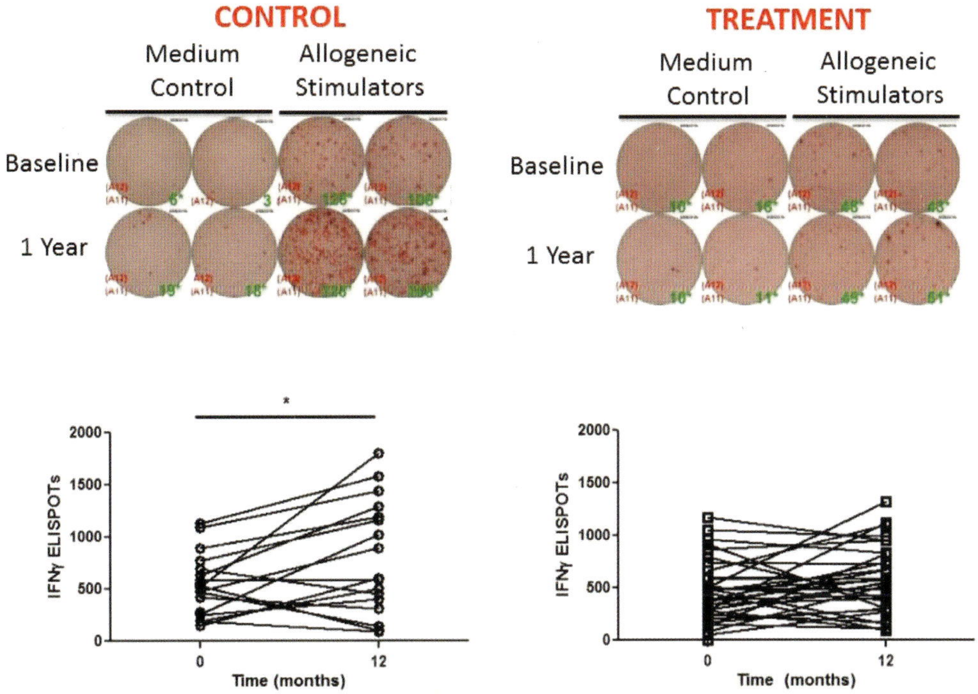

Figure 5. Vitamin D supplementation may prevent the time-dependent increase in PRT. (A) Representative ELISPOT PRT wells in duplicate at baseline and one year with no stimulation (media control) or response to allogeneic B cells. (B) Quantified results reveal a significant increase in the number of IFNγ ELISPOTs over time in the control group (517.4+/−280.8 to 797.8+/−542.3 spots, p = 0.03), but the comparison of "delta" PRT (1 year – baseline) in the treatment vs control group did not reach statistical significance (104.8+/−330.8 in treatment vs 252.9+/−431.3 in control, p = 0.25).

cells in each patient. In this assay, PBMC are stimulated with a panel of HLA-typed allogeneic B cell lines inducing alloreactive memory, but not naïve, T-cells to produce IFNγ [3]. Our previously published work showed that the summed responses to a randomly selected panel of 6 primary B cell lines is sufficient to provide reproducible and interpretable information [19], and that subjects with the highest PRT results were at an elevated risk for developing post-transplant acute rejection and inferior one year kidney function [5].

The PRT results were similar in the active treatment and control groups at baseline (450.9+/−301.2 vs 517.4+/−280.8 spots, p = 0.41) (**Figure 5**). Whereas the PRT did not change over 1 year study in the patients treated with oral D_3, the PRT increased significantly in the controls (517.4+/−280.8 to 797.8+/−542.3 spots, p = 0.03) (**Figure 5**). However, when comparing the "delta" PRT (1 year – baseline) in the treatment vs control group, this comparison did not reach statistical significance (delta PRT in treatment 104.8+/−330.8 vs 252.9+/−431.3 in control, p = 0.25). D_3 supplementation did not alter the development of new alloantibodies (**Figure 6**).

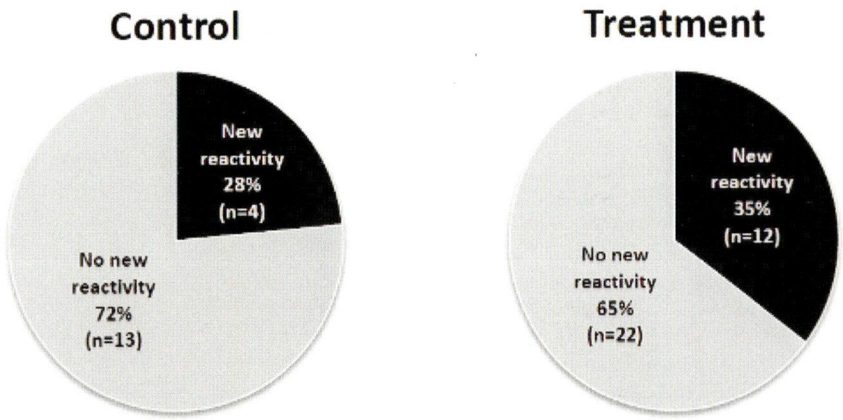

Figure 6. Vitamin D supplementation does not alter anti-HLA antibodies. Pie charts depicting the percentages of patients in each group that developed new anti-HLA antibodies between entry and 1 year (p = 0.393). A new reactivity was defined as having a MFI <1000 at baseline and > 5000 at one year using the LuminexPRA assay.

Effect of D_3 supplementation on peripheral pro-inflammatory monocytes

Peripheral blood monocytes are a heterogenous population of mononuclear cells capable of modulating inflammation and activating T cells, regulating expression of MHC, co-stimulatory molecules, and cytokines. Previous work by others showed that "non-classical" $CD14^{lo}/CD16+$ monocytes produce higher amounts of pro-inflammatory cytokines and express more cell surface HLA-DR than their classical $CD14{+}{+}/CD16^{neg}$ monocyte counterparts [30]. We did not observe differences in either of these monocyte subsets, either between groups at baseline and 1 year, or between groups over time (**Table 4**).

The $CD14^{lo}/CD16+$ non-classical monocyte population is comprised of two subgroups: M-DC8+ and $M\text{-}DC8^{neg}$ cells. The M-DC8+ subset has been shown to express two-fold more HLA class I and II molecules, to produce higher amounts of IL-12, and to induce more potent Th1 immune responses for the priming of cord blood T cells versus the M-DC8- population [31]. While there appeared to be a time-dependent, 50% decrease in M-DC8+ monocytes in the treatment group (**Table 4**), this change over time was not statistically significantly different from changes in the control group over time.

Discussion

In this pilot RCT of D_3 supplementation in vitamin D-deficient hemodialysis (HD) patients, we demonstrate safety and efficacy of D_3 in the setting of concurrent therapy with activated vitamin D analogs. Subjects randomized to D_3 therapy did not experience sustained hypercalcemia or other adverse events. While our study was not powered to examine mortality, the overall mortality of the cohort did not exceed that of the dialysis population in general [29] and published data show a survival benefit from vitamin D supplementation in other populations [32].

We newly show that D_3 supplementation may inhibit the expansion of alloreactive T-cell memory over 1 year on dialysis. Although the comparison of "delta" PRT (1 year – baseline) in the treatment vs control group did not reach statistical significance, (delta PRT in treatment group: 104.8+/−330.8 vs 252.9+/−431.3 in control group, $p=0.25$), this pilot study provides important data on standard deviation and effect size that can be used to design and power a larger clinical trial. If confirmed in a larger RCT, this would be the first demonstration of a potentially clinically relevant effect of nutritional vitamin D supplementation (D_3) that could impact standard of practice. These data expand upon our prior cross-sectional observations [19] and suggest that vitamin D supplements may prevent the induction of environmentally driven, heterologous (cross-reactive) cellular alloimmunity. The results support the therapeutic use of nutritional vitamin D (D_2 or D_3) in all hemodialysis patients, especially those on the transplant waiting list who may benefit from vitamin D's inhibitory effects on alloimmunity. We demonstrated potential effects of D_3 supplementation on cellular alloresponses in just one year; as most HD patients on the deceased-donor waiting list wait from 2–7 years for a transplant, and the risk for developing cross-reactive anti-donor T-cell immunity increases with longer HD vintage [33], the impact of vitamin D deficiency on heterologous immunity over time may be even greater, and needs to be evaluated in larger prospective multi-center longitudinal studies.

Our findings are consistent with emerging evidence in the literature that deficiency of 25(OH)D (despite exogenous $1{,}25(OH)_2D$ therapy) reduces local immune cell production of active vitamin D, and thereby promotes inflammation [16,34]. While hemodialysis patients are commonly treated with $1{,}25(OH)_2D$ analogs for the prevention of renal osteodystrophy, there are currently no recommendations for the regular surveillance or repletion of the precursor, 25(OH)D, and the prevalence of vitamin D deficiency in this population is high [20]. Vitamin D has been reported to inhibit dendritic cell (DC) differentiation and maturation and impair DC antigen presentation to attenuate the alloreactive T-cell response [10,11]. Consistent with these observations, we noted fewer proinflammatory monocytes in the treatment arm over time (**Table 4**), suggestive of an inhibitory effect on APCs, but the difference in this change between treatment and control groups was not statistically significant. Vitamin D has also been reported to promote Th2 immunity while limiting Th1 responses and to inhibit antigen-induced T-cell activation [12,13], which could prevent induction of cross-reactive alloimmunity. We acknowledge that results from this limited RCT do not reveal the mechanisms that underlie our findings; however, they suggest that vitamin D supplementation impacts alloreactive memory formation through a process that is likely to involve local production of $1{,}25(OH)_2D$ and provide a foundation for future detailed mechanistic studies by our group and others.

Observational studies in the kidney transplant population show an association between 25(OH)D deficiency and inferior graft outcomes [24,25,35]. In addition, a functional polymorphism in the vitamin D receptor (VDR) (*FokI*, rs10735810) leading to increased transcriptional activity has been shown to correlate with improved renal allograft survival [36]. Results of our immunological studies are consistent with these clinical observations, and highlight the need for prospective trials of vitamin D therapy in kidney transplant candidates and recipients with a focus on graft and patient outcomes, possibly stratifying by polymorphisms in the VDR and other genes involved in vitamin D metabolism and function.

Significant limitations of our study include the un-blinded nature and lack of a placebo control, thus introducing the possibility of study subject and investigator bias. However, all laboratory-based assays were performed by technicians unaware of study subject treatment assignment in an effort to minimize investigator bias. Because patients were aware of group assignment, we cannot exclude the possibility that some patients assigned to the control group obtained vitamin D supplements elsewhere. However, as 25(OH)D concentrations remained stable over time in the control group, it is unlikely that these patients were taking clinically significant doses of any vitamin D supplements.

In conclusion, the results of this pilot RCT show that nutritional vitamin D (D_3) supplementation is safe and effective in vitamin D-deficient HD patients concurrently treated with $1{,}25(OH)_2D$, and may prevent time-dependent increases in memory T-cell alloreactivity. Because memory T-cell alloreactivity pre-transplantation negatively affects post-transplant outcomes, and because vitamin D deficiency is associated with higher rates of acute rejection in kidney transplant recipients [35], treatment with vitamin D has the potential to improve kidney transplant outcomes and needs to be evaluated prospectively in transplant candidates/recipients. Given the apparent safety and low cost of vitamin D supplements, routine screening and correction of 25(OH)D deficiency should be considered in all dialysis units, with monitoring and reporting of the risks and benefits observed in a larger population.

Supporting Information

Adverse Events Table S1 Tabular view of adverse events.

CONSORT Checklist S1 Completed CONSORT checklist for randomized controlled trials referencing the manuscript.

Foxp3stainingeBioscience S1 Instructions for Foxp3 intracellular staining.

Protocol S1 IRB-approved study protocol detailing all study-related procedures.

Raw Data S1 Excel spreadsheet of raw data from the study.

Sample Case Report Form S1 Sample case report form from the trial used for data collection.

Acknowledgments

The authors thank the physicians, staff, and patients at the Mount Sinai 94th Street and Terrence Cardinal Cooke hemodialysis units in New York City for their participation in this study.

Author Contributions

Conceived and designed the experiments: AM PSH. Performed the experiments: LL ML MK KO AB. Analyzed the data: LL AM. Contributed reagents/materials/analysis tools: AG-S RA. Contributed to the writing of the manuscript: LL AM ADB JU PSH. Study subject recruitment: JT SL BR VL.

References

1. Schenk AD, Nozaki T, Rabant M, Valujskikh A, Fairchild RL (2008) Donor-reactive CD8 memory T cells infiltrate cardiac allografts within 24-h posttransplant in naive recipients. American journal of transplantation: official journal of the American Society of Transplantation and the American Society of Transplant Surgeons 8: 1652–1661.
2. Valujskikh A, Pantenburg B, Heeger PS (2002) Primed allospecific T cells prevent the effects of costimulatory blockade on prolonged cardiac allograft survival in mice. American journal of transplantation: official journal of the American Society of Transplantation and the American Society of Transplant Surgeons 2: 501–509.
3. Heeger PS, Greenspan NS, Kuhlenschmidt S, Dejelo C, Hricik DE, et al. (1999) Pretransplant frequency of donor-specific, IFN-gamma-producing lymphocytes is a manifestation of immunologic memory and correlates with the risk of posttransplant rejection episodes. Journal of immunology (Baltimore, Md: 1950) 163: 2267–2275.
4. Hricik DE, Rodriguez V, Riley J, Bryan K, Tary-Lehmann M, et al. (2003) Enzyme linked immunosorbent spot (ELISPOT) assay for interferon-gamma independently predicts renal function in kidney transplant recipients. American journal of transplantation: official journal of the American Society of Transplantation and the American Society of Transplant Surgeons 3: 878–884.
5. Poggio ED, Augustine JJ, Clemente M, Danzig JM, Volokh N, et al. (2007) Pretransplant cellular alloimmunity as assessed by a panel of reactive T cells assay correlates with acute renal graft rejection. Transplantation 83: 847–852.
6. Nadazdin O, Boskovic S, Murakami T, Tocco G, Smith R-N, et al. (2011) Host alloreactive memory T cells influence tolerance to kidney allografts in nonhuman primates. Science translational medicine 3.
7. Adams AB, Williams MA, Jones TR, Shirasugi N, Durham MM, et al. (2003) Heterologous immunity provides a potent barrier to transplantation tolerance. The Journal of clinical investigation 111: 1887–1895.
8. Wu Z, Bensinger SJ, Zhang J, Chen C, Yuan X, et al. (2004) Homeostatic proliferation is a barrier to transplantation tolerance. Nature medicine 10: 87–92.
9. Hewison M, Burke F, Evans KN, Lammas DA, Sansom DM, et al. (2007) Extra-renal 25-hydroxyvitamin D3-1alpha-hydroxylase in human health and disease. The Journal of steroid biochemistry and molecular biology 103: 316–321.
10. Piemonti L, Monti P, Sironi M, Fraticelli P, Leone BE, et al. (2000) Vitamin D3 affects differentiation, maturation, and function of human monocyte-derived dendritic cells. Journal of Immunology 164: 4443–4451.
11. Penna G, Adorini L (2000) 1 Alpha,25-dihydroxyvitamin D3 inhibits differentiation, maturation, activation, and survival of dendritic cells leading to impaired alloreactive T cell activation. Journal of Immunology (Baltimore, Md: 1950) 164: 2405–2411.
12. Boonstra A, Barrat FJ, Crain C, Heath VL, Savelkoul HF, et al. (2001) 1alpha,25-Dihydroxyvitamin d3 has a direct effect on naive CD4(+) T cells to enhance the development of Th2 cells. Journal of immunology (Baltimore, Md: 1950) 167: 4974–4980.
13. Bhalla AK, Amento EP, Serog B, Glimcher LH (1984) 1,25-Dihydroxyvitamin D3 inhibits antigen-induced T cell activation. J Immunol 133: 1748–1754.
14. Adorini L, Penna G, Casorati M, Davalli AM, Gregori S (2001) Induction of transplantation tolerance by 1,25-dihydroxyvitamin D(3). Transplantation proceedings 33: 58–59.
15. Liu PT, Stenger S, Li H, Wenzel L, Tan BH, et al. (2006) Toll-like receptor triggering of a vitamin D-mediated human antimicrobial response. Science (New York, NY) 311: 1770–1773.
16. Jeffery LE, Wood AM, Qureshi OS, Hou TZ, Gardner D, et al. (2012) Availability of 25-hydroxyvitamin D(3) to APCs controls the balance between regulatory and inflammatory T cell responses. Journal of immunology (Baltimore, Md: 1950) 189: 5155–5164.
17. Looker AC, Johnson CL, Lacher DA, Pfeiffer CM, Schleicher RL, et al. (2011) Vitamin D status: United States, 2001–2006. NCHS data brief: 1–8.
18. Pramyothin P, Holick MF (2012) Vitamin D supplementation: guidelines and evidence for subclinical deficiency. Curr Opin Gastroenterol 28: 139–150.
19. Sawinski D, Uribarri J, Peace D, Yao T, Wauhop P, et al. (2010) 25-OH-vitamin D deficiency and cellular alloimmunity as measured by panel of reactive T cell testing in dialysis patients. Am J Transplant 10: 2287–2295.
20. Jean G, Terrat JC, Vanel T, Hurot JM, Lorriaux C, et al. (2008) Daily oral 25-hydroxycholecalciferol supplementation for vitamin D deficiency in haemodialysis patients: effects on mineral metabolism and bone markers. Nephrology, dialysis, transplantation: official publication of the European Dialysis and Transplant Association - European Renal Association 23: 3670–3676.
21. Matias PJ, Jorge C, Ferreira C, Borges M, Aires I, et al. (2010) Cholecalciferol supplementation in hemodialysis patients: effects on mineral metabolism, inflammation, and cardiac dimension parameters. Clin J Am Soc Nephrol 5: 905–911.
22. Wasse H, Huang R, Long Q, Singapuri S, Raggi P, et al. (2012) Efficacy and safety of a short course of very-high-dose cholecalciferol in hemodialysis. The American journal of clinical nutrition 95: 522–528.
23. Saab G, Young DO, Gincherman Y, Giles K, Norwood K, et al. (2007) Prevalence of vitamin D deficiency and the safety and effectiveness of monthly ergocalciferol in hemodialysis patients. Nephron Clin Pract 105: c132–138.
24. Bienaimé F, Girard D, Anglicheau D, Canaud G, Souberbielle JC, et al. (2013) Vitamin D Status and Outcomes After Renal Transplantation. Journal of the American Society of Nephrology: JASN.
25. Kim H, Kang S-W, Yoo T-H, Kim MS, Kim SI, et al. (2012) The impact of pretransplant 25-hydroxy vitamin D deficiency on subsequent graft function: an observational study. BMC nephrology 13.
26. Saghaei M (2004) Random allocation software for parallel group randomized trials. BMC Med Res Methodol 4: 26.
27. Zand MS, Bose A, Vo T, Coppage M, Pellegrin T, et al. (2005) A renewable source of donor cells for repetitive monitoring of T- and B-cell alloreactivity. American journal of transplantation: official journal of the American Society of Transplantation and the American Society of Transplant Surgeons 5: 76–86.
28. Nair V, Sawinski D, Akalin E, Friedlander R, Ebcioglu Z, et al. (2012) Effect of high-dose intravenous immunoglobulin on anti-HLA antibodies in sensitized kidney transplant candidates. Clin Transplant 26: E261–268.
29. Goodkin DA, Bragg-Gresham JL, Koenig KG, Wolfe RA, Akiba T, et al. (2003) Association of comorbid conditions and mortality in hemodialysis patients in Europe, Japan, and the United States: the Dialysis Outcomes and Practice Patterns Study (DOPPS). Journal of the American Society of Nephrology: JASN 14: 3270–3277.
30. Ziegler-Heitbrock L (2007) The CD14+ CD16+ blood monocytes: their role in infection and inflammation. Journal of leukocyte biology 81: 584–592.
31. de Baey A, Mende I, Riethmueller G, Baeuerle PA (2001) Phenotype and function of human dendritic cells derived from M-DC8(+) monocytes. European journal of immunology 31: 1646–1655.
32. Bjelakovic G, Gluud LL, Nikolova D, Whitfield K, Wetterslev J, et al. (2011) Vitamin D supplementation for prevention of mortality in adults. Cochrane Database Syst Rev: CD007470.
33. Augustine JJ, Poggio ED, Clemente M, Aeder MI, Bodziak KA, et al. (2007) Hemodialysis vintage, black ethnicity, and pretransplantation antidonor cellular immunity in kidney transplant recipients. Journal of the American Society of Nephrology: JASN 18: 1602–1606.
34. Hewison M (2011) Vitamin D and innate and adaptive immunity. Vitamins and hormones 86: 23–62.
35. Lee JR, Dadhania D, August P, Lee JB, Suthanthiran M, et al. (2014) Circulating levels of 25-hydroxyvitamin d and acute cellular rejection in kidney allograft recipients. Transplantation 98: 292–299.
36. Lavin PJ, Laing ME, O'Kelly P, Moloney FJ, Gopinathan D, et al. (2007) Improved renal allograft survival with vitamin D receptor polymorphism. Renal failure 29: 785–789.

Risk Factors for the First Episode of Peritonitis in Southern Chinese Continuous Ambulatory Peritoneal Dialysis Patients

Xiaoguang Fan[1,3], Rong Huang[1,2], Juan Wang[1,2], Hongjian Ye[1,2], Qunying Guo[1,2], Chunyan Yi[1], Jianxiong Lin[1], Qian Zhou[1,2], Fengmin Shao[3], Xueqing Yu[1,2], Xiao Yang[1,2]*

1 Department of Nephrology, The First Affiliated Hospital, Sun Yat-sen University, Guangzhou, People's Republic of China, **2** Key Laboratory of Nephrology, Ministry of Health, Guangzhou, People's Republic of China, **3** Department of Nephrology, Zhengzhou University People's Hospital, Zhengzhou, People's Republic of China

Abstract

Background: The first episode of peritonitis affects survival of the peritoneal membrane as a medium for dialysis as well as survival of patients. The aim of this study is to investigate risk factors associated with the first episode of peritonitis in Southern Chinese continuous ambulatory peritoneal dialysis (CAPD) patients.

Methods: This is a single-center, retrospective, cohort study. All incident CAPD patients from 1 January 2006 to 31 December 2010 were recruited, and followed up until their first episode of peritonitis or 31 December, 2012. Baseline demographic, socioeconomic, clinical and laboratory data were collected. Cox proportional model was used to determine the factors associated with the first episode of peritonitis.

Results: In a cumulative 30756.5 patient-months follow-up (the median vintage 26.1 months) of 1117 CAPD patients, 309(27.7%) patients presented the first episodes of peritonitis. The cumulative peritonitis-free survival was 86.2%, 78.1%, 71.4% and 57.8% at 1, 2, 3 and 5 year, respectively. The multivariate analysis showed that factors associated with risk for the first episode of peritonitis were elderly patients (>65 years) [hazard ratio (HR) = 1.427, 95% confidence interval (CI) = 1.051 to 1.938, P = 0.023], male(HR = 1.315, 95% CI = 1.028 to 1.684, P = 0.030), lower education level (HR = 1.446, 95% CI: 1.127 to 1.855, P = 0.004) and albumin <38g/L (HR = 1.425, 95% CI: 1.112 to 1.825, P = 0.005).

Conclusions: Older age, male, lower educational level and hypoalbuminemia at the commencement of PD were the risk factors associated with the first episode of peritonitis in Southern Chinese CAPD patients.

Editor: Zhanjun Jia, University of Utah School of Medicine, United States of America

Funding: This study is supported by the U.S Baxter's Renal Discoveries Extramural Grant Program, Key Clinical Program of the Ministry of Health of China (2010439); the National Basic Research Program of China (Grant No 2011CB504000) and the National Key Technology R&D Program (No. 2011BAI10B08).The funders had no role in study design, data collection and analysis, decision to publish, or preparation of the manuscript.

Competing Interests: The authors have the following interests: this work was supported in part by the U.S Baxter's Renal Discoveries Extramural Grant Program. There are no patents, products in development or marketed products to declare.

* Email: yangxsysu@126.com

Introduction

Peritonitis is one of the most common and severe complications associated with peritoneal dialysis (PD), constituting the primary cause of catheter loss and exit from the dialysis technique [1]. It has reported that the first episode of peritonitis affects survival of peritoneal membrane as a medium for dialysis as well as survival of the PD patients [2]. A study identified that the time interval until the first episode of peritonitis was shorter in PD patients coming from hemodialysis (HD) as compared to those with no previous experience on renal replacement therapy (RRT) [3]. Another study confirmed the aboriginal and obese PD patients have a higher rate of peritonitis and a shorter time to the first episode of peritonitis [4]. Moreover, the incidence and etiology of peritonitis episodes vary based on geographical region, and change over time [5].

However, to our knowledge, there were fewer studies about the risk factors associated with the first episode of peritonitis in Chinese PD patients. Therefore, we conducted this study, to get an improved understanding of the risk factors associated with the development of the first episode of peritonitis.

Materials and Methods

Patient Population

This single-center retrospective cohort study included all incident CAPD patients followed up in the PD center, The First Affiliated Hospital of Sun Yat-sen University, from 1 January 2006 to 31 December 2010. To satisfy the study protocol, all patients had to have received at least 3 consecutive months of PD therapy, and the exclusion criteria was the patients who were not maintained on PD more than 90 days, younger than 18 years old, or began PD in other centers and exchanged to follow up in our center. The dataset in the study are derived from included patient's files in our PD center. The study was conducted in compliance with the ethical principles of the Helsinki Declaration (http://www.wma.net/en/30publications/10policies/b3/index.html) and approved by the Human Ethics Committees of Sun Yat-sen University. Written informed consent was obtained from all participants.

The baseline characteristics of all patients within 1–3 months of the start of PD therapy were collected, including demographic data [age (years), gender, education level (senior middle school or above, junior high school or below), region where patients live(urban, rural), family incomes (thousand RMB/per year) (0 to 50, 50 and above), cause of end-stage renal disease (ESRD), previous hemodialysis, previous kidney transplant, major comorbidities (cardiovascular disease, such as myocardial infarction, angina, or history of congestive heart failure, cerebrovascular event, and peripheral vascular disease with or without amputation), hypertension, diabetes, malignancy, Charlson comorbidity index (CCI) score at the start of PD [6], body mass index (BMI) (kg/m^2), type of catheter, operator], biochemical data [white blood cell (WBC), hemoglobin levels (g/l), hypersensitivity C-reactive protein(HsCRP) (mg/l), serum albumin levels (g/l), potassium (mmol/l), calcium(mmol/l), phosphate(mmol/l), calcium-phosphate product (Ca×P), blood urea nitrogen(BUN) (mmol/l), serum creatinine (umol/l),intact parathyroid hormone(iPTH) (pg/ml)], PD adequacy indices [renal and peritoneal Kt/V(urea clearance index) urea, residual urine volume(ml/24 h), baseline dialysate-to-plasma ratio of creatinine(D/Pcr)] and indices of nutrition [normalized protein catabolic rate (nPCR) (g/kg/d)], microbiological characteristics of the first episode of peritonitis, and total follow-up period (months). A standard peritoneal equilibration test was performed within the first 1–3 months after PD initiation. Patients were followed up until the primary end point, namely, the first episode of peritonitis. Those lost to follow-up were coded as censored observations, including death, transplantation, transfer to hemodialysis for reasons other than peritonitis and spontaneous recovery of renal function,or on 31 December 2012.

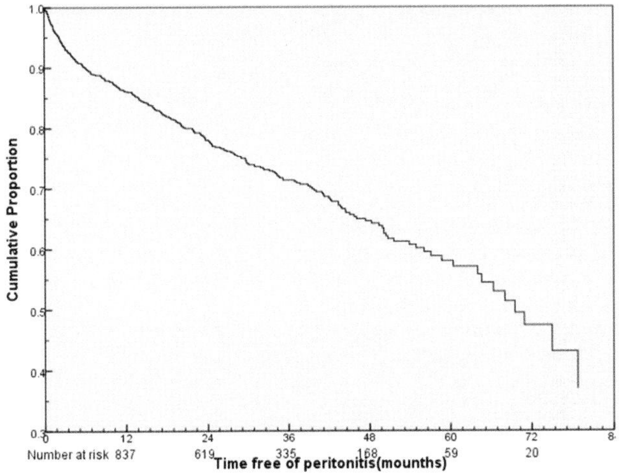

Figure 1. Peritonitis-free survival of 1117 incident peritoneal dialysis patients.

Definition of Peritonitis and the First Episode of Peritonitis

Recorded episodes of peritonitis met at least 2 of the following 3 criteria from the 2010 International Society for Peritoneal Dialysis (ISPD) guideline recommendations [7]: 1. Symptoms of peritoneal inflammation such as abdominal pain; 2. An effluent white blood cell count exceeding 100/ml after a dwell time of at least 2 hours, with at least 50% polymorphonuclear neutrophilic cells; 3. Presence of organisms on Gram stain or subsequent culturing of PD fluid.

The first episode of peritonitis was defined as the first case in which cloudy peritoneal fluid was observed, with a leukocyte count equal to or greater than 100 cells/mm^3, and with >50% polymorphonuclear cells.

Prescription of antibiotics was based on the patient's clinical conditions according to the guideline of ISPD combined with our center's experience. Patients were hospitalized whenever necessary.

Statistical Analyses

Continuous data that are normally distributed are termed "parametric data," and those that are not normally distributed, "nonparametric data." Parametric data are presented as mean ± standard deviation. Nonparametric data are presented as median values with the interval from the 25th to the 75th percentile. Categorical variables are expressed as a percentage or ratio. Parametric data were compared by independent sample T-test or rank sum test. Nonparametric data were compared by the chi-square test. Demographic, socioeconomic, clinical data and PD adequacy variables were included in peritonitis risk analysis. Peritonitis-free survival curve was constructed according to Kaplan–Meier method. Univariate Cox proportional hazard regression was used to select variables associated with the first episode of peritonitis to the final multivariate Cox model and the elimination criterion for them was $P>0.20$. Collinearity among variables was tested and if statistically significant interactions were presented, one of them was excluded. All of the reported p-values are two-tailed, statistical significance was defined as $P<0.05$. All statistical analyses were performed using SPSS 18.0 (SPSS Inc.) software.

Results

In a total of 1252 incident CAPD patients, 1117 patients 18 years or older who remained at least 90 days on PD were eligible for the study, whereas 62 were excluded for not completing 90 days on PD, 14 patients were younger than 18 years old and 59 patients began PD in other centers and exchanged to follow up in our center. The study population was followed up for a median of 26.1 months [interquartile range (IQR) 12.0–39.5 months]. Mean age at commencement of CAPD was 48.3±15.5 years (range 18–84 years). Elder (>65 years) and male patients comprised of a proportion of 16.5% and 58.6%, respectively. Etiologies of ESRD were chronic glomerulonephritis (58.7%), diabetic nephropathy (21.9%), hypertensive nephrosclerosis (6.2%), and other renal disease (13.2%).

Three hundred and nine (27.7%) patients presented total 513 episodes of peritonitis during a cumulative follow-up period of 30,756.5 patient-months, whereas the remaining 808(72.3%) patients had no peritonitis. The overall peritonitis rate was 1/60 patient-months. The cumulative peritonitis-free survival was 86.2%, 78.1%, 71.4% and 57.8% at 1, 2, 3 and 5 year, respectively (Figure 1). Compared with the peritonitis-free patients, the patients with the first episode of peritonitis had

Table 1. Baseline clinical characteristics and laboratory biochemistry data.

	Peritonitis-free group		first peritonitis group		P-value
	N	**mean±SD, medain**	**N**	**mean±SD, medain**	
Age(years)	808	47.1±15.5	309	51.8±14.9	**0.000**
Men (%)	475	58.8%	181	58.6%	0.738
Diabetes (%)	186	23.0%	67	21.7%	0.633
CCI score	808	3.51±1.81	309	4.10±2.21	**0.000**
BMI(kg/m^2)	761	21.4±3.1	301	21.3±2.9	0.660
eGFR(ml/min1.73 m^2)	592	3.71±2.96	222	3.64±2.62	0.756
Residual urine(ml/24 h)	596	736±489	231	723±510	0.732
D/P cr	460	0.71±0.12	172	0.71±0.12	0.957
Weekly Kt/V	592	2.39±0.68	223	2.36±0.67	0.553
nPCR(g/kg/d)	590	0.96±0.27	223	0.94±0.27	0.469
WBC(10^{12}/L)	786	6.77±2.05	307	6.98±2.28	0.140
Hemoglobin(g/L)	786	103±20	306	101±22	0.157
Prealbumin(g/L)	554	337±101	195	322±102	0.080
AST(U/L)	765	23.7±14.2	299	25.0±17.1	0.233
ALT(U/L)	765	15(11, 23)	299	16(11, 23)	0.342
ALP(U/L)	764	77.3±35.3	298	88.6±61.2	**0.003**
Serum albumin(g/L)	768	37.8±5.1	299	36.4±5.5	**0.000**
HsCRP(mg/L)	545	1.60(0.58,5.93)	200	2.71(0.88, 9.17)	**0.002**
Sodium(mmol/L)	783	140±4	306	140±4	0.204
Potassium(mmol/L)	782	3.79±0.74	304	3.72±0.70	0.138
Calcium(mmol/L)	782	2.27±0.22	305	2.26±0.34	0.671
Phosphorus(mmol/L)	759	1.46±0.44	297	1.41±0.44	0.091
Glucose(mmol/L)	781	5.32±2.44	306	5.34±2.42	0.889
Total cholesterol(mmol/L)	702	5.10±1.33	283	5.09±1.31	0.949
HDL-C(mmol/L)	698	1.31±0.46	282	1.27±0.41	0.307
Urea nitrogen(mmol/L)	784	17.2±7.9	306	17.4±15.8	0.737
Creatinine (umol/L)	785	761±277	306	738±279	0.176
Uric acid(umol/L)	749	421±89	291	419±99	0.813
iPTH (pg/ml)	688	216(88, 408)	280	224(83,395)	0.942
Serum iron((umol/L)	596	8.20(5.70,12.0)	217	8.8(6.0,12.1)	0.220

CCI: Charlson comorbidity index; BMI: body mass index; eGFR: estimated glomerular filtration rate; D/P cr: dialysate-to-plasma ratio of creatinine; Kt/V: urea clearance index; nPCR: normalized protein catabolic rate; WBC: white blood cell; AST: Aspartate aminotransferase; ALT: Alanine aminotransferase; ALP: Alkaline phosphatase; HsCRP: high sensitivity C-reactive protein; HDL-C: High-density lipoprotein cholesterol; iPTH: intact parathyroid hormone.

advanced age, higher levels of CCI score, ALP, HsCRP ($P<0.05$) and lower levels of serum albumin ($P<0.05$) (Table 1).

Causative organisms of the first episode of peritonitis of the cohorts are summarized in following: 99 (32%) were due to gram-

Table 2. Outcome of the different organisms infection for the first episode of peritonitis (n = 309).

Causative organisms	Sample size (n)	Cure (n, %)	Transfer to hemodialysis (n, %)	Death (n, %)	Average time to death (d)
Gram-positive organism	99	95 (96.0%)	2 (2.0%)	2 (2.0%)	25
Gram-negative organisms	70	66 (94.2%)	2 (2.9%)	2 (2.9%)	25
Fungi	18	1 (5.5%)	14 (77.8%)	3 (16.7%)	13
Multiple organisms	3	3 (100%)	0	0	0
Negative culture	77	72 (93.5%)	4 (5.2%)	1 (1.3%)	41
No microbiological information	42	40 (95.2%)	0	2 (4.8%)	32.5

Table 3. Frequency and median time to the first episode of peritonitis according to demographic factors.

Variable	N	First Peritonitis Frequency (%)	Median Time to the First Episode of Peritonitis (months)	P value
Age (years)				
≤65	934	250(26.8)	13.9	
>65	183	59(32.2)	10.2	**0.009**
Gender				
Women	461	128(27.8)	18.3	
Men	656	181(27.6)	10.2	0.166
Educational level				
≥Senior middle school	514	126(24.5)	13.0	
≤Junior high school	533	169(31.7)	15.7	**0.017**
Income (thousand RMB/per year)				
≤50	786	218(27.7)	16.0	
>50	162	43(26.5)	6.2	0.631
Region where patients live				
Urban	713	203(28.5)	14.2	
Rural	393	102(26.0)	10.9	0.865
Catheter type, tip				
Straight	961	263(27.4)	11.8	
Coiled	149	44(29.5)	18.2	0.279
Previous hemodialysis				
Yes	39	9(23.1)	11.0	
No	1078	300(27.8)	13.4	0.593
Previous Kidney transplantation				
Yes	9	3(33.3)	14.6	
No	1108	306(27.6)	13.2	0.971
Operator				
Self	1045	290(27.8)	13.8	
Else	71	18(25.4)	5.9	0.527

positive agents, 70 (22.7%) to gram-negative germs, and 18 (5.8%) to fungi. Among the gram-positive organisms, the most frequent was Streptococcus (11.7%), followed by Coagulase-negative staphylococci (11.3%), Staphylococcus aureus (4.2%) and Enterococcus (1.0%), the other gram-positive organisms (3.9%). Among the gram-negative organisms, Escherichia coli was the main gram-negative germ causing 12.9% of the cases, followed by Klebsiella pneumoniae (4.5%), Pseudomonas aeruginosa (0.3%), other gram-negative organisms(4.9%). Microbiological information was not reported in 42 (13.6%) episodes and negative culture was observed in 77 (24.9%). For the outcome of the first episode of peritonitis, 277 (89.6%) patients were cured, 22(7.1%) transferred to hemodialysis, 10 (3.2%) death, and the average time to death was 24.5 days (range: 3 to 53 days), and the outcome of the different organisms infection for the first episode of peritonitis in detail are showed in Table 2.

The frequency of the first episode of peritonitis and the median time to the first episode of peritonitis according to demographic, socioeconomic, dialysis-related, clinical and PD adequacy variables are expressed in Tables 3 and 4. Age, educational level, and albumin were associated with risk for the first episode of peritonitis in univariate Cox analysis (Tables 3 and 4), and were entered in the multivariate Cox proportional hazard model. Gender, hemoglobin and potassium were also entered in the multivariate Cox proportional hazard model because their P value were <0.20 in univariate analysis. For the collinearity among variables, no significant interaction was found between variables.

The multivariate analysis by using independent variables as categorical data demonstrated that factors independently associated with increased hazard risk (HR) for the first episode of peritonitis were old age(>65 years versus ≤65 years: HR = 1.427, 95% CI = 1.051 to 1.938, P = 0.023), male(male versus female: HR = 1.315, 95% CI = 1.028 to 1.684, P = 0.030), lower education level (≤ junior high school versus ≥senior middle school: HR = 1.446, 95% CI: 1.127 to 1.855, P = 0.004) and serum albumin (<38 g/L versus ≥38 g/L: HR = 1.425, 95% CI: 1.112 to 1.825, P = 0.005) (Table 5). The result by using independent variables as continuous data showed that factors associated with risk for the first episode of peritonitis were advanced age (HR = 1.016, 95% CI = 1.007 to 1.024, P = 0.000), male (HR = 1.376, 95% CI = 1.079 to 1.756, P = 0.010) and lower albumin level (HR = 0.961, 95% CI = 0.937 to 0.985, P = 0.002), which was similar with the results analyzed with categorical data.

Table 4. Frequency and median time to the first episode of peritonitis according to clinical factors.

Variable	N	First Peritonitis Frequency (%)	Median Time to the First Episode of Peritonitis (months)	P value
Diabetes				
No	864	242(28.0)	13.0	
Yes	253	67(26.5)	15.3	0.959
Cardiovascular disease				
No	819	222(27.1)	13.4	
Yes	298	87(29.2)	13.1	0.357
Hypertension				
No	797	216(27.1)	13.4	
Yes	320	93(29.1)	13.1	0.374
Malignancy				
No	1092	301(27.6)	13.4	
Yes	25	8(32.0)	7.0	0.406
BMI(kg/m^2)				
<18.5	177	52(29.4)	22.5	0.962
18.5–24.9	761	215(28.3)	11.6	
25–29.9	110	32(29.1)	8.0	0.704
≥30	14	2(14.3)	12.7	0.341
Ca×P				
<55	930	260(28.0)	14.0	
≥55	143	42(29.4)	5.9	0.827
Hemoglobin(g/l)				
≥110	400	100(25.0)	15.9	
<110	679	194(28.6)	13.1	0.081
Potassium (mmol/L)				
≥3.5	686	177(25.8)	11.8	
<3.5	400	127(31.8)	16.0	0.123
Serum albumin(g/L)				
≥38	567	139(24.5)	13.4	
<38	500	160(32.0)	13.8	**0.000**
Residual urine				
≥100	797	221(27.7)	15.3	
<100	31	11(35.5)	14.6	0.201
nPCR(g/kg/d)				
≥0.8	581	158(27.2)	16.1	
<0.8	232	65(28.0)	11.1	0.632
Weekly Kt/V				
≥1.7	720	201(27.9)	14.2	
<1.7	95	22(23.2)	23.7	0.653

Discussion

Our retrospective cohort study showed that the proportion of patients with the first episode of peritonitis was 27.7%. The cumulative peritonitis-free survival was 86.2%, 78.1%, 71.4% and 57.8% at 1, 2, 3 and 5 year, respectively. Older age, male, lower educational level and hypoalbuminemia were associated with the first episode of peritonitis.

Our result identified that the elderly patients (>65 years) was a risk factor for the first episode of peritonitis. The result was in accordance with the ANZDATA [4] analysis, which identified Aboriginal race, obesity, and older age as predictors of peritonitis. On the contrary, the USRDS results [8] and a multicenter observational study in BRAZPD [9] showed that older age was not a predictor of peritonitis risk. Recently, a single-center study manifested elderly patients were at higher risk of peritonitis episodes [10]. This finding could be explained by the decreased dexterity and vision in elderly patients, which can be a hindrance to proper aseptic technique. Moreover, it can be explained by the association between the older age and comorbidities [3].

Table 5. Cox proportional hazards regression model.

Variable	HR	95% CI		P value
		Lower	Upper	
Age >65 years	1.427	1.051	1.938	**0.023**
Gender: male	1.315	1.028	1.684	**0.030**
Educational level ≤ junior high school	1.446	1.127	1.855	**0.004**
Serum albumin <38 g/L	1.425	1.112	1.825	**0.005**
Hemoglobin <110 g/L	1.184	0.916	1.529	0.198
Potassium <3.5 mmol/L	1.154	0.906	1.470	0.245

Cox proportional hazards regression model (n = 309 episodes in 1117 patients).

Several studies have observed a higher rate of peritonitis in women, and most caused by gram-negative bacilli derived from vaginal contamination [11]. However, an interesting finding of the present study was that men were associated with the high risk for the first episode of peritonitis as compared to women. So the reason for our result may be as follow: firstly, this maybe because the obedience of men was not better than women; Secondly, it may due to the more social interaction needs for men than women, and some men even still insist on working during the dialysis interphase, which may cause the fluctuations of patient's living environment and thus may be impacted by the poor environmental in surrounding. One point that what we should not ignore was women maybe more careful and had better personal hygiene condition than men in the daily life. Last but not the least, it is possible that men comprised 58.7% of our study group.

Regarding educational level, Martin *et al.* [9] reported that the influence of educational level on peritonitis risk was observed after adjustment for the socioeconomic and demographic characteristics as well as relevant coexisting medical factors and comorbidities, showing the strong influence of educational level on peritonitis risk. A similar result reported by Chern *et al* [12], showed that a lower education level was a major risk factor for peritonitis, independent of age, sex, hypoalbuminemia, and comorbidities. We also found an association between lower education level and the first episode of peritonitis which was in accordance with these reports. Lower education level maybe associated with the decreased ability to learn the operation procedure and associated knowledge about CAPD, so to build a comprehensive and long-time CAPD education program according to the patients' different educational level is more important, especially for CAPD patients with lower education level.

Hypoalbuminemia in baseline was a strong risk factor for the first episode of peritonitis in the present study. The influence of hypoalbuminemia on peritonitis risk has been previously reported. Studies in the United States [13] and Hong Kong [14] found that every 1 g/dL decrease of serum albumin concentration increased the risk of peritonitis by 74% and 67% respectively. In our study, compared with the patients with a baseline serum albumin level of 38 g/L or greater, patients with a baseline serum albumin level less than 38 g/L had a hazard ratio of 1.406(HR = 1.406) for the first episode of peritonitis. It was well known that hypoalbuminemia is the result of malnutrition and inflammatory response and may lead to susceptibility to infection. Therefore, the intervention measures should be given to improve of patients' nutritional status to prevent malnutrition in CAPD patients.

Actually, in contrast to the previous studies, diabetes, socioeconomic status, transferring from HD to PD, and BMI did not influence the first episode of peritonitis in our study. Data on diabetes have been conflicting, but the majority of authors have reported that presence of diabetes is associated with higher peritonitis risk. For our center, diabetes was not the major cause of ESRD, and the technique survival in CAPD patients with diabetes was similar to those without diabetes [15]. Regarding socioeconomic status, Chow *et al.* [16] showed that the need for social security assistance and illiteracy were the only statistically significant factors associated with time to the first episode of peritonitis, after adjustment for age and medical factors, such as diabetes and serum albumin. However, Andrade, B. K *et al.* [17] reported that economic status is not independently associated with survival in a large cohort and should not be considered a barrier for PD indication, and our result was in line with the latter.

In this study there was a high proportion of culture-negative episodes. The antibiotic drugs used in the local hospital before they transferred to our hospital may resulted in higher culture-negative rate. In addition, we should review the laboratory methods currently utilized and generate new protocols to improve the results in our center.

The main strength of this study is the fact that it was a large single-center cohort study of incident CAPD patients, incorporating several potentially important demographic, socioeconomic, PD adequacy, residual renal function, and educational factors. Moreover, this is the first Southern China study designed to address whether these factors are predictors for the first episode of peritonitis risk. However, our study has several limitations. First, this single-center study was based on retrospective data and the data of some induces was missing, and this may lead to the biased results. Moreover, our data set did not include the data on dedicated room to dialysis operate, exit site catheter care, whether wearing a face mask, patient's hand hygiene condition and patients' compliance, all the factors that could represent peritonitis risk factors. In addition, it has been reported [18] that fluid excess associated with protein-energy wasting, old age, and decreased residual urine output. But the relationship between the volume status and peritonitis is worth for further study. Hence, further studies with more complete data collection and multicenter involvement will be needed to identify the factors associated with PD-related peritonitis in Southern China.

Conclusions

Older age, male, lower educational level and hypoalbuminemia at initiation of PD were related to the first episode of peritonitis, independent of hemoglobin and potassium. These results may be helpful in identifying the patients starting PD treatment who are at the highest risk for the first episode of peritonitis, and could help to take intervention to prevent and improve CAPD outcomes.

Acknowledgments

We thank all doctors and nurses in our PD center for their patient care and data collection.

Author Contributions

Performed the experiments: XGF XY. Analyzed the data: RH JW QZ. Contributed reagents/materials/analysis tools: XQY QYG HJY CYY JXL. Contributed to the writing of the manuscript: XGF XY. Contributed to discussions: XQY FMS XY.

References

1. Woodrow G, Turney JH, Brownjohn AM (1997) Technique failure in peritoneal dialysis and its impact on patient survival. Perit Dial Int 17: 360–364.
2. Brown MC, Simpson K, Kerssens JJ, Mactier RA (2011) Peritoneal dialysis-associated peritonitis rates and outcomes in a national cohort are not improving in the post-millennium (2000–2007). Perit Dial Int 31: 639–650.
3. Portoles J, Janeiro D, Lou-Arnal LM, Lopez-Sanchez P, Ortega M, et al. (2013) First episodes of peritoneal infection: description and prognostic factors. Nefrologia 33: 316–324.
4. Lim WH, Johnson DW, McDonald SP (2005) Higher rate and earlier peritonitis in Aboriginal patients compared to non-Aboriginal patients with end-stage renal failure maintained on peritoneal dialysis in Australia: analysis of ANZDATA. Nephrology (Carlton) 10: 192–197.
5. Remon C, Quiros PL, Perez BV, Toran D, Tejuca F, et al. (2006) [Report of the Andalusian registry of patients with end stage renal disease in treatment with peritoneal dialysis: period 1999–2004]. Nefrologia 26: 45–55.
6. Charlson ME, Pompei P, Ales KL, MacKenzie CR (1987) A new method of classifying prognostic comorbidity in longitudinal studies: development and validation. J Chronic Dis 40: 373–383.
7. Li PK, Szeto CC, Piraino B, Bernardini J, Figueiredo AE, et al. (2010) Peritoneal dialysis-related infections recommendations: 2010 update. Perit Dial Int 30: 393–423.
8. Oo TN, Roberts TL, Collins AJ (2005) A comparison of peritonitis rates from the United States Renal Data System database: CAPD versus continuous cycling peritoneal dialysis patients. Am J Kidney Dis 45: 372–380.
9. Martin LC, Caramori JC, Fernandes N, Divino-Filho JC, Pecoits-Filho R, et al. (2011) Geographic and educational factors and risk of the first peritonitis episode in Brazilian Peritoneal Dialysis study (BRAZPD) patients. Clin J Am Soc Nephrol 6: 1944–1951.
10. Hsieh YP, Chang CC, Wen YK, Chiou PF, Yang Y (2014) Predictors of peritonitis and the impact of peritonitis on clinical outcomes of continuous ambulatory peritoneal dialysis patients in Taiwan-10 years' experience in a single center. Perit Dial Int 34: 85–94.
11. Kotsanas D, Polkinghorne KR, Korman TM, Atkins RC, Brown F (2007) Risk factors for peritoneal dialysis-related peritonitis: can we reduce the incidence and improve patient selection? Nephrology (Carlton) 12: 239–245.
12. Chern YB, Ho PS, Kuo LC, Chen JB (2013) Lower education level is a major risk factor for peritonitis incidence in chronic peritoneal dialysis patients: A retrospective cohort study with 12-year follow-up. Perit Dial Int.; 33: 552–558.
13. Wang Q, Bernardini J, Piraino B, Fried L (2003) Albumin at the start of peritoneal dialysis predicts the development of peritonitis. Am J Kidney Dis 41: 664–669.
14. Chow KM, Szeto CC, Leung CB, Kwan BC, Law MC, et al. (2005) A risk analysis of continuous ambulatory peritoneal dialysis-related peritonitis. Perit Dial Int 25: 374–379.
15. Yang X, Yi C, Liu X, Guo Q, Yang R, et al. (2013) Clinical outcome and risk factors for mortality in Chinese patients with diabetes on peritoneal dialysis: a 5-year clinical cohort study. Diabetes Res Clin Pract 100: 354–361.
16. Chow KM, Szeto CC, Leung CB, Law MC, Li PK (2005) Impact of social factors on patients on peritoneal dialysis. Nephrol Dial Transplant 20: 2504–2510.
17. de Andrade BK, Qureshi AR, Lopes AA, Fernandes N, Barbosa LM, et al. (2011) Family income and survival in Brazilian Peritoneal Dialysis Multicenter Study Patients (BRAZPD): time to revisit a myth? Clin J Am Soc Nephrol 6: 1676–1683.
18. Guo Q, Yi C, Li J, Wu X, Yang X, et al. (2013) Prevalence and risk factors of fluid overload in Southern Chinese continuous ambulatory peritoneal dialysis patients. PLoS One 8: e53294.

Recipient-Related Risk Factors for Graft Failure and Death in Elderly Kidney Transplant Recipients

Xingqiang Lai, Guodong Chen, Jiang Qiu, Changxi Wang, Lizhong Chen*

Organ Transplant Center, The First Affiliated Hospital, Sun Yat-sen University, Guangzhou, China

Abstract

Background: Elderly patients with end-stage renal disease have become the fastest growing population of kidney transplant candidates in recent years. However, the risk factors associated with long-term outcomes in these patients remain unclear.

Methods: We retrospectively analyzed 166 recipients aged 60 years or older who underwent primary deceased kidney transplantation between 2002 and 2013 in our center. The main outcomes included 1-, 3- and 5-year patient survival as well as overall and death-censored graft survival. The independent risk factors affecting graft and patient survival were analyzed using Cox regression analysis.

Results: The 1-, 3-, 5-year death-censored graft survival rates were 93.6%, 89.4% and 83.6%, respectively. Based on the Cox multivariate analysis, panel reactive antibody (PRA)>5% [hazard ratio (HR) 4.295, 95% confidence interval (CI) 1.321–13.97], delayed graft function (HR 4.744, 95% CI 1.611–13.973) and acute rejection (HR 4.971, 95% CI 1.516–16.301) were independent risk factors for graft failure. The 1-, 3-, 5-year patient survival rates were 84.8%, 82.1% and 77.1%, respectively. Longer dialysis time (HR 1.011 for 1-month increase, 95% CI 1.002–1.020), graft loss (HR 3.501, 95% CI 1.559–7.865) and low-dose ganciclovir prophylaxis (1.5 g/d for 3 months) (HR 3.173, 95% CI 1.063–9.473) were risk factors associated with patient death.

Conclusions: The five-year results show an excellent graft and patient survival in elderly kidney transplant recipients aged ≥ 60 years. PRA>5%, delayed graft function, and acute rejection are risk factors for graft failure, while longer duration of dialysis, graft loss and low-dose ganciclovir prophylaxis are risk factors for mortality in elderly recipients. These factors represent potential targets for interventions aimed at improving graft and patient survival in elderly recipients.

Editor: Stanislaw Stepkowski, University of Toledo, United States of America

Funding: This study was supported by the 5010 Clinical Research Project of Sun Yat-sen University (2007003) and the National Natural Science Fund Youth Science project (81302549). The funders had no role in study design, data collection and analysis, decision to publish, or preparation of the manuscript.

Competing Interests: The authors have declared that no competing interests exist.

* Email: clz@medmail.com.cn

These authors contributed equally to this work.

Introduction

Kidney transplantation is considered to be the best treatment option for patients with end-stage renal disease (ESRD), regardless of their age. Currently, the mean age of patients undergoing renal transplantation has increased. This trend is observed not only in western countries such as America but also in Asian countries. Patients ≥60 years with ESRD have become the fastest growing population of wait-listed individuals and kidney transplant candidates [1,2]. Over the last decade, both the absolute number and percent of transplants performed in patients aged ≥65 years have approximately doubled [1]. Previous studies have reported that elderly ESRD patients after kidney transplantation have lower mortality rates and improved quality of life compared with those who remain on dialysis treatment [3,4,5].

However, despite the known benefits of kidney transplantation over dialysis in the elderly patients, long-term outcomes of the recipients and their grafts are still limited [6]. Given the rapid increase in the number of senior renal transplant candidates combined with a growing shortage of donor kidneys, it is increasingly important to optimize the long-term outcomes in the elderly recipients. The characteristics of the elderly patients at transplantation may have an important impact on graft and patient survival. Published studies regarding the recipient factors that predict outcomes in elderly recipients are limited, especially in China. Accurately determining the possible predictors involved in graft and patient survival is crucial for improving long-term outcomes in elderly recipients.

Therefore, the aim of this study was to evaluate graft and patient survival in kidney transplant recipients aged ≥60 years and to determine the possible recipient-related risk factors associated with clinical outcome.

Patients and Methods

This retrospective cohort study was approved by the Institutional Review Board/Ethics Committee of The First Affiliated Hospital of Sun Yat-sen University, and all aspects of the study complied with the Helsinki Declaration of 1975. The Ethics Committee of The First Affiliated Hospital of Sun Yat-sen University specifically approved that not informed consent was required because all data were going to be analyzed anonymously. All of the organs were from donation after brain death (DBD) or donation after cardiac death (DCD), and all of the organ donors had provided informed written consent. No prisoner organs were used in this study.

All patients aged 60 years or older who underwent first-time kidney transplantation from deceased donors in our center between January 2002 and June 2013 were collected. We excluded patients who had received another organ besides the kidney. The recipient characteristics included age, gender, causes of ESRD, pre-transplant comorbidities [including diabetes mellitus, hypertension, coronary artery disease (CAD)], type and time on dialysis, and panel reactive antibody (PRA) level at transplantation. The induction agents, basic maintained immunosuppressive regimens, and regimens for cytomegalovirus (CMV) prophylaxis were also recorded. After surgery, the number and frequency of adverse events including delayed graft function (DGF), acute rejection (AR) and chronic rejection (CR) at any time, leucopenia, infectious events, graft loss and patient death, malignancy and other new onset diseases were recorded. The causes of graft failure and mortality were also recorded.

Patients received IL-2 receptor antagonist (IL2RA, including basiliximab or daclizumab) or rabbit anti-thymocyte globulin (rATG) as induction agents. The maintained immunosuppressive regimens consisted of cyclosporine or tacrolimus, mycophenolate mofetil (MMF) and prednisone. From 2002 to 2006, most of the recipients received a low-dose ganciclovir (1.5 g/d for 3 months) for CMV prophylaxis, whereas patients mainly received a high-dose ganciclovir (3.0 g/d for 3 months) since 2007. Sulfamethoxazole was administered orally for 3 months for Pneumocystis jirovecii pneumonia prophylaxis.

DGF was defined as the need for dialysis in the first week after transplantation. AR was diagnosed based on clinical manifestations such as fever, oliguria, and serum creatinine elevation of > 25% from the baseline value and was confirmed by a subsequent renal allograft biopsy. Biopsy-proven acute rejections (BPAR) included all acute rejections which were graded borderline or higher by Banff'97 criteria. CR was diagnosed by clinical findings with a decrease in kidney function and developing a gradual rise in serum creatinine, and was confirmed by renal allograft biopsy with histological features including thickening of the intima of arterioles and arteries, sclerosis of glomeruli, and tabular atrophy.

Statistical analysis

All data were analyzed by SPSS for Windows Version 19.0 (SPSS, Chicago, Illinois, USA). Continuous variables are expressed as counts and percentages, and categorical variables are expressed as the means with standard deviations (mean ± SD). Actuarial graft and patient survival were calculated using Kaplan–Meier analysis. To assess variables associated with transplant outcome, univariate and multivariate Cox proportional hazards regression models were employed. The association between outcomes and all co-variables were tested separately in univariate Cox analyses. To evaluate the potential independent risk factors for transplant outcomes, all variables associated with graft loss or patient death at a $P<0.2$ level in the univariate Cox analysis were included in the final multivariate model. A P-value <0.05 was considered to indicate statistical significance.

Results

Patient characteristics

We collected data from 166 primary deceased kidney transplant recipients aged 60 or older between January 2002 and June 2013. The demographic and baseline characteristics of these elderly patients are shown in Table 1. The mean recipient age was 64.6±3.8 years, and 109 (65.7%) recipients were male. The main cause of ESRD was chronic glomerulonephritis, followed by diabetes mellitus. Hypertension was the most prevalent comorbidity in these aged recipients. The mean duration of dialysis was 18.6±22.1 months. Initial immunosuppressive induction therapy based on IL2RA was 68.1% and that based on rATG was 31.9%. At baseline, 56.6% and 43.4% of patients were on cyclosporine-based and tacrolimus-based immunosuppression, respectively; for CMV prophylaxis, 101 (60.8%) recipients received low-dose ganciclovir (1.5 g/d for 3 months), and 65 (39.2%) received high-dose ganciclovir (3.0 g/d for 3 months).

Graft and patient survival

The adverse events during the 5-year follow-up are shown in Table 2. The incidence of DGF, AR and chronic rejection (CR) was 9%, 16.9% and 8.3%, respectively. Infection was the most common adverse event in the elderly patients, with an incidence of 55.4%. The incidence of CMV infection was 17.5%, and most of which occurred in the first year post-transplantation. A total of 36 patients experienced graft loss and 29 patients died within 5-year follow-up. Overall and death-censored graft survival and patient survival are shown in Figure 1. The 1-, 3-, 5-year overall graft survival was 84.3%, 78% and 70.6%, respectively. However, when patient death was not considered as graft loss (death-censored), the 1-, 3-, 5-year graft survival reached 93.6%, 89.4% and 83.6%, respectively. Patient survival was 84.8% at 1 year, 82.1% at 3 year and 77.1% at 5 year. The causes of graft loss and patient death are shown in Table 3. The main causes of graft loss were patient death (52.8%) and AR (16.7%). Most of the patients died of infection (55.2%) and CAD (17.2%). In addition, among the infectious mortality, there were 11 deaths due to severe CMV disease.

Risk factors for graft loss

During a 5-year follow-up, there were 36 cases of graft loss in the cohort. More than half of the graft losses (52.8%) were due to patient death. Univariate analysis showed that longer dialysis time, PRA>5%, DGF and AR were risk factors for death-censored graft loss. Based on the Cox multivariate models, a PRA>5% [hazard ratio (HR) 4.295, 95% confidence interval (CI) 1.321–13.97], DGF (HR 4.744, 95% CI 1.611–13.973) and AR (HR 4.971, 95% CI 1.516–16.301) remained independent risk factors for death-censored graft loss, except for longer dialysis time (Table 4). The status of comorbidities, including diabetes mellitus, hypertension and CAD were not associated with shorter graft survival.

Risk factors for patient death

There were 29 deaths during the 5-year follow-up. The risk factors for patient death were shown in Table 5. Univariate analysis showed that longer dialysis time, AR, graft loss and low-dose ganciclovir prophylaxis were risk factors for patient death. However, when data was analysis by final Cox multivariate model, we found that longer dialysis time (HR 1.011 for 1-month increase, 95% CI 1.002–1.020), graft loss (HR 3.501, 95% CI 1.559–7.865) and low-dose ganciclovir prophylaxis (HR 3.173,

Table 1. Recipient baseline characteristics (N = 166).

Recipient age, yr (mean±SD)	64.6±3.8	Dialysis, n (%)	
Male recipients, n (%)	109 (65.7)	Nondialysis	46 (27.7)
Cause of ESRD, n (%)		Hemodialysis	87 (52.4)
Chronic glomerulonephritis	73 (44)	Peritoneal dialysis	33 (19.9)
Diabetes mellitus	51 (30.7)	Time on dialysis, months (mean±SD)	18.6±22.1
Hypertension	19 (11.4)	PRA>5%, n (%)	16 (9.6)
Obstructive nephropathy	7 (4.2)	IL2RA, n (%)	113 (68.1)
Polycystic kidney	6 (3.6)	rATG, n (%)	53 (31.9)
Others or unknown	10 (6)	Cyclosporine, n (%)	94 (56.6)
Comorbidities, n (%)		Tacrolimus, n (%)	72 (43.4)
Diabetes mellitus	70 (42.1)	Low-dose ganciclovir (1.5 g/d), n (%)	101 (60.8)
Hypertension	120 (72.3)	High-dose ganciclovir (3.0 g/d), n (%)	65 (39.2)
Coronary artery disease (CAD)	24 (14.5)		

95% CI 1.063–9.473) remained significant independent risk factors for mortality. AR, diabetes mellitus, hypertension, CAD, and DGF were not significantly associated with patient death.

Discussion

The rapid increase in elderly patients with ESRD has raised an important issue regarding the optimization of long-term outcomes in this population. Despite a higher percentage of cadaveric kidney donors being allocated to older patients, the short-term graft survival is excellent in the majority of these patients. However, longer-term graft survival in the elderly recipients is less than expected due to death with a functioning graft, which is the major cause of graft loss. Elderly renal transplant recipients are at increased risk of graft loss and death compared with younger cohorts [7,8]. Considering the rapid growth of an aging ESRD population and the shortage of donor kidneys, identifying the possible risk factors of graft and patient survival in elderly recipients is crucial for improving their long-term outcome.

In this study, we retrospectively analyzed 166 cases of renal transplantation from deceased donors in recipients aged ≥60 years and identified the possible risk factors predicting poor clinical outcome. Consistent with previous studies, death with a functioning graft is the leading cause of graft loss in elderly patients, with a percentage of more than 50% [9]. When patient death was not considered as the cause of graft loss, the 1-, 3-, 5-year graft survival reached 93.6%, 89.4% and 83.6%, respectively. Similar to previous studies, a PRA>5% at the time of transplantation was

Table 2. Adverse events in 5-year follow-up.

Adverse events	n (%)
DGF	15 (9)
AR	28 (16.9)
CR	3 (8.3)
Leukopenia	9 (5.4)
All infections	92 (55.4)
Urinary tract	7 (4.2)
Probable bacterial or other	35 (21.1)
Confirmed bacterial	64 (38.6)
CMV	29 (17.5)
BK polyoma virus	1 (0.6)
Fungal	10 (6)
Liver impairment	39 (23.5)
New onset diabetes mellitus	18 (10.8)
Congestive heart failure	8 (4.8)
Cerebrovascular accident	4 (2.4)
Malignancy	9 (5.4)
Graft loss	36 (21.7)
Death	29 (17.5)

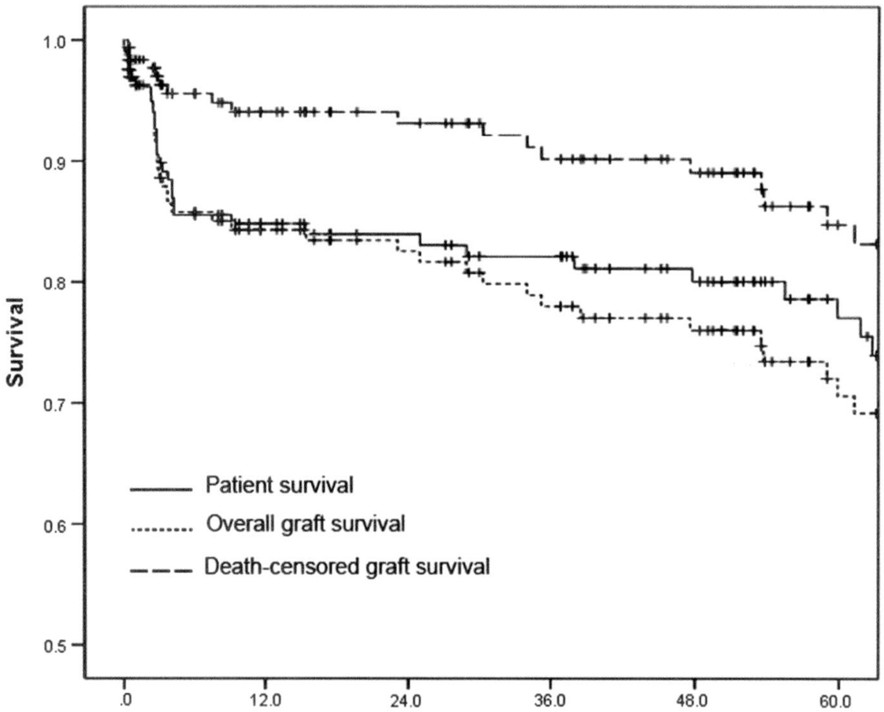

Number at risk					
Patient survival	144	143	141	139	137
Overall graft survival	143	141	136	134	130
Death-censored graft survival	157	156	153	152	149

Figure 1. Patient survival, overall and death-censored graft survival.

a significant independent risk factor for graft loss in recipients aged ≥60 years. Heldal et al. [10] reported a PRA>5% as a risk factor for graft loss in patients aged ≥70 years, whereas Faravardeh et al. [11] demonstrated that a PRA>10% was a risk factor for graft failure in recipients aged ≥65 years.

In our study, we found that patients aged ≥60 years experienced a low incidence of AR episodes, which were similar to previous findings [12]. Although the incidence of AR was lower in the elderly transplant recipients, the impact of AR episodes was far more severe than in the young recipients [13]. We found that both DGF and AR were risk factors for graft loss in recipients aged ≥60 years. Heldal et al. [10] reported that DGF was an independent predictor for death-censored graft loss in the elderly recipients aged 60 years or older. Similarly, in the study by Faravardeh et al. [11], DGF and AR were risk factors for graft failure not only in younger recipients but also in elderly cohorts aged ≥65 years. In a multicenter case-control study in Spain, Moreso et al. [14] also confirmed that AR was an independent predictor of death-censored graft failure in adult renal transplant recipients. However, in another prospective multicenter study performed in Spain, the authors did not find any significant association between AR and allograft loss in neither recipients

Table 3. Causes of graft loss and mortality (5 years).

Graft loss (N = 36)	n (%)	Mortality (N = 29)	n (%)
Patient death	19 (52.8)	Infection	16 (55.2)
AR	6 (16.7)	CAD	5 (17.2)
CR	3 (8.3)	Cerebrovascular accident	2 (6.9)
Chronic allograft nephropathy	4 (11.1)	Malignancy	3 (10.3)
Recurrence	1 (2.8)	Liver disease	1 (3.5)
ARF	1 (2.8)	Hemorrhage	1 (3.5)
PNF	1 (2.8)	Unknown	1 (3.5)
Technical failure	1 (2.8)		

ARF, acute renal failure; PNF, primary no function.

Table 4. Risk factors for death-censored graft loss (5 years).

Variables	Univariate analysis			Cox multivariate analysis		
	HR	95% CI	P value	HR	95% CI	P value
Age (1-year increase)	1.059	0.95–1.179	0.3	—	—	—
Gender (male vs female)	1.255	0.464–3.397	0.655	—	—	—
Dialysis time (1-month increase)	1.013	1.001–1.026	0.028	1.014	0.999–1.029	0.061
Diabetes mellitus	0.624	0.231–1.691	0.354	—	—	—
Hypertension	2.016	0.458–8.866	0.353	—	—	—
CAD	0.638	0.146–2.795	0.551	—	—	—
PRA>5%	10.503	4.037–27.325	<0.001	4.295	1.321–13.97	0.015
Induction (IL2RA vs rATG)	0.553	0.156–1.959	0.359	—	—	—
Cyclosporin vs tacrolimus	2.05	0.778–5.396	0.146	1.322	0.495–3.534	0.577
DGF	5.908	2.059–16.954	0.001	4.744	1.611–13.973	0.005
AR	6.782	2.612–17.609	<0.001	4.971	1.516–16.301	0.008

HR, hazard ratio; CI, confidence interval.

aged ≥60 years nor in younger recipients [15]. Nevertheless, AR and DGF can result in functional and structural damage to the graft, which leads to late poor graft outcomes. Therefore, a decrease in the incidence of AR or DGF may result in an improvement of late graft outcome.

The literature on the association between duration of dialysis and transplant outcome is rich and at times inconsistent. Most of the studies reported that longer duration of dialysis was associated with poorer patient and graft outcome in kidney transplant recipients [16,17,18], whereas some other studies didn't find any association between dialysis duration and patient or graft survival [15]. In addition, there are also some studies reported that longer time on dialysis was independent risk factor only for patient death, but not for graft loss [9,19]. In the study by Faravardeh et al. [11], the authors reported that longer dialysis time was a risk factor for graft loss and mortality in recipients aged <50 years, but not in those aged ≥50 years. Therefore, the risk of transplant outcome associated with increased dialysis duration time may differ between various countries and populations. In this retrospective study, we demonstrated that increased time on dialysis was an independent risk factor for patient death. Since the maintenance of dialysis status may accelerate cardiovascular changes, including vascular calcification, left ventricular hypertrophy and congestive heart failure [20], longer time on dialysis may result in an increased risk of death, especially in the elderly with a higher incidence of vascular complications. In the current study, we did not find longer duration of dialysis to be a significant independent risk factor for graft failure in multivariate Cox regression model. This finding may be explained by the fact that the elderly may differ somewhat from the younger population, since the incidence of acute rejection appears to steadily reduce with increased age [1]. In addition, the mean duration of pretransplant dialysis in our cohort is 18.6 months, which is relatively short compared to previous studies. Furthermore, the relatively small sample may somewhat weaken the impact of dialysis time on graft survival.

Table 5. Risk factors for patient death (5 years).

Variables	Univariate analysis			Cox multivariate analysis		
	HR	95% CI	P value	HR	95% CI	P value
Age (1-year increase)	1.068	0.974–1.171	0.16	1.081	0.985–1.186	0.1
Gender (male vs female)	1.243	0.577–2.675	0.579	—	—	—
Dialysis time (1-month increase)	1.013	1.004–1.022	0.004	1.011	1.002–1.020	0.02
Diabetes mellitus	0.713	0.336–1.51	0.377	—	—	—
Hypertension	0.924	0.393–2.171	0.856	—	—	—
CAD	1.412	0.574–3.47	0.452	—	—	—
Induction (IL2RA vs rATG)	0.438	0.166–1.155	0.095	1.627	0.38–6.966	0.512
CsA vs FK506	1.627	0.777–3.407	0.197	1.554	0.735–3.289	0.249
DGF	2.345	0.889–6.185	0.085	2.303	0.856–6.196	0.098
AR	3.595	1.697–7.617	0.001	1.91	0.715–5.101	0.197
Graft loss	4.571	2.073–10.081	<0.001	3.501	1.559–7.865	0.002
Ganciclovir (1.5 g/d vs 3 g/d)	3.947	1.366–11.401	0.011	3.173	1.063–9.473	0.039

Graft failure was a significant risk factor for mortality for patients aged ≥60 years in our study, which was confirmed in previous studies [11]. The increased death rate was partly due to the potential immediate complications of graft loss and longer-term worse survival of returning to dialysis.

CMV infection is a common problem in immunocompromised hosts and an important cause of morbidity and mortality in kidney transplant recipients [21]. Previous studies had demonstrated that CMV infection was associated with acute and chronic graft rejection [22], increased incidence of opportunistic infection [23], graft loss and decreased recipient survival [24]. Universal prophylaxis with effective antiviral agents is one of the possible approaches for prevention of CMV infection. In China, ganciclovir remains the preferred agent for prophylaxis and treatment of CMV infection due to its effectiveness and affordable price to most patients. The study by Ahmed and colleagues demonstrated that low-dose ganciclovir (1.0 g/d for 3 months) was as effective at decreasing the incidence of clinical CMV disease as high-dose ganciclovir (3.0 g/d for 3–6 months) in renal transplant recipients [25]. However, in the present study, we found that a low-dose ganciclovir (1.5 g/d for 3 months) was significantly associated with shorter patient survival in elderly recipients. This difference could be explained by the fact that the mean age of Ahmed's recipients was 46.1±2.2 years, which was much lower than those in our study. Elderly patients are thought to generate a less robust immune response due to a decreased immunogenicity with increased age [26] combined with more pre-transplant comorbidities, which may increase the overall risk of infectious death in elderly transplant recipients [27,28]. Low-dose ganciclovir may be not as effective as high-dose ganciclovir for CMV prophylaxis in elderly recipients. Therefore, it is important to widely use a high-dose ganciclovir to decrease the incidence of CMV infection in the more susceptible population such as the elderly renal transplant recipients.

CAD was one of the most common comorbidities and causes of death in elderly recipients. Faravardeh et al. [11] reported that CAD was a risk factor for mortality in both recipients aged ≥65 years and the younger cohort aged <50 years, while Heldal et al. [10] found that CAD increased mortality in transplant recipients up to 70 years but not in older recipients. However, in our study, we did not find CAD to be a risk factor for mortality in patients aged ≥60 years at transplantation, which was consistent with Doyle's finding [29]. The lower prevalence of CAD in the elderly recipients may be a likely explanation for our finding because there were fewer patients with CAD in our cohort and this likely led to a loss of some power to detect the significance of this factor. This is not surprising, as China is known traditionally for low incidence of CAD and low plasma cholesterol levels due to the Chinese diet and lifestyle [30,31]. Although the incidence of CAD has increased in the last 2 decades, the incidence attained is still significantly lower than that in the Western countries [32]. Furthermore, the morbidity and mortality of CAD is much lower in south China compared with in the north [30]. Since all of the patients included were from south of China, it is reasonable that the number and proportion of CAD was low in our study. Similar to previous studies, we did not find an association between diabetes and patient survival [9,29,33]. We also did not find hypertension as a significant risk factor for graft failure or patient death.

Our study has certain limitations inherent in its retrospective nature because data were collected from patients transplanted from 2002 to June 2013. There were certain patients missing in the follow-up (10.5% of the overall cohort), which may reduce potential adverse effects of various risk factors that would be observed over a longer-term. In addition, the relatively small sample size might have less power to detect the effect of variables that have a smaller impact on the poor clinical outcome.

In conclusion, the transplant outcomes are excellent among recipients aged 60 years or older. We found that PRA>5%, DGF and AR were risk factors for graft failure, while longer time on dialysis, failed grafts and low-dose ganciclovir prophylaxis were risk factors for mortality in recipients aged ≥60 years. These factors represent potential targets for interventions aimed at improving graft and patient survival in elderly recipients. Therefore, reducing PRA level and decreasing the incidence of DGF and AR may result in longer graft survival, while shortening the duration of dialysis may lead to longer patient survival. In addition, high-dose ganciclovir prophylaxis should be widely used in elderly recipient to decrease the incidence of CMV infection. Nevertheless, further prospective, randomized and multicenter studies are needed to confirm these findings.

Author Contributions

Conceived and designed the experiments: XQL GDC. Performed the experiments: XQL GDC. Analyzed the data: XQL GDC. Contributed reagents/materials/analysis tools: GDC JQ CXW LZC. Wrote the paper: XQL GDC. Finalized the manuscript: XQL GDC. Read and approved the final manuscript: LZC.

References

1. Danovitch GM, Gill J, Bunnapradist S (2007) Immunosuppression of the elderly kidney transplant recipient. Transplantation 84: 285–291.
2. McCullough KP, Keith DS, Meyer KH, Stock PG, Brayman KL, et al. (2009) Kidney and pancreas transplantation in the United States, 1998–2007: access for patients with diabetes and end-stage renal disease. Am J Transplant 9: 894–906.
3. Wolfe RA, Ashby VB, Milford EL, Ojo AO, Ettenger RE, et al. (1999) Comparison of mortality in all patients on dialysis, patients on dialysis awaiting transplantation, and recipients of a first cadaveric transplant. N Engl J Med 341: 1725–1730.
4. Johnson DW, Herzig K, Purdie D, Brown AM, Rigby RJ, et al. (2000) A comparison of the effects of dialysis and renal transplantation on the survival of older uremic patients. Transplantation 69: 794–799.
5. Oniscu GC, Brown H, Forsythe JL (2004) How great is the survival advantage of transplantation over dialysis in elderly patients? Nephrol Dial Transplant 19: 945–951.
6. Meier-Kriesche HU, Schold JD, Srinivas TR, Kaplan B (2004) Lack of improvement in renal allograft survival despite a marked decrease in acute rejection rates over the most recent era. Am J Transplant 4: 378–383.
7. Roodnat JI, Zietse R, Mulder PG, Rischen-Vos J, van Gelder T, et al. (1999) The vanishing importance of age in renal transplantation. Transplantation 67: 576–580.
8. Meier-Kriesche H, Ojo AO, Arndorfer JA, Port FK, Magee JC, et al. (2001) Recipient age as an independent risk factor for chronic renal allograft failure. Transplant Proc 33: 1113–1114.
9. Cardinal H, Hebert MJ, Rahme E, Houde I, Baran D, et al. (2005) Modifiable factors predicting patient survival in elderly kidney transplant recipients. Kidney Int 68: 345–351.
10. Heldal K, Hartmann A, Leivestad T, Svendsen MV, Foss A, et al. (2009) Clinical outcomes in elderly kidney transplant recipients are related to acute rejection episodes rather than pretransplant comorbidity. Transplantation 87: 1045–1051.
11. Faravardeh A, Eickhoff M, Jackson S, Spong R, Kukla A, et al. (2013) Predictors of graft failure and death in elderly kidney transplant recipients. Transplantation 96: 1089–1096.
12. Patel SJ, Knight RJ, Suki WN, Abdellatif A, Duhart BJ, et al. (2011) Rabbit antithymocyte induction and dosing in deceased donor renal transplant recipients over 60 yr of age. Clin Transplant 25: E250–E256.
13. Meier-Kriesche HU, Srinivas TR, Kaplan B (2001) Interaction between acute rejection and recipient age on long-term renal allograft survival. Transplant Proc 33: 3425–3426.
14. Moreso F, Alonso A, Gentil MA, Gonzalez-Molina M, Capdevila L, et al. (2010) Improvement in late renal allograft survival between 1990 and 2002 in Spain: results from a multicentre case-control study. Transpl Int 23: 907–913.

15. Morales JM, Marcen R, Del CD, Andres A, Gonzalez-Molina M, et al. (2012) Risk factors for graft loss and mortality after renal transplantation according to recipient age: a prospective multicentre study. Nephrol Dial Transplant 27 Suppl 4: v39–v46.
16. Meier-Kriesche HU, Port FK, Ojo AO, Rudich SM, Hanson JA, et al. (2000) Effect of waiting time on renal transplant outcome. Kidney Int 58: 1311–1317.
17. Goldfarb-Rumyantzev A, Hurdle JF, Scandling J, Wang Z, Baird B, et al. (2005) Duration of end-stage renal disease and kidney transplant outcome. Nephrol Dial Transplant 20: 167–175.
18. Remport A, Keszei A, Vamos EP, Novak M, Jaray J, et al. (2011) Association of pre-transplant dialysis duration with outcome in kidney transplant recipients: a prevalent cohort study. Int Urol Nephrol 43: 215–224.
19. Helantera I, Salmela K, Kyllonen L, Koskinen P, Gronhagen-Riska C, et al. (2014) Pretransplant dialysis duration and risk of death after kidney transplantation in the current era. Transplantation 98: 458–464.
20. Himmelfarb J, Ikizler TA (2010) Hemodialysis. N Engl J Med 363: 1833–1845.
21. Brennan DC (2001) Cytomegalovirus in renal transplantation. J Am Soc Nephrol 12: 848–855.
22. Cainelli F, Vento S (2002) Infections and solid organ transplant rejection: a cause-and-effect relationship? Lancet Infect Dis 2: 539–549.
23. George MJ, Snydman DR, Werner BG, Griffith J, Falagas ME, et al. (1997) The independent role of cytomegalovirus as a risk factor for invasive fungal disease in orthotopic liver transplant recipients. Boston Center for Liver Transplantation CMVIG-Study Group. Cytogam, MedImmune, Inc. Gaithersburg, Maryland. Am J Med 103: 106–113.
24. De Keyzer K, Van Laecke S, Peeters P, Vanholder R (2011) Human cytomegalovirus and kidney transplantation: a clinician's update. Am J Kidney Dis 58: 118–126.
25. Ahmed J, Velarde C, Ramos M, Ismail K, Serpa J, et al. (2004) Outcome of low-dose ganciclovir for cytomegalovirus disease prophylaxis in renal-transplant recipients. Transplantation 78: 1689–1692.
26. Martins PN, Pratschke J, Pascher A, Fritsche L, Frei U, et al. (2005) Age and immune response in organ transplantation. Transplantation 79: 127–132.
27. Meier-Kriesche HU, Ojo AO, Hanson JA, Kaplan B (2001) Exponentially increased risk of infectious death in older renal transplant recipients. Kidney Int 59: 1539–1543.
28. Kauffman HM, McBride MA, Cors CS, Roza AM, Wynn JJ (2007) Early mortality rates in older kidney recipients with comorbid risk factors. Transplantation 83: 404–410.
29. Doyle SE, Matas AJ, Gillingham K, Rosenberg ME (2000) Predicting clinical outcome in the elderly renal transplant recipient. Kidney Int 57: 2144–2150.
30. Tao SC, Huang ZD, Wu XG, Zhou BF, Xiao ZK, et al. (1989) CHD and its risk factors in the People's Republic of China. Int J Epidemiol 18: S159–S163.
31. Campbell TC, Parpia B, Chen J (1998) Diet, lifestyle, and the etiology of coronary artery disease: the Cornell China study. Am J Cardiol 82: 18T–21T.
32. Ueshima H, Sekikawa A, Miura K, Turin TC, Takashima N, et al. (2008) Cardiovascular disease and risk factors in Asia: a selected review. Circulation 118: 2702–2709.
33. Fabrizii V, Winkelmayer WC, Klauser R, Kletzmayr J, Saemann MD, et al. (2004) Patient and graft survival in older kidney transplant recipients: does age matter? J Am Soc Nephrol 15: 1052–1060.

Acinetobacter Peritoneal Dialysis Peritonitis: A Changing Landscape over Time

Chia-Ter Chao[1,2], Szu-Ying Lee[3], Wei-Shun Yang[4], Huei-Wen Chen[5], Cheng-Chung Fang[6], Chung-Jen Yen[7], Chih-Kang Chiang[8], Kuan-Yu Hung[5], Jenq-Wen Huang[5]*

1 Division of Nephrology, Department of Internal Medicine, National Taiwan University Hospital Jin-Shan Branch, New Taipei City, Taiwan, **2** Graduate Institute of Toxicology, National Taiwan University, Taipei, Taiwan, **3** Division of Nephrology, Department of Internal Medicine, National Taiwan University Hospital Yun-Lin Branch, Yun-Lin County, Taiwan, **4** Division of Nephrology, Department of Internal Medicine, National Taiwan University Hospital Hsin-Chu Branch, Hsin-Chu County, Taiwan, **5** Division of Nephrology, Department of Internal Medicine, National Taiwan University Hospital, Taipei, Taiwan, **6** Department of Emergency Medicine, National Taiwan University Hospital, Taipei, Taiwan, **7** Department of Geriatrics and Gerontology, National Taiwan University Hospital, Taipei, Taiwan, **8** Department of Integrative diagnostics and Therapeutics, National Taiwan University Hospital, Taipei, Taiwan

Abstract

Background: *Acinetobacter* species are assuming an increasingly important role in modern medicine, with their persistent presence in health-care settings and antibiotic resistance. However, clinical reports addressing this issue in patients with peritoneal dialysis (PD) peritonitis are rare.

Methods: All PD peritonitis episodes caused by *Acinetobacter* that occurred between 1985 and 2012 at a single centre were retrospectively reviewed. Clinical features, microbiological data, and outcomes were analysed, with stratifications based upon temporal periods (before and after 2000).

Results: *Acinetobacter* species were responsible for 26 PD peritonitis episodes (3.5% of all episodes) in 25 patients. *A. baumannii* was the most common pathogen (54%), followed by *A. iwoffii* (35%), with the former being predominant after 2000. Significantly more episodes resulted from breaks in exchange sterility after 2000, while those from exit site infections decreased ($P = 0.01$). The interval between the last and current peritonitis episodes lengthened significantly after 2000 (5 vs. 13.6 months; $P = 0.05$). All the isolates were susceptible to cefepime, fluoroquinolone, and aminoglycosides, with a low ceftazidime resistance rate (16%). Nearly half of the patients (46%) required hospitalisation for their *Acinetobacter* PD-associated peritonitis, and 27% required an antibiotic switch. The overall outcome was fair, with no mortality and a 12% technique failure rate, without obvious interval differences.

Conclusions: The temporal change in the microbiology and origin of *Acinetobacter* PD-associated peritonitis in our cohort suggested an important evolutional trend. Appropriate measures, including technique re-education and sterility maintenance, should be taken to decrease the *Acinetobacter* peritonitis incidence in PD patients.

Editor: Shamala Devi Sekaran, University of Malaya, Malaysia

Funding: This study is financially supported by National Taiwan University Hospital intramural fund (project NO. 102-N2249). The funders had no role in study design, data collection and analysis, decision to publish, or preparation of the manuscript.

Competing Interests: The authors have declared that no competing interests exist.

* Email: 007378@ntuh.gov.tw

Introduction

The utilisation of peritoneal dialysis (PD) in end-stage renal disease (ESRD) has been long purported for its economical advantage and similar effects on patient outcomes compared with haemodialysis (HD) [1,2]. However, the underuse of PD in most countries could be attributable to several factors, including the infectious complications [1,3]. Among these complications, PD-associated peritonitis is the most dreadful, accounting for 8% to 21% of infection-related mortality and 30% of technique failures [4,5]. Gram-negative bacteria (GNB) cause 25% to 40% of PD peritonitis episodes worldwide, secondary to gram-positive bacteria, and the number is still increasing [6,7].

Among GNB peritonitis, the acronym SPICE (*Serratia*, *Providencia*, indole-positive *Proteus/Acinetobacter/Morganella*, *Citrobacter*, *Enterobacter*, or *Hafnia*) denotes a spectrum of organisms with an intrinsic tendency for antibiotic resistance [8]. These pathogens demonstrate inducible beta-lactamase during initial therapy, potentially leading to empirical regimen failure, prolonged peritoneal damage, and worse outcomes [9]. In the ANZDATA registry, the SPICE group of pathogens accounts for 26.9% of all non-*Pseudomonas* GNB PD-associated peritonitis, and *Acinetobacter* species are responsible for <20% of these cases [10,11]. Intuitively thinking, patients with *Acinetobacter* PD-associated peritonitis might have poorer prognoses compared with the other Enterobacteriaceae members, owing to their high antibiotic resistance rates. However, past reports suggested just the opposite, with technique failure rates of 9% [12] and 9.2% [13] in several studies. In addition, several researchers proposed that *Acinetobacter* peritonitis might occur with an immunocompromised status [12,14]. These reports were all published nearly 2 decades ago, and the temporal changes of clinical characteristics, microbiologic features, and outcomes of patients with *Acinetobacter* PD peritonitis are unknown. Utilising a longitudinal PD registry of more than 2 decades in a single centre, we conducted the present study to explore the transition of these parameters over different time periods.

Subjects and Methods

Ethical considerations

The ethics committee of the NTUH approved the current study (No. 201212165RINC). The local institutional review board did not mandate patient consent, as no interventions were performed and patient privacy was not breached. The local institutional review board waived the need for written informed consent from the participants.

Study design and setting

In 1985, the National Taiwan University Hospital (NTUH) PD program was established [9,15]. Patients with ESRD who underwent PD for >3 months were eligible for the present study. Patients with episodes of culture-confirmed *Acinetobacter* species PD peritonitis between 1985 and 2012 were selected. Peritonitis was diagnosed according to the presence of symptomatology and cloudy effluent, with a white blood cell count >100/μL and neutrophil percentage >50% [5].

Clinical data collection

All enrolees' demographic profiles, including age, sex, and comorbidities (diabetes mellitus [DM], heart failure [HF], and autoimmune diseases), were reviewed [16,17]. The aetiologies of their ESRD were also documented. Through a chart review, patients' medications, including steroid, immunosuppressant, and antibiotic use, within 1 month before the selected peritonitis episodes were recorded, along with laboratory data.

For each peritonitis episode caused by *Acinetobacter*, we documented the PD vintage and modality (continuous ambulatory peritoneal dialysis [CAPD] or automated peritoneal dialysis [APD]) and the initial symptoms. Laboratory data during the peritonitis episodes were obtained. Pathogen species and the corresponding antibiogram were identified. The presumptive origins of each peritonitis episode were divided into a break in sterility during the exchange procedure, gastrointestinal (GI) microflora transmural migration, exit site infection/tunnel infection, or undetermined, according to past reports [18,19]. Empirical antibiotic regimens for PD peritonitis in our institute were as follows: first-generation cephalosporin with aminoglycoside before 1998 and first-generation cephalosporin with third-generation cephalosporin after 1998, according to the recommendations of the International Society for Peritoneal Dialysis (ISPD), unless otherwise indicated [5,9,15,20,21].

Outcome variables

The outcome measures in the present study consisted of primary response, antibiotic switch (secondary response), relapse peritonitis, repeat peritonitis, Tenckhoff catheter removal, and patient death. The primary response was defined as symptomatic improvement of the patient within 3 days of receiving empirical antibiotics, accompanied by effluent leukocyte count <100/μL. The secondary response was defined as a response to the second-line antibiotics when effluent did not turn clear after first-line antibiotic use [9,15]. If an antibiotic switch occurred, the duration of empirical antibiotic use was also recorded. Repeat peritonitis was defined as peritonitis recurring 4 weeks after the previous episode, whereas relapse peritonitis was defined as peritonitis recurring within 4 weeks after the treatment of the previous episode, both involving the same pathogen [5,21]. Peritonitis-related death was considered if the patient's death occurred within 1 month of the peritonitis episode and was attributable to peritonitis [9,15].

Results

During the study period, 369 of 1278 chronic PD patients developed 744 episodes of PD-related peritonitis over 40,499 patient-months, with an overall peritonitis incidence of 1 per 54 patient-months (before 2000, 1 per 37 patient-months; after 2000, 1 per 64 patient-months). Among the 744 episodes of PD-related peritonitis, 25 patients developed 26 peritonitis episodes from *Acinetobacter* species (3.5% of all episodes), with an incidence of 1 per 1558 patient-months. One patient developed 2 separate episodes of *Acinetobacter* peritonitis, and the remaining patients each experienced 1 episode. To delineate the temporal changes of their clinical features, we divided the *Acinetobacter* peritonitis cohort into 2 phases, those that occurred before 2000 and those that occurred during or after 2000.

Clinical features of Acinetobacter PD-associated peritonitis

The demographic profiles and clinical characteristics of the patients who developed PD-related peritonitis caused by *Acinetobacter* are listed in Table 1, according to the time of onset. Overall, the mean age and PD vintage of the patients with *Acinetobacter* peritonitis were 52 years and 29 months, respectively, without differences between phases. Three-fourths of the patients chose CAPD as their dialysis modality. One-third of *Acinetobacter* peritonitis patients had DM, but only 12% of patients had HF.

The most common aetiologies of ESRD in the *Acinetobacter* peritonitis patients included DM (31%) and chronic glomerulonephritis (31%), followed by lupus (4%) and hypertension (4%). No significant difference was found between those that occurred before 2000 and those that occurred after 2000. Only 1 patient had undergone intra-abdominal surgery (cholecystitis with open cholecystectomy) before developing *Acinetobacter* peritonitis. Another patient received an antibiotic within the month before the current peritonitis episode (cephalexin for cellulitis for 1 week), and still another lupus patient was receiving prednisolone 10 mg daily.

Table 2 shows the relevant features of the current *Acinetobacter* peritonitis episodes. The current peritonitis episode represented the first peritonitis episode in 62% of the patients, and for those who had already developed peritonitis, there were on average 2 episodes before the *Acinetobacter* episodes (Table 2). No significant difference in past peritonitis episode counts was observed between those that occurred before 2000 and those that occurred after 2000, but it was interesting to note that the time from the last peritonitis episode was borderline significantly longer in the after-2000 group ($P = 0.07$; Table 2). To verify this result, we further constructed a diagram comparing latency between the last peritonitis and *Acinetobacter* episodes within the historic cohorts and ours. We observed a temporal evolution of this feature, with lengthening of such latency (Figure 1; $P < 0.01$).

The presenting symptoms of PD-related peritonitis caused by *Acinetobacter* were abdominal pain (85%), followed by nausea/vomiting (31%), fever (27%), and diarrhoea (15%). All the patients exhibited a turbid dialysate. The mean effluent leukocyte count

Table 1. Baseline features of patients with *Acinetobacter* PD-associated peritonitis.

Characteristics	*Total (n = 26)*	*Before 2000 (n = 12)*	*After 2000 (n = 14)*	*P value**
Incidence (one episode per patient-months)	1558	805	2053	<0.01
Age (years)	52 (23–84)	48 (37–71)	55 (23–84)	0.11
Gender (male %)	11 (42)	4 (33)	7 (50)	0.32
Vintage (months)	29 (1–80)	27 (1–80)	31 (3–60)	0.45
Modality (CAPD %)	19 (73)	10 (83)	9 (64)	0.29
Comorbidities				
DM	8 (31)	2 (16)	6 (43)	0.12
Heart failure	3 (12)	3 (25)	0 (0)	0.08
Autoimmune disorders	2 (8)	1 (8)	1 (7)	0.96
ESRD aetiology				0.15
DM	8 (31)	2 (16)	6 (43)	
CGN	8 (31)	4 (33)	4 (29)	
Hypertension	1 (4)	0 (0)	1 (7)	
Lupus	1 (4)	1 (8)	0 (0)	
Congenital renal dysplasia	1 (4)	0 (0)	1 (7)	
Unknown	7 (23)	5 (42)	2 (7)	
Laboratory data				
Albumin (mg/dL)	3.7 (2.5–4.2)	3.6 (2.5–4.2)	3.7 (2.6–4.2)	0.36
Hemoglobin (g/dL)	9.6 (6.3–13.8)	8.4 (6.3–13.8)	10.6 (8.4–11.7)	0.01
Creatinine (mg/dL)	11 (7.1–16.1)	12.2 (8.8–16.1)	10 (7.1–14.4)	0.07
Total cholesterol (mg/dL)	187.8 (113–321)	198 (124–321)	179.1 (113–267)	0.38

*Comparison between before-2000 group and after-2000 group.
Continuous variables are expressed in mean (ranges), while categorical variables are expressed in number (percentage in parentheses).
Abbreviations: CAPD, continuous ambulatory peritoneal dialysis; CGN, chronic glomerulonephritis; DM, diabetes mellitus; ESRD, end-stage renal disease.

was 5296/μL (range, 148–13,300/μL), with 95% neutrophils (range, 90–98%). The initial blood leukocyte levels were 8094/μL (range, 3400–15,930/μL), with 82% neutrophils (range, 55–94%). The most common species from the effluent was *Acinetobacter baumannii* (54%), followed by *A. iwoffii* (35%), *A. ursingii* (4%), and *A. junii* (4%). *A. baumannii* was the predominant pathogen after 2000, while *A. iwoffii* outnumbered the others before 2000 ($P = 0.01$; Table 2). Two episodes (8%) showed polymicrobial growth (both involved *A. baumannii* and occurred after 2000). Coagulase-negative staphylococci and *Acremonium* species were each responsible for 1 episode of polymicrobial growth. None of the patients had concomitant *Acinetobacter* bacteremia.

The most common identifiable causes of PD-related peritonitis caused by *Acinetobacter* were a break in exchange sterility (19%) and translocation of GI microflora (19%), followed by exit site infection/tunnel infection (8%; Table 2). Approximately half of the episodes did not have an identifiable origin. It is interesting to speculate that an exchange sterility break emerged as the predominant origin of *Acinetobacter* peritonitis after 2000, while the proportions of causes related to exit site infection/tunnel infection and unidentified peritonitis declined significantly after 2000 ($P<0.01$).

The antibiotic susceptibilities of the *Acinetobacter* species are shown in Table 2. All the identified *Acinetobacter* species were susceptible to aminoglycosides (including gentamicin and amikacin), fluoroquinolones, and a fourth-generation cephalosporin (cefepime) after 1995. Approximately 16% of *Acinetobacter* species were non-susceptible to ceftazidime, among which three-fourths were resistant. In addition, 8% of isolates showed intermediate resistance to piperacillin, while 4% were resistant to ticarcillin. Intraperitoneal cefazolin/ceftazidime was initially used in 12 episodes (46%), and intraperitoneal cefazolin/aminoglycosides were used in another 12 episodes (46%; all before 1998). Two patients (8%) were initially treated with intravenous vancomycin/ceftazidime for septic shock. Antibiotics were shifted to intravenous ceftazidime and intraperitoneal gentamicin in 1 patient and intraperitoneal ceftazidime/gentamicin in the other after the patients stabilised with fair responses.

Outcomes of Acinetobacter PD-associated peritonitis

Table 3 lists the clinical outcomes of the patients with PD-related peritonitis caused by *Acinetobacter*. A primary response was achieved in 16 episodes (62%), and after antibiotics, a secondary response was obtained in another 7 episodes (27%). There was no difference between time groups regarding antibiotic response percentage. The average time to antibiotic switch was 4 days (range, 2–9 days), and episodes that occurred after 2000 presented a significantly shorter time to antibiotic switch ($P<0.01$). Those responding to antibiotics were maintained on susceptible antibiotics for an average of 17 days (range, 12–21 days). About half of the episodes (46%) required hospitalisation, with more patients in the after-2000 group admitted ($P = 0.01$) but no significant difference in hospitalisation duration. A total of 3 patients (12%) with PD-related peritonitis caused by *Acinetobacter* had technique failure with catheter removal. The overall outcome was fair. None of the patients with *Acinetobacter* PD-associated

Table 2. Features of *Acinetobacter* PD-associated peritonitis episodes.

Clinical features	*Total (n = 26)*	*Before 2000 (n = 12)*	*After 2000 (n = 14)*	*P value**
Parameters regarding previous episodes				
Previous peritonitis episodes numbers (if present)	2.1 (n = 10)	2 (n = 5)	2.2 (n = 5)	0.77
Time to last peritonitis (months)	9.3 (1–27)	5 (1–13)	13.6 (3–27)	0.05
Most recent PD peritonitis pathogen	Culture-negative (6) Coagulase-negative staphylococci (2) *Enterococcus fecalis* (1) MRSA (1)	Culture-negative (4) Coagulase-negative staphylococci (1)	Culture-negative (2) Coagulase-negative staphylococci (1) *Enterococcus fecalis* (1) MRSA (1)	
Parameters of current episode				
Pathogen				0.01
Acinetobacter baumannii	14 (54)	5 (42)	9 (64)	
Acinetobacter iwoffii	9 (35)	6 (50)	3 (21)	
Acinetobacter ursingii	1 (4)	0 (0)	1 (7)	
Acinetobacter junii	1 (4)	1 (8)	0 (0)	
Unspecified *Acinetobacter*	1 (4)	0 (0)	1 (7)	
Presumed peritonitis origin				<0.01
Break in exchange sterility	5 (19)	0 (0)	5 (36)	
Gastrointestinal bacterial translocation	5 (19)	1 (8)	4 (29)	
Exit site infection or tunnel infection	2 (8)	2 (16)	0 (0)	
Un-identified	14 (54)	9 (75)	5 (36)	
Antibiotic susceptibilities				
Aminoglycosides (gentamicin/amikacin)	**S** 26 (100)	**S** 26 (100)	**S** 26 (100)	
Ceftazidime	**S** 22 (84)	**S** 9 (76)	**S** 13 (93)	
	I 1 (4)	**I** 1 (8)	**I** 0 (0)	
	R 3 (12)	**R** 2 (16)	**R** 1 (7)	
Cefepime	**S** 26 (100)	**S** 26 (100)	**S** 26 (100)	
Ticarcillin	**S** 24 (92)	**S** 10 (84)	**S** 26 (100)	
	I 1 (4)	**I** 1 (8)		
	R 1 (4)	**R** 1 (8)		
Piperacillin	**S** 24 (92)	**S** 10 (84)	**S** 26 (100)	
	I 2 (8)	**I** 2 (16)		
Fluoroquinolone (ciprofloxacin, levofloxacin)	**S** 26 (100)	**S** 26 (100)	**S** 26 (100)	
Carbapenem	**S** 26 (100)	**S** 26 (100)	**S** 26 (100)	

*Comparison between before-2000 group and after-2000 group.
Continuous variables are expressed in mean (ranges), while categorical variables are expressed in number (percentage in parentheses).
Abbreviations: MRSA, methicillin-resistant *Staphylococcus aureus*; PD, peritoneal dialysis.

peritonitis developed relapse or repeat peritonitis, and there was no mortality from such peritonitis.

Discussion

In the present study of *Acinetobacter* peritonitis episodes over more than 20 years, we found that *A. baumannii* was the most common species identified from the effluent, and the leading causes of infection were sterility break and GI microflora translocation. Nearly half required hospitalisation, but the outcome was good, with only 12% of technique failure and no mortality cases. In addition, temporal differences in the clinical features, including the interval between the last and current peritonitis episodes, increased significantly after 2000, along with more episodes from sterility break and less from exit site infection/tunnel infection. However, the fair outcome of *Acinetobacter* peritonitis surprisingly did not change with time.

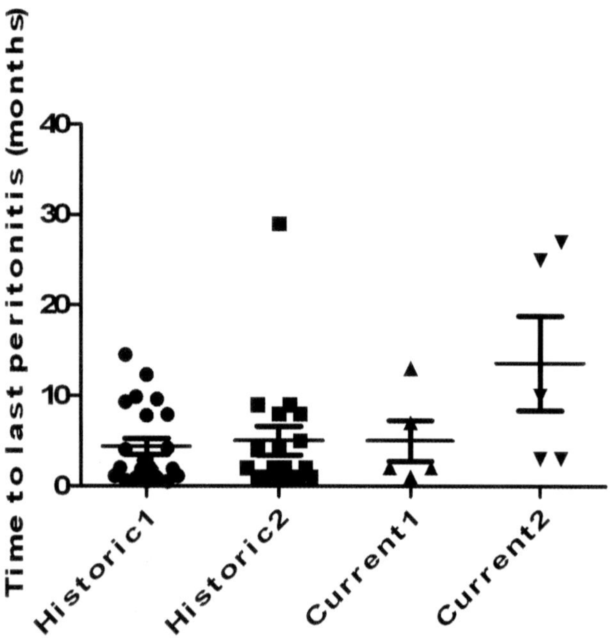

Figure 1. Diagram plotting the distribution of time between the last and current peritonitis episodes in different reports. Our contemporary cohort demonstrated a significantly longer latency compared with the others ($P<0.01$ between the after-2000 cohort and the historic 1 and 2 cohorts). Historic 1 cohort, data derived from *Am J Kidney Dis* 1989; 14(2): 101–4 Historic 2 cohort, data derived from *Perit Dial Int* 1994; 14(2): 174–7.

Compared with past reports of *Acinetobacter* peritonitis, our patients (before 2000) were of similar age and carried a similar percentage of comorbidities (DM and autoimmune disorders; Tables 1 and 4). However, the mean age of the patients with *Acinetobacter* peritonitis seemed to be younger than the others with peritonitis from different pathogens (mean age: historic cohort, 41 years; our cohort, 52 years; ANZDATA, 61–64 years) [7,10]. This might account for the fact that these patients manifested a milder comorbidity profile than the others with peritonitis (Table 1).

Acinetobacter species are strictly aerobic, pleomorphic, and non-motile GNB. To date, 26 named species and 9 genomic species have been identified, among which *A. baumannii* and *Acinetobacter* genomic species 3 and 13TU are collectively referred to as the *A. baumannii* complex [22,23]. Towner and colleagues identified 3 major overlapping populations of *Acinetobacter* species, each with different epidemiologic and microbiologic features [24]. First, *A. baumannii* complex species are prone to develop antibiotic resistance and frequently cause nosocomial outbreaks through their persistent presence in health-care facilities. Second, *A. iwoffii* and *A. johnsonii* are antibiotic-susceptible skin commensal flora of animals and humans, mostly resulting in food spoilage. Finally, *A. calcoaceticus* and other *Acinetobacter* members are ubiquitous colonisers in soil and wastewater, with low virulence and high antibiotic sensitivity. In our PD peritonitis series, the predominant pathogen differed with time; *A. iwoffii* was the predominant offender before 2000 but was replaced by *A. baumannii* after 2000 (Table 2). This seems to suggest that the ecology of *Acinetobacter* breaching the peritoneum has changed temporally, from common skin flora (*A. iwoffii*) to colonisers of health-care settings (*A. baumannii*). This transition might reflect the improvement of exchange systems and increased utilisation of health-care resources as time passed.

Galvao *et al.* proposed that *Acinetobacter* PD peritonitis often occurred during a "vulnerable period, when hosts were immunocompromised," especially in the months immediately following another PD peritonitis episode [12]. This theory was subsequently embraced by other researchers, and the average period between the last peritonitis and *Acinetobacter* episodes was 4 to 5 months at that time (Table 4) [13,14]. However, from our findings (Figure 1), the formerly recognised susceptible period of developing *Acinetobacter* peritonitis seemed vanishing in the modern PD era, and now most episodes did not follow the previous peritonitis as closely as they did in the past. Furthermore, the proportion of PD peritonitis cases from sterility breaks in our cohort also increased significantly after 2000, with a decrease in peritonitis originating

Table 3. Outcomes of *Acinetobacter* PD-associated peritonitis.

Variables	*Total (n = 26)*	*Before 2000 (n = 12)*	*After 2000 (n = 14)*	*P value**
Antibiotics				
Primary response	16 (62)	7 (58)	9 (64)	0.76
Secondary response	7 (27)	3 (25)	4 (29)	0.62
Time to antibiotic switch (days)	4 (2–9)	6 (2–14)	3 (3–5)	<0.01
Total antibiotic duration (days)	17 (12–21)	16 (12–21)	18 (14–21)	0.28
Hospitalization	12 (46)	3 (25)	9 (64)	0.01
Length of stay	13 (5–23)	13 (10–14)	14 (5–23)	0.77
Tenckhoff catheter removal	3 (12)	2 (17)	1 (7)	0.47
Relapse peritonitis	0 (0)	0 (0)	0 (0)	
Repeat peritonitis	0 (0)	0 (0)	0 (0)	
Mortality	0 (0)	0 (0)	0 (0)	

*Comparison between before-2000 group and after-2000 group.
Continuous variables are expressed in mean (ranges), while categorical variables are expressed in number (percentage in parentheses).
Abbreviations: PD, peritoneal dialysis.

from unidentified sources (Tables 2 and 4). We proposed that the development of *Acinetobacter* peritonitis in the modern era might not result from a dysregulated host immune status in PD patients (as before), but more from the hygiene breaks and failure to perform sterile exchange procedures. This phenomenon could be reminiscent of the routes of staphylococci infections.

The choice of treatment for *Acinetobacter* PD-associated peritonitis is contrary to what we might expect if extrapolating from the experiences of hospital-acquired *Acinetobacter* species infections [25]. In our cohort, all isolates were susceptible to aminoglycosides, fourth-generation cephalosporins (available after 1995), and fluoroquinolones, whilst only 10% to 20% were non-susceptible to third-generation cephalosporins or anti-pseudomonal penicillins (Table 2). However, strains with resistance to aminoglycosides or fluoroquinolones did exist (Table 4). Based on the findings of past reports and ours, we propose that fourth-generation cephalosporins might be a more suitable choice for *Acinetobacter* PD peritonitis, followed by aminoglycosides or fluoroquinolones. Empirical use of ceftazidime might carry a 10% to 30% risk for treatment failure.

An interesting issue among our findings is that the outcomes of *Acinetobacter* peritonitis remained fair throughout the follow-up period, despite the increase in *A. baumannii* percentage. *A. baumannii* infections are reportedly associated with 10% to 20% higher attributable mortality and longer length of hospital stay [2,26,27], and inappropriate antibiotic regimens further increase the risk [28]. Thus, the observed fair outcome in this series of predominantly *A. baumannii* PD-associated peritonitis is unusual. We proposed several reasons for this finding. First, the overall antibiotic resistance rate in our *Acinetobacter* effluent isolates is quite low (including *A. baumannii*), and this phenomenon holds true in other major PD peritonitis series as well (Table 4) [8,12,14]. Second, the empirical antibiotic regimens recommended by the ISPD for peritonitis invariably contain aminoglycosides or ceftazidime, both with fair efficacy against *Acinetobacter* isolates [5,20,21]. Consequently, the chance of treatment failure would be expectedly low; therefore, clinical outcomes would be better in this specific type of *Acinetobacter* infection than in the other types. Finally, as we explained, the origin of *Acinetobacter* PD peritonitis has gradually shifted from poor host immunity to

Table 4. Comparison between the current (after-2000) and the historic cohort.

Characteristics	*Historic 1 (n = 23, 1989)*[#]	*Historic 2 (n = 28, 1994)*[&]	*Current (after 2000) (n = 14)*
Age (years)	41 (9–66)	NA	55 (23–84)
Gender (male %)	16 (70)	NA	7 (50)
Comorbidities			
DM	5 (22)	NA	6 (43)
Autoimmune disorders	2 (9)	NA	1 (7)
Time to last peritonitis (months)	4 (0.5–14.5)	5 (1–29)	13.6 (3–27)
Pathogen			
Acinetobacter baumannii	8 (35)	27 (96)	9 (64)
Acinetobacter iwoffii	3 (13)	1 (4)	3 (21)
Acinetobacter ursingii	0 (0)	0 (0)	1 (7)
Unspecified Acinetobacter	12 (52)	0 (0)	1 (7)
Presumed peritonitis origin			
Break in exchange sterility	4 (17)	NA	5 (36)
Gastrointestinal bacterial translocation	3 (13)		4 (29)
Exit site infection or tunnel infection	0 (0)		0 (0)
Un-identified	16 (70)		5 (36)
Antibiotic susceptibilities			
Aminoglycoside	**S** 20 (87)	NA	**S** 14 (100)
	I 3 (13)		
Ceftazidime	**S** 23 (100)	**S** 19 (69)	**S** 13 (93)
		R 9 (31)	**R** 1 (7)
Cefepime	NA	NA	**S** 14 (100)
Fluoroquinolone	**S** 23 (100)	**S** 22 (79)	**S** 14 (100)
		R 6 (21)	
Outcomes			
Tenckhoff catheter removal	2 (9)	10 (36)	1 (7)
Recurrent peritonitis	1 (4)	0 (0)	0 (0)
Mortality	0 (0)	1 (4)	0 (0)

NA, not available.
[#]Adapted from Galvao C et al. *Am J Kidney Dis* 1989; 14(2): 101–4.
[&]Adapted from Lye WC et al. *Perit Dial Int* 1994; 14(2): 174–7.

sterility break. This might also play a role in the relatively fair outcome of *Acinetobacter* peritonitis.

To our knowledge, this study is the most up-to-date and comprehensive report of PD-associated peritonitis caused by *Acinetobacter*, with focused descriptions of their clinical features. The temporal changes in the characteristics of patients with *Acinetobacter* peritonitis include an increasing proportion of *A. baumannii*, more cases from breaks in exchange sterility, fewer cases from catheter infections, and an increasing interval between the previous and the present peritonitis episodes. These features might have important epidemiologic meanings in the PD field and warrant our continuous attention.

Acknowledgments

We are grateful to the staffs of the Center of Peritoneal Dialysis in National Taiwan University Hospital (NTUH) for their contributions, the staffs of the Second core lab of the department of Medical Research of NTUH for their technical support.

Author Contributions

Conceived and designed the experiments: CTC JWH. Performed the experiments: CTC SYL WSY HWC CCF CJY CKC KYH JWH. Analyzed the data: CTC SYL WSY HWC CCF CJY CKC KYH JWH. Contributed reagents/materials/analysis tools: CTC JWH. Wrote the paper: CTC SYL WSY HWC CCF CJY CKC KYH JWH.

References

1. Li PK-T, Chow KM (2013) Peritoneal Dialysis–First Policy Made Successful: Perspectives and Actions. Am J Kidney Dis 62: 993–1005.
2. Baboolal K, McEwan P, Sondhi S, Spiewanowski P, Wechowski J, et al (2008) The cost of renal dialysis in a UK setting–a multicentre study. Nephrol Dial Transplant 23: 1982–1989.
3. Lafrance JP, Rahme E, Iqbal S, Elftouh N, Vallee M, et al (2012) Association of Dialysis Modality with Risk for Infection-Related Hospitalization: A Propensity Score–Matched Cohort Analysis. Clin J Am Soc Nephrol 7: 1598–1605.
4. Najafi I, Alatab S, Atabak S, Majelan NN, Sanadgol H, et al (2013) Seventeen years' experience of peritoneal dialysis in Iran: first official report of the Iranian peritoneal dialysis registry. Perit Dial Int June 3 [Epub].
5. Li PK-T, Szeto CC, Piraino B, Bernadini J, Figueiredo AE, et al (2010) Peritoneal dialyusis-related infections recommendations: 2010 update. Perit Dial Int 30: 393–423.
6. Zelenitsky S, Barns L, Findlay I, Alfa M, Ariano R, et al (2000) Analysis of microbiological trends in peritoneal dialysis–related peritonitis from 1991 to 1998. Am J Kidney Dis 36: 1009–1013.
7. Barraclough K, Hawley CM, McDonald SP, Brown FG, Rosman JB, et al (2010) Polymicrobial Peritonitis in Peritoneal Dialysis Patients in Australia: Predictors, Treatment, and Outcomes. Am J Kidney Dis 55: 121–131.
8. Friedman O, Jassal SV, Bargman JM (2008) Acinetobacter Peritoneal Dialysis Peritonitis: Description and Relation to the SPICE Family of Organisms. Perit Dial Int 28: 195–197.
9. Chao CT, Lee SY, Yang WS, Chen HW, Fang CC, et al (2013) Citrobacter peritoneal dialysis peritonitis: rare occurrence with poor outcomes. Int J Med Sci 10: 1092–1098.
10. Jarvis EM, Hawley CM, McDonald SP, Brown FG, Rosman JB, et al (2010) Predictors, treatment, and outcomes of non-Pseudomonas Gram-negative peritonitis. Kidney Int 78: 408–414.
11. Szeto CC, Leung CB, Chow KM, Kwan BC, Law MC, et al (2005) Change in bacterial aetiology of peritoneal dialysis-related peritonitis over 10 years: experience from a centre in south-east Asia. Clin Microbiol Infect 11: 837–839.
12. Galvao C, Swartz R, Rocher L, Reynolds J, Starmann B, et al (1989) Acinetobacter peritonitis during chronic peritoneal dialysis. Am J Kidney Dis 14: 101–104.
13. Lye WC, Lee EJ, Ang KK (1991) Acinetobacter peritonitis in patients on CAPD: characteristics and outcome. Adv Perit Dial 7: 176–179.
14. Lye W, Lee EJ, Leong S, Kumarasinghe G (1994) Clinical characteristics and outcome of Acinetobacter infections in CAPD patients. Perit Dial Int 14: 174–177.
15. Chao CT, Lee SY, Yang WS, Chen HW, Fang CC, et al (2013) Peritoneal dialysis peritonitis by anaerobic pathogens: a retrospective case series. BMC Nephrol 14: 111.
16. Chao CT, Wu VC, Lai CF, Shiao CC, Huang TM, et al (2012) Advanced age affects the outcome-predictive power of RIFLE classification in geriatric patients with acute kidney injury. Kidney Int 82: 920–927.
17. Chao CT, Lin YF, Tsai HB, Wu VC, Ko WJ (2013) Acute kidney injury network staging in geriatric postoperative acute kidney injury patients: shortcomings and improvements. J Am Coll Surg 217: 240–250.
18. Prowant B, Nolph K, Ryan L, Twardowski Z, Khanna R (1986) Peritonitis in continuous ambulatory peritoneal dialysis: analysis of an 8-year experience. Nephron 43: 105–109.
19. Kern E, Newman L, Cacho C, Schulak JA, Weiss MF (2002) Abdominal catastrophe revisited: the risk and outcome of enteric peritoneal contamination. Perit Dial Int 22: 323–334.
20. Keane WF, Bailie GR, Boeschoten E, Gokal R, Golper TA, et al (2000) Adult peritoneal dialysis-related peritonitis treatment recommendations: 2000 update. Perit Dial Int 20: 396–411.
21. Piraino B, Bailie G, Bernardini J, Boeschoten E, Gupta A, et al (2005) Peritoneal dialysis-related infections recommendations: 2005 update. Perit Dial Int 25: 107–131.
22. Gerner-Smidt P, Tjernberg I, Ursing J (1991) Reliability of phenotypic tests for identification of Acinetobacter species. J Clin Microbiol 29: 277–282.
23. McConnell MJ, Actis L, Pachón J (2013) Acinetobacter baumannii: human infections, factors contributing to pathogenesis and animal models. FEMS Microbiol Rev 37: 130–155.
24. Towner KJ (2009) Acinetobacter: an old friend, but a new enemy. J Hosp Infect 73: 355–363.
25. Zarrilli R, Pournaras S, Giannouli M, Tsakris A (2013) Global evolution of multidrug-resistant Acinetobacter baumannii clonal lineages. Int J Antimicrob Agent 41: 11–19.
26. Falagas M, Bliziotis I, Siempos I (2006) Attributable mortality of Acinetobacter baumannii infections in critically ill patients: a systematic review of matched cohort and case-control studies. Crit Care 10: R48.
27. Abbo A, Carmeli Y, Navon-Venezia S, Siegman-Igra Y, Schwaber MJ (2007) Impact of multi-drug-resistant Acinetobacter baumannii on clinical outcomes. Eur J Clin Microbiol Infect Dis 26: 793–800.
28. Falagas ME, Kasiakou SK, Rafailidis PI, Zouglakis G, Morfou P (2006) Comparison of mortality of patients with Acinetobacter baumannii bacteraemia receiving appropriate and inappropriate empirical therapy. J Antimicrob Chemother 57: 1251–1254.

Association of Angiopoietin-2 with Renal Outcome in Chronic Kidney Disease

Yi-Chun Tsai[1,2,3], Yi-Wen Chiu[2,3], Jer-Chia Tsai[2,3], Hung-Tien Kuo[2,3], Su-Chu Lee[2], Chi-Chih Hung[2,3], Ming-Yen Lin[3], Shang-Jyh Hwang[1,2,3,4], Mei-Chuan Kuo[1,2,3]*, Hung-Chun Chen[2,3]

1 Graduate Institute of Clinical Medicine, Kaohsiung Medical University, Kaohsiung, Taiwan, **2** Division of Nephrology, Department of Internal Medicine, Kaohsiung Medical University Hospital, Kaohsiung, Taiwan, **3** Faculty of Renal Care, College of Medicine, Kaohsiung Medical University, Kaohsiung, Taiwan, **4** Institute of Population Sciences, National Health Research Institutes, Miaoli, Taiwan

Abstract

Background: The pathophysiological mechanisms of renal function progression in chronic kidney disease (CKD) have still not been completely explored. In addition to well-known traditional risk factors, non-traditional risk factors, such as endothelial dysfunction, have gradually attracted physicians' attention. Angiopoietin-2 (Ang-2) impairs endothelial function through preventing angiopoietin-1 from binding to Tie2 receptor. Whether Ang-2 is associated with renal function progression in CKD is unknown.

Methods: This study enrolled 621 patients with stages 3–5 CKD to assess the association of circulating Ang-2 with commencing dialysis, doubling creatinine and rapid decline in renal function (the slope of estimated glomerular filtration rate (eGFR) greater than 5 ml/min per 1.73 m^2/y) over follow-up of more than 3 years.

Results: Of all patients, 224 patients (36.1%) progressed to commencing dialysis and 165 (26.6%) reached doubling creatinine. 85 subjects (13.9%) had rapid decline in renal function. Ang-2 quartile was divided at 1494.1, 1948.8, and 2593.1 pg/ml. The adjusted HR of composite outcomes, either commencing dialysis or doubling creatinine was 1.53 (95% CI: 1.06–2.23) for subjects of quartile 4 compared with those of quartile 1. The adjusted OR for rapid decline in renal function was 2.96 (95% CI: 1.13–7.76) for subjects of quartile 4 compared with those of quartile 1. The linear mixed-effects model shows a more rapid decrease in eGFR over time in patients with quartile 3 or more of Ang-2 than those with the lowest quartile of Ang-2.

Conclusions: Ang-2 is an independent predictor of adverse renal outcome in CKD. Further study is needed to identify the pathogenic role of Ang-2 in CKD progression.

Editor: Effie C. Tsilibary, National Center for Scientific Research Demokritos, Greece

Funding: These authors have no support or funding to report.

Competing Interests: The authors have declared that no competing interests exist.

* Email: mechku@cc.kmu.edu.tw

Introduction

Chronic kidney disease (CKD) has been recognized as a worldwide health issue [1]. The pathophysiological mechanisms of renal function progression in CKD have still not been completely explored. In addition to well-known traditional risk factors, non-traditional risk factors, such as endothelial dysfunction, which might lead to cell apoptosis, vascular regression and renal fibrosis, have gradually attracted physicians' attention [2].

The angiopoietin (Ang)/Tie ligand-receptor system tightly controls the endothelial phenotype during angiogenesis and vascular inflammation [3]. Among the members of Ang family, Ang-1 and Ang-2 have attracted much attention [4]. Ang-1-driven Tie2 phosphorylation maintains structure integrity of vasculature, and protects the endothelium from excessive activation by cytokines and growth factors [5]. On the other hand, Ang-2 is expressed in endothelial cells, and stored in Weibel-Palade bodies (WPB) [6]. The rapid release of Ang-2 from endothelial cells upon activation of the endothelium by hypoxia, histamine, and thrombin would disrupt the protective, constitutive Ang-1/Tie2 signaling by preventing Ang-1 from binding to the receptor [5,7]. Consequently, the loss of Tie2 signaling destabilizes the endothelium and contributes to angiogenic or inflammatory response to cytokines and growth factors [8].

Increased circulating Ang-2 has been found in diabetes mellitus [9], arterial hypertension [10], congestive heart failure [11], peripheral artery disease [12], coronary artery disease [13], sepsis [14], critical illness [15], and acute kidney injury [16]. Additionally, accumulating evidence shows that circulating Ang-2 is also markedly elevated in CKD and dialysis patients [17]. Elevated Ang-2 levels are also correlated with long-term mortality in patients with CKD stage 4 and on dialysis [18]. Although Ang-2 is associated with microalbuminuria [19], a clinical marker of renal injury, the relationship between Ang-2 and renal progression has not been well-explored in CKD patients not on dialysis. This study tries to analyze whether Ang-2 is associated with renal outcome, including reaching commencing dialysis and rapid decline in renal function (estimated glomerular filtration rate (eGFR) decline per year), in patients with CKD stages 3–5.

Materials and Methods

Study Participants

This observational study was conducted at a tertiary hospital in Southern Taiwan. Six hundred and twenty-one patients with CKD stages 3–5, who had follow-up for one year at least in our integrated CKD program, were enrolled in the study from January 2006 to December 2011. CKD was staged according to K/DOQI definitions and the eGFR was calculated using the equation of the 4-variable Modification of Diet in Renal Disease (MDRD) Study (CKD stage 3, eGFR: 30–59 ml/min/1.73 m^2; CKD stage 4, eGFR: 15–29 ml/min/1.73 m^2; CKD stage 5, eGFR <15 ml/min/1.73 m^2) [20].

Ethics Statement

The study protocol was approved by the Institutional Review Board of the Kaohsiung Medical University Hospital (KMUH-IRB-990198). Informed consents were obtained in written form from patients and all clinical investigations were conducted according to the principles expressed in the Declaration of Helsinki.

Data Collection

Demographic and clinical data were obtained from medical records and interviews with patients at enrollment. The participant was asked to fast for at least 12 hours before blood sample collection for the biochemistry study and protein in urine was measured using urine protein-creatinine ratio. Patients were classified as diabetic by history and blood glucose values using the American Diabetes Association criteria, oral hypoglycemia agent use, or insulin use. Hypertension was defined as those with a history, or antihypertensive drugs use. Heart disease was defined as a history of heart failure, acute or chronic ischemic heart disease, or myocardial infarction. Cerebrovascular disease was defined as a history of cerebral infarction or hemorrhage. Information regarding patient medications including β-blocker, calcium channel blockers, angiotensin converting enzyme inhibitors (ACEI), and angiotensin II receptor blockers (ARB) before and after enrollment was obtained from medical records.

Quantification of circulating Angiopoietin-2

Plasma Angiopoietin-2 was measured in duplicate using commercial enzyme-linked immunosorbent assays (R&D Systems Inc, Minneapolis, MN) according to the instructions of the manufacturer. The sensitivity of Ang-2 assay was 1.20 pg/ml. Intraassay and interassay coefficients of variation of Ang-2 were 1.8% and 1.2%, respectively.

Renal Outcomes

Patients were contacted at outpatient clinics at 3-month intervals to ascertain the clinical status. Renal outcomes included commencing dialysis, doubling creatinine and rapid decline in renal function. Commencing dialysis was defined as requiring maintenance hemodialysis and peritoneal dialysis and confirmed by reviewing medical charts or catastrophic illness certificate (issued by the Bureau of National Health Insurance in Taiwan). The timing for commencing dialysis was considered according to the regulations of the Bureau of the National Health Insurance of Taiwan regarding eGFR, uremic status, nutritional status, and the laboratory data. The timing for doubling creatinine was considered based on all creatinine values from enrollment to the end of the observation period. The decline in renal function was assessed by the eGFR slope, defined as the regression coefficient between eGFR and time in units of ml/min per 1.73 m^2 per year. All eGFR values available from enrollment to the end of the observation period were included for calculation. At least three eGFR values were required to estimate the eGFR slope. Rapid decline in renal function was defined as the eGFR slope greater than 5 ml/min/1.73 m^2 per year based on Kidney Disease: Improving Global Outcomes (KDIGO) suggestion [21]. Patients were censored at death, last contact, or the end of observation in October 2013.

Statistical Analysis

Baseline characteristics of all subjects were stratified by quartiles of Ang-2, cut at 1494.1, 1948.8, and 2593.1 pg/ml. Continuous variables were expressed as mean ±SD or median (25th, 75th percentile), as appropriate, and categorical variables were expressed as percentages. Skewed distribution continuous variables were log-transformed to approximate normal distribution. The significance of differences in continuous variables between groups was tested using one-way analysis of variance (ANOVA) or the Kruskal-Wallis H test, as appropriate. The difference in the distribution of categorical variables was tested using the Chi-square test. Kaplan-Meier survival analysis was used to test Ang-2 as a predictor of the risk of composite outcomes either commencing dialysis or doubling creatinine. Cox regression models were applied to examine the relationship between Ang-2 and composite outcomes either commencing dialysis or doubling creatinine. Multivariable logistic regression models were also used to evaluate the association of Ang-2 with rapid decline in renal function. A linear mixed-effects model analysis was used to identify the factors associated with a change of eGFR, with control for internal correlations and other covariates. All the variables in Table 1 were tested by univariate analysis and those variables with P-value less than 0.05, including diabetes, heart disease, eGFR, urine protein-creatinine ratio cut at 1 g/g, serum albumin, phosphate, calcium, hemoglobin and cholesterol levels, and age, gender, and ACEI/ARB use were selected for multivariate cox and logistic analyses and linear mixed-effects model analysis. Statistical analyses were conducted using SPSS 18.0 for Windows (SPSS Inc., Chicago, Illinois). Statistical significance was set at a two-sided p-value of less than 0.05.

Results

Characteristics of Entire Cohort

A total of 621 participants with CKD stages 3 to 5 were analyzed (mean eGFR 21.8 ml/min/1.73 m^2, 146 in stage 3, 243 in stage 4, 232 in stage 5). The mean age was 65.3±12.7 years and 55.4% were male. Table 1 shows the baseline clinical characteristics stratified by quartiles of Ang-2, divided at 1494.1, 1948.8, and 2593.1 pg/ml. Of all patients, 532 (85.7%) were hypertensive and 239(38.5%)were diabetic mellitus. Pre-existing and documented heart disease and cerebral vascular disease were noted in 111(17.9%) and 55(8.9%) of patients respectively. The proportion of diabetes and β-blocker, serum blood urea nitrogen, phosphate and high-sensitivity C-reactive protein levels, and urine protein-creatinine ratio increased and eGFR, serum hemoglobin, calcium, and albumin levels decreased with Ang-2 quartiles.

Table 1. The clinical characteristics of study subjects stratified by angiopoietin-2 quartile.

		Angiopoietin-2[a]				
	Entire Cohort N=621	**Quartile 1 N=151**	**Quartile 2 N=157**	**Quartile 3 N=157**	**Quartile 4 N=156**	**P-trend**
Demographics						
Age (year)	65.3±12.7	62.2±13.6#	67.1±11.0*	65.9±12.2	66.0±13.2	0.005
Sex (male), n(%)	344(55.4)	98(64.9)	89(56.7)	83(52.9)	74(47.4)*	0.01
Smoke, n(%)	120(19.4)	36(23.8)	22(14.0)	26(17.0)	36(23.1)	0.1
Alcohol,n(%)	49(7.9)	20(13.2)†	13(8.3)	7(4.6)*	9(5.8)	0.03
Cardiovascular disease, n(%)	111(17.9)	27(17.9)	20(12.7)	33(21.0)	31(19.9)	0.2
Cerebral vascular disease,n(%)	55(8.9)	11(7.3)	19(12.1)	15(9.6)	10(6.4)	0.2
Hypertension, n(%)	532(85.7)	133(88.1)	138(87.9)	129(82.2)	132(84.6)	0.3
Diabetes mellitus, n(%)	239(38.5)	48(31.8)	57(36.3)	60(38.2)	74(47.4)	0.03
Hyperlipidemia, n(%)	272(43.8)	66(43.7)	77(49.0)	65(41.4)	64(41.0)	0.4
CKD cause, n(%)						
Chronic glomerulonephritis	232(37.4)	57(37.7	55(35.0)	61(38.9)	59(37.8)	0.6
Diabetic nephropathy	180(29)	41(27.2)	41(26.1)	47(29.9)	51(32.7)*	
Others	209(33.7)	53(35.1)	61(38.9)	49(31.2)	46(29.5)	
CKD stage 3 n(%)	146(23.5)	45(29.8)	37(23.6)	37(23.6)	27(17.3)	0.003
4 n(%)	243(39.1)	62(41.1)	72(45.9)	57(36.3)	52(33.3)	
5 n(%)	232(37.4)	44(29.1)	48(30.6)	63(40.1)	77(49.4)	
Medications						
Calcium channel blocker, n (%)	341(54.9)	80(53.0)	89(56.7)	78(49.7)	94(60.3)	0.3
β-blocker, n (%)	147(23.7)	26(17.2)	28(17.8)	45(28.7)	48(30.8)*#	0.005
ACEI/ARB, n (%)	353(56.8)	89(58.9)	90(57.3)	85(54.1)	89(57.1)	0.8
Statin, n(%)	170(27.4)	40(26.5)	47(29.9)	40(25.5)	43(27.6)	0.8
Laboratory parameters						
Blood urea nitrogen (mg/dl)	41.1(30.0,60.0)	34.9(26.9,52.8)	38.7(29.5,55.1)	41.5(30.9,60.1)	50.6(35.5,66.1)*#	<0.001
Creatinine (mg/dl)	2.9(2.1,5.0)	2.8(1.9,4.4)	2.8(2.0,4.6)	3.0(2.2,5.6)	3.6(2.3,5.6)	0.005
eGFR (ml/min/1.73 m^2)	21.8±12.6	24.7±13.9†	22.7±11.8	20.7±12.3*	18.9±11.9*#	<0.001
Fasting sugar (g/dl)	101(92,117)	99(91,111)	100(94,119)	100(91,117)	102(92,126)* †	0.3
Glycated hemoglobin (%)	5.8(5.5,6.7)	5.7(5.4,6.4)	5.9(5.6,6.8)	5.7(5.4,6.4)	6.1(5.5,7.2)*†	0.01
Hemoglobin (g/dl)	10.9±2.1	11.7±2.1#†	11.0±2.1*	10.7±2.1*	10.4±1.9*#	<0.001
Albumin (g/dl)	4.1(3.9,4.3)	4.2(4.0,4.4)†	4.2(3.9,4.3)†	4.0(3.8,4.3)*#	4.0(3.7,4.2)*#	<0.001
Phosphate (mg/dl)	4.1(3.6,4.8)	4.0(3.5,4.6)	4.0(3.6,4.6)	4.1(3.7,4.8)	4.3(3.8,5.1)	0.02
Calcium (mg/dl)	8.9±0.6	9.1±0.6†	9.0±0.6	8.8±0.6*	8.8±0.8*	<0.001
Uric acid (mg/dl)	7.6±1.9	7.5±1.9	7.6±1.8	7.4±1.5	7.8±2.1	0.2
Cholesterol (mg/dl)	187±45	192±47	190±40	182±45	188±46	0.2
Triglyceride (mg/dl)	115(78,173)	115(78,181)	112(82,172)	108(76,162)	126(79,181)	0.6
hsCRP (mg/L)	1.6(0.6,4.2)	1.4(0.7,3.5)	1.5(0.5,3.7)	1.5(0.6,3.5)	2.2(0.8,6.5)*# †	0.03
Parathyroid hormone (pg/ml)	72(37,157)	62(36,142)	63(35,120)	76(40,190)	106(33,191)	0.2
Urine protein-creatinine ratio >1 g/g n (%)	275(49.3)	57(41.0)	66(46.8)	70(49.6)	82(59.9)*#	0.01

Data are expressed as number (percentage) for categorical variables and mean±SD or median (25th, 75th percentile) for continuous variables, as appropriate. Conversion factors for units: eGFR in mL/min/1.73 m^2 to mL/s/1.73 m^2, ×0.01667 ; hemoglobin in g/dL to g/L, ×10; albumin in g/dL to g/L, ×10; calcium-phosphate product in mg^2/dL^2 to $mmol^2/L^2$, ×0.0806; cholesterol in mg/dL to mmol/L, ×0.02586; triglyceride in mg/dL to mmol/L, ×0.01129; uric acid in mg/dL toμmol/L, ×59.48. Abbreviations: CKD, chronic kidney disease; ECW, extracellular water; ICW, intracellular water; TBW, total body water; ACEI, angiotensin converting enzyme inhibitors; ARB, angiotensin II receptor blockers; eGFR, estimated glomerular filtration rate; hsCRP, high-sensitivity C-reactive protein.

*$P<0.05$ compared with quartile 1; #$P<0.05$ compared with quartile 2; †$P<0.05$ compared with quartile 3.

[a]Angiopoietin-2 quartile cut at 1494.1, 1948.8, and 2593.1 pg/ml.

(A) Composite outcomes

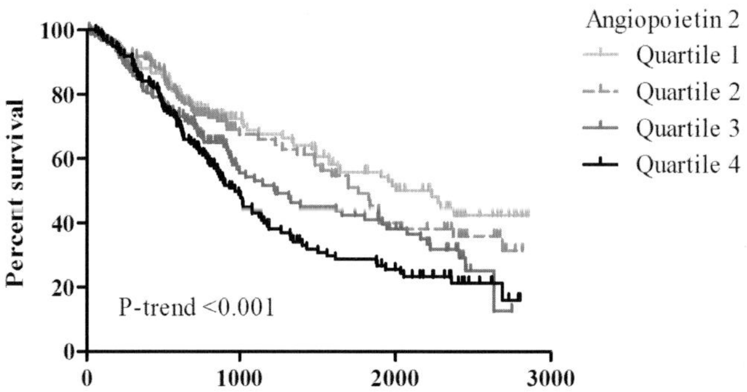

Quartile 1	151	64	37	(No. Patients at Risk)
Quartile 2	157	43	22	
Quartile 3	157	43	26	
Quartile 4	156	50	22	

(B) Commencing dialysis

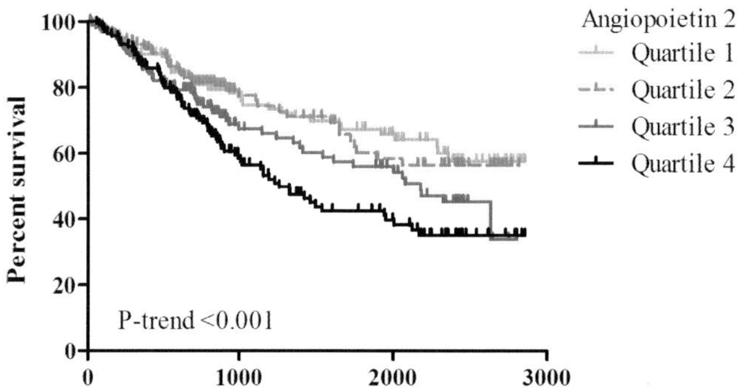

Quartile 1	151	66	42	(No. Patients at Risk)
Quartile 2	157	48	31	
Quartile 3	157	49	34	
Quartile 4	156	56	27	

(C) Doubing creatinine

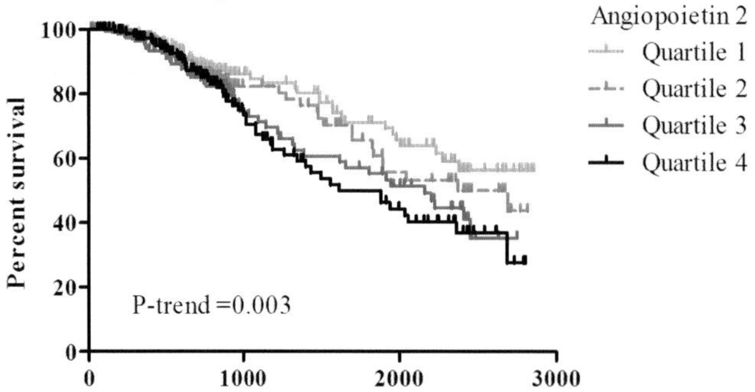

Quartile 1	151	64	37	(No. Patients at Risk)
Quartile 2	157	43	22	
Quartile 3	157	43	26	
Quartile 4	156	50	22	

Figure 1. Kaplan-Meier survival curve for composite outcomes, either commencing dialysis or doubling creatinine of all subjects stratified by angiopoietin-2 quartile.

Ang-2 and composite outcomes, either commencing dialysis or doubling creatinine

Over a mean follow-up period of 38.2±26.3 months, 224 patients (36.1%) progressed to commencing dialysis (198 hemodialysis and 26 peritoneal dialysis, Table 2). Seventy-one (11.4%) had mortality before reaching commencing dialysis. 18 (2.9%) were lost to follow-up (the mean follow-up period: 19.7±10.9 months), and no significant difference of proportion from quartile 1 to quartile 4 was found. A stepwise increase in the proportion of commencing dialysis from quartile 1 to quartile 4 was found (P-trend <0.001). Of all subjects, 165 (26.6%) reached doubling creatinine during follow-up period, but there was no significant difference among Ang-2 quartiles. Kaplan-Meier survival curve showed a significant correlation between quartiles of Ang-2 and composite outcomes, either commencing dialysis or doubling creatinine (Figure 1). Table 3 presents the longitudinal associations between stepwise increases in Ang-2 levels and composite outcomes, either commencing dialysis or doubling creatinine. The unadjusted hazard ratio (HR) of composite outcomes was 1.96 (95% Confidence interval (CI): 1.43–2.69) for subjects of quartile 4 compared with those of quartile 1. The adjusted HR of composite outcomes was 1.53 (95% CI: 1.06–2.23) for subjects of quartile 4 compared with those of quartile 1. The longitudinal association between composite outcomes and stepwise increases in Ang-2 levels (P-trend = 0.03).

The unadjusted risk for commencing dialysis increased 2 fold (HR: 2.01, 95% CI: 1.39–2.90) for subjects of quartile 4 compared with those of quartile 1. The adjusted risk for commencing dialysis increased 85% (HR: 1.85, 95% CI: 1.20–2.85) for subjects of quartile 4 compared with those of quartile 1. The longitudinal association between commencing dialysis and stepwise increases in Ang-2 levels (P-trend = 0.005). The unadjusted risk for doubling creatinine increased 89% (HR: 1.89, 95% CI: 1.21–2.93) for subjects of quartile 4 compared with those of quartile 1. However, there was no significant association of doubling creatinine with Ang-2 quartiles in adjusted model.

Ang-2, rapid decline in renal function and change in eGFR

Eighty-five subjects (13.9%) had rapid decline in renal function. Patients of progressive decline in renal function (eGFR slope greater than 5 ml/min/1.73 m^2/yr) were more likely to have higher level of Ang-2 than those of non-progressive decline in renal function (eGFR slope less than 5 ml/min/1.73 m^2/yr) (median: 1944.9 *v.s.* 2066.0 pg/ml, P = 0.01). No significant different in baseline eGFR was found between the two groups. The adjusted risk for rapid decline in renal function increased 2.9 folds (OR: 2.96, 95% CI: 1.13–7.76) for subjects of quartile 4 compared with those of quartile 1 (Table 4). Table 4 also shows the effect of study group on the change in eGFR in the linear mixed-effects model. The highest quartile of Ang-2 was associated with a significant decrease in eGFR over time as compared with the lowest quartile of Ang-2 (unstandardized coefficient $\beta = -1.73$, 95% CI: −3.34, −0.11, P = 0.03).

Discussion

To our knowledge, this study is the first to evaluate the association of Ang-2 with adverse renal outcome in patients with stages 3–5 CKD over an observation period of 3 years. Ang-2 is associated with composite renal outcomes, either commencing dialysis or doubling creatinine after adjustment of baseline renal function and associated risk factors. Patients with quartile 3 or more of Ang-2 have more than 1.7 and 3.0-fold increase in risk for commencing dialysis and rapid decline in renal function respectively. Additionally, the linear mixed-effects model shows a more rapid decrease in eGFR over time in patients with quartile 3 or more of Ang-2 than those with quartile 1 of Ang-2. CKD patients with quartile 3(1948.8 pg/ml) or more of Ang-2 are more likely to reach the plateau of adverse renal outcome.

With regard to glomerular diseases, studies by Belinda et al. [22] pointed out that increased glomerular expression of Ang-2 would tend to antagonize Ang-1-induced Tie-2 activation and destabilize capillaries and glomerular endothelia in podocin/Ang-2 transgene mice. There were significant increases in albuminuria and glomerular endothelial apoptosis, with significant decreases of both nephrin proteins and vascular endothelial growth factor A (VEGF-A), which were critical for maintenance of glomerular endothelia and glomerular filtration barrier integrity [23–25]. Besides, Seron et al. [26] indicated a chronic loss of renal interstitial capillaries in human nephropathy, and Futrakul et al. [27] suggested that an "anti-angiogenic environment" may exist in long-standing nephropathies. In clinical views, accumulating evidence shows that circulating Ang-2 is inversely related to eGFR and increases with advanced CKD and Ang-2 level is still increasing even after entering maintenance of dialysis [17]. However, little is known about a clinical relationship between Ang-2 and adverse renal outcome. The present study identifies that increased circulating Ang-2 is associated with risks for commencing dialysis and rapid decline in renal function in patients not on dialysis, and Ang-2 is an independent predictor of adverse renal outcome in CKD cohort.

Consistent with reports by Chang et al. [19], our results also showed a significant association of circulating Ang-2 with hypoalbuminemia and high-sensitivity C-reactive protein (hs-CRP), as indicators of malnutrition-inflammation. Fiedler et al. identified Ang-2 as an autocrine regulator of endothelial cell inflammatory responses and Ang-2 acts as a switch of vascular responsiveness exerting a permissive role for the activities of proinflammatory cytokines [11]. Ang-2 serves the link between angiogenic and inflammatory pathway, Ang-2 signaling between cellular elements in renal fibrosis, including endothelial cells, pericytes, myofibroblasts, and macrophages [23]. Meanwhile, CKD has been regarded as a disease with persistent and low-grade inflammation, and our previous study indicated that inflammation is an independent predictor of rapid decline in renal function in CKD cohort [28]. Hence, there might be an interaction among Ang-2, inflammation and rapid decline in renal function. The findings of our subgroup analysis show that elevated Ang-2 is independently associated with risk for maintenance dialysis in subjects of less than the median of hsCRP (1.56 mg/l; HR for log Ang-2: 4.80, 95%CI: 1.68–13.76). In addition, there is a significant association between Ang-2 and maintenance dialysis in subjects of serum albumin above 3.5 g/dl (HR for log Ang-2: 2.15, 95%CI: 1.05–4.38). Thus, circulating Ang-2 is possibly a significant risk factor for adverse renal outcome independent of malnutrition-inflammation.

Increased endothelial Ang-2 secretion is stimulated by exogenous stimuli such as angiotensin II, tumor necrosis factor-α, hypoxia, and reactive oxygen species, which are characteristics in

Table 2. Renal outcome of all subjects stratified by Angiopoietin-2 quartile.

	Entire Cohort N = 621	Angiopoietin-2[a]				
		Quartile 1 N = 151	Quartile 2 N = 157	Quartile 3 N = 157	Quartile 4 N = 156	P-trend
Follow-up time (month)	38.2±26.3	43.8±28.1	30.0±25.9	35.7±26.0	35.5±24.6	0.02
No. of SCr measurement	17 (9,27)	18(8, 27)	15(9,23)	15(9,24)	20(12,28)	0.01
Doubling creatinine (n,%)	165(26.6)	35(23.2)	37(23.6)	45(28.7)	48(30.8)	0.3
eGFR decline (mL/min/1.73 m^2/year)	−1.6(−3.3,−0.4)	−1.3(−2.8,0.1)	−1.8(−3.6,−0.9)	−1.8(−3.8,−0.6)	−1.5(−3.1,−0.2)	0.01
Commencing dialysis (n,%)	224(36.1)	45(29.8)	43(27.4)	59(37.6)	77(49.4)	<0.001

Data are expressed as number (percentage) for categorical variables and median (25th, 75th percentile) for continuous variables, as appropriate.
Conversion factors for units: eGFR in mL/min/1.73 m^2 to mL/s/1.73 m^2, ×0.01667.
Abbreviations: eGFR, estimated glomerular filtration rate.
[a]Angiopoietin-2 quartile cut at 1494.1, 1948.8, and 2593.1 pg/ml.

CKD progression [5]. Endothelial injury in glomerular vasculature may induce endothelial Ang-2 secretion, and meanwhile, increased Ang-2 may lead to glomerular albuminuria through endothelial injury. It is difficult to evaluate whether increased Ang-2 is a cause or consequence of CKD progression [5]. Because of this complicated interaction among Ang-2, traditional risk factors, and CKD, we adjusted associated risk factors for rapid decline in renal function in multivariate analysis. We also performed subgroup analysis in different CKD stages, but the results did not consistent at all (Figure S1–S3). It is probably related to relative small number of subgroup and short observation period. We need further study to evaluate whether these risk factors are modifiers or confounders in association of Ang-2 and commencing dialysis. Besides, to consider the influence of competing risk of death on commencing dialysis, we performed further analysis, and the results are consistent (HR for quartile 4 compared with quartile 1: 1.85 (95% CI: 1.20–2.86). Our findings show a strong association of Ang-2 and adverse renal outcome and emphasize its importance as a predictor in CKD cohort.

Despite exogenous stimuli, Ang-2 was excreted by factors influencing the exocytosis of Weibel-Palade body, including thrombin, histamine, serotonin, vascular endothelial growth factor (VEGF) and epinephrine [29]. Therefore, it could be influenced by medication. In this study, no significant difference of medication was found among Ang-2 quartiles except for β-blocker. In post hoc multiple comparisons, subjects of Ang-2 quartile 4 had higher proportion of using β-blocker than those of Ang-2 quartile 1 and 2. The reason might be related to blood pressure control or arrhythmia. The present study has a limitation that we did not record blood pressure and arrhythmia at enrollment. In late CKD, patients usually need three or more kinds of anti-hypertension medicines to keep adequate blood pressure and use β-blocker for arrhythmia. It is probably the reason for the different proportion of β-blocker usage. Contrarily, β-blocker promotes cardiac angiogenesis in heart failure via activation of VEGF signaling pathway [30]. Hence, higher level of Ang-2 in late CKD patients may be partially related to long term usage of β-blocker. We also add β-blocker usage into multivariate analysis, and Ang-2 is still associated with adverse renal outcome. Further study is needed to investigate the relationship of ang-2 and β-blocker.

Ang-2 is usually elevated in diabetes and associated with endothelial dysfunction, which leads to microvascular and macrovascular complications [9,31,32]. The pathophysiological mechanisms by which Ang-2 participates in rapid decline in renal function are complicated and include various pathways, such as arterial stiffness or oxidative stress [17,19]. Our results show an association of Ang-2 quartiles with the proportion of diabetes, but no correlation between Ang-2 quartiles and glycated hemoglobin in patients with integrated CKD care program. Although average sugar level is under strict control, some patients still reach adverse renal outcome. Accumulating evidence indicates that strict glycemic control might not be enough to prevent rapid decline in renal function in late CKD [33]. It is probably that Ang-2 is

Table 3. The adjusted risks for composite outcomes, either commencing dialysis or doubling creatinine according to Angiopoietin-2 quartile.

Angiopoietin-2[a]	Composite outcomes		Commencing dialysis		Double creatinine	
	Hazard ratio (95% CI)	P-value	Hazard ratio (95% CI)	P-value	Hazard ratio (95% CI)	P-value
Quartile 1	Reference		Reference		Reference	
Quartile 2	1.42(0.95–2.13)	0.08	1.50(0.92–2.44)	0.01	1.43(0.83–2.47)	0.1
Quartile 3	1.54(1.05–2.27)	0.02	1.73(1.10–2.71)	0.02	1.47(0.87–2.48)	0.1
Quartile 4	1.53(1.06–2.23)	0.02	1.85(1.20–2.85)	0.02	1.47(0.87–2.45)	0.1

Abbreviations: CI, Confidence Interval; eGFR, estimated glomerular filtration rate.
Adjusted model: age, sex, cardiovascular disease, diabetes mellitus, angiotensin converting enzyme inhibitors/angiotensin II receptor blockers use, estimated glomerular filtration rate, hemoglobin, serum calcium and cholesterol levels, log serum albumin and phosphate, and urine protein-creatinine ratio cut at 1 g/g.
[a]Angiopoietin-2 quartile cut at 1494.1, 1948.8, and 2593.1 pg/ml.

Table 4. The adjusted risks for rapid decline in renal function and change of eGFR according to Angiopoietin-2 quartile.

Angiopoietin-2[a]	Rapid decline in renal function		Change of eGFR	
	Odds ratio (95% CI)	P-value	Unstandardized coefficient β^b (95% CI)	P-value
Quartile 1	Reference		Reference	
Quartile 2	3.40(1.32–8.75)	0.01	−1.03(−2.63,0.57)	0.1
Quartile 3	3.04(1.18–7.82)	0.02	−1.66(−3.25,−0.07)	0.03
Quartile 4	2.96(1.13–7.76)	0.02	−1.73(−3.33,−0.11)	0.03

Abbreviations: CI, Confidence Interval; eGFR, estimated glomerular filtration rate.
Adjusted model: age, sex, cardiovascular disease, diabetes mellitus, angiotensin converting enzyme inhibitors/angiotensin II receptor blockers use, estimated glomerular filtration rate, hemoglobin, serum calcium and cholesterol levels, log serum albumin and phosphate, , and urine protein-creatinine ratio cut at 1 g/g.
[a]Angiopoietin-2 quartile cut at 1494.1, 1948.8, and 2593.1 pg/ml.
[b]β expressed as ml/min/1.73 m^2/year in eGFR.

associated with adverse renal outcome beyond the effects of diabetes. Additionally, patients with cardiovascular disease, cerebrovascular disease or hypertension are more likely to have higher circulating Ang-2 level [10,11,13,34]. Ang-2 has been associated with cardiovascular markers, such as cell adhesion molecules and inflammation [35], and increases endothelial apoptosis, enhances myocardial microvascular inflammation, and promotes cardiac fibrosis [31]. Although there was no different proportion of cardiovascular disease, cerebrovascular disease and hypertension in Ang-2 quartiles at baseline in our cohort, Ang-2 might be probably associated with cardiovascular events in the future. Thus, further study is needed to evaluate the relationship between Ang-2 and cardiovascular outcome.

On the other hand, previous study reported a significant correlation between Ang-2 and asymmetric dimethylarginine (ADMA), as the nitric oxide (NO) synthase inhibitor [17]. CKD has been regarded as a NO-deficient state, and the oxidative stress leads to not only renal function decline, but also adverse cardiovascular sequelae [36,37]. Thus, ADMA is not only a uremic toxin, but also a strong marker of endothelial dysfunction and atherosclerosis [38]. Sascha et al. speculated that the increased Ang-2 levels might reveal excess Weibel-Palade body exocytosis as a consequence of decreased NO bioavailability in the presence of high ADMA levels [17]. Although further in vivo and in vitro studies are needed to evaluate the interaction between Ang-2 and NO bioavailability, it could possibly explain one of the potential mechanisms responsible for the association between Ang-2 and adverse renal outcome.

This study has some limitations that must be considered. The major uncertainty is whether circulating Ang-2 is biologically active in CKD patients. The biological implication of Ang-2 changes in the range observed in our patients is still unknown. Besides, Ang-2 was measured once at enrollment. The effect of the time-varying Ang-2 levels might be underestimated. Additionally, the mechanism contributing to the association between increased circulating Ang-2 and rapid decline in renal function has not been well-explored. Further study is needed to investigate the pathogenic link between Ang-2 and rapid decline in renal function.

In conclusion, our study demonstrates that elevated circulating Ang-2 is associated with increased risks for adverse renal outcome in stages 3–5 CKD patients. Future studies will be necessary to evaluate the pathogenic role of Ang-2 in renal progression, and to establish the beneficial renal function by targeting Ang-2.

Supporting Information

Figure S1 Adjusted hazard ratios (HRs) of commencing dialysis for Angiopoietin-2 (Ang-2) quartile 4 compared with Ang-2 quartile 1 in CKD stages 3–5 subjects stratified by proteinuria, high sensitivity c-reactive protein (hsCRP), serum albumin and angiotensin converting enzyme inhibitors (ACEI)/angiotensin II receptor blockers (ARB) usage. Ratios were adjusted for age, sex, cardiovascular disease, diabetes mellitus, ACEI/ARB usage, estimated glomerular filtration rate, hemoglobin, serum calcium and cholesterol levels, log serum albumin and phosphate, and urine protein-creatinine ratio cut at 1 g/g. The median values of serum albumin and hsCRP are 3.8 g/dl and 1.5 mg/l respectively.

Figure S2 Adjusted hazard ratios (HRs) of commencing dialysis for Angiopoietin-2 (Ang-2) quartile 4 compared with Ang-2 quartile 1 in CKD stages 3–4 subjects stratified by proteinuria, high sensitivity c-reactive protein (hsCRP), serum albumin and angiotensin converting enzyme inhibitors (ACEI)/angiotensin II receptor blockers (ARB) usage. Ratios were adjusted for age, sex, cardiovascular disease, diabetes mellitus, ACEI/ARB usage, estimated glomerular filtration rate, hemoglobin, serum calcium and cholesterol levels, log serum albumin and phosphate, and urine protein-creatinine ratio cut at 1 g/g. The median values of serum albumin and hsCRP are 3.8 g/dl and 1.5 mg/l respectively.

Figure S3 Adjusted hazard ratios (HRs) of commencing dialysis for Angiopoietin-2 (Ang-2) quartile 4 compared with Ang-2 quartile 1 in CKD stage 5 subjects stratified by proteinuria, high sensitivity c-reactive protein (hsCRP), serum albumin and angiotensin converting enzyme inhibitors (ACEI)/angiotensin II receptor blockers (ARB) usage. Ratios were adjusted for age, sex, cardiovascular disease, diabetes mellitus, ACEI/ARB usage, estimated glomerular filtration rate, hemoglobin, serum calcium and cholesterol levels, log serum albumin and phosphate, and urine protein-creatinine ratio cut at 1 g/g. The median values of serum albumin and hsCRP are 3.8 g/dl and 1.5 mg/l respectively.

Acknowledgments

The authors thank the help from the Statistical Analysis Laboratory, Department of Medical Research, Kaohsiung Medical University Hospital, Kaohsiung Medical University. ***Support***: Dr. Tsai's research was supported by the Kaohsiung Medical University Faculty of Renal Care.

Author Contributions

Conceived and designed the experiments: Y-CT M-CK. Performed the experiments: S-CL M-CK. Analyzed the data: Y-CT C-CH M-YL. Contributed reagents/materials/analysis tools: Y-WC J-CT H-TK S-JH M-CK H-CC. Wrote the paper: Y-CT M-CK.

Reference

1. Nugent RA, Fathima SF, Feigl AB, Chyung D (2011) The burden of chronic kidney disease on developing nations: a 21st century challenge in global health. Nephron Clin Pract 118: 269–277.
2. Chang FC, Lin SL (2013) The role of angiopoietin-2 in progressive renal fibrosis. J Formos Med Assoc 112: 175–176.
3. Brindle NP, Saharinen P, Alitalo K (2006) Signaling and functions of angiopoietin-1 in vascular protection. Circ Res 98: 1014–1023.
4. Fam NP, Verma S, Kutryk M, Stewart DJ (2003) Clinician guide to angiogenesis. Circulation 108: 2613–2618.
5. Fiedler U, Augustin HG (2006) Angiopoietins: a link between angiogenesis and inflammation. Trends Immuno 27: 552–558.
6. Fiedler U, Scharpfenecker M, Koidl S, Hegen A, Grunow V, et al. (2004) The Tie-2 ligand angiopoietin-2 is stored in and rapidly released upon stimulation from endothelial cell Weibel-Palade bodies. Blood 103: 4150–4156.
7. Huang YQ, Li JJ, Hu L, Lee M, Karpatkin S (2002) Thrombin induces increased expression and secretion of angiopoietin-2 from human umbilical vein endothelial cells. Blood 99: 1646–1650.
8. Fiedler U, Reiss Y, Scharpfenecker M, Grunow V, Koidl S, et al. (2006) Angiopoietin-2 sensitizes endothelial cells to TNF-alpha and has a crucial role in the induction of inflammation. Nat Med 12: 235–239.
9. Lim HS, Lip GY, Blann AD (2005) Angiopoietin-1 and angiopoietin-2 in diabetes mellitus: relationship to VEGF, glycaemic control, endothelial damage/dysfunction and atherosclerosis. Atherosclerosis 180: 113–118.
10. Nadar SK, Blann A, Beevers DG, Lip GY (2005) Abnormal angiopoietins 1&2, angiopoietin receptor Tie-2 and vascular endothelial growth factor levels in hypertension: relationship to target organ damage [a sub-study of the Anglo-Scandinavian Cardiac Outcomes Trial (ASCOT)]. J Intern Med 258: 336–343.
11. Chong AY, Caine GJ, Freestone B, Blann AD, Lip GY (2004) Plasma angiopoietin-1, angiopoietin-2, and angiopoietin receptor tie-2 levels in congestive heart failure. J Am Coll Cardiol 43: 423–428.
12. David S, Kumpers P, Hellpap J, Horn R, Leitolf H, et al. (2009) Angiopoietin-2 and cardiovascular disease in dialysis and kidney transplantation. Am J Kidney Dis 53: 770–778.
13. Lee KW, Lip GY, Blann AD (2004) Plasma angiopoietin-1, angiopoietin-2, angiopoietin receptor tie-2, and vascular endothelial growth factor levels in acute coronary syndromes. Circulation 110: 2355–2360.
14. Parikh SM, Mammoto T, Schultz A, Yuan HT, Christiani D, et al. (2006) Excess circulating angiopoietin-2 may contribute to pulmonary vascular leak in sepsis in humans. PLoS Med 3: e46.
15. Kumpers P, Lukasz A, David S, Horn R, Hafer C, et al. (2008) Excess circulating angiopoietin-2 is a strong predictor of mortality in critically ill medical patients. Crit Care, 12: R147.
16. Kumpers P, Hafer C, David S, Hecker H, Lukasz A, et al. (2010) Angiopoietin-2 in patients requiring renal replacement therapy in the ICU: relation to acute kidney injury, multiple organ dysfunction syndrome and outcome. Intensive Care Med 36: 462–470.
17. David S, Kumpers P, Lukasz A, Fliser D, Martens-Lobenhoffer J, et al. (2010) Circulating angiopoietin-2 levels increase with progress of chronic kidney disease. Nephrol Dial Transplant 25: 2571–2576.
18. David S, John SG, Jefferies HJ, Sigrist MK, Kumpers P, et al. (2012) Angiopoietin-2 levels predict mortality in CKD patients. Nephrol Dial Transplant 27: 1867–1872.
19. Chang FC, Lai TS, Chiang CK, Chen YM, Wu MS, et al. (2013) Angiopoietin-2 is associated with albuminuria and microinflammation in chronic kidney disease. PloS One, 8: e54668.
20. Levey AS, Bosch JP, Lewis JB, Greene T, Rogers N, et al. (1999) A more accurate method to estimate glomerular filtration rate from serum creatinine: a new prediction equation. Modification of Diet in Renal Disease Study Group. Ann Intern Med 130: 461–470.
21. Levin A, Stevens PE (2014) Summary of KDIGO 2012 CKD Guideline: behind the scenes, need for guidance, and a framework for moving forward. Kidney Int 85: 49–61.
22. Davis B, Dei Cas A, Long DA, White KE, Hayward A, et al. (2007) Podocyte-specific expression of angiopoietin-2 causes proteinuria and apoptosis of glomerular endothelia. J Am Soc Nephrol 18: 2320–2329.
23. Woolf AS, Gnudi L, Long DA (2009) Roles of angiopoietins in kidney development and disease. J Am Soc Nephrol 20: 239–244.
24. Tryggvason K, Patrakka J, Wartiovaara J (2006) Hereditary proteinuria syndromes and mechanisms of proteinuria. N Engl J Med 354: 1387–1401.
25. Eremina V, Sood M, Haigh J, Nagy A, Lajoie G, et al. (2003) Glomerular-specific alterations of VEGF-A expression lead to distinct congenital and acquired renal diseases. J Clin Invest 111: 707–716.
26. Seron D, Alexopoulos E, Raftery MJ, Hartley B, Cameron JS (1990) Number of interstitial capillary cross-sections assessed by monoclonal antibodies: relation to interstitial damage. Nephrol dial transplant 5: 889–893.
27. Futrakul N, Butthep P, Futrakul P (2008) Altered vascular homeostasis in chronic kidney disease. Clin Hemorheol Microcirc 38: 201–207.
28. Tsai YC, Hung CC, Kuo MC, Tsai JC, Yeh SM, et al. (2012) Association of hsCRP, white blood cell count and ferritin with renal outcome in chronic kidney disease patients. PloS One, 7: e52775.
29. Rondaij MG, Bierings R, Kragt A, van Mourik JA, Voorberg J (2006) Dynamics and plasticity of Weibel-Palade bodies in endothelial cells. Arterioscler Thromb Vasc Biol 26: 1002–1007.
30. Rengo G, Cannavo A, Liccardo D, Zincarelli C, de Lucia C, et al. (2013) CVascular endothelial growth factor blockade prevents the beneficial effects of β-blocker therapy on cardiac function, angiogenesis, and remodeling in heart failure. Circ Heart Fail 6: 1259–67.
31. Chen JX, Zeng H, Reese J, Aschner JL, Meyrick B (2012) Overexpression of angiopoietin-2 impairs myocardial angiogenesis and exacerbates cardiac fibrosis in the diabetic db/db mouse model. Am J Physiol Heart Circ Physiol 302: 1003–1012.
32. Anuradha S, Mohan V, Gokulakrishnan K, Dixit M (2010) Angiopoietin-2 levels in glucose intolerance, hypertension, and metabolic syndrome in Asian Indians (Chennai Urban Rural Epidemiology Study-74). Metabolism Clinical and Experimental 59: 774–779.
33. Shurraw S, Hemmelgarn B, Lin M, Majumdar SR, Klarenbach, et al. (2011) SAssociation between glycemic control and adverse outcomes in people with diabetes mellitus and chronic kidney disease: a population-based cohort study. Arch Intern Med 171: 1920–1927.
34. Cui X, Chopp M, Zacharek A, Ye X, Roberts C, et al (2011) Angiopoietin/Tie2 pathway mediates type 2 diabetes induced vascular damage after cerebral stroke. Neurobiol Dis 43: 285–292.
35. Shroff RC, Price KL, Kolatsi-Joannou M, Todd AF, Wells D, et al (2013) Circulating angiopoietin-2 is a marker for early cardiovascular disease in children on chronic dialysis. PLOS one 8: e56273.
36. Wever R, Boer P, Hijmering M, Stroes E, Verhaar M, et al. (1999) Nitric oxide production is reduced in patients with chronic renal failure. Arterioscler Thromb Vasc Biol 19: 1168–1172.
37. Baylis C (2012) Nitric oxide synthase derangements and hypertension in kidney disease. Curr Opin Nephrol Hypertens 21: 1–6.
38. Kielstein JT, Zoccali C (2005) Asymmetric dimethylarginine: a cardiovascular risk factor and a uremic toxin coming of age? Am J Kidney Dis 46: 186–202.

Hyponatremia as a Predictor of Mortality in Peritoneal Dialysis Patients

Tae Ik Chang[1], Yung Ly Kim[2], Hyungwoo Kim[2], Geun Woo Ryu[2], Ea Wha Kang[1], Jung Tak Park[2], Tae-Hyun Yoo[2], Sug Kyun Shin[1], Shin-Wook Kang[2,3], Kyu Hun Choi[2], Dae Suk Han[2], Seung Hyeok Han[2]*

1 Department of Internal Medicine, NHIS Medical Center, Ilsan Hospital, Goyangshi, Gyeonggi-do, Republic of Korea, **2** Department of Internal Medicine, College of Medicine, Yonsei University, Seoul, Republic of Korea, **3** Brain Korea 21 for Medical Science, Severance Biomedical Science Institute, Yonsei University, Seoul, Republic of Korea

Abstract

Background and Aim: Hyponatremia is common in patients with chronic kidney disease and is associated with increased mortality in hemodialysis patients. However, few studies have addressed this issue in peritoneal dialysis (PD) patients.

Methods: This prospective observational study included a total of 441 incident patients who started PD between January 2000 and December 2005. Using time-averaged serum sodium (TA-Na) levels, we aimed to investigate whether hyponatremia can predict mortality in these patients.

Results: Among the baseline parameters, serum sodium level was positively associated with serum albumin ($\beta = 0.145$; $p = 0.003$) and residual renal function (RRF) ($\beta = 0.130$; $p = 0.018$) and inversely associated with PD ultrafiltration ($\beta = -0.114$; $p = 0.024$) in a multivariable linear regression analysis. During a median follow-up of 34.8 months, 149 deaths were recorded. All-cause death occurred in 81 (55.9%) patients in the lowest tertile compared to 37 (25.0%) and 31 (20.9%) patients in the middle and highest tertiles, respectively. After adjusting for multiple potentially confounding covariates, increased TA-Na level was associated with a significantly decreased risk of all-cause (HR per 1 mEq/L increase, 0.79; 95% CI, 0.73–0.86; $p < 0.001$) and infection-related (HR per 1 mEq/L increase, 0.77; 95% CI, 0.70–0.85; $p < 0.001$) deaths.

Conclusions: This study showed that hyponatremia is an independent predictor of mortality in PD patients. Nevertheless, whether correcting hyponatremia improves patient survival is unknown. Future interventional studies should address this question more appropriately.

Editor: Pasqual Barretti, Sao Paulo State University, Brazil

Funding: This work was supported by the Brain Korea 21 Project for Medical Science, Yonsei University, by a National Research Foundation of Korea (NRF) grant funded by the Korean government (MEST) (No. 2011-0030711), and by a grant of the Korea Healthcare Technology R&D Project, Ministry of Health and Welfare, Republic of Korea (A102065). The funders had no role in study design, data collection and analysis, decision to publish, or preparation of the manuscript.

Competing Interests: The authors have declared that no competing interests exist.

* Email: hansh@yuhs.ac

Introduction

Electrolyte handling is universally impaired in patients with chronic kidney disease (CKD) because of failing kidney function. Therefore, these patients are vulnerable to complications caused by electrolyte imbalance. Although this issue is partly resolved by dialysis treatment, patients with end-stage renal disease (ESRD) commonly suffer from electrolyte disturbances [1].

Hyponatremia, usually defined as a serum sodium concentration <135 mEq/L, is one of the most common electrolyte disorders and is believed to be an important risk factor for mortality in patients with many serious medical conditions including advanced heart failure or liver cirrhosis [2–5]. In these conditions, it is generally assumed that hyponatremia reflects the severity of the underlying disease rather than directly contributing to mortality. Hyponatremia is also common in CKD patients [1]. Moreover, recent studies have shown that lower serum sodium concentrations are associated with increased mortality in maintenance hemodialysis (HD) patients and CKD patients prior to dialysis therapy [6–10]. However, the underlying mechanisms are complex and still need to be clarified. In addition, it is still uncertain whether hyponatremia itself can contribute to mortality or merely represents a surrogate marker for other unknown risk factors in chronic maintenance dialysis patients.

Although peritoneal dialysis (PD) is an established therapeutic modality in ESRD, characteristics of dialysis treatment clearly differ between PD and HD. In particular, serum levels of electrolytes fluctuate between dialysis sessions in patients receiving HD due to the intermittent nature of HD treatment, while these levels remain relatively stable in PD patients. This unique feature led us to investigate which factors are associated with hyponatremia and its clinical outcomes in patients chronic PD. To date, few studies have addressed this issue, in particular the relationship between serum sodium level and risk of death, in PD patients [11–15]. Therefore, the purpose of this study was to investigate whether hyponatremia can predict mortality in a large prospective cohort of incident patients undergoing PD.

Methods

Ethics statement

The study was carried out in accordance with the Declaration of Helsinki and approved by the Institutional Review Board of Ilsan Hospital Clinical Trial Center. We obtained informed written consent from all participants involved in our study.

Patients

The study population included 549 ESRD patients who started PD at Yonsei University Severance Hospital or NHIS Ilsan Hospital between January 2000 and December 2005. Exclusion criteria were 1) <18 years of age at initiation of PD, 2) follow-up duration less than 6 months, 3) prior history of HD or a kidney transplant before the initiation of PD, 4) recovery of kidney function, or 5) initiation of PD for other reasons such as acute renal failure or congestive heart failure. Therefore, this prospective observational study included a total of 441 incident patients (Figure 1).

Data collection

Demographic and clinical data were collected at the beginning of PD including age, gender, body mass index (BMI) calculated as weight/(height)^2, cause of ESRD, and presence of diabetes and coronary artery disease. Each subject was scored using the Charlson Comorbidity Index at the start of PD. This index is a scoring system that includes weight factors for important concomitant diseases [16,17]. All patients underwent urea kinetic studies within three months of PD initiation including Kt/V urea, normalized protein catabolic rate (nPCR), percentage of lean body mass (%LBM), PD ultrafiltration, and residual glomerular filtration rate (GFR). Residual GFR was calculated as the average urea and creatinine clearance from a 24-h urine collection [18]. nPCR was calculated by the methods described by Randerson et al. [19] and normalized to standard body weight (total body water/0.58). Total body water was estimated by Watson formula [20]. The %LBM was determined from creatinine kinetics according to Keshaviah et al. [21]. Laboratory data obtained at the time of dialysis adequacy measurement were considered baseline values and included serum sodium, potassium, and bicarbonate concentrations, serum albumin, ferritin, and serum C-reactive protein (CRP) levels. All laboratory parameters were recorded longitudinally throughout the follow-up period, and were calculated as an average of the mean of measurements every 3-month period. Because dialysis adequacy is generally measured within the first month after starting dialysis therapy and every 6 month thereafter in our centers, time-averaged dialysis adequacy parameters were determined as an average of the mean of the measurements in every 6-month period. Serum sodium concentration was measured by an electrode-based method (UniCel DXC 800; Beckman Coulter, Inc., CA, USA) and was corrected for serum glucose level (in such a case of serum glucose above a normal of 100 mg/dL) using the following formula: Corrected sodium = measured sodium+0.016×(serum glucose−100) [22].

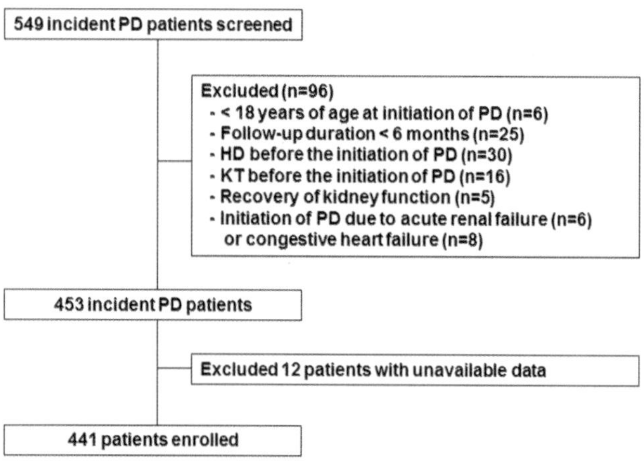

Figure 1. Flow chart of participants in the cohort. PD, peritoneal dialysis; HD, hemodialysis; KT, kidney transplant.

Study outcomes

Study participants were followed until December 31, 2011. The primary outcome parameters were all-cause, cardiovascular, and infection-related mortality.

Statistical analysis

All values are expressed as the mean ± standard deviation or percentages. Statistical analyses were performed using SPSS for Windows version 13.0 (SPSS, Inc., Chicago, IL, USA) and the software packages R version 3.0.2. Data were analyzed using Student's *t*–test and the Chi-square test, and ANOVA was used for multiple comparisons. The Kolmogorov-Smirnov test was used to determine the normality of the distribution of parameters. If data were not normally distributed, they were expressed as the median and interquartile range (or after log-transformation) and were compared using the Mann–Whitney test or Kruskal-Wallis test. Relationships between serum sodium and continuous variables were assessed using Pearson's correlation coefficient, and categorical variables were evaluated using Spearman's R test. Multiple linear regression analysis was performed to identify the determinants of serum sodium level.

Under conditions of competing risk, Kaplan-Meier analyses and traditional Cox regression models can produce misleading results, so corresponding competing risk methods were used [23–25]. The cumulative incidence of death was compared among 3 groups based on tertile of time-averaged serum sodium (TA-Na) levels (< 137, 137 to 139, and ≥139 mEq/L) using the K-sample test developed by Gray [23]. Data for switch to HD, kidney transplantation, and loss to follow-up were censored in the analysis. Patients who died within the first 3 months after converting to HD or receiving a kidney graft were considered deaths related to PD. To determine risk factors for mortality, multivariate Cox regression using methods of Fine and Gray [24] was performed, and four different models were constructed; Model 1 adjusted for epidemiologic parameters including age, sex, BMI, and Charlson Comorbidity Index score. Model 2 adjusted for all parameters in model 1 plus medication use including dose of furosemide, use of icodextrin, and use of high-glucose dialysate. Model 3 adjusted for all parameters in model 2 plus dialysis dose including PD ultrafiltration and total Kt/Vurea. Model 4 adjusted for all parameters in model 3 plus malnutrition-inflammatory parameters including serum potassium, serum bicarbonate, serum albumin, serum ferritin, CRP, residual GFR, nPCR, and %LBM. The results are expressed as a hazard ratio (HR) and 95% confidence interval (CI). First-order interaction terms between covariates were examined for all models, but there was no evidence of an interaction between those covariates. A p–value less than 0.05 was considered statistically significant.

Table 1. Clinical characteristics of the study subjects stratified by time-averaged serum sodium level.

	Time-averaged serum sodium (mEq/L; number of subjects)				
	Total (n = 441)	**<137 (n = 145)**	**137 to <139 (n = 148)**	**≥139 (n = 148)**	***p* for trend**
Age (years)	59.2±13.8	60.6±13.4	58.3±14.2	58.8±13.8	0.251
Gender (male)	240 (54.4)	76 (52.4)	79 (53.4)	85 (57.4)	0.388
Body mass index (kg/m^2)	22.9±6.7	22.4±2.6	23.5±7.7	22.6±3.3	0.846
Presence of diabetes mellitus	227 (51.5)	73 (50.3)	73 (49.3)	81 (54.7)	0.446
Presence of coronary artery disease	70 (15.9)	27 (18.6)	24 (16.2)	19 (12.8)	0.176
Charlson Comorbidity Index score	3.0±1.0	3.2±1.0	3.0±1.1	3.0±0.9	0.065
Laboratory findings*					
Serum sodium (mEq/L)	137.7±2.7	134.5±2.1	138.0±0.6	140.3±0.9	<0.001
Serum potassium (mEq/L)	4.1±0.7	4.2±0.8	4.1±0.6	4.1±0.7	0.274
Serum bicarbonate (mEq/L)	25.9±2.4	25.7±2.3	26.1±2.3	26.0±2.5	0.206
Serum albumin (g/dL)	3.1±0.5	2.9±0.5	3.1±0.6	3.2±0.5	<0.001
Serum ferritin (ng/mL)	274.3 [52–521]	294.7 [52–509]	258.3 [59–521]	271.2 [56–514]	0.314
C-reactive protein (mg/dL)	0.7 [0.01–16.2]	0.8 [0.01–14.2]	0.4 [0.01–6.3]	0.8 [0.01–16.2]	0.623
Residual GFR (mL/min/1.73m^2)*	4.0 [0.2–29.3]	3.9 [0.2–18.9]	4.0 [0.3–29.3]	4.4 [0.3–19.0]	0.004
Daily ultrafiltration (mL)*					
Peritoneal dialysis	731.6±569.3	811.2±601.6	751.2±563.1	634.1±531.4	0.008
Total	1827.6±691.4	1847.6±706.0	1794.2±700.2	1841.4±671.3	0.943
Automated peritoneal dialysis	5 (1.1)	1 (0.7)	2 (1.4)	2 (1.4)	0.594
Icodextrin use daily	35 (7.9)	25 (17.2)	10 (6.8)	0 (0.0)	<0.001
2.5% and/or 4.25% dialysate use daily	105 (23.8)	38 (26.2)	41 (27.7)	26 (17.6)	0.081
Total weekly Kt/V urea*	2.3±0.8	2.2±0.7	2.3±0.9	2.4±0.8	0.061
nPCR (g/Kg/day)*	0.9±0.3	0.9±0.3	0.9±0.3	1.0±0.2	0.012
Lean body mass (% body weight)*	66.4±12.4	61.4±11.9	66.8±13.8	67.4±14.2	<0.001
Anti-hypertensive medications					
ACE inhibitor or ARB	302 (68.5)	98 (67.6)	104 (70.3)	100 (67.6)	0.995
Alpha and/or beta blocker	217 (49.2)	72 (49.7)	78 (52.7)	67 (45.3)	0.450
Calcium channel blocker	265 (60.1)	86 (59.3)	91 (61.5)	88 (59.5)	0.981

Table 1. Cont.

	Time-averaged serum sodium (mEq/L; number of subjects)				
	Total (n = 441)	**<137 (n = 145)**	**137 to <139 (n = 148)**	**≥139 (n = 148)**	***p* for trend**
Thiazide or thiazide-like diuretics	48 (10.9)	19 (13.1)	13 (8.8)	16 (10.8)	0.534
Lasix or other loop diuretics	200 (45.4)	64 (44.1)	71 (48.0)	65 (43.9)	0.966
Dose of furosemide (mg/day)	46.8±61.6	48.7±63.5	52.4±66.1	39.4±54.4	0.192

Values for categorical variables are given as number (percentage); values for continuous variables are given as mean ± standard deviation or median [interquartile range].
*Laboratory and dialysis-specific parameters are given as time-averaged values. GFR, glomerular filtration rate; nPCR, normalized protein catabolic rate; ACE, angiotensin converting enzyme; ARB, angiotensin receptor blocker.

Results

Patient characteristics

The mean age of the patients was 59.2 years (range, 22 to 85 years), 54.4% were males, and patients were on PD for a mean duration of 43.2 months (range, 6 to 142 months). The mean baseline and TA-Na levels were 138.2±3.7 mEq/L and 137.7±2.7 mEq/L (median, 138.1 mEq/L; range, 126.2 to 143.1 mEq/L) respectively. Table 1 details the baseline characteristics of the 441 patients categorized by tertile of TA-Na level. Serum albumin (p for trend <0.001), residual GFR (p for trend $= 0.004$), nPCR (p for trend $= 0.012$), and %LBM (p for trend <0.001) were higher at higher TA-Na level, whereas PD ultrafiltration (p for trend $= 0.008$) and use of icodextrin (p for trend <0.001) were lower at higher TA-Na level. However, we observed no significant differences in the types of antihypertensive agents, dosage of furosemide used, or use of high-glucose dialysate according to TA-Na level.

Factors associated with baseline serum sodium

Correlation analyses were performed to identify factors associated with baseline serum sodium level (Table 2). There was no correlation between age, gender, BMI, Charlson Comorbidity Index score, serum potassium, serum CRP, total Kt/V urea, nPCR and serum sodium. In contrast, baseline serum sodium level positively correlated with serum albumin ($\rho = 0.177$; $p<0.001$), residual GFR ($\rho = 0.211$; $p<0.001$), and %LBM ($\rho = 0.109$; $p = 0.022$), whereas it inversely correlated with serum ferritin level ($\rho = -0.133$; $p = 0.005$) and PD ultrafiltration ($\rho = -0.169$; $p< 0.001$). A multivariate linear regression analysis that was adjusted for these factors revealed that serum albumin ($\beta = 0.145$; $p = 0.003$), residual GFR ($\beta = 0.130$; $p = 0.018$), and PD ultrafiltration ($\beta = -0.114$; $p = 0.024$) were independently associated with baseline serum sodium.

Hyponatremia as a predictor of mortality

During follow-up, 149 deaths were recorded, and the median survival period was 34.8 months (range, 6.0 to 142.2 months). Infection (37.6%) was the most common cause of death in this study, followed by cardiovascular disease (36.2%). All-cause death occurred in 81 (55.9%) patients in the lowest tertile compared with 37 (25.0%) and 31 (20.9%) patients in the middle and highest tertiles ($p<0.001$), respectively. Similar findings were observed for cardiovascular and infection-related deaths (data not shown).

Higher TA-Na was associated with lower mortality (Table 3). Even after adjusting for various parameters, the association between the two was significant and consistent. Using serum TA-Na as a continuous variable, the HR for all-cause mortality was 0.79 for every 1 mEq/L increase in TA-Na (95% CI, 0.73–0.86; $p<0.001$), indicating that higher TA-Na was significantly associated with decreased risk of mortality. Moreover, the increased mortality risk associated with lower TA-Na was similar for infection-related (HR, 0.77 per 1 mEq/L higher TA-Na; 95% CI, 0.70–0.85; $p<0.001$) death. In addition, patients with TA-Na<137 mEq/L conferred a 3.35- and 3.18-fold increased risk of all-cause and infection-related mortality, respectively, compared with patients with TA-Na≥139 mEq/L. However, the risk for cardiovascular death was not associated with TA-NA levels. The cumulative incidence of death was significantly lower in patients with higher TA-Na level compared to patients with a TA-Na level <137 mEq/L (Figure 2).

Discussion

In this study, we sought to delineate the relationship between serum sodium level and mortality in our ESRD cohort of patients with PD. We showed that serum sodium level exhibited a significant positive association with serum albumin and residual renal function (RRF), while it inversely correlated with PD ultrafiltration. In addition, low TA-Na level independently predicted all-cause mortality, suggesting that hyponatremia is a potential predictor of adverse outcomes in these patients.

Serum sodium concentration in humans is tightly regulated and the presence of hypotonic hyponatremia implies that the extracellular fluid compartment contains water in excess of sodium. Interestingly, the kidneys' ability to dilute urine, that is to elaborate urine with minimal osmolality, is generally preserved even in advanced CKD. However, its ability to concentrate is, indeed, severely limited in these patients [26]. Furthermore, in ESRD patients, water and sodium removal are almost exclusively determined by dialysis procedure, particularly when accompanied by complete loss of RRF. Therefore, dialysis-dependent patients are vulnerable to develop dysnatremia. However, the clinical impact of hyponatremia in these patients has been inadequately studied.

Table 2. Cross-sectional correlation analyses between baseline serum sodium level and patient characteristics.

		Serum Na	Age	BMI	CCI	K	Albumin	Ferritin*	CRP*	Residual GFR*	PD UF	Total Kt/Vurea	nPCR	LBM
Serum Na	ρ	1	−0.047	0.072	−0.058	0.022	0.177	−0.133	0.006	0.211	−0.169	0.068	0.054	0.109
	p	-	0.329	0.129	0.223	0.640	<0.001	0.005	0.909	<0.001	<0.001	0.156	0.260	0.022
Age	ρ		1	−0.019	0.041	−0.133	−0.230	0.266	0.261	−0.058	−0.026	0.033	−0.165	−0.458
	p		–	0.695	0.695	0.005	<0.001	<0.001	<0.001	0.222	0.590	0.489	<0.001	<0.001
BMI	ρ			1	0.083	−0.007	0.021	0.024	−0.070	−0.039	0.026	−0.013	0.227	−0.046
	p			–	0.082	0.880	0.661	0.609	0.161	0.419	0.588	0.780	<0.001	0.333
CCI.	ρ				1	0.021	−0.058	0.032	0.030	−0.044	0.126	−0.019	−0.020	0.021
	p				–	0.659	0.226	0.508	0.542	0.360	0.008	0.697	0.675	0.660
K	ρ					1	0.031	−0.140	−0.070	−0.003	0.121	−0.074	0.152	0.098
	p					-	0.510	0.003	0.162	0.958	0.574	<0.001	0.001	0.039
Albumin	ρ						1	-0.094	−0.096	0.145	−0.015	0.147	0.271	0.269
	p						-	0.048	0.053	0.002	0.754	0.002	<0.001	<0.001
Ferritin*	ρ							1	0.243	−0.246	0.129	−0.088	−0.152	−0.218
	p							-	<0.001	<0.001	0.007	0.066	0.001	<0.001
CRP*	ρ								1	-0.070	0.096	0.047	−0.114	−0.193
	p								-	).158	0.055	0.342	0.022	<0.001
Residual GFR*	ρ									1	−0.365	0.533	0.238	0.376
	p									-	<0.001	<0.001	<0.001	<0.001
PD UF	ρ										1	0.065	0.067	0.027
	p										-	0.171	0.157	0.577
Total Kt/Vurea	ρ											1	0.451	0.293
	p											-	<0.001	<0.001
nPCR	ρ												1	0.464
	p												-	<0.001
LBM	ρ													1
	p													-

*Data for ferritin, CRP, and residual GFR were log-transformed.
BMI, body mass index; CCI, Charlson Comorbidity Index score; Na, sodium; K, serum potassium; tCO2, serum bicarbonate; CRP, C-reactive protein; GFR, glomerular filtration rate; PD UF, peritoneal dialysis ultrafiltration; nPCR, normalized protein, LBM, percentage of lean body mass.

Table 3. Multivariable Cox regression analyses for all-cause, cardiovascular, and infection-related mortality.

	Model 1			Model 2			Model 3			Model 4		
	HR	**(95% CI)**	*p*	**HR**	**(95% CI)**	*p*	**HR**	**(95% CI)**	*p*	**HR**	**(95% CI)**	*p*
Continuous model												
(per 1mEq/L TA-Na increase)												
All-cause mortality	0.78	(0.73–0.84)	<0.001	0.77	(0.72–0.83)	<0.001	0.78	(0.73–0.84)	<0.001	0.79	(0.73–0.86)	<0.001
Cardiovascular mortality	0.93	(0.84–1.02)	0.100	0.91	(0.82–1.00)	0.043	0.93	(0.84–1.02)	0.120	0.95	(0.84–1.08)	0.440
Infection-related mortality	0.78	(0.72–0.85)	<0.001	0.78	(0.72–0.85)	<0.001	0.78	(0.71–0.85)	<0.001	0.77	(0.70–0.85)	<0.001
Categorical (tertile) model												
All-cause mortality												
TA-Na<137 mEq/L	3.35	(2.15–5.24)	<0.001	3.70	(2.34–5.85)	<0.001	3.53	(2.23–5.60)	<0.001	3.35	(2.01–5.60)	<0.001
137 mEq/L≤TA-Na<139 mEq/L	1.13	(0.67–1.91)	0.640	1.16	(0.69–1.96)	0.570	1.12	(0.67–1.88)	0.660	1.17	(0.66–2.07)	0.600
TA-Na≥139 mEq/L	1.00	(reference)		1.00	(reference)		1.00	(reference)		1.00	(reference)	
Cardiovascular mortality												
TA-Na<137 mEq/L	1.82	(0.93–3.55)	0.079	2.09	(1.06–4.10)	0.033	1.90	(0.96–3.77)	0.067	1.70	(0.78–3.71)	0.180
137 mEq/L≤TA-Na<139 mEq/L	1.29	(0.64–2.61)	0.480	1.29	(0.63–2.61)	0.480	1.20	(0.59–2.45)	0.610	1.37	(0.64–2.92)	0.420
TA-Na≥139 mEq/L	1.00	(reference)		1.00	(reference)		1.00	(reference)		1.00	(reference)	
Infection-related mortality												
TA-Na<137 mEq/L	2.94	(1.65–5.26)	<0.001	3.05	(1.68–5.51)	<0.001	2.94	(1.60–5.41)	<0.001	3.18	(1.58–6.41)	0.0012
137 mEq/L≤TA-Na<139 mEq/L	0.79	(0.36–1.74)	0.560	0.81	(0.36–1.76)	0.570	0.79	(0.36–1.76)	0.570	0.78	(0.31–2.02)	0.610
TA-Na≥139 mEq/L	1.00	(reference)		1.00	(reference)		1.00	(reference)		1.00	(reference)	

TA-Na, time-averaged serum sodium; HR, hazard ratio; CI, confidence interval. Model 1 adjusted for epidemiologic parameters including age, sex, body mass index, and Charlson Comorbidity Index score. Model 2 adjusted for all model 1 parameters plus medication including dose of furosemide, use of icodextrin, and use of high glucose dialysate. Model 3 adjusted for all model 2 parameters plus dialysis dose including peritoneal dialysis ultrafiltration (PDUF) and total Kt/V urea. Model 4 adjusted for all model 3 parameters plus malnutrition-inflammatory parameters including serum potassium, serum bicarbonate, serum albumin, serum ferritin, C-reactive protein (CRP), residual glomerular filtration rate (GFR), normalized protein catabolic rate (nPCR), and percentage of lean body mass (%LBM). Laboratory (serum sodium, potassium, bicarbonate, albumin, ferritin, and CRP) and dialysis-specific (PDUF, Kt/V urea, residual GFR, nPCR, %LBM) parameters are given as time-averaged values.

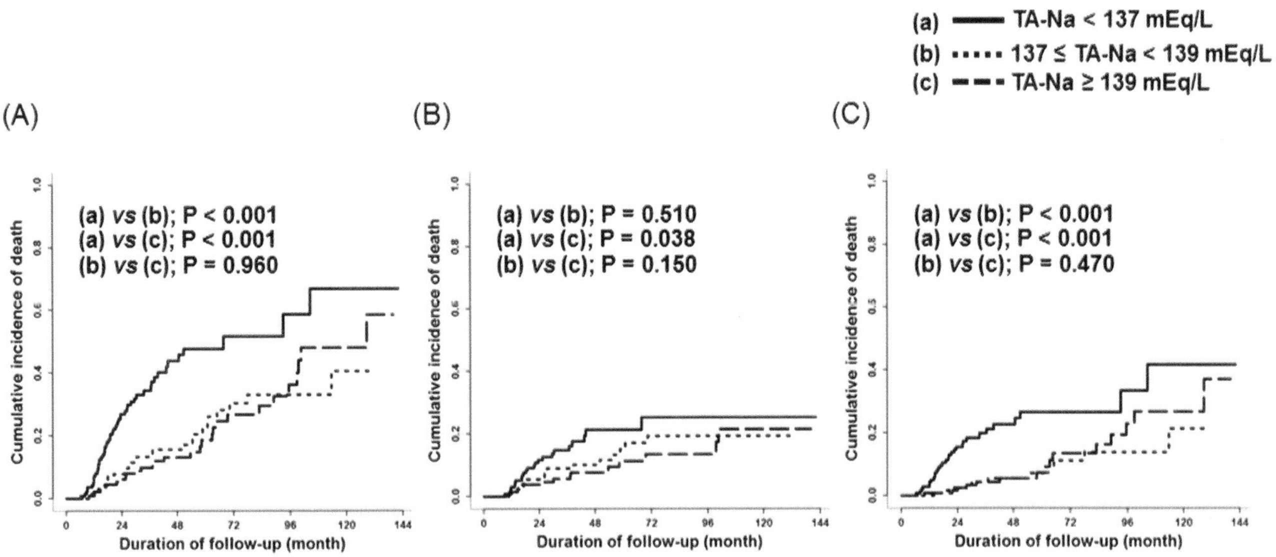

Figure 2. The Cumulative incidence of all-cause (A), cardiovascular (B), and infection-related (C) mortality based on the level of time-averaged serum sodium (TA-Na).

In our study, hyponatremia (defined as <135 mEq/L) was present in 58 patients (13.2%) at the initiation of PD. However, previous studies of PD patients have used a more strict definition of hyponatremia (defined as ≤130 mEq/L on 2 consecutive measurements) [13–15]. When we use this definition, 11 patients (2.5%) presented with hyponatremia at the start of PD. In addition, 21 patients (4.8%) developed hyponatremia during follow-up, which was comparable with the 5.2% of patients reported in a previous study by Zevallos *et al.* [13] but much lower than the 14.5% of patients observed in a recent study by Dimitriadis *et al* [14]. However, when we defined hyponatremia as <135 mEq/L, which is the threshold generally accepted in clinical practice, 115 patients (26.1%) developed hyponatremia during the follow-up period. These findings suggest that hyponatremia is common in PD patients, although the incidence may differ depending on the chosen definition.

The underlying mechanisms for hyponatremia in PD patients are complex and unclear. In general, as suggested by Edelman *et al.* [27], serum sodium concentration is determined by rapidly exchangeable body sodium, potassium, and total body water. Thus, hypotonic hyponatremia typically develops due to decrease in the fraction of body sodium and potassium over body water. Such reduction is potentially caused by various combinations of changes in body cations and water. In particular, the cation fraction can be often decreased in patients on dialysis because these patients are prone to fluid overload. In addition to this mechanism, dialysis-specific conditions should be taken into to explain hyponatremia in dialysis patients. Of note, therapeutic modality itself such as diffusive transport, convective transport, and ultrafiltration can induce the changes of body cations and water and thus results in altered serum sodium concentrations in PD patients [28]. Therefore, in patients on PD, alterations in serum sodium concentrations can occur as a result of the dialytic and nondialytic changes in the mass balance of body sodium, body potassium, and body water.

In addition, osmotic shift of water from the intracellular into the extracellular compartment and intracellular entry of sodium are putative mechanisms of PD-associated hyponatremia in certain clinical states, including potassium deficit, protein-energy wasting (PEW) and use of icodextrin solutions as PD dialysate [13,29–31]. However, although there is evidence suggesting that entry of extracellular sodium into the cells causes hyponatremia in various settings [13,29–31], hyponatremia is unlikely to occur unless such a shift is accompanied by imbalances of monovalent cations and water that decrease the cation fraction as aforementioned.

The most important finding in this study is the strong and significant association between lower serum sodium concentration and mortality in PD patients. This association has previously been shown in maintenance dialysis patients and CKD patients prior to dialysis therapy [6–10,12,15]. In keeping with these, our robust finding supports evidence that hyponatremia portends a poor prognosis in these patients. In multivariate models with rigorous adjustments, low serum sodium concentration remained an independent predictor of mortality. In addition, patients with TA-Na level <137 mEq/L had adjusted HRs for all-cause, and infection-related mortality of 3.35 and 3.18, respectively, compared to the reference group with TA-Na level ≥139 mEq/L, indicating that higher serum sodium level is associated significantly with lower mortality risk. Relevant to our finding is a recent observation in HD patients based on data from the Dialysis Outcomes and Practice Pattern Study, showing that patients with mean serum sodium level <137 mEq/L had a 45% higher risk of death compared with patients with serum sodium ≥140 mEq/L [7].

The underlying mechanisms for increased mortality in advanced CKD patients with lower serum sodium level are also unclear. In severely ill patients without CKD, vasopressin is secreted in response to neurohormonal activation. Whether vasopressin contributes to the development of hyponatremia in patients with CKD is largely unknown. Possibly, vasopressin could explain the association between hyponatremia and mortality in this population if it acts in the same manner as in non-CKD patients with serious underlying conditions [32]. In addition, hyponatremia is related to other adverse features. In particular, reduced RRF may limit free water clearance, resulting in hyponatremia. Interestingly, RRF was identified as a significant factor associated with baseline serum sodium in this study; higher residual GFR was independently associated with a higher serum sodium concentration. This finding suggests that residual kidney function even in the advanced stage can contribute to sodium handling and prevent hyponatremia by excreting relatively more water than sodium. Conversely, loss of RRF in the end may result in inability to control excess water, leading to hyponatremia. Furthermore, PEW status may affect sodium level by depleting intracellular potassium and solutes [13,29]. In the present study, there were significant associations between serum sodium level and some nutritional markers such as serum albumin and %LBM. If this is the case, low sodium level can represent underlying unfavorable conditions. Finally, inflammatory response has recently been suggested as a cause of hyponatremia [33–35]. Among many inflammatory markers, interleukin-6 is reported to induce central vasopressin secretion [35]. Of note, loss of RRF, PEW, and inflammation are established predictors of mortality in patients on dialysis [36–38], and all of the aforementioned mechanisms together may account for the association between hyponatremia and mortality in these patients.

There are several limitations to the present study. This was an observational study with a relatively small sample size. Hence, causality of our findings needs further confirmation. In particular, there has been much concern about whether hyponatremia directly causes death or is merely a marker of disease severity. Furthermore, it is unknown whether correcting hyponatremia can improve clinical outcomes in CKD patients. A detailed discussion about these issues is beyond our scope. However, it is likely that hyponatremia can occur in severe underlying conditions and may itself further increase the risk of adverse outcomes. Lack of information to further explain hyponatremia is another drawback. Because this was an observational study, we could not collect data describing the amount of sodium removed by PD or the amount being ingested in the diet. Other data representing overall volume status such as body weight changes, dietary water intake, and a bioelectrical impedance analysis were not available for analysis. Despite these limitations, this study showed that low TA-Na level independently predicted all-cause and infection-related mortality, even after extensive adjusting for demographic, clinical, laboratory, and dialysis-specific covariates. Our robust findings suggest that hyponatremia portends a poor prognosis, and thus physicians should be more meticulous in clinical practice with respect to correcting both this electrolyte imbalance and underlying disease.

Conclusion

This study showed that a low serum sodium concentration was an independent predictor of mortality in PD patients. The relationship between low serum sodium level and adverse outcomes may be attributed to loss of RRF and underlying conditions such as PEW. Whether correcting hyponatremia improves patient survival requires further investigations.

Author Contributions

Conceived and designed the experiments: TIC THY SKS SWK KHC DSH SHH. Performed the experiments: TIC YLK HWK GWR EWK JTP. Analyzed the data: TIC SHH. Contributed to the writing of the manuscript: TIC SHH.

References

1. Combs S, Berl T (2014) Dysnatremias in patients with kidney disease. Am J kidney Dis 63: 294–303.
2. Adrogue HJ, Madias NE (2000) Hyponatremia. N Engl J Med 342: 1581–1589.
3. Upadhyay A, Jaber BL, Madias NE (2006) Incidence and prevalence of hyponatremia. Am J Med 119 (suppl 1): S30–S35.
4. Arroyo V, Rodes J, Gutierrez-Lizarraga MA, Revert L (1976) Prognostic value of spontaneous hyponatremia in cirrhosis with ascites. Am J Dig Dis 21: 249–256.
5. Bettari L, Fiuzat M, Shaw LK, Wojdyla DM, Metra M, et al. (2012) Hyponatremia and long-term outcomes in chronic heart failure–an observational study from the Duke Databank for Cardiovascular Diseases. J Card Fail 18: 74–81.
6. Waikar SS, Curhan GC, Brunelli SM (2011) Mortality associated with low serum sodium concentration in maintenance hemodialysis. Am J Med 124: 77–84.
7. Hecking M, Karaboyas A, Saran R, Sen A, Hörl WH, et al. (2012) Predialysis serum sodium level, dialysate sodium, and mortality in maintenance hemodialysis patients: the Dialysis Outcomes and Practice Patterns Study (DOPPS). Am J Kidney Dis 59: 238–248.
8. Mc Causland FR, Brunelli SM, Waikar SS (2012) Dialysate sodium, serum sodium and mortality in maintenance hemodialysis. Nephrol Dial Transplant 27: 1613–1618.
9. Nigwekar SU, Wenger J, Thadhani R, Bhan I (2013) Hyponatremia, mineral metabolism, and mortality in incident maintenance hemodialysis patients: a cohort study. Am J Kidney Dis 62: 755–762.
10. Kovesdy CP, Lott EH, Lu JL, Malakauskas SM, Ma JZ, et al. (2012) Hyponatremia, hypernatremia, and mortality in patients with chronic kidney disease with and without congestive heart failure. Circulation 125: 677–684.
11. Lee HH, Choi SJ, Lee HN, Na SY, Chang JH, et al. (2010) De novo hyponatremia in patients undergoing peritoneal dialysis: A 12-month observational study. Korean J Nephrol 29: 31–37.
12. Kang SH, Cho KH, Park JW, Yoon KW, Do JY (2013) Characteristics and clinical outcomes of hyponatraemia in peritoneal dialysis patients. Nephrology (Carlton) 18: 132–137.
13. Zevallos G, Oreopoulos DG, Halperin ML (2001) Hyponatremia in patients undergoing CAPD: Role of water gain and/or malnutrition. Perit Dial Int 21: 72–76.
14. Dimitriadis C, Sekercioglu N, Pipili C, Oreopoulos DG, Bargman JM (2014) Hyponatraemia in peritoneal dialysis: Epidemiology in a single center and correlation with clinical and biochemical parameters. Perit Dial Int 34: 260–270.
15. Tseng MH, Cheng CJ, Sung CC, Chou YC, Chu P, et al. (2014) Hyponatremia is a surrogate marker of poor outcome in peritoneal dialysis-related peritonitis. BMC nephrol 15: 113.
16. Charlson ME, Pompei P, Ales KL, MacKenzie CR (1987) A new method of classifying prognostic comorbidity in longitudinal studies: development and validation. J Chronic Dis 40: 373–383.
17. Charlson M, Szatrowski TP, Peterson J, Gold J (1994) Validation of a combined comorbidity index. J Clin Epidemiol 47: 1245–1251.
18. Nolph KD, Moore HL, Prowant B, Meyer M, Twardowski ZJ, et al. (1993) Cross sectional assessment of weekly urea and creatinine clearances and indices of nutrition in continuous ambulatory peritoneal dialysis patients. Perit Dial Int 13: 178–183.
19. Randerson DH, Chapman GV, Farrell PC (1981) Amino acid and dietary status in CAPD patients, in Peritoneal Dialysis, edited by Atkins RC, Farrell PC, Thomson N, Edinburgh, Churchill- Livingstone. 180–191.
20. Watson PE, Watson ID, Batt RD (1980) Total body water volumes for adult males and females estimated from simple anthropometric measurements. Am J Clin Nutr 33: 27–39.
21. Keshaviah PR, Nolph KD, Moore HL, Prowant B, Emerson PF, et al. (1994) Lean body mass estimation by creatinine kinetics. J Am Soc Nephrol. 4: 1475–1485.
22. Katz MA (1973) Hyperglycemia-induced hyponatremia–calculation of expected serum sodium depression. N Engl J Med 289: 843–844.
23. Kim HT (2007) Cumulative incidence in competing risks data and competing risks regression analysis. Clin Cancer Res 13: 559–565.
24. Fine J, Gray R (1999) A proportional hazards model for the subdistribution of a competing risk. J Am Stat Assoc 94: 496–509.
25. Verduijn M1, Grootendorst DC, Dekker FW, Jager KJ, le Cessie S (2011) The analysis of competing events like cause-specific mortality–beware of the Kaplan-Meier method. Nephrol Dial Transplant 26: 56–61.
26. Hoorn EJ, Zietse R (2008) Hyponatremia revisited: translating physiology to practice Nephron Physiol 108: 46–59.
27. Edelman IS, Leibman J, O'Meara MP, Birkenfeld LW (1958) Interrelations between serum sodium concentration, serum osmolality and total exchangeable sodium, total exchangeable potassium and total body water. J Clin Invest 37: 1236–1256.
28. Nguyen MK, Kurtz I (2005) A new formula for predicting alterations in plasma sodium concentration in peritoneal dialysis. Am J Physiol Renal Physiol 288: F1113–F1117.
29. Cherney DZ, Zevallos G, Oreopoulos D, Halperin ML (2001) A physiological analysis of hyponatremia: implications for patients on peritoneal dialysis. Perit Dial Int 21: 7–13.
30. Posthuma N, ter Wee PM, Donker AJ, Oe PL, van Dorp W, et al. (1997) Serum disaccharides and osmolality in CCPD patients using icodextrin or glucose as daytime dwell. Perit Dial Int 17: 602–607.
31. Gokal R, Moberly J, Lindholm B, Mujais S (2002) Metabolic and laboratory effects of icodextrin. Kidney Int Suppl 81: S62–S71.

32. Hoorn EJ, Zietse R (2013) Hyponatremia and mortality: moving beyond associations. Am J Kidney Dis 62: 139–149.
33. Mandai S, Kuwahara M, Kasagi Y, Kusaka K, Tanaka T, et al. (2013) Lower serum sodium level predicts higher risk of infection-related hospitalization in maintenance hemodialysis patients: an observational cohort study. BMC Nephrol 14: 276.
34. Beukhof CM, Hoorn EJ, Lindemans J, Zietse R (2007) Novel risk factors for hospital-acquired hyponatraemia: a matched case-control study. Clin Endocrinol (Oxf) 66: 367–372.
35. Swart RM, Hoorn EJ, Betjes MG, Zietse R (2011) Hyponatremia and inflammation: the emerging role of interleukin-6 in osmoregulation. Nephron Physiol 118: 45–51.
36. Vilar E, Farrington K (2011) Emerging importance of residual renal function in end-stage renal failure. Semin Dial 24: 487–494.
37. Han SH, Han DS (2014) Nutrition in patients on peritoneal dialysis. Nat Rev Nephrol 8: 163–175.
38. Wang AY (2011) Consequences of chronic inflammation in peritoneal dialysis. Semin Nephrol 31: 159–171.

Pioglitazone Improves Fat Distribution, the Adipokine Profile and Hepatic Insulin Sensitivity in Non-Diabetic End-Stage Renal Disease Subjects on Maintenance Dialysis: A Randomized Cross-Over Pilot Study

Anne Zanchi[1,3]*, Luc Tappy[2,3], Kim-Anne Lê[2], Murielle Bortolotti[2], Nicolas Theumann[4], Georges Halabi[1], Thierry Gauthier[1], Claudine Mathieu[1], Sylvie Tremblay[1], Pauline Coti Bertrand[3], Michel Burnier[1], Daniel Teta[1]

1 Service of Nephrology, Department of Medicine, Lausanne University Hospital, Centre Hospitalier Universitaire Vaudois, Lausanne, Switzerland, **2** Department of Physiology, University of Lausanne, Lausanne, Switzerland, **3** Service of Endocrinology, Diabetes and Metabolism, Department of Medicine, Lausanne University Hospital, Centre Hospitalier Universitaire Vaudois, Lausanne, Switzerland, **4** Department of Radiology, Lausanne University Hospital, Centre Hospitalier Universitaire Vaudois, Lausanne, Switzerland

Abstract

Background: Fat redistribution, increased inflammation and insulin resistance are prevalent in non-diabetic subjects treated with maintenance dialysis. The aim of this study was to test whether pioglitazone, a powerful insulin sensitizer, alters body fat distribution and adipokine secretion in these subjects and whether it is associated with improved insulin sensitivity.

Trial Design: This was a double blind cross-over study with 16 weeks of pioglitazone 45 mg vs placebo involving 12 subjects.

Methods: At the end of each phase, body composition (anthropometric measurements, dual energy X-ray absorptometry (DEXA), abdominal CT), hepatic and muscle insulin sensitivity (2-step hyperinsulinemic euglycemic clamp with 2H2-glucose) were measured and fasting blood adipokines and cardiometabolic risk markers were monitored.

Results: Four months treatment with pioglitazone had no effect on total body weight or total fat but decreased the visceral/sub-cutaneous adipose tissue ratio by 16% and decreased the leptin/adiponectin (L/A) ratio from 3.63×10^{-3} to 0.76×10^{-3}. This was associated with a 20% increase in hepatic insulin sensitivity without changes in muscle insulin sensitivity, a 12% increase in HDL cholesterol and a 50% decrease in CRP.

Conclusions/Limitations: Pioglitazone significantly changes the visceral-subcutaneous fat distribution and plasma L/A ratio in non diabetic subjects on maintenance dialysis. This was associated with improved hepatic insulin sensitivity and a reduction of cardio-metabolic risk markers. Whether these effects may improve the outcome of non diabetic end-stage renal disease subjects on maintenance dialysis still needs further evaluation.

Editor: Stephen L. Atkin, Weill Cornell Medical College Qatar, Qatar

Funding: Funding of this study was internal to the Service of Nephrology at the Lausanne University Hospital. The funders had no role in study design, data collection and analysis, decision to publish, or preparation of the manuscript. Investigators performed completely the study design, data collection and analysis and prepared the manuscript.

Competing Interests: The authors have declared that no competing interests exist.

* Email: Anne.Zanchi@chuv.ch

Introduction

Patients with ESRD on maintenance dialysis are prone to body fat redistribution with an excess of visceral adipose tissue (VAT), relative to subcutaneous adipose tissue (SAT). This pattern of fat distribution is associated with dyslipidemia [1] and inflammatory cytokine production [2], all intimately linked with insulin resistance (IR). Abdominal obesity, as well as truncal fat distribution without obesity, predict all cause and cardiovascular mortality in patients with ESRD [3].

Furthermore, adipose tissue accumulation coupled with low glomerular filtration rate may lead to the accumulation of plasma adipokines. Among adipokines, lower levels of adiponectin have been associated with the development of IR, whereas leptin is directly correlated with body fat and nutritional intake [4,5]. In ESRD, leptin accumulates to a much larger extent than adiponectin, thus producing an elevated plasma leptin to adiponectin (L/A) ratio [6]. Plasma L/A ratio is identified as the best correlate of IR measured by the hyperinsulinemic euglycemic clamp (HEGC) in African American patients with ESRD on maintenance hemodialysis [7]. The L/A plasma ratio is also considered as an atherogenic index in the general population [8], and in patients with type 2 diabetes (T2DM) [9]. Thus, a high L/A ratio in ESRD may play a pivotal role in the pathogenesis of both IR and cardiovascular complications in ESRD.

Glitazones are effective insulin sensitizers available in clinical practice and their use is associated with significant and favourable changes in body fat distribution and adipokine profile in subjects with T2DM [10]. Furthermore, glitazones have also been shown to improve glucose metabolism in diabetic and non diabetic ESRD subjects [11–13]. Whether these effects are related to glitazone-induced changes in body fat distribution or to changes in blood L/A ratio is not known.

The aim of this study was to evaluate whether pioglitazone alters body fat distribution and the L/A ratio in non diabetic subjects on maintenance dialysis, and whether this was associated with alterations in insulin sensitivity. Pioglitazone significantly changed the visceral-subcutaneous fat distribution and plasma L/A while improving hepatic insulin sensitivity.

Subjects and Methods

The study design was double blind randomized cross-over with 2 phases (Figure 1) and conducted at the University Hospital of Lausanne, Switzerland (CHUV). In 2007, it received the approvals from the local Ethics Committee (Human Research Ethics Committee, Lausanne) and from Swissmedic (Swiss Agency for Therapeutic Products) according to the principles expressed in the declaration of Helsinki. At the time of the submission, the local ethics committee did not require the registration in ClinicalTrial.-gov. For this reason, the trial was registered only while it was ongoing in 2010 under ClinicalTrial.gov NCT01253928. The protocol for this trial and supporting CONSORT checklist are available as supporting information; see Checklist S1 and Protocol S1 and S2. This manuscript focuses exclusively on data of body composition, adipokines, glucose metabolism and insulin resistance. Non diabetic patients with ESRD treated for more than 3 months in the dialysis centre of the CHUV and in related centers of the Canton de Vaud, were recruited after informed and written consent. Recruitment took place between 2008–2010 and followed up until 2011. Diabetic patients were excluded to prevent the confounding factor of insulin treatment on IR assessment. Other exclusion criteria were: estimated survival less than 6 months, active infection, hospitalization within 1 month before the study, congestive heart failure NYHA class III–IV and abnormal liver function tests. The sample size chosen for this pilot study was consistent with other studies having used this technique in this population [7,14,15]. For this study, twelve subjects were included, of which 8 were on hemodialysis (HD; age: 59.6±4.4 years) and 4 on peritoneal dialysis (PD, age: 43.5±3.6 years). The average body mass index (BMI) was of 27.2±0.74 kg/m^2 (range: 24.0–30.5 kg/m^2).

Each subject underwent the 2 treatment phases lasting 16 weeks each, separated by a wash-out period of at least 2 weeks (Figure 1). The sequence of treatment was randomized following allocation to random numbers with the objective to have an equal number of individuals starting with pioglitazone or placebo. The medical staff providing the random allocation sequence differed from those blinded for the treatment allocation involved in the recrutement, and interventions. For those starting with the pioglitazone phase, the following 18 week period without treatment (washout and placebo phase) was considered sufficient to avoid a significant carry-over effect of the pioglitazone phase. A similar design was used recently in a study examining the effects of pioglitazone on insulin sensitivity and sub-cutaneous adipose cell morphology [16]. The primary outcome was changes in visceral/subcutaneous abdominal fat distribution. Secondary outcomes were changes in the L/A ratio, in hepatic and muscle insulin sensitivity and in biochemical cardiovascular risk markers.

At the end of each treatment, subjects underwent anthropometric [17] and DEXA measurements and an abdominal CT scan at the level of L4–L5 for the measurement of abdominal fat distribution. For HD patients, these measurements were performed immediately after an HD session, whereas for PD patients, they were performed after the morning PD effluent drainage.

During the whole study, subjects were followed by their nephrologist. For HD patients, dry body weight and ultrafiltration rates (UF) were recorded at each HD session. A clinical examination was performed once a week with special focus on the presence of lower extremity edema and on other signs of fluid overload. For PD patients, dry weight was recorded each morning at bedside and daily UF rates were registered. Patients were instructed to report each PD exchange and solutions on a flow sheet. Patients were seen every 4 weeks by their nephrologist who performed a clinical examination with special focus on the presence of lower extremity edema and on other signs of fluid overload. In addition, a weekly phone call was made to the subject to check for potential side-effects and/or signs of fluid overload.

Metabolic investigations

Subjects reported at 0700 am to the metabolic unit, after a 10 h overnight fast. HD patients were investigated in the metabolic unit the day following an HD session. PD patients were investigated after their first PD exchange in the morning. On arrival, subjects were asked to empty their bladder and body composition was estimated from subcutaneous skin-fold measurements at the biceps, triceps, subscapular and suprailiac sites [17]. An indwelling catheter was inserted into an antecubital vein of the right wrist for repeated blood sampling. A second indwelling catheter was inserted into an antecubital vein of the other arm for glucose, insulin and tracer infusions. If the patient had an arteriovenous fistula placed on the upper limb, this was accessed using a 16 gauge fistula needle for infusions of glucose, insulin and tracers, and the blood sampling catheter was placed on the other side. Blood was collected at baseline for the measurement of plasma concentrations of glucose, insulin, total, HDL and LDL cholesterol, triglycerides, CRP, IL-6, leptin and adiponectin. Monthly measurements of serum albumin (immunonephelemetry), creatinine, and normalized protein catabolic rate (nPCR) were provided by the dialysis centers in order to complete the assessment of nutritional status and to estimate daily protein intake.

Methods for the 2-step hyperinsulinemic euglycemic clamp. Liver and muscle IS were measured for 3 h after the initial 2 h tracer infusion. A 2-step hyperinsulinemic euglycemic clamp (0.03 mU · kg^{-1} · min^{-1} and 1 mU · kg^{-1} · min^{-1}, 90 min each), was performed and aimed to achieve a glycemia of 5.5 mmol/l, regardless of the patients' fasting blood glucose. Blood samples were collected every 5 min during the clamp to monitor plasma glucose concentration and at 30 min intervals for the analysis of tracers and insulin. Glucose metabolism was assessed during the 2-step clamp with the continuous infusion of 6,6-[$^2H_2$]glucose infusion (Cambridge Isotope Laboratories, Inc. Andover, MA; bolus: 2 mg/kg; continuous 20 µg · kg^{-1} · min^{-1}) and the plasma measurements of 6,6-[$^2H_2$]glucose. Substrate

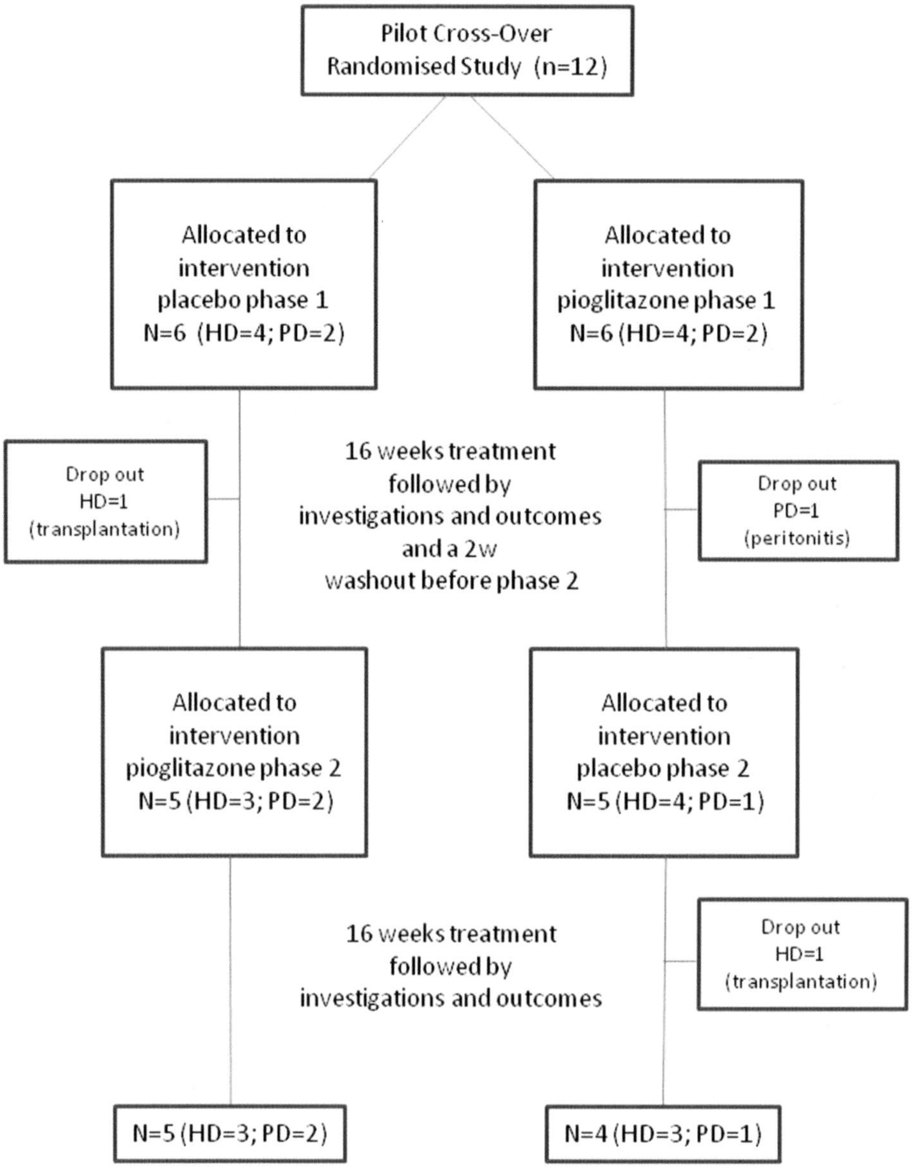

Figure 1. Flow chart of the double blinded cross-over study.

oxidation was measured by indirect calorimetry (ventilated canopy) from 0800 to 1300 [18] by using the equations of Livesey and Elia [19].

Glucose appearance rates were calculated at baseline and during moderate and high insulinemia from plasma 6,6 $^2H_2$ glucose Steele's equations for steady state conditions [20]. Endogenous glucose production (EGP) was identical with glucose appearance rate in fasting conditions. During hyperinsulinemia, EGP was computed as (glucose appearance rate) - (glucose infusion rate). Since all measurements were done under steady state conditions, total glucose disposal rate was considered as equal to glucose appearance.

Analytical determinations

Plasma was immediately separated from blood by centrifugation at 4°C for 10 min at 3600 rpm and stored at −20°C. Commercial radioimmunoassy kits were used to measure plasma insulin, leptin, and adiponectin (LINCO Research, St Charles, MO). During the clamp, plasma glucose concentrations were measured by the glucose oxidase method with a Beckman glucose analyzer II (Beckman Instruments, Fullerton, CA). Plasma 6,6-[$^2H_2$]glucose isotopic enrichment was measured by gas chromatography-mass spectrometry (Hewlett-Packard Instruments), as previously described [21]. Breath $^{13}CO_2$ isotopic enrichment was determined by Isotope Ratio Mass Spectrometry (IR/MS) on a Tracermass C/N (SerCon Ltd, Crewe, Cheshire, UK). The homeostatic model assessment of insulin resistance index (HOMA-IR) and the HOMA corrected by adiponectin index (HOMA-AD) were calculated according to published formulas [7].

Statistical Analysis

Because dialysis patients are heterogeneous, we chose to perform a cross-over design instead of a case-control study. This design increases the power of the study as each individual examined serves as their own control. Taking into account the within patient standard deviation and expected differences between treatments for body fat distribution and for adiponectin plasma levels based on previous studies using the same dosage of pioglitazone and same duration of study [10,22], a sample size of 12 individuals was chosen with a projected drop-out rate of 10–20% to reach the respectively 10 and 7 patients required to detect a treatment difference for body fat distribution (primary end point) and adiponectin plasma levels. At the end of each period (pioglitazone and placebo), absolute values of parameters were paired and compared as in previous publications using the same design [16,23,24]. Data were expressed as mean ± SEM. The statistical differences between the 2 periods of treatment (placebo and pioglitazone) were analysed by the paired Student's t test using the Minitab software. A level of $p<0.05$ was considered statistically significant. The analysis of variance (ANOVA) for paired comparisons was performed to examine an overall effect of treatment during the clamp studies and whether the sequence of treatments influenced the response to treatment (carry over effect). The residual method was used when examining the effects of pioglitazone while adjusting for co-variables. Briefly, this procedure uses a linear regression to assess the effect of confounders on the dependent variable, and then computes the residual (difference between observed and predicted value). The residuals were then compared using a standard paired t-test.

Results

Nine subjects completed both phases of the study (**Table 1**). Two HD subjects dropped out of the study due to kidney transplantation. One PD subject dropped out because of peritonitis and subsequently switched to HD.

Body Composition

The body composition of subjects, at termination of each phase, is presented in **Table 2**. Pioglitazone had no effect on total body weight, but significantly decreased abdominal VAT and the VAT/SAT ratio (mean ± SEM; n = 9, placebo: 0.69±0.09, pioglitazone: 0.58±0.09, p = 0.002). After stratification for dialysis modality, in HD patients VAT/SAT ratio was of (mean ± SEM; n = 6) placebo: 0.84±0.06, pioglitazone: 0.72±0.07, p = 0.01. In PD patients VAT/SAT ratio was of (mean ± SEM; n = 3) placebo: 0.37±0.1, pioglitazone: 0.29±0.04, p = 0.2. These changes were similar in both dialysis modalities although it did not reach a significant level in PD because of the small number of observations. Subscapular subcutaneous fat deposition significantly increased. In contrast, there was no effect on lean mass, and on bone mineral density (BMD).

Fasting blood chemistry

Table 3 summarizes the biochemical analysis at termination of each phase. Plasma albumin, creatinine and nPCR were not affected by pioglitazone. HDL cholesterol increased significantly with pioglitazone. There was a trend toward a decrease in CRP and IL-6 plasma levels in accordance with a study performed in hemodialysis patients [25,26]. Under pioglitazone, plasma leptin concentrations significantly decreased, whereas plasma adiponectin significantly increased, thus resulting in a dramatically suppressed L/A ratio (**Figure 2**; mean ± SEM; n = 9, placebo: 3.63±1.04, pioglitazone: 0.76±0.25, p = 0.008). These effects remained significant when adjusting the L/A ratio to visceral fat, total glucose disposal rate (GDR), or hepatic glucose output. After stratification for dialysis modality, in HD patients L/A ratio was of (mean ± SEM; n = 6) placebo: 3.85±1.37, pioglitazone: 0.79±0.32, p = 0.039. In PD patients L/A ratio was of (mean ± SEM; n = 3) placebo: 3.18±1.88, pioglitazone: 0.69±0.5, p = 0.2. These changes were similar in both dialysis modalities although it did not reach a significant level in PD patients because of the small number of observations.

Glucose homeostasis (Table 3, Figure 3)

Pioglitazone significantly decreased fasting blood glucose and HOMA-IR was lower with pioglitazone than with placebo (resp. 1.75±0.2 vs 2.3±0.3; p = 0.05). Hepatic glucose output (endogenous glucose production) was significantly decreased (−20.6%, Figure 3a) with pioglitazone at baseline, demonstrating an improvement in hepatic IS with pioglitazone. This difference was maintained, although not significantly, at low and high dose insulin infusion rates. There was a trend towards an increase in the hepatic insulin sensitivity index (HISI, +56.8%, p = 0.06). As at baseline, GDR is equivalent to hepatic glucose production, the effects of insulin on GDR are only presented during the insulin infusion steps (Figure 3b). At low dose and high dose insulin infusion rates, pioglitazone did not significantly improve GDR. As expected, glucose oxidation was increased with insulin infusion (Figure 3c). Pioglitazone did not influence glucose oxidation at baseline or during insulin infusions.

In order to evaluate a possible carry-over effect, we compared the values of VAT and L/A ratio among subjects starting with the

Table 1. Characteristics of subjects enrolled and having completed both phases.

Subject	Age	Sex	Ethnicity	Cause of ESRD	Duration of dialysis (months)	Dialysis modality
1	68	M	W	Ischemic nephropathy and renal cholesterol emboli	52	HD
2	71	M	W	IgA nephropathy	61	HD
3	53	M	A	Obstructive uro-nephropathy	17	HD
4	79	M	W	Hypertensive nephroangiosclerosis	49	HD
5	57	M	W	Post-streptococcal Glomerulo-nephritis	124	HD
6	40	M	W	Polycystic kidney disease	42	HD
7	39	F	W	Reflex uro-nephropathy	35	PD
8	42	F	W	Membrano-proliferative glomerulonephritis	37	PD
9	54	M	W	Hypertensive nephroangiosclerosis	40	PD

M: male, F: female, W:White, A: African, HD: hemodialysis, PD: peritoneal dialysis.

Table 2. Body composition measurements at termination of placebo and pioglitazone phases.

	Placebo	Pioglitazone	*Diff (95%CI)*	*P*
Weight (kg)	78.4±2.2	78.1±2.4	0.35 (−0.7;1.4)	
Delta weight from start to end of phase	0.51±0.48	0.69±0.35	−0.18 (−1.7;1.3)	
BMI (kg/m^2)	27±0.8	26.7±0.8	0.2 (−0.3;0.8)	
Waist circumference (cm)	103.6±2.9	103.6±3.3	0 (−1.2;1.2)	
Subscapular skinfold (cm)	16±1.2	19.1±1.5	−3.1 (−6.0;−0.2)	0.04
Biceps skinfold (cm)	9.3±1.6	8.0±1.6	1.39 (−1.2;4.0)	
Triceps skinfold (cm)	20.6±2.7	19.1±2.5	1.6 (−1.0;4.1)	
Brachial muscular circumference (mm)	272.2±4.6	271±4.8	1.3 (−4.6;7.1)	
DEXA measurements				
DEXA fat (kg)	26.1±2.1	25.7±2.2	0.4 (−1.1;1.8)	
DEXA fat (%)	33.3±2.5	33.1±2.8	0.2 (−1.5;1.9)	
DEXA leg fat (kg)	7.8±0.9	8.1±1.0	−0.2 (−0.7;0.3)	
DEXA arm fat (kg)	2.9±0.4	3.1±0.4	−0.17 (−0.5;0.12)	
Lean mass (kg)	49.9±2.3	49.8±2.4	0.2(−1.0;1.4)	
Lean mass: leg (kg)	15.4±0.9	15.1±0.9	0.3 (−0.2;0.7)	
Lean mass: arm (kg)	4.7±0.6	5.3±0.4	−0.7 (−1.9;0.6)	
BMD (g/cm2)	1.09±0.03	1.09±0.03	0 (−0.02;0.01)	
BMD spine (g/cm2)	0.92±0.03	0.94±0.05	−0.01 (−0.10;0.07)	
BMD pelvis (g/cm2)	1.08±0.06	1.08±0.05	0 (−0.03;0.03)	
BMD arm (g/cm2)	1.44±0.16	1.63±0.05	−0.20 (−0.65;0.26)	
Abdominal CT scan measurements				
VAT (cm2)	18.3±2.8	15.9±2.8	2.3 (0.9;3.8)	0.005
SAT (cm2)	27.6±2.4	28.5±2.7	−0.9 (−2.3;0.6)	
VAT/SAT ratio	0.69±0.09	0.58±0.09	0.11 (0.05;0.12)	0.002

VAT: visceral adipose tissue area; SAT: subcutaneous adipose tissue area, DEXA: dual energy X-ray absorptiometry, BMD: bone mineral density.

Table 3. Biochemistry values at termination of placebo and pioglitazone phases.

	Placebo	Pioglitazone	*Diff (95%CI)*	*P*
Cholesterol (mmol/l)	3.99±0.21	3.99±0.21	−0.03 (−0.43;0.37)	
HDLcholesterol (mmol/l)	0.65±0.06	0.73±0.04	−0.09 (−0.17;0)	0.047
Triglyceride (mmol/l)	1.47±0.17	1.67±0.18	−0.19(−0.62;0.23)	
LDL cholesterol (mmol/l)	2.81±0.25	2.53±0.29	0.28 (−0.1;0–65)	
Albumine (g/l)	40.0±2.2	39.1±1.9	1.0 (−3.7;5.6)	
nPCR (g/kg/day)	0.99±0.10	1.03±0.12	−0.04 (−0.16;0.08)	
Creatinine (μmol/l)	800±64	819±63	−19 (−92;54)	
CRP (mg/l)	7.88±2.56	3.96±1.44	3.92 (−0.44;8.28)	0.07
IL-6 (pg/ml)	6.11±4.4	3.6±2.5	2.52 (−2.34;7.39)	
Glucose (mmol/l)	5.1±0.2	4.8±0.1	0.3 (0.03;0.6)	0.04
Insulin (μU/ml)	9.8±1.3	8.1±0.8	1.8 (−0.2;3.8)	
HOMA-IR	2.3±0.3	1.75±0.2	0.5 (0;1)	0.05
HOMA-AD	120±35	46±14	74.7 (−18.7;168.1)	
Leptin (ng/ml)	54.0±16.5	36.7±15.9	17.3 (0.87;33.7)	0.04
Adiponectin (μg/ml)	22.6±5.1	49.1±9.0	−26.5 (−51.8;1.2)	0.04
Leptin/Adiponectin ratio	$3.63\times10^{-3}\pm1.04\times10^{-3}$	$0.76\times10^{-3}\pm0.25\times10^{-3}$	2.87 (1.0;4.8)	0.008

nPCR: normalized protein catabolic rate, HOMA-IR: Homeostatic model assessment of insulin resistance, HOMA-AD: HOMA corrected by adiponectin, NEFA: non-esterified fatty acids.

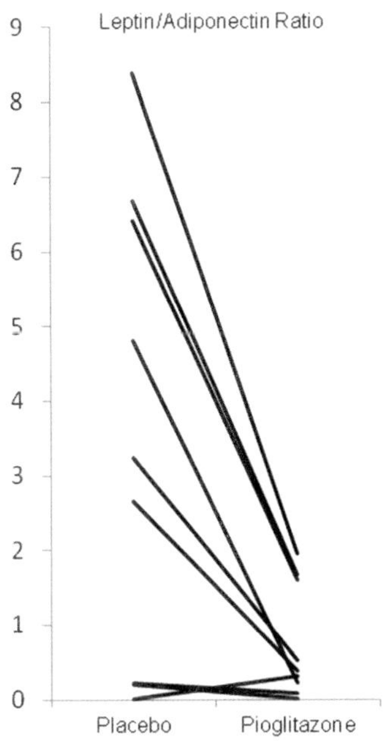

Figure 2. Individual changes in the leptin/adiponectin ratio.

placebo phase (n = 5) versus subjects starting with the pioglitazone phase (n = 4). The difference of pioglitazone-induced changes in VAT for placebo vs pioglitazone starters was respectively of (mean±SEM) −2.5 cm^2±0.8 (−13.7%±3.6; p = 0.033)) and −2.1 cm^2±0.8 (−15.7% cm^2±6.6; p = 0.147) suggesting that there may be a carry-over effect of pioglitazone on VAT with a consequent decreased difference in pioglitazone starters. The differences of pioglitazone-induced changes in L/A ratio for placebo or pioglitazone starters was respectively of (mean±SEM) −2.03±0.87; p = 0.081 and −3.93±1.5; p = 0.075. Thus, for these parameters, having started with pioglitazone or placebo did not have a significant impact on the pioglitazone-induced changes compared to placebo. The numbers are indeed low and a much larger study would be required to explore a possible carry-over effect.

Safety

No significant side effects were observed during pioglitazone therapy. Three patients were hospitalized for reasons unrelated with the use of pioglitazone (see above) and were dropped out. None of the patients developed signs of fluid retention and interdialytic weight gains and UF volumes were comparable between 2 phases.

Discussion

Insulin resistance is common in subjects with chronic kidney disease and ESRD [27,28] and is associated with worse cardiovascular outcomes [29]. Mechanisms involved in the "uremic IR state" are multiple [28]. Among them, increase in visceral fat, change in adipokines, chronic inflammation, are modified by the IS properties of pioglitazone in patients with normal renal function [22]. Yet, these effects have not been studied in ESRD patients. We therefore assessed whether pioglitazone alters the body fat distribution in non diabetic ESRD subjects and whether it is associated with an improvement in insulin sensitivity and cardiometabolic risk factors.

We show that the short term use of pioglitazone is safe in ESRD patients treated by maintenance dialysis and leads to a change in body fat distribution. Although total body fat did not change, there was a significant decrease in the VAT abdominal area, and in the VAT/SAT ratio, indicating a redistribution of visceral fat toward the subcutaneous area as demonstrated by the significant increase in fat at the subscapular site. These changes in fat distribution were associated with significant metabolic changes. The adipokine profile changed favourably with a strong suppression of the high L/A ratio to levels close to those found in the general population [30]. HDL-cholesterol increased and there was a decrease in inflammation. Hepatic insulin sensitivity significantly improved, as documented by a lower fasting hepatic glucose production and an increase in the hepatic insulin sensitivity index. This is consistent with visceral fat playing a key role in the development of hepatic insulin resistance and inflammation.

This study is the first to examine the effects of glitazones on insulin sensitivity in ESRD subjects, using the HEGC technique. HEGC is certainly the gold standard but is a complicated procedure and in general, only surrogate indicators of IR have been studied in previous reports. In non ESRD T2DM subjects, pioglitazone primarily suppresses endogenous glucose production (EGP) and some studies show an enhancement of insulin-induced GDR [22,31,32]. Our study population differs from these studies as none were T2DM, and all were on HD or PD and presented with only slight or moderate IR [7,27]. Our results show that the uremic state did not interfere with the favorable effects of pioglitazone on body fat redistribution, adiponectin levels, EGP and on inflammation. However, there were no alterations of insulin-mediated glucose disposal. Since this is known to be essentially mediated at high insulinemia, it indicates either no effect of pioglitazone on muscle sensitivity in these patients, or more likely, these non diabetic individuals have a smaller degree of muscle insulin resistance compared to hepatic insulin resistance.

Pioglitazone lead to a suppression of the L/A ratio close to levels found in the general population. The respective contribution from subcutaneous and visceral fat to plasma leptin and adiponectin levels is difficult to assess because many factors other than fat mass may determine plasma leptin and adiponectin, especially in dialysis patients. Furthermore a direct effect of pioglitazone on the gene expression of adipokines has been demonstrated [33–35] and may contribute to the observed findings in this study. Although the relationship between adiponectin levels and visceral fat mass is less clear in patients with chronic kidney disease than in the general population, adiponectin has been inversely associated with visceral fat in a cohort of patients with ESRD [36]. The pioglitazone-induced increase in adiponectin found in this study confirms previous findings [26,37,38] and could be related to the decrease in visceral fat. This effect indeed can be considered as positive as high stable adiponectin levels were found to be associated with more favorable cardiovascular outcomes in patients with ESRD [39]. The decrease in leptin with pioglitazone is a new finding. Glitazones suppress leptin rodent gene expression [33,34] and decrease by 40% leptin production from human adipocyte cultures [40], but have no effect on plasma levels of leptin [22]. However, the absence of an increase in plasma leptin in those studies despite fat gain may mask a glitazone-induced decrease in leptin production per unit of fat mass. In the current study, the absence of gain in total fat mass with pioglitazone may have facilitated the observed decrease in plasma leptin due to downregulation of leptin gene expression. Indeed, the decrease in plasma leptin is interesting, since leptin may be considered as a uremic toxin in ESRD [41].

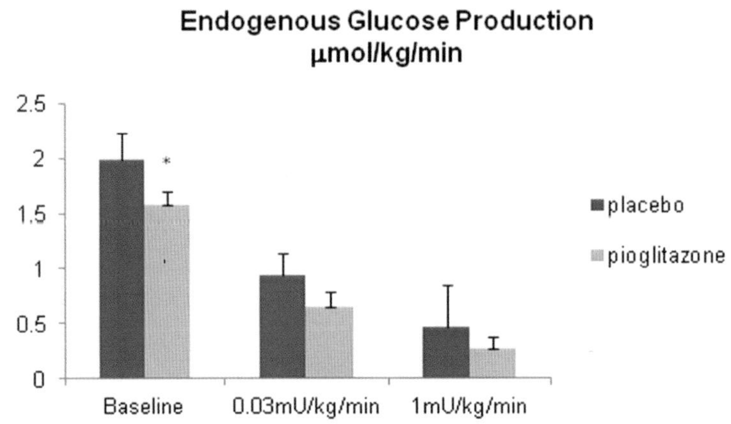

Figure 3a

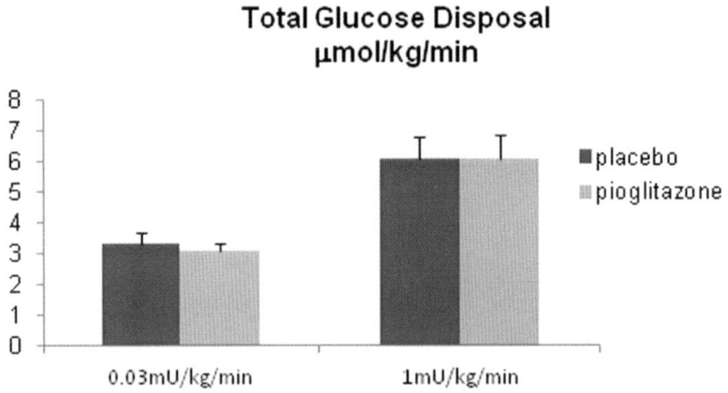

Figure 3b

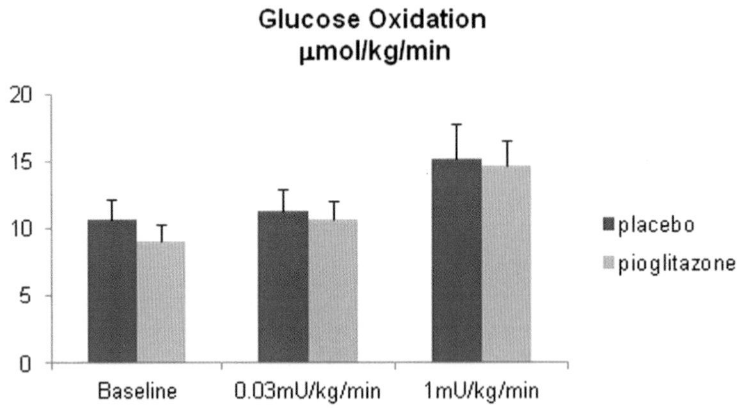

Figure 3c

Figure 3. Glucose metabolism during a 2-step HEGC, values at baseline and during insulin infusion rates of 0.03 mU/kg/min and 1 mU/kg/min. * $p<0.05$.

While stratifying for dialysis modality, similar changes for body composition and adipokines were observed in HD and PD patients. These changes were significant for HD patients but not for PD patients because of the small number of observations. These results show that the effects of pioglitazone are independent from dialysis modality.

This study has several strengths. First, we used the gold standard methods to measure abdominal body fat distribution and insulin sensitivity. Second, we used a double-blinded randomized design, which enabled to compare the effects of pioglitazone versus placebo in the same patient. The limitations of the study include the small number of patients studied due to the complexity and laborious nature of the procedure. However the sample size is consistent with other studies having used this technique in this population [7,14,15]. In addition, a possible carry-over effect cannot be excluded. If all subjects had started with the placebo phase, the effects of pioglitazone may have been even greater than observed with this cross-over design.

In conclusion, 16 week treatment of pioglitazone in non diabetic ESRD subjects on maintenance dialysis is well tolerated, reduces visceral fat and improves the adipokine profile with a decrease in hepatic insulin resistance. Whether these effects may improve the outcome of non diabetic ESRD patients still needs further evaluation.

Acknowledgments

We thank T. Alp Ikizler for his helpful comments and contribution in revising this manuscript.

Author Contributions

Conceived and designed the experiments: AZ LT MB DT. Performed the experiments: LT KAL MB NT ST. Analyzed the data: AZ LT DT. Contributed reagents/materials/analysis tools: NT TG CM GH PCB. Wrote the paper: AZ LT DT.

References

1. Odamaki M, Furuya R, Ohkawa S, Yoneyama T, Nishikino M, et al. (1999) Altered abdominal fat distribution and its association with the serum lipid profile in non-diabetic haemodialysis patients. Nephrol Dial Transplant 14: 2427–2432.
2. Axelsson J, Rashid Qureshi A, Suliman ME, Honda H, Pecoits-Filho R, et al. (2004) Truncal fat mass as a contributor to inflammation in end-stage renal disease. Am J Clin Nutr 80: 1222–1229.
3. Postorino M, Marino C, Tripepi G, Zoccali C, Group CW (2009) Abdominal obesity and all-cause and cardiovascular mortality in end-stage renal disease. J Am Coll Cardiol 53: 1265–1272.
4. Weigle DS, Duell PB, Connor WE, Steiner RA, Soules MR, et al. (1997) Effect of fasting, refeeding, and dietary fat restriction on plasma leptin levels. J Clin Endocrinol Metab 82: 561–565.
5. Considine RV, Sinha MK, Heiman ML, Kriauciunas A, Stephens TW, et al. (1996) Serum immunoreactive-leptin concentrations in normal-weight and obese humans. N Engl J Med 334: 292–295.
6. Teta D, Maillard M, Halabi G, Burnier M (2008) The leptin/adiponectin ratio: potential implications for peritoneal dialysis. Kidney Int Suppl: S112–118.
7. Hung AM, Sundell MB, Egbert P, Siew ED, Shintani A, et al. (2011) A comparison of novel and commonly-used indices of insulin sensitivity in African American chronic hemodialysis patients. Clinical journal of the American Society of Nephrology: CJASN 6: 767–774.
8. Norata GD, Raselli S, Grigore L, Garlaschelli K, Dozio E, et al. (2007) Leptin:adiponectin ratio is an independent predictor of intima media thickness of the common carotid artery. Stroke 38: 2844–2846.
9. Satoh N, Naruse M, Usui T, Tagami T, Suganami T, et al. (2004) Leptin-to-adiponectin ratio as a potential atherogenic index in obese type 2 diabetic patients. Diabetes Care 27: 2488–2490.
10. Miyazaki Y, Mahankali A, Matsuda M, Mahankali S, Hardies J, et al. (2002) Effect of pioglitazone on abdominal fat distribution and insulin sensitivity in type 2 diabetic patients. J Clin Endocrinol Metab 87: 2784–2791.
11. Lin SH, Lin YF, Kuo SW, Hsu YJ, Hung YJ (2003) Rosiglitazone improves glucose metabolism in nondiabetic uremic patients on CAPD. Am J Kidney Dis 42: 774–780.
12. Wong TY, Szeto CC, Chow KM, Leung CB, Lam CW, et al. (2005) Rosiglitazone reduces insulin requirement and C-reactive protein levels in type 2 diabetic patients receiving peritoneal dialysis. Am J Kidney Dis 46: 713–719.
13. Manley HJ, Allcock NM (2003) Thiazolidinedione safety and efficacy in ambulatory patients receiving hemodialysis. Pharmacotherapy 23: 861–865.
14. DeFronzo RA, Tobin JD, Rowe JW, Andres R (1978) Glucose intolerance in uremia. Quantification of pancreatic beta cell sensitivity to glucose and tissue sensitivity to insulin. J Clin Invest 62: 425–435.
15. Barazzoni R, Zanetti M, Stulle M, Mucci MP, Pirulli A, et al. (2008) Higher total ghrelin levels are associated with higher insulin-mediated glucose disposal in non-diabetic maintenance hemodialysis patients. Clin Nutr 27: 142–149.
16. Koenen TB, Tack CJ, Kroese JM, Hermus AR, Sweep FC, et al. (2009) Pioglitazone treatment enlarges subcutaneous adipocytes in insulin-resistant patients. J Clin Endocrinol Metab 94: 4453–4457.
17. Durnin JV, Womersley J (1974) Body fat assessed from total body density and its estimation from skinfold thickness: measurements on 481 men and women aged from 16 to 72 years. The British journal of nutrition 32: 77–97.
18. Jallut D, Tappy L, Kohut M, Bloesch D, Munger R, et al. (1990) Energy balance in elderly patients after surgery for a femoral neck fracture. JPEN Journal of parenteral and enteral nutrition 14: 563–568.
19. Livesey G, Elia M (1988) Estimation of energy expenditure, net carbohydrate utilization, and net fat oxidation and synthesis by indirect calorimetry: evaluation of errors with special reference to the detailed composition of fuels. The American journal of clinical nutrition 47: 608–628.
20. Debodo RC, Steele R, Altszuler N, Dunn A, Bishop JS (1963) On the Hormonal Regulation of Carbohydrate Metabolism; Studies with C14 Glucose. Recent Prog Horm Res 19: 445–488.
21. Schneiter P, Gillet M, Chiolero R, Jequier E, Tappy L (1999) Hepatic nonoxidative disposal of an oral glucose meal in patients with liver cirrhosis. Metabolism: clinical and experimental 48: 1260–1266.
22. Miyazaki Y, Mahankali A, Wajcberg E, Bajaj M, Mandarino LJ, et al. (2004) Effect of pioglitazone on circulating adipocytokine levels and insulin sensitivity in type 2 diabetic patients. The Journal of clinical endocrinology and metabolism 89: 4312–4319.
23. Zanchi A, Chiolero A, Maillard M, Nussberger J, Brunner HR, et al. (2004) Effects of the peroxisomal proliferator-activated receptor-gamma agonist pioglitazone on renal and hormonal responses to salt in healthy men. J Clin Endocrinol Metab 89: 1140–1145.
24. Zanchi A, Maillard M, Jornayvaz FR, Vinciguerra M, Deleaval P, et al. (2010) Effects of the peroxisome proliferator-activated receptor (PPAR)-gamma agonist pioglitazone on renal and hormonal responses to salt in diabetic and hypertensive individuals. Diabetologia 53: 1568–1575.
25. Abe M, Okada K, Maruyama T, Maruyama N, Soma M, et al. (2010) Clinical effectiveness and safety evaluation of long-term pioglitazone treatment for erythropoietin responsiveness and insulin resistance in type 2 diabetic patients on hemodialysis. Expert Opin Pharmacother 11: 1611–1620.
26. Li Y, Xie QH, You HZ, Tian J, Hao CM, et al. (2012) Twelve weeks of pioglitazone therapy significantly attenuates dysmetabolism and reduces inflammation in continuous ambulatory peritoneal dialysis patients–a randomized crossover trial. Perit Dial Int 32: 507–515.
27. Kobayashi S, Maesato K, Moriya H, Ohtake T, Ikeda T (2005) Insulin resistance in patients with chronic kidney disease. American journal of kidney diseases: the official journal of the National Kidney Foundation 45: 275–280.
28. Hung AM, Ikizler TA (2011) Factors determining insulin resistance in chronic hemodialysis patients. Contributions to nephrology 171: 127–134.
29. Shinohara K, Shoji T, Emoto M, Tahara H, Koyama H, et al. (2002) Insulin resistance as an independent predictor of cardiovascular mortality in patients with end-stage renal disease. Journal of the American Society of Nephrology: JASN 13: 1894–1900.
30. Yun JE, Won S, Mok Y, Cui W, Kimm H, et al. (2011) Association of the leptin to high-molecular-weight adiponectin ratio with metabolic syndrome. Endocr J 58: 807–815.
31. Basu R, Shah P, Basu A, Norby B, Dicke B, et al. (2008) Comparison of the effects of pioglitazone and metformin on hepatic and extra-hepatic insulin action in people with type 2 diabetes. Diabetes 57: 24–31.
32. Tonelli J, Li W, Kishore P, Pajvani UB, Kwon E, et al. (2004) Mechanisms of early insulin-sensitizing effects of thiazolidinediones in type 2 diabetes. Diabetes 53: 1621–1629.
33. Kallen CB, Lazar MA (1996) Antidiabetic thiazolidinediones inhibit leptin (ob) gene expression in 3T3-L1 adipocytes. Proc Natl Acad Sci U S A 93: 5793–5796.
34. Saraf N, Sharma PK, Mondal SC, Garg VK, Singh AK (2012) Role of PPARg2 transcription factor in thiazolidinedione-induced insulin sensitization. J Pharm Pharmacol 64: 161–171.
35. Maeda N, Takahashi M, Funahashi T, Kihara S, Nishizawa H, et al. (2001) PPARgamma ligands increase expression and plasma concentrations of adiponectin, an adipose-derived protein. Diabetes 50: 2094–2099.
36. Stenvinkel P, Marchlewska A, Pecoits-Filho R, Heimburger O, Zhang Z, et al. (2004) Adiponectin in renal disease: relationship to phenotype and genetic variation in the gene encoding adiponectin. Kidney Int 65: 274–281.
37. Bajaj M, Suraamornkul S, Piper P, Hardies LJ, Glass L, et al. (2004) Decreased plasma adiponectin concentrations are closely related to hepatic fat content and hepatic insulin resistance in pioglitazone-treated type 2 diabetic patients. J Clin Endocrinol Metab 89: 200–206.
38. van Wijk JP, de Koning EJ, Cabezas MC, op't Roodt J, Joven J, et al. (2005) Comparison of rosiglitazone and metformin for treating HIV lipodystrophy: a randomized trial. Ann Intern Med 143: 337–346.
39. Diez JJ, Estrada P, Bajo MA, Fernandez-Reyes MJ, Grande C, et al. (2009) High stable serum adiponectin levels are associated with a better outcome in prevalent dialysis patients. Am J Nephrol 30: 244–252.
40. Nolan JJ, Olefsky JM, Nyce MR, Considine RV, Caro JF (1996) Effect of troglitazone on leptin production. Studies in vitro and in human subjects. Diabetes 45: 1276–1278.
41. Teta D (2012) Adipokines as uremic toxins. J Ren Nutr 22: 81–85.

Permissions

All chapters in this book were first published in PLOS ONE, by The Public Library of Science; hereby published with permission under the Creative Commons Attribution License or equivalent. Every chapter published in this book has been scrutinized by our experts. Their significance has been extensively debated. The topics covered herein carry significant findings which will fuel the growth of the discipline. They may even be implemented as practical applications or may be referred to as a beginning point for another development.

The contributors of this book come from diverse backgrounds, making this book a truly international effort. This book will bring forth new frontiers with its revolutionizing research information and detailed analysis of the nascent developments around the world.

We would like to thank all the contributing authors for lending their expertise to make the book truly unique. They have played a crucial role in the development of this book. Without their invaluable contributions this book wouldn't have been possible. They have made vital efforts to compile up to date information on the varied aspects of this subject to make this book a valuable addition to the collection of many professionals and students.

This book was conceptualized with the vision of imparting up-to-date information and advanced data in this field. To ensure the same, a matchless editorial board was set up. Every individual on the board went through rigorous rounds of assessment to prove their worth. After which they invested a large part of their time researching and compiling the most relevant data for our readers.

The editorial board has been involved in producing this book since its inception. They have spent rigorous hours researching and exploring the diverse topics which have resulted in the successful publishing of this book. They have passed on their knowledge of decades through this book. To expedite this challenging task, the publisher supported the team at every step. A small team of assistant editors was also appointed to further simplify the editing procedure and attain best results for the readers.

Apart from the editorial board, the designing team has also invested a significant amount of their time in understanding the subject and creating the most relevant covers. They scrutinized every image to scout for the most suitable representation of the subject and create an appropriate cover for the book.

The publishing team has been an ardent support to the editorial, designing and production team. Their endless efforts to recruit the best for this project, has resulted in the accomplishment of this book. They are a veteran in the field of academics and their pool of knowledge is as vast as their experience in printing. Their expertise and guidance has proved useful at every step. Their uncompromising quality standards have made this book an exceptional effort. Their encouragement from time to time has been an inspiration for everyone.

The publisher and the editorial board hope that this book will prove to be a valuable piece of knowledge for researchers, students, practitioners and scholars across the globe.

List of Contributors

Jonathan A. Lorch
Department of Medicine, Weill Cornell Medical College and The Rogosin Institute, New York, New York, United States of America

Victor E. Pollak
Department of Medicine, University of Colorado Health Sciences Center, Aurora, Colorado, United States of America
MIQS, Inc., Boulder, Colorado, United States of America

Wim Van Biesen
Renal Division, Ghent University Hospital, Ghent, Belgium

Sabine N. van der Veer
Department of Medical Informatics, Academic Medical Center, Amsterdam, The Netherlands

Mark Murphey
Irish Kidney Association, Dublin, Ireland

Olga Loblova
A and R Edelman, London, United Kingdom
Department of Public Policy, Central European University, Budapest, Hungary

Simon Davies
Department of Nephrology, University Hospital of North Staffordshire, Stoke on Trent, United Kingdom

Yuan-Chi Shen
Department of Urology, Kaohsiung Chang Gung Memorial Hospital, Kaohsiung, Taiwan, 2 Cheng Shiu University, Kaohsiung, Taiwan
Department of Medical Research, Chi Mei Medical Center, Tainan, Taiwan

Jhi-Joung Wang
Department of Medical Research, Chi Mei Medical Center, Tainan, Taiwan

Shih-Feng Weng
Department of Medical Research, Chi Mei Medical Center, Tainan, Taiwan
Department of Hospital and Health Care Administration, Chia Nan University of Pharmacy and Science, Tainan, Taiwan

Kai-Jen Tien
Division of Endocrinology and Metabolism, Department of Internal Medicine, Chi Mei Medical Center, Tainan, Taiwan
The Center of General Education, Chia Nan University of Pharmacy and Science, Tainan, Taiwan

Hung-Ta Wo, Po-Cheng Chang, Chun-Chieh Wang, Ming-Shien Wen and Chung-Chuan Chou
Department of Cardiology, Chang-Gung Memorial Hospital, Linko, Taiwan

Tien-Hsing Chen
Department of Cardiology, Chang-Gung Memorial Hospital, Linko, Taiwan
Department of Cardiology, Chang-Gung Memorial Hospital, Xiamen, China, Chang Gung University College of Medicine, Kaohsiung, Taiwan

Marine L. Croze and Christophe O. Soulage
Université de Lyon, F-69600, Oullins, France
INSERM, U1060, CarMeN, INSA-Lyon, Univ. Lyon-1, Villeurbanne, France

Caroline C. Pelletier, Laetitia Koppe, Pascaline M. Alix, Emilie Kalbacher and Fitsum Guebre-Egziabher
Université de Lyon, F-69600, Oullins, France
INSERM, U1060, CarMeN, INSA-Lyon, Univ. Lyon-1, Villeurbanne, France
Hospices Civils de Lyon, Service de Ne´phrologie, Hôpital E Herriot, Lyon, France

Denis Fouque
Université de Lyon, F-69600, Oullins, France
INSERM, U1060, CarMeN, INSA-Lyon, Univ. Lyon-1, Villeurbanne, France
Hospices Civils de Lyon, Service de Néphrologie, Centre Hospitalier Lyon-SUD, Pierre-Bénite, France

Aoumeur Hadj-Aissa
Université de Lyon, F-69600, Oullins, France
Hospices Civils de Lyon, Exploration Fonctionnelle Re´nale et Me´tabolique, Hôpital E Herriot, Lyon, France

Jeonghwan Lee
Department of Internal Medicine, Hallym University Hangang Sacred Heart Hospital, Seoul, Korea
Clinical Research Center for End Stage Renal Disease (CRC for ESRD), Daegu, Korea

Jung Pyo Lee
Clinical Research Center for End Stage Renal Disease (CRC for ESRD), Daegu, Korea

Department of Internal Medicine, Seoul National University Boramae Medical Center, Seoul, Korea

Chun Soo Lim
Clinical Research Center for End Stage Renal Disease (CRC for ESRD), Daegu, Korea
Department of Internal Medicine, Seoul National University Boramae Medical Center, Seoul, Korea
Department of Internal Medicine, Seoul National University College of Medicine, Seoul, Korea

Ji In Park and Yon Su Kim
Clinical Research Center for End Stage Renal Disease (CRC for ESRD), Daegu, Korea
Department of Internal Medicine, Seoul National University College of Medicine, Seoul, Korea

Jin Ho Hwang
Clinical Research Center for End Stage Renal Disease (CRC for ESRD), Daegu, Korea
Department of Internal Medicine, Chung-Ang University Hospital, Seoul, Korea

Hye Min Jang
Clinical Research Center for End Stage Renal Disease (CRC for ESRD), Daegu, Korea
Department of Statistics, Kyungpook National University, Daegu, Korea

Ji-Young Choi and Yong-Lim Kim
Clinical Research Center for End Stage Renal Disease (CRC for ESRD), Daegu, Korea
Department of Internal Medicine, Kyungpook National University School of Medicine, Daegu, Korea

Chul Woo Yang
Clinical Research Center for End Stage Renal Disease (CRC for ESRD), Daegu, Korea
Department of Internal Medicine, The Catholic University of Korea College of Medicine, Seoul, Korea

Shin-Wook Kang
Clinical Research Center for End Stage Renal Disease (CRC for ESRD), Daegu, Korea
Department of Internal Medicine, Yonsei University College of Medicine, Seoul, Korea

Nam-Ho Kim
Clinical Research Center for End Stage Renal Disease (CRC for ESRD), Daegu, Korea
Department of Internal Medicine, Chonnam National University Medical School, Gwangju, Korea

Khalid Bashar, Donagh Healy, Elrasheid A. H. Kheirelseid, Mary Clarke - Moloney, Paul E. Burke and Eamon G. Kavanagh
Department of vascular surgery, University Hospital Limerick, Limerick, Ireland

Leonard D. Browne and Michael T. Walsh
Centre for Applied Biomedical Engineering Research (CABER), Department of Mechanical, Aeronautical and Biomedical Engineering, Materials and Surface Science Institute, University of Limerick, Limerick, Ireland

Stewart Redmond Walsh
Department of surgery, National University of Ireland, Galway, Ireland

Ping Wen, Hong Ye, Xiaochun Wu, Lei Jiang, Bing Tang, Yang Zhou, Li Fang, Hongdi Cao, Weichun He, Chunsun Dai and Junwei Yang
Center for Kidney Disease, Second Affiliated Hospital, Nanjing Medical University, Nanjing, China

Yafang Yang
Department of Radiology, Second Affiliated Hospital, Nanjing Medical University, Nanjing, China

Dan Song
Department of Nephrology, Affiliated Wuxi Hospital, Nanjing Medical University, Wuxi, China

Sarah J. Ramer
Rutgers New Jersey Medical School, Newark, New Jersey, United States of America

Elan D. Cohen
Division of General Internal Medicine, Department of Medicine, University of Pittsburgh School of Medicine, Pittsburgh, Pennsylvania, United States of America

Chung-Chou H. Chang
Division of General Internal Medicine, Department of Medicine, University of Pittsburgh School of Medicine, Pittsburgh, Pennsylvania, United States of America
Department of Biostatistics, University of Pittsburgh Graduate School of Public Health, Pittsburgh, Pennsylvania, United States of America

Amber E. Barnato
Division of General Internal Medicine, Department of Medicine, University of Pittsburgh School of Medicine, Pittsburgh, Pennsylvania, United States of America
Department of Clinical and Translational Science, University of Pittsburgh School of Medicine, Pittsburgh, Pennsylvania, United States of America
Department of Health Policy and Management, University of Pittsburgh Graduate School of Public Health, Pittsburgh, Pennsylvania, United States of America
The CRISMA Laboratory (Clinical Research, Investigation, and Systems Modeling of Acute Illness), Department of Critical Care Medicine, University of Pittsburgh, Pittsburgh, Pennsylvania, United States of America

Mark L. Unruh
Division of Nephrology, Department of Internal Medicine, University of New Mexico School of Medicine, Albuquerque, New Mexico, United States of America

Evelyn C. Nieves Torres, Binxia Yang, Rajiv Janardhanan and Akshaar Brahmbhatt
Vascular and Interventional Radiology Translational Laboratory, Department of Radiology, Mayo Clinic, Rochester, Minnesota, United States of America

Sanjay Misra
Vascular and Interventional Radiology Translational Laboratory, Department of Radiology, Mayo Clinic, Rochester, Minnesota, United States of America,
Department of Biochemistry and Molecular Biology, Mayo Clinic, Rochester, Minnesota, United States of America

Ed Leof and Debabrata Mukhopadhyay
Department of Biochemistry and Molecular Biology, Mayo Clinic, Rochester, Minnesota, United States of America

Deborah L. Zimmerman and Marcel Ruzicka
Associate Professor of Medicine, Division of Nephrology, Ottawa Hospital, Kidney Research Centre of the Ottawa Hospital Research Institute, University of Ottawa, Ottawa, Ontario, Canada

Paul Hebert
Professor of Medicine, Surgery, Anesthesia and Epidemiology, University of Ottawa; Senior Scientist, Clinical Epidemiology, Ottawa Hospital Research Institute, Ottawa, Ontario, Canada

Dean Fergusson
Associate Professor, Departments of Medicine, Surgery, Epidemiology and Community Medicine, Senior Scientist and Director, Clinical Epidemiology Program, Ottawa Hospital Research Institute, Ottawa, Ontario, Canada

Rhian M. Touyz
Institute of Cardiovascular and Medical Sciences, BHF Glasgow Cardiovascular Research Centre, University of Glasgow, Glasgow, United Kingdom

Kevin D. Burns
Professor of Medicine, Division of Nephrology, Senior Scientist, Kidney Research Centre of the Ottawa Hospital Research Institute, University of Ottawa, Ottawa, Ontario, Canada

Jun-qing Yang, Peng Ran, Ji-yan Chen, Li-wen Li, Ning Tan, Guang Li, Shuo Sun, Yong Liu, Jia-xin Zhan, Jian-yi Zheng and Ying-ling Zhou
Department of Cardiology, Guangdong Cardiovascular Institute, Guangdong General Hospital, Guangdong Academy of Medical Sciences, Guangzhou, Guangdong, China

Yi-ting He
Department of Cardiology, Shunde first hospital, Foshan, Guangdong, China

Bruno Guéry, Aude Servais, Elarbi Harrami, Lynda Bererhi, Brigitte Zins and Malik Touam
Université Paris-Descartes, Faculté de Médecine, Assistance Publique-Hôpitaux de Paris, Service de Néphrologie, Hôpital Necker-Enfants Malades, Paris, France

Dominique Joly
Université Paris-Descartes, Faculté de Médecine, Assistance Publique-Hôpitaux de Paris, Service de Néphrologie, Hôpital Necker-Enfants Malades, Paris, France
Institut National de la Santé et de la Recherche Médicale U845, Hôpital Necker-Enfants Malades, Paris, France

Corinne Alberti
Université Denis Diderot, Assistance Publique-Hôpitaux de Paris, Hôpital Robert Debré, Unité d'Epidémiologie Clinique et Institut National de la Santé et de la Recherche Médicale CIE 5, Paris, France

Albina Nowak
Division of Internal Medicine, University Hospital Zürich, Zürich, Switzerland

Ferruh Artunc
Department of Internal Medicine, Division of Endocrinology, Diabetology, Vascular Disease, Nephrology and Clinical Chemistry, University of Tübingen, Tübingen, Germany

Björn Friedrich
Department of Internal Medicine, Division of Endocrinology, Diabetology, Vascular Disease, Nephrology and Clinical Chemistry, University of Tübingen, Tübingen, Germany
Dialysis center Leonberg, Leonberg, Germany

Andreas L. Serra
Division of Nephrology, University Hospital Zürich, Zürich, Switzerland

Tobias Breidthardt
Division of Nephrology, University Hospital Basel, Basel, Switzerland

Raphael Twerenbold, Myriam Peter and Christian Mueller
Division of Cardiology, University Hospital Basel, Basel, Switzerland

Peter Biesenbach, Kurt Derfler, Wilfred Druml and Marcus D. Säemann
Internal Medicine III/Clinical Division of Nephrology and Dialysis, Medical University of Vienna, Vienna, Austria

Renate Kain, Afschin Soleiman, Alexandra Benharkou and Andrew Rees
Clinical Institute of Pathology, Medical University of Vienna, Vienna, Austria

Thomas Perkmann
Department of Laboratory Medicine, Medical University of Vienna, Vienna, Austria

Hsin-Bang Leu
Cardiovascular center, National Taiwan University Hospital, Hsinchu Branch, Hsinchu, Taiwan
Healthcare and Management Center, Taipei Veterans General Hospital, Taipei, Taiwan
Cardiovascular Research Center, National Yang-Ming University, Taipei, Taiwan

Chao-Lun Lai
Cardiovascular center, National Taiwan University Hospital, Hsinchu Branch, Hsinchu, Taiwan
School of Medicine, National Taiwan University, Taipei, Taiwan

Chih-Cheng Wu
Cardiovascular center, National Taiwan University Hospital, Hsinchu Branch, Hsinchu, Taiwan
School of Medicine, National Taiwan University, Taipei, Taiwan
School of Medicine, National Yang-Ming University, Taipei, Taiwan

Shing-Jong Lin
Division of Cardiology, Taipei Veterans General Hospital, Taipei, Taiwan
Department of Medical Research and Education, Taipei Veterans General Hospital, Taipei, Taiwan
Department of Medicine, National Yang-Ming University, Taipei, Taiwan
Institute of Clinical Medicine, National Yang-Ming University, Taipei, Taiwan
School of Medicine, National Yang-Ming University, Taipei, Taiwan
Cardiovascular Research Center, National Yang-Ming University, Taipei, Taiwan

Jaw-Wen Chen
Division of Cardiology, Taipei Veterans General Hospital, Taipei, Taiwan
Department of Medical Research and Education, Taipei Veterans General Hospital, Taipei, Taiwan
Cardiovascular Research Center, National Yang-Ming University, Taipei, Taiwan
Institute and Department of Pharmacology, National Yang-Ming University, Taipei, Taiwan

Po-Hsun Huang
Division of Cardiology, Taipei Veterans General Hospital, Taipei, Taiwan
Department of Medicine, National Yang-Ming University, Taipei, Taiwan
Institute of Clinical Medicine, National Yang-Ming University, Taipei, Taiwan
School of Medicine, National Yang-Ming University, Taipei, Taiwan
Cardiovascular Research Center, National Yang-Ming University, Taipei, Taiwan

Frances E. Tiffin-Richards, Ana S. Costa, Karl Kuckuck and Jörg B. Schulz
Department of Neurology, RWTH Aachen University Hospital, Aachen, Germany
Jülich Aachen Research Alliance (JARA) - Translational Brain Medicine, Aachen and Jülich, Germany

Kathrin Reetz
Department of Neurology, RWTH Aachen University Hospital, Aachen, Germany
Jülich Aachen Research Alliance (JARA) - Translational Brain Medicine, Aachen and Jülich, Germany
Institute of Neuroscience and Medicine (INM-4), Research Center Jülich GmbH, Jülich, Germany

Bernhard Holschbach
KfH Curatorship for Dialysis and Kidney Transplant e.V., KfH-Nephrology Center, Stolberg, Germany

Rolf D. Frank
Department of Internal Medicine, St.-Antonius-Hospital Eschweiler, Eschweiler, Germany

Athina Vassiliadou
Dialysis Center Aachen, Dialysis Center, Aachen, Germany

Thilo Krüger and Jürgen Floege
Division of Nephrology and Clinical Immunology, RWTH Aachen University, Aachen, Germany

Theresa Gross
Division of Nephrology and Clinical Immunology, RWTH Aachen University, Aachen, Germany
Department of Internal Medicine, Dresden-Friedreichstadt Hospital, Dresden, Germany

Frank Eitner
Division of Nephrology and Clinical Immunology, RWTH Aachen University, Aachen, Germany
Bayer Pharma AG, Global Drug Development, Kidney Diseases Research, Wuppertal, Germany

Dongsheng Cheng, Yang Fei, Yumei Liu, Junhui Li, Yuqiang Chen, Xiaoxia Wang and Niansong Wang
Department of Nephrology and Rheumatology, Shanghai Jiaotong University Affiliated Sixth People's Hospital, Shanghai, P.R. China

Ping-Fang Chiu, Chirn-Bin Chang and Chia-Chu Chang
Division of Nephrology, Department of Internal Medicine, Changhua Christian Hospital, Changhua, Taiwan
School of Medicine, Chung-Shan Medical University, Taichung, Taiwan

Chia-Lin Wu
Division of Nephrology, Department of Internal Medicine, Changhua Christian Hospital, Changhua, Taiwan
School of Medicine, Chung-Shan Medical University, Taichung, Taiwan
Institute of Clinical Medicine, National Yang-Ming University, Taipei, Taiwan

Der-Cherng Tarng
Institute of Clinical Medicine, National Yang-Ming University, Taipei, Taiwan
Division of Nephrology, Department of Medicine, Taipei Veterans General Hospital, Taipei, Taiwan
Department and Institute of Physiology, National Yang-Ming University, Taipei, Taiwan

Hung-Ming Wu
Inflammation Research and Drug Development Center, Changhua Christian Hospital, Changhua, Taiwan

Hung-Hsiang Liou
Division of Nephrology, Department of Internal Medicine, Hsin Jen Hospital, Taipei, Taiwan

Naya Huang, Li Fan, Qingdong Xu, Ricong Xu, Liping Xiong, Xueqing Yu and Haiping Mao
Department of Nephrology, The First Affiliated Hospital, Sun Yat-sen University, Key Laboratory of Nephrology, Ministry of Health of China, Guangdong Provincial Key Laboratory of Nephrology, Guangzhou, Guangdong, China

Jiehui Chen
Department of Nephrology, The First Affiliated Hospital, Sun Yat-sen University, Key Laboratory of Nephrology, Ministry of Health of China, Guangdong Provincial Key Laboratory of Nephrology, Guangzhou, Guangdong, China
Department of Nephrology, The Sixth People's Hospital of Shenzhen, Shenzhen, Guangdong, China

Qian Zhou
Epidemiology Research Unit, Translational Medicine Research Center, The First Affiliated Hospital, Sun Yat-sen University, Guangzhou, Guangdong, China

Federica Genovese, Morten A. Karsdal and Diana J. Leeming
Nordic Bioscience, Fibrosis Biology and Biomarkers, Herlev, Denmark

Alexandra Scholze and Martin Tepel
Odense University Hospital, Department of Nephrology, Institute for Molecular Medicine, Cardiovascular and Renal Research, Institute of Clinical Research, University of Southern Denmark, Odense, Denmark

Meilan Zhou, Guoshang Xu, Lijuan Zhao, Chen Huang and Rong Li
Department of Nephrology, Xijing Hospital, the Fourth Military Medical University, Xi'an, Shaan xi, China

Lijie He, Weijuan Lou and Hanmin Wang and Shiren Sun
Department of Nephrology, Xijing Hospital, the Fourth Military Medical University, Xi'an, Shaan xi, China
State Key Laboratory of Cancer Biology, Xijing Hospital, the Fourth Military Medical University, Xi'an, Shaan xi, China

Lihua Ji
Department of Nephrology, Xijing Hospital, the Fourth Military Medical University, Xi'an, Shaan xi, China
State Key Laboratory of Cancer Biology, Xijing Hospital, the Fourth Military Medical University, Xi'an, Shaan xi, China
Department of Nephrology, Xingyuan Hospital, the Fourth Hospital of Yulin, Yulin, Shaan xi, China

Wei Liang
Department of Nephrology, Xijing Hospital, the Fourth Military Medical University, Xi'an, Shaan xi, China
State Key Laboratory of Cancer Biology, Xijing Hospital, the Fourth Military Medical University, Xi'an, Shaan xi, China
Department of Nephrology, the Ninth Hospital of Xi'an, Xi'an, Shaan xi, China

Xiangmei Chen
Department of Nephrology, Xijing Hospital, the Fourth Military Medical University, Xi'an, Shaan xi, China
Department of Nephrology, State Key Laboratory of Kidney Diseases, Chinese PLA General Hospital and Medical College, Beijing, China

Alferso C. Abrahams, Jan Willem van der Veer, Marianne C. Verhaar and Walther H. Boer
Department of Nephrology and Hypertension, University Medical Center Utrecht, Utrecht, The Netherlands

Sayed M. Habib and Michiel G. H. Betjes
Department of Internal Medicine, Division of Nephrology and Transplantation, Erasmus Medical Center, Rotterdam, The Netherlands

Amélie Dendooven and Tri Q. Nguyen
Department of Pathology, University Medical Center Utrecht, Utrecht, The Netherlands

Bruce L. Riser
Department of Physiology and Biophysics, Rosalind Franklin University of Medicine and Science, IL, United States of America

Raechel J. Toorop
Department of Vascular Surgery, University Medical Center Utrecht, Utrecht, The Netherlands

Christopher J. E. Watson
Department of Surgery, Addenbrooke's Hospital, and Cambridge NIHR Biomedical Research Centre, Cambridge, United Kingdom

Chun-Tai Mao, Ming- Jui Hung and Chao-Hung Wang
Heart Failure Center, Division of Cardiology, Department of Internal Medicine, Chang Gung Memorial Hospital, Keelung, Taiwan
College of Medicine, Chang Gung University, Taoyuan, Taiwan

Tien-Hsing Chen
Division of Cardiology, Department of Internal Medicine, Chang Gung Memorial Hospital, Taipei, Taiwan
Department of cardiology, Chang Gung Memorial Hospital, Xiamen, China
College of Medicine, Chang Gung University, Taoyuan, Taiwan

Ming-Lung Tsai, Chao-Yung Wang, Ming-Shien Wen, I-Chang Hsieh and Chun-Chi Chen
Division of Cardiology, Department of Internal Medicine, Chang Gung Memorial Hospital, Taipei, Taiwan
College of Medicine, Chang Gung University, Taoyuan, Taiwan

Yu-Jen Yu, I-Wen Wu, Chin-Chan Lee, Chio-Yin Sun and Heng-Jung Hsu
Department of Nephrology, Chang Gung Memorial Hospital, Keelung, Taiwan
College of Medicine, Chang Gung University, Tao-Yuan, Taiwan

Mai-Szu Wu
Department of Nephrology, Chang Gung Memorial Hospital, Keelung, Taiwan
Division of Nephrology, Taipei Medical University Hospital, Taipei, Taiwan
School of Medicine, Taipei Medical University, Taipei, Taiwan

Chun-Yu Huang and Kuang-Hung Hsu
Laboratory for Epidemiology, Department of Health Care Management, Chang Gung University, Tao-Yuan, Taiwan

Lily Li, Marvin Lin, Maria Krassilnikova, Katya Ostrow, Amanda Bader, Brian Radbill, Jaime Uribarri, Joji Tokita, Staci Leisman, Vijay Lapsia and Anita Mehrotra
Division of Nephrology, Icahn School of Medicine at Mount Sinai, New York, New York, United States of America
Department of Medicine, Icahn School of Medicine at Mount Sinai, New York, New York, United States of America

Peter S. Heeger
Division of Nephrology, Icahn School of Medicine at Mount Sinai, New York, New York, United States of America
Department of Medicine, Icahn School of Medicine at Mount Sinai, New York, New York, United States of America
Recanati Miller Transplantation Institute, Icahn School of Medicine at Mount Sinai, New York, New York, United States of America
Immunology Institute, Icahn School of Medicine at Mount Sinai, New York, New York, United States of America

Adolfo García- Sastre
Department of Medicine, Icahn School of Medicine at Mount Sinai, New York, New York, United States of America
Department of Microbiology, Icahn School of Medicine at Mount Sinai, New York, New York, United States of America
Global Health and Emerging Pathogens Institute, Icahn School of Medicine at Mount Sinai, New York, New York, United States of America

Andrea D. Branch
Department of Medicine, Icahn School of Medicine at Mount Sinai, New York, New York, United States of America
Division of Liver Diseases, Icahn School of Medicine at Mount Sinai, New York, New York, United States of America

Randy A. Albrecht
Department of Microbiology, Icahn School of Medicine at Mount Sinai, New York, New York, United States of America
Global Health and Emerging Pathogens Institute, Icahn School of Medicine at Mount Sinai, New York, New York, United States of America

Chunyan Yi and Jianxiong Lin
Department of Nephrology, The First Affiliated Hospital, Sun Yat-sen University, Guangzhou, People's Republic of China

Rong Huang, Juan Wang, Hongjian Ye, Qunying Guo, Qian Zhou, Xueqing Yu and Xiao Yang
Department of Nephrology, The First Affiliated Hospital, Sun Yat-sen University, Guangzhou, People's Republic of China
Key Laboratory of Nephrology, Ministry of Health, Guangzhou, People's Republic of China

Xiaoguang Fan
Department of Nephrology, The First Affiliated Hospital, Sun Yat-sen University, Guangzhou, People's Republic of China
Department of Nephrology, Zhengzhou University People's Hospital, Zhengzhou, People's Republic of China

Fengmin Shao
Department of Nephrology, Zhengzhou University People's Hospital, Zhengzhou, People's Republic of China

Xingqiang Lai, Guodong Chen, Jiang Qiu, Changxi Wang and Lizhong Chen
Organ Transplant Center, The First Affiliated Hospital, Sun Yat-sen University, Guangzhou, China

Chia-Ter Chao
Division of Nephrology, Department of Internal Medicine, National Taiwan University Hospital Jin-Shan Branch, New Taipei City, Taiwan
Graduate Institute of Toxicology, National Taiwan University, Taipei, Taiwan

Szu-Ying Lee
Division of Nephrology, Department of Internal Medicine, National Taiwan University Hospital Yun-Lin Branch, Yun-Lin County, Taiwan

Wei-Shun Yang
Division of Nephrology, Department of Internal Medicine, National Taiwan University Hospital Hsin-Chu Branch, Hsin-Chu County, Taiwan

Kuan-Yu Hung, Jenq-Wen Huang and Huei-Wen Chen
Division of Nephrology, Department of Internal Medicine, National Taiwan University Hospital, Taipei, Taiwan

Cheng-Chung Fang
Department of Emergency Medicine, National Taiwan University Hospital, Taipei, Taiwan

Chung-Jen Yen
Department of Geriatrics and Gerontology, National Taiwan University Hospital, Taipei, Taiwan

Chih-Kang Chiang
Department of Integrative diagnostics and Therapeutics, National Taiwan University Hospital, Taipei, Taiwan

Yi-Chun Tsai and Mei-Chuan Kuo
Graduate Institute of Clinical Medicine, Kaohsiung Medical University, Kaohsiung, Taiwan
Division of Nephrology, Department of Internal Medicine, Kaohsiung Medical University Hospital, Kaohsiung, Taiwan
Faculty of Renal Care, College of Medicine, Kaohsiung Medical University, Kaohsiung, Taiwan

Shang-Jyh Hwang
Graduate Institute of Clinical Medicine, Kaohsiung Medical University, Kaohsiung, Taiwan
Division of Nephrology, Department of Internal Medicine, Kaohsiung Medical University Hospital, Kaohsiung, Taiwan
Faculty of Renal Care, College of Medicine, Kaohsiung Medical University, Kaohsiung, Taiwan
Institute of Population Sciences, National Health Research Institutes, Miaoli, Taiwan

Su-Chu Lee
Division of Nephrology, Department of Internal Medicine, Kaohsiung Medical University Hospital, Kaohsiung, Taiwan

Yi-Wen Chiu, Jer-Chia Tsai, Hung-Tien Kuo, Chi-Chih Hung and Hung-Chun Chen
Division of Nephrology, Department of Internal Medicine, Kaohsiung Medical University Hospital, Kaohsiung, Taiwan
Faculty of Renal Care, College of Medicine, Kaohsiung Medical University, Kaohsiung, Taiwan

Ming-Yen Lin
Faculty of Renal Care, College of Medicine, Kaohsiung Medical University, Kaohsiung, Taiwan

Tae Ik Chang, Ea Wha Kang and Sug Kyun Shin
Department of Internal Medicine, NHIS Medical Center, Ilsan Hospital, Goyangshi, Gyeonggi-do, Republic of Korea

Yung Ly Kim, Hyungwoo Kim, Geun Woo Ryu, Kyu Hun Choi, Dae Suk Han, Seung Hyeok Han, Jung Tak Park and Tae-Hyun Yoo
Department of Internal Medicine, College of Medicine, Yonsei University, Seoul, Republic of Korea

Shin-Wook Kang
Department of Internal Medicine, College of Medicine, Yonsei University, Seoul, Republic of Korea
Brain Korea 21 for Medical Science, Severance Biomedical Science Institute, Yonsei University, Seoul, Republic of Korea

Georges Halabi, Thierry Gauthier, Claudine Mathieu, Sylvie Tremblay, Michel Burnier and Daniel Teta
Service of Nephrology, Department of Medicine, Lausanne University Hospital, Centre Hospitalier Universitaire Vaudois, Lausanne, Switzerland

Anne Zanchi
Service of Nephrology, Department of Medicine, Lausanne University Hospital, Centre Hospitalier Universitaire Vaudois, Lausanne, Switzerland
Service of Endocrinology, Diabetes and Metabolism, Department of Medicine, Lausanne University Hospital, Centre Hospitalier Universitaire Vaudois, Lausanne, Switzerland

Kim-Anne Lê and Murielle Bortolotti
Department of Physiology, University of Lausanne, Lausanne, Switzerland

Luc Tappy
Department of Physiology, University of Lausanne, Lausanne, Switzerland
Service of Endocrinology, Diabetes and Metabolism, Department of Medicine, Lausanne University Hospital, Centre Hospitalier Universitaire Vaudois, Lausanne, Switzerland

Pauline Coti Bertrand
Service of Endocrinology, Diabetes and Metabolism, Department of Medicine, Lausanne University Hospital, Centre Hospitalier Universitaire Vaudois, Lausanne, Switzerland

Nicolas Theumann
Department of Radiology, Lausanne University Hospital, Centre Hospitalier Universitaire Vaudois, Lausanne, Switzerland

Index